Principles of Molecular Oncology

Principles of
Molecular Oncology

Edited by

Miguel H. Bronchud, MD, PhD

Hospital General of Granollers, Barcelona, Spain

MaryAnn Foote, PhD

Amgen Inc., Thousand Oaks, CA

William P. Peters, MD, PhD

Barbara Ann Karmanos Cancer Institute, The Detroit Medical Center
Wayne State University, Detroit, MI

Murray O. Robinson, PhD

Amgen Inc., Thousand Oaks, CA

Forewords by
E. Donnall Thomas, MD
and
David J. Weatherall, MD, FRS

Humana Press ✳ **Totowa, New Jersey**

For additional copies, pricing for bulk purchases, and/or information about other Humana titles, contact Humana at the above address or at any of the following numbers: Tel.: 973-256-1699; Fax: 973-256-8341; E-mail: humana@humanapr.com

This publication is printed on acid-free paper. ∞
ANSI Z39.48-1984 (American Standards Institute) Permanence of Paper for Printed Library Materials.

Due diligence has been taken by the publishers, editors, and authors of this book to assure the accuracy of the information published and to describe generally accepted practices. The contributors herein have carefully checked to ensure that the drug selections and dosages set forth in this text are accurate and in accord with the standards accepted at the time of publication. Notwithstanding, as new research, changes in government regulations, and knowledge from clinical experience relating to drug therapy and drug reactions constantly occurs, the reader is advised to check the product information provided by the manufacturer of each drug for any change in dosages or for additional warnings and contraindications. This is of utmost importance when the recommended drug herein is a new or infrequently used drug. It is the responsibility of the treating physician to determine dosages and treatment strategies for individual patients. Further it is the responsibility of the health care provider to ascertain the Food and Drug Administration status of each drug or device used in their clinical practice. The publisher, editors, and authors are not responsible for errors or omissions or for any consequences from the application of the information presented in this book and make no warranty, express or implied, with respect to the contents in this publication.

Printed in the United States of America. 10 9 8 7 6 5 4 3 2 1

Library of Congress Cataloging-in-Publication Data

Principles of molecular oncology / edited by Miguel H. Bronchud ... [et al.].
        p.   cm.
    Includes bibliographical references and index.
    ISBN 0-89603-581-6 (alk. paper)
    1. Carcinogenesis. 2. Cancer—Molecular aspects. I. Bronchud, Miguel H.
    [DNLM: 1. Medical Oncology. 2. Molecular Biology. 3. Neoplasms—genetics. QZ 200 P9575 2000]
    RC268.5.P75   2000
    616.99'2—dc21
    DNLM/DLC   99-16733
    for Library of Congress   CIP

Foreword

At the midpoint of the 20th century, our knowledge of cancer was based on epidemiology and pathology, and treatment consisted of surgery and radiation therapy. At mid-century, Medawar and colleagues initiated the understanding of transplantation immunology, Farber described the first use of an antifolic drug to treat leukemia, and Jacobson and coworkers described the irradiation-protection effect of spleen cells. These observations opened the door to the development of chemotherapy and transplantation in the treatment of cancer. Despite the rapid development of these new disciplines, progress was usually based on empiric observations and clinical trials.

The rapid advances in molecular biology at the end of the 20th century mark a new era in our knowledge of cancer. Molecular immunology, molecular genetics, molecular pharmacology, and the Human Genome Project are in the process of providing a level of understanding of cancer undreamed of in the past. Optimism is based on the firm belief that understanding at the molecular level will lead to better and earlier diagnosis, to new forms of treatment, and, most importantly, eventually to prevention of many types of cancer.

Principles of Molecular Oncology provides a bold new look at the evolution of our knowledge of cancer. Authors from many disciplines are bringing together the facets that provide a comprehensive view of the whole. In a field progressing as rapidly as the understanding of cancer at the molecular level, any book must be regarded as a report of work in progress. The reader will enjoy the opportunity to pause and look at the whole field as it stands today. This book will prove both informative and intellectually satisfying.

E. Donnall Thomas, MD
Fred Hutchinson Cancer Research Center
Nobel Laureate in Medicine/Physiology, 1990

v

Foreword

A famous London surgeon is quoted as saying that a cure for cancer would not be discovered by people in white coats working in laboratories, but rather by somebody leaning over a fence watching workmen digging a hole in the ground. Indeed, the idea that malignant disease might have a single cause, bred no doubt from the remarkable successes at the turn of the century in relating some of the major successes in relating some of the major killers of humankind to infectious agents, was rife until quite recently. But until the era of molecular biology, and the remarkable insights into cell biology that followed, the cancer field was in the doldrums. Viruses as the cause of human cancer had come and gone, chemical carcinogens and exposure to ionizing radiation seemed to be unlikely causes of the bulk of human cancers, and it was not at all clear where to turn in cancer research. However, in the 1960s, two fields of investigation started to yield results that at least held some promise. Epidemiological studies showed quite unequivocally that there is a relationship between the development of certain cancers and cigaret smoking. And at least some forms of leukemia appeared to be associated with specific chromosomal changes. However, until the advent of recombinant DNA technology, there was no indication as to how these observations might be connected or about the cellular mechanisms of malignant transformation.

When historians of science look back on the close of the 20th century and try to evaluate the fruits of the application of molecular and cell biology to the study of human disease, it is likely that they will pinpoint the better understanding of the biology of cancer as one of the highlights of this period. The discovery of oncogenes, together with improvements in cytogenetics, resulted in an amalgamation of these two fields of research and led to the dawning of an understanding of how cancers might result from the breakdown of normal cellular homeostatic mechanisms. Subsequently, the elucidation of the genetic control of the cell cycle, and how certain oncogenes monitor different aspects of cellular activity, allowing cells to go into cycle or directing them toward apoptosis, has started to provide some insights into the cellular mechanisms of malignant disease. Almost overnight, cancer has become less mysterious. It is clear that in many cases it results from the acquisition of mutations in one or more oncogenes that we acquire during our lifetime. Since at least some of these may result from specific chromosomal changes, or from the action of environmental carcinogens, these observations provide an elegant synthesis of several different fields of research. So although the final details of how a cell becomes cancerous still remain to be worked out, at last we have a blueprint of where to go in the future.

Although it is true to say that the clinical impact of the remarkable advances in molecular medicine of the last few years may still be some time in the future, and that their immediate benefits have been oversold to the public, there seems little doubt that these new discoveries will play a major role in the cancer field in the future. The molecular approach is likely to provide a wide range of extremely valuable diagnostic agents for both the early recognition and assessment of the prognosis of different forms of cancer. It also seems likely that gene therapy, something that has been "just around the corner" for far too long, will find some of its early applications in cancer treatment. Thus, although molecular biology has shown us that cancer is an extremely complex disease, and that there are multiple routes to the neoplastic phenotype, there is little doubt that much of this work will find application in the clinic in the not too distant future.

All these aspects of this complex and rapidly moving field are covered in this excellent book, *Principles of Molecular Oncology*. Clinical oncologists will find a series of balanced reviews of the current state-of-the-art of the diagnosis and treatment of cancer based on molecular technology, and, since cancer touches almost every field of clinical practice, specialists in other disciplines will find a very lucid and readable account of what is happening in one of the genuine success stories of today's molecular medicine.

Writing a foreword for a book for one of one's former students, while a constant reminder of the closeness of personal dissolution, is still an enormous pleasure. If nothing else, it is reassuring to see that at least a few resistant human lines can survive all the potential damage of medical education and emerge relatively unscathed. I wish the editors and the excellent team of authors that they have brought together all the success with this book that it deserves. In a field that is moving so rapidly it is vital to have a bird's eye view of the state of the art: I am sure that readers will obtain a balanced view of the potential and limitations of this exciting field.

Professor Sir David J. Weatherall, FRS
Regius Professor of Medicine
University of Oxford

Preface

Thomas Hodgkin's (1796–1866) criteria for determining a cancer's malignancy would still stand today: appearance of the tumor, tendency to spread, enlargement of neighboring lymph nodes, general symptoms of wasting. Until the late 18th century, medicine was symptom oriented. Toward the early 19th century, the French clinico-pathological school stressed symptoms of diagnostic significance and the primacy of physical signs. Louis Pasteur (1822–1895) did much to solve the problem of correlating microbes and disease, and Robert Koch formulated the now famous postulates to prove the pathogenicity of microorganisms. In spite of extremely important therapeutic advances (such as antimicrobials, endocrine agents, and drugs based on receptor–ligand interactions of inhibition of enzyme catalytic sites), our diagnostic skills today appear to be more potent than our ability to cure. X-rays, CT scans, NMR, ultrasounds, radioisotopes, PET scans, endoscopies, and other high-tech procedures have gradually increased our diagnostic abilities and have decreased our strict dependence on the skilled elucidation of clinical physical signs. After the important discoveries of molecular biology and genetics in the second half of the 20th century, molecular medicine is seen as the main promise for medical progress in the coming century, but it will probably come at the inevitable price of increasing complexity.

Leibniz (1646–1716) argued that Nature obeys a principle of "simplicity" or "least action." This concept has been often associated with "positivism," to the effect that one should choose the "simplest hypothesis" fitting the facts. Simplicity, however, has been criticized on the grounds that for any given problem there can still be several possible explanations of equal simplicity. In other words, simplicity is elegant, but it can also be deceiving. The history of science reveals progressively more complex, rather than simpler, laws and theories. In some of the most advanced sciences (for example, physics), the 20th century has brought us extremely complex theories, such as quantum mechanics or the general theory of relativity, fully understandable only to a few gifted minds.

Similarly, cancer is also turning out to be a more complex phenomenon than originally thought by many. This is why a realistic approach is a common denominator to all of the chapters of this book. Nevertheless, the search for esthetic formal simplicity and a general model pervades most of the text, together with a firm belief that even cancer can be understood and eventually defeated. The book is written by a combination of basic scientists and clinical researchers, and it is meant for practicing clinicians (such as medical oncologists, radiotherapists, hematologists, internists, general surgeons, urologists, gynecologists, thoracic surgeons, orthopedic surgeons), pharmacologists, and advanced medical students. The emphasis is not on biological mechanisms or pathology, but on prevention, early diagnosis, prognosis, and treatment.

The first chapter of *Principles of Molecular Oncology* presents the conceptual framework applicable to the rest of the book. Cancer is approached not from a specific disease-oriented point of view (e.g., lung cancer, breast cancer) nor from a selective therapeutic point of view (e.g., surgery, radiotherapy, chemotherapy). Instead, we have focused the problem starting from the hypothesis that cancer can be regarded as a "disease of key regulatory pathways." Pathways involved, for example, in the homeostatic regulation of cell growth, differentiation, and death. Carcinogenesis, as it is understood today, involves several cumulative genetic changes that, in at least some instances, can lead to the acquisition of a malignant phenotype. At the same time, these successive molecular changes can provide us with "markers" of malignant or premalignant lesions at genetic or cellular levels or circulating in the extracellular fluids. Some can even be inherited, leading to a genetic predisposition to malignant disease. The picture is still incomplete, but it seems reasonable to propose that each individual cancer has its own natural history, genetic makeup, and clonal evolution. Each individual cancer, therefore, may provide a particular "matrix of targets" for therapeutic intervention, conditioned by the regulatory networks of the tissue of origin. Moreover, even transformed cells are liable to modulation by their own microenvironment and the immune system of the host, and therapies can be directed not only to the cancer cells themselves, but also to the immune system of the patient and the specific microenvironment (e.g., to delay or prevent angiogenesis, tissue invasion, and metastasis).

There are still many gaps in our knowledge, both in terms of biological mechanisms and new effector molecules. These "blank spaces" in the matrix will eventually be filled by rapidly accumulating knowledge, just as new atoms gradually filled the chemical periodic table at the turn of the century. It seems likely that most of these key regulatory cascades will converge into a limited number of key regulatory events: the coordinated expression or suppression of a battery of genes, the initiation of normal DNA replication at multiple different sites in the genome, the culmination of the developmental history, and cell fate, of any given clone.

The future of molecular oncology is exciting. It will have profound implications in the prevention, early detection, and treatment of cancer. It might also help to change some of our unhealthy life habits for healthier ones, estimate individual vulnerability to environmental carcinogens, or allow the development of effective anticarcinogenic diets. Cancers do not happen overnight, and the often protracted lag periods of cancer growth should allow opportunities for chemoprevention or new methods of screening and early detection. Nuclear magnetic devices of the future might help to detect "in vivo" areas of genomic instability or chromosomal "disorder" by focusing on abnormal DNA patterns. The ultimate outcomes of basic research (and early clinical research) are seldom identifiable while the research is in progress. Better coordination of all research efforts by university, government agencies, pharmaceutical corporations, and international scientific societies will lead to success. Medicine is evolving at a more rapid pace than ever before, with the increasing specialization and integration of parts, learning through the association of ideas and the natural equilibration of interests. *Principles of Molecular Oncology*, and the preceding *Principles of Molecular Medicine* by Larry Jameson et al. (Humana Press, 1998) are good examples of what has already been achieved.

I am indebted to the generous contribution of all authors, from both sides of the Atlantic; and to the constant support of the other editors (Murray Robinson and William Peters), and MaryAnn Foote, in particular. Many thanks are due to Thomas Lanigan, Jr. and to Paul Dolgert at Humana Press, for believing in the project even when it looked implausible. My gratitude also to the European School of Oncology (Milan) and to Gonville and Caius College at the University of Cambridge, for allowing me to direct a course on "Molecular Biology for Cancer Clinicians" in 1996 and in 1998, which led me to propose the writing of this book. On a more personal note, I take particular pleasure in acknowledging the stimulating influence of all of my mentors and teachers, and, especially of Max Perutz, who taught me how to enjoy the beauty of a hemoglobin molecule in three dimensions; David Weatherall, who pioneered the concept of molecular medicine and taught me how to make sense of gene defects (as well as how to palpate an enlarged spleen); and Mike Dexter, who insisted on looking at live cells with respect for the unknown, but through the eyes of a child.

Miguel H. Bronchud, MD, PhD

Contents

Contributors

ANTONELLA AIELLO, PhD • *Division of Experimental Oncology, National Cancer Institute, Milan, Italy*

CAROLINE ARCHER, MD • *The Institute of Cancer Research, Royal Cancer Hospital, London, UK*

GUNNAR ÅSTRÖM, MD, PhD • *Department of Oncology, University of Uppsala, Uppsala, Sweden*

MARIA ROSA BANI, PhD • *Mario Negri Institute for Pharmacological Research, Milan, Italy*

C. JONAS BERGH, MD, PhD • *Department of Oncology, University of Uppsala, Uppsala, Sweden*

SARAH BIRINDELLI, PhD • *Division of Experimental Oncology, National Cancer Institute of Milan, Italy*

LEONARDO BRIZUELA, PhD • *Mitotix Inc., Cambridge, MA*

MIGUEL H. BRONCHUD, MD, PhD • *Division of Medical Oncology, Hospital General de Gran Ollers, Barcelona, Spain*

ANGELO A. CARDOSA, MD • *Dana-Farber Cancer Institute, Boston, MA*

MITCHELL DOWSET, PhD • *The Institute of Cancer Research, Royal Cancer Hospital, London, UK*

CARLOS FERREIRA, MD • *Department of Oncology, Free University Hospital, Amsterdam, The Netherlands*

MARYANN FOOTE, PhD • *Amgen Inc., Thousand Oaks, CA*

GIUSEPPE GIACCONE, MD, PhD • *Department of Oncology, Free University Hospital, Amsterdam, The Netherlands*

RAFFAELLA GIAVAZZI, MD • *Mario Negri Institute for Pharmacological Research, Milan, Italy*

JENO GYURIS, PhD • *Mitotix Inc., Cambridge, MA*

DANIEL F. HAYES, MD • *Lombardi Cancer Center, Georgetown University Medical Center, Washington, DC*

ALAN HORWICH, MD, PhD • *The Institute of Cancer Research, Royal Cancer Hospital, London, UK*

V. CRAIG JORDAN, PhD, DSc • *Robert H. Lurie Cancer Center, Northwestern University Medical School, Chicago, IL*

DANIEL KALDERON, PhD • *Department of Biological Sciences, Columbia University, New York, NY*

CINZIA LAVARINO, PhD • *Division of Experimental Oncology, National Cancer Institute, Milan, Italy*

THOMAS LINDAHL • *Department of Oncology, University of Uppsala, Uppsala, Sweden*

HONG LIU, MD, PhD • *Robert H. Lurie Cancer Center, Northwestern University Medical School, Chicago, IL*

MUZAMMIL M. MANSURI, PhD • *Mitotix Inc., Cambridge, MA*

MATTHEW MOYLE, PhD • *Amgen Inc., Thousand Oaks, CA*

FRANCESC MITJANS, PhD • *Merck Research Laboratories, Barcelona, Spain*

TORBJÖN NORBERG, Fil Lic • *Department of Oncology, University of Uppsala, Uppsala, Sweden*

MICHAEL PALAZZOLO, MD, PhD • *Amgen Inc., Thousand Oaks, CA*

WILLIAM P. PETERS, MD, PhD • *Barbara Ann Karmanos Cancer Institute, Detroit, MI*

MARCO ALESSANDRO PIEROTTI, PhD • *Division of Experimental Oncology, National Cancer Institute, Milan, Italy*

SILVANA PILOTTI, MD • *Division of Experimental Oncology, National Cancer Institute, Milan, Italy*

HERBERT M. PINEDO, MD, PhD • *Department of Oncology, Free University Hospital, Amsterdam, The Netherlands*

JAUME PIULATS, MD • *Merck Research Laboratories, Barcelona, Spain*

MURRAY O. ROBINSON, PhD • *Amgen Inc., Thousand Oaks, CA*

GILLIAN ROSS, BM, PhD • *The Institute of Cancer Research, Royal Cancer Hospital, London, UK*

KAROL SIKORA, MD • *Department of Clinical Oncology, Hammersmith Hospital, London, UK*

SIGRID SJÖGREN (KLAAR), MD, PhD • *Department of Oncology, University of Uppsala, Uppsala, Sweden*

GABRIELLA SOZZI, PhD • *Division of Experimental Oncology, National Cancer Institute, Milan, Italy*

E. DONNALL THOMAS, MD • *Fred Hutchinson Cancer Research Center, Seattle, WA*

CHRISTOS TOLIS, MD • *Department of Oncology, Free University Hospital, Amsterdam, The Netherlands*

PETER TROTT, MD • *The Institute of Cancer Research, Royal Cancer Hospital, London, UK*

DAVID J. WEATHERALL, MD, FRS • *Department of Medicine, University of Oxford, Oxford, UK*

PAUL WORKMAN, PhD • *The Institute of Cancer Research, CRC Centre for Cancer Therapeutics, Surrey, UK*

I

MOLECULAR MARKERS

1

Selecting the Right Targets for Cancer Therapy

Miguel H. Bronchud and William P. Peters

Introduction

It will surely be through science and hard work, rather than some peculiar trick of magic or mere luck, that cancer will finally be defeated. To understand the prospects of cancer research, practicing clinicians and the public in general should have some idea of the present state of our knowledge on the subject. In the past two decades there has been an explosion of knowledge in the molecular aspects of cancer: some 200 genes and their respective protein products have been described as directly or indirectly linked to cancer. There are so many trees that there is a real risk of missing the forest. Cancer clinicians (medical oncologists, hematologists, general surgeons, gynecologists, urologists, etc.) find it increasingly more difficult to stay abreast of knowledge in the molecular aspects of these complex diseases. Indeed, some believe that in the not too distant future, relevant information will pass from the molecular pathology laboratory to the busy cancer clinical units only with the help of clever computer programs. Before clinicians can determine the curability or incurability of any given cancer, and to decide which sequence and combination of drugs to use to treat a patient, they will need to consult a computer program and the molecular pathology laboratory.

An important objective of this book was not only to discuss the almost 200 molecular markers of malignant disease (the trees), but also to explain their potential clinical roles in the diagnosis, prognosis, and treatment of cancer. We believe all authors have succeeded in accomplishing this, and should be congratulated. In this initial chapter, we shall try to see the forest, even if, in light of present knowledge, it remains difficult to bridge the vast gulfs that open up on closer examination, and that cannot yet be spanned by the most audacious hypothesis.

Hereditary tumors and nonhereditary tumors, cellular and tissue markers, and circulating cancer markers have genetic markers. Some of these markers are already used routinely in clinical practice (e.g., several circulating cancer markers are useful for the diagnosis, prognosis, and follow-up of some cancer types). Others are being investigated as a source of important prognostic information or even as predictors of response to chemotherapy or radiotherapy (e.g., several cellular and tissue markers), and still others are being explored in the context of genetic counseling, as potentially useful to screen for hereditary cancer predisposition.

From: *Principles of Molecular Oncology*
Edited by: M. H. Bronchud, M. A. Foote, W. P. Peters, and M. O. Robinson © Humana Press Inc., Totowa, NJ

Regulatory pathways involved in the complex regulation of cell growth, differentiation, senescence, and cell death are being gradually understood, although we are still largely unable to draw schematically precise cell-type specific regulatory pathways. In contrast, the classical metabolic regulatory pathways have been known for many years. Pathways such as the citric acid cycle (postulated by Krebs in 1937), the central role of ATP in the energy transfer cycles (postulated mainly by Lipmann in 1939–41), or the intriguing hypothesis to explain the mechanism of oxidative and photosynthetic phosphorylation (postulated by Mitchell in 1961), to name but a few examples, have been part of biochemistry textbooks for decades. Twenty years ago, the structure of DNA had already been known for two decades and yet eminent scientists were pessimistic about real therapeutic progress in oncology. John Cairns, for example, admitted that "at present so little is known about the control of cell growth that there is no way of guessing when we will arrive at the necessary understanding—it could be in the next 10 or 20 years, or not for another century" *(1)*. It was so difficult to visualize the discovery of new revolutionary cancer treatments that it did not even enter into the speculative, day-to-day conversation of people engaged in cancer research.

This book is a good demonstration that things have changed. Although there is still no treatment for any of the major lethal cancers that is as effective as the antibiotics are for infections, the knowledge that has accumulated on the fine regulatory mechanisms that are deranged in cancer cells is vast and undoubtedly promises new therapeutic insights. In contrast to the situation 20 yr ago, not only do we know many molecular targets for which to design new drugs for the chemoprevention or treatment of cancer, but, paradoxically, we have an apparent excess of targets for our current resources of drug development worldwide. The Human Genome Project is in progress, should complete its first objectives by the year 2005, and it is likely to give us further insights and more potential targets. In other words, the rate-limiting step in progress against cancer is the amount of resources we can spend and the optimization and coordination of this huge research process, rather than a lack of therapeutic targets.

Selecting the right targets for cancer therapy can make a big difference. If, for example, we were clever or lucky enough to guess correctly the right targets for the main human cancers, and if large multinational pharmaceutical companies agreed to focus their efforts and enormous resources on these right targets, then revolutionary new cancer treatments might become available for clinical testing within 5–10 yr. But, if we were wrong, or not enough importance was given to this war against cancer by politicians or business people, then it might take another 20 or 30 yr, or even longer.

The object of all cancer research is simply to stop cancer from being a major cause of death and human suffering, and it is in this light that all new research must ultimately be judged. In this chapter, we review some new prospects in the prevention, early detection, and treatment of cancer, based on four basic truths of oncology:

1. Cancer can be prevented.
2. Cancer can be diagnosed, and the earlier the diagnosis the higher the chances of curative treatment.
3. Cancer can be cured (by local or systemic therapies, or a combination of both), but the impact on mortality of present therapies is limited.

4. Cancer cannot always be cured, and it seems reasonable to predict that even in the year 2040 there will still be many cancers that are incurable at the time of clinical presentation.

Cancer Can Be Prevented

Trends in Mortality Due to Cancer

About 200 distinct varieties of cancer are recognized, but fortunately most of these are very rare, and most cancer mortality falls within a much smaller list. In the Western world cancer is the second largest cause of mortality, after cardiovascular disease. Infectious disease, which once ruled supreme, now causes only about 1–2% of all deaths. In our industrialized countries, approx 1% of the population dies every year, and there is a clear trend toward stabilization in the population growth, because of an important reduction in birth rate. In the United States, age-adjusted mortality due to cancer in 1994 was 6% higher than in 1970. After decades of steady increases, the age-adjusted mortality due to all cancers plateaued, then decreased by about 1% from 1991 to 1994.

Observed changes in mortality due to cancer primarily reflect changing incidence or early detection, rather than more effective therapies. This small recent decline in mortality because of cancer in the United States was greatest among black men and among persons 55 yr of age. Mortality among white men 55 yr or older has also declined recently. These trends *(2)* reflect a combination of changes in death rates from specific types of cancer, with important declines due to reduced cigarette smoking or improved screening methods and a mixture of increases and decreases in the incidence of types of cancer not directly linked to tobacco use. The use of mortality as the chief measure of progress against cancer, rather than incidence or survival, stresses the outcome that is most reliably reported and is of greatest concern to the public. Adjustment for age (age-adjusted mortality) removes the effects of changes in the age distribution of the population, and with it the effect of changing mortality from causes other than cancer.

Trends in incidence, although important, are not quite so reliable, because of the variability in the precision of diagnostic information, the trends in screening and early detection, and the criteria for reporting cancer. For example, the development and commercial promotion of the prostate-specific antigen (PSA) test probably contributed to the doubling of the reported incidence of cancer of the prostate between 1974 and 1990.

In their 1997 article, Bailar and Gornik *(2)* admit that in the past two or three decades there have been significant improvements in the treatment of children and young adults with cancer, in the management of Hodgkin's disease (HD), and in the palliation of symptoms of advanced cancer. They concluded that the effect of primary prevention (an observed trend toward a reduction in smoking in the United States) and secondary prevention (e.g., the Papanicolaou smear) are more important and support the view that the dominant research strategies of the past 40 yr, particularly the emphasis on improving treatments, should be redirected toward prevention (primary or secondary) to achieve a significant reduction in age-adjusted mortality due to cancer.

The long latency periods that commonly occur between the first exposure to the carcinogenic agent and the appearance of clinical disease should also, at least theoretically, be seen as a window of opportunity for early diagnostic and therapeutic intervention, and possibly cure. This latent period usually lasts for 20–40 yr, although it may be as short as 1 or as long as 60. The interval is subject to random factors, partly because few cancers are induced by a single brief exposure, and partly because there are still relatively few data with detailed reliable information about the exact dates when exposure began and ended. After the nuclear bombing of Hiroshima and Nagasaki, the incidence of leukemia peaked about 5 yr after exposure, but the incidence of solid tumors increased for 15–20 yr. The evidence that many of the common cancers are preventable can be derived by four main groups of observations: differences in the incidence of a particular type of cancer between different settled communities, differences between migrants from a community and those who remained behind, variation with time within particular communities, and the actual identification of a large number of specific and controllable causes *(3)*.

Diet and Cancer

Epidemiology and laboratory research should complement each other and both are needed to understand the important causes of cancer and to learn how to prevent it. With at least 10,000 trace chemicals detectable sometime in our bodies, the task of relating cause and effect is not easy.

Consider, for example, diet. For several decades there has been suggestive evidence that the incidence of many of the common cancers could be decreased by modification of our diet; but, with few exceptions, there is still little reliable evidence as to what modifications would be of major importance. Epidemiological data suggest that people with diets rich in β-carotene have lower cancer rates, particularly of lung cancer, than people with β-carotene-poor diets. However, in the α-tocopherol, β-carotene cancer prevention trial (ATBC) and the β-carotene and retinol efficacy trial (CARET), both of which included smokers, there were surprisingly more new cancers and deaths in the treatment cohorts than in the placebo cohorts. Recent studies in animal models *(4)* suggest that a diet very rich in β-carotene may be enough to promote squamous metaplasia in the lungs, a precancerous stage, probably because of increased expression of tumor promoters such as c-*jun* and c-*fos*, and decreased expression of tumor-suppressor retinoic acid-receptor-β. This example is a good illustration of the difficulties associated with any experimental manipulation of diet.

Consumption of alcohol has been shown to potentiate the effects of tobacco smoke on cancers of the mouth, pharynx, esophagus, and larynx *(5)*. In combination with smoking, the risks can multiply 35-fold among heavy consumers of both products, and the rate of cancer associated with alcohol could be higher than the 3% previously estimated.

The retinoids, synthetic and natural derivatives of vitamin A, are agents active in cancer therapy and prevention. Advances in the understanding of which nuclear retinoid receptors or coregulators transmit the appropriate growth and differentiation signals *(6)* have led to hopes that diet supplementation with the adequate types and amounts of these substances may contribute to chemoprevention of cancer *(7)*.

A consistent finding in epidemiological studies on cancer and diet is the protective effect of fresh fruits and vegetables. Besides carotenoids, some studies have suggested that vitamins C and E and allium vegetables may protect against stomach cancer *(8)*, whereas intake of fiber may lower the risk of colon cancer *(9)*. Few things are probably as important to our health as the food that we eat. Eating the wrong sort of food increases one's likelihood of developing one or both of the two biggest killers of the 20th century (cancer and heart disease). During the last few decades, an enormous amount of money has been spent on research to find out which foodstuffs are responsible for which diseases. As far as the consumer is concerned, there is still a good deal of confusion and controversy: Are animal fats bad? Does salt cause high blood pressure? How much fiber should the average daily diet contain? What is the best way to avoid high cholesterol? Are vitamin supplements needed? How can caloric input be tailored to consumption of calories? What is a "healthy diet"?

In the case of animal fats, if one looks at the independent scientific evidence, there is no doubt that most people in the Western countries eat too much animal fat. The amount of fat, especially saturated fat, consumed by thc average citizen of the United States or northern European countries (e.g., Germany, Britain, and The Netherlands) is highly dangerous. The incidence of heart disease is increasing. Indeed, Britain, where animal fat consumption is high, has one of the highest rates of heart attack.

Fraumeni admits that in view of the limitations of nutritional methods in epidemiology, further progress is likely to depend on innovative analytical studies using biochemical assays, as well as intervention studies involving dietary supplements and modifications *(10)*. Intermediate endpoint markers are promising but often not sufficiently specific.

Viruses and Cancer

Another example of potential preventability of cancer comes from virus-related carcinogenesis. Cancer once was more common in women than in men in nearly all countries because of the great frequency of carcinoma of the cervix uteri and the rarity of smoking-related cancers (such as lung, bladder, or head and neck cancers), and this frequency remains in populations in several Latin American countries. Elsewhere, cancer is now more common in men. Cervical cancer in women is still prevalent all over the world (with nearly half a million cases reported each year) and it is the leading cause of cancer mortality and morbidity in countries such as Mexico, Colombia, and Ecuador. The evidence is now very strong that human papilloma viruses (HPVs) are etiological agents associated with the majority of cervical cancer types (both squamous and adenocarcinomas). HPVs are small DNA viruses that usually cause warts (epidermal papillomas) in the skin, but some can also infect the genital tract. More than 30 HPVs have been identified in the female genital tract. Four of these viruses (HPV-16, HPV-18, HPV-31, and HPV-45) probably account for 80% of cervical cancers and code for at least two oncogenes (*E6* and *E7*) which are expressed once the viral genome integrates into the host's DNA, disrupting some of the key pathways of cell-cycle control. The retinoblastoma protein (Rb) is a 928-residue nuclear protein that exists as a differentially phosphorylated family of regulatory polypeptides. In spite of extensive research, relatively little is known about how this protein might operate in vivo in molecular terms, although it is an important tumor-suppressor molecule, and the state of Rb phosphorylation changes dramatically at key check points in the cell cycle *(11)*. Rb protein can form specific complexes with each of a series of three transforming products of DNA tumor viruses: adenovirus E1A, papovaviral large T antigen (Ag), and the E7 product of several HPVs.

The detection of HPV infection using molecular diagnostic methods such as the polymerase chain reaction (PCR) is now used, together with the traditional cytological Papanicolaou smear analysis, in screening programs of early detection of cervical cancers. Theoretically, HPV vaccines should be able to prevent infection and protect against malignant transformation. No effective vaccines have yet been developed, partly because of the multiple serological subtypes, partly because the main protective immunity agent active in mucosal membranes (such as the cervix uteri) is immunoglobulin A (IgA), which is only temporarily induced so that a putative HPV vaccine would have to be administered repeatedly to maintain an effective level of immunity. However, a live attenuated virus vaccine, modeled on the successful control of smallpox, yellow fever, and polio viruses by such vaccines, could offer several advantages: infection of the female genital tract might confer long-lasting immunity, similar to that after natural infections and could prevent reinfection. In addition, live attenuated viral vaccines are good candidates for inexpensive mass immunization in underdeveloped countries (where the prevalence is highest) without the need for sterile equipment. Costs of anticancer vaccination programs are likely to increase dramatically. For example, hepatitis B virus (HBV) vaccination has been called the world's second best cancer control program, after the campaign against cigarette smoking. The association between hepatocellular carcinoma and HBV in some countries (e.g., Taiwan and Gambia) is very strong, and the implementation of HBV vaccination programs in neonates and children has already reduced, according to World Health Organization (WHO) figures, the occurrence of hepatocellular carcinomas in the first decade of life. In contrast to HPV, there is no evidence that the HBV genome carries a true oncogene, and the carcinogenic activity of the virus is thought to be due to indirect effects through chronic liver damage: hepatocellular injury, necrosis, inflammation, and liver degeneration.

Epstein–Barr virus (EBV) is a highly B lymphotropic virus, targeting B lymphocytes through a specific interaction between their major envelope glycoprotein and a complement receptor molecule. EBV is a herpesvirus widespread in human populations, carried by most individuals as an asymptomatic lifelong infection, probably the result of millions of years of virus–host coevolution. However, this same virus is associated with several malignancies, including endemic Burkitt's lymphoma (BL), nasopharyngeal carcinomas, the so-called "midline lethal granulomas" (a particularly aggressive form of non-Hodgkin's lymphomas [NHL]), many cases of HD and a relatively new entity which has attracted considerable attention: posttransplant lymphoproliferative disease (12). The expression of viral Ags in EBV-positive HD raises the possibility of developing tumor immunotherapy. Virus-related malignancies are, at least theoretically, ideal targets for immunotherapy, because the viral proteins in the tumor cells provide unique targets for antibodies (Abs) or cytotoxic T lymphocytes (CTLs). Autologous EBV-specific CTLs infusions have been shown to be safe and to protect bone marrow transplant recipients from posttransplant lymphoproliferative disease (13).

An interesting, nonviral, association between an infectious agent and cancer is the case of *Helicobacter pylori* infection. The eradication of *H. pylori* leads to remission induction in most patients with low-grade gastric mucosa-associated lymphoid tissue

(MALT) lymphomas in limited stages, which supports the view that *H. pylori*-induced gastritis somehow lead to clonal evolution of CD5- and CD10-B lymphocytes and, finally, malignant transformation *(14)*. However, even after removal of the underlying stimulus (*H. pylori*) by appropriate antibiotic therapy, an ongoing process of somatic hypermutation of B cells and Ag selection can be detected, challenging the view that these lymphomas can be entirely cured by the elimination of *H. pylori* infection *(15)*.

Nicotine and Tobacco

Smoking is so widespread that it is rarely viewed as a form of drug abuse or as an addiction, even though it fits all of the accepted criteria for drug dependence *(16)*. The potential adverse effects of tobacco use, unlike other addictive disorders, are associated with chronic rather than experimental or occasional use. Much has been written on the links between smoking and serious health problems (chronic respiratory problems, cancer, and cardiovascular disease) and repetition here would be tedious. If there is one carcinogen the importance of which has been unshakably established, it is cigarette smoke. It has been estimated that if smoking was abolished, the number of people dying from lung cancer would in due time decrease by 80%. It has been calculated that one's life is shortened 14 min for every cigarette smoked. However, in spite of public awareness of the serious health consequences of smoking, the worldwide incidence and prevalence of cigarette smoking is increasing. In some areas of the United States and Europe, the number of women who die of smoking-related cancer of the lung is now higher than the number of women who die of breast cancer. Although there is considerable evidence that nicotine is the reinforcing constituent that gives tobacco its universal popularity, it is still uncertain why it creates so enduring a pattern of self-administration. Smokers may continue to smoke for enjoyment or social reinforcement, to alleviate anxiety, or because it is fashionable; environmental stimuli and social reinforcers interact with pharmacological factors. However, it is clear that the rate of relapse among compulsive smokers (who report irritability, depression, and autonomic function changes when they cease smoking) is discouragingly high, with only 10–25% remaining smoke-free for more than 2 yr.

Specific treatments, such as nicotine skin patches or chewing gum with or without supportive psychotherapy, have only marginally improved these results. Although preventive measures targeted at young people (such as educating children at school about the risks) remain promising, results so far have not had any dramatic effect. In general, most smokers initiate their habit before they are 20 yr old. A vaccine against nicotine (if at all possible) might induce an immune response (cellular and/or humoral) with both specificity and memory. For example, an adequate Ab response to nicotine might neutralize its pharmacological properties and abolish the reinforcing constituent responsible, at least in part, for addiction to tobacco smoking. Alternatively, a cellular immune response might induce a local inflammatory reaction in the lips, tongue, or oropharyngeal mucosa and discourage people from smoking. Nicotinic esters can produce nonimmunologic contact urticaria *(17)* (at least in some animal models), but the potential allergenic nature of nicotine has not been fully investigated.

The percentage of nicotine in tobacco varies considerably and may range from 0.5% to 8.0%. The smoke of the average cigarette may yield 6–8 mg, and that of a cigar may contain from 15 mg to more than 40 mg of nicotine. Some 90% of the nicotine in inhaled smoke is absorbed compared with only 25–50% of that in smoke that is drawn into the mouth and then expelled. Nearly 500 other compounds have been identified in the particulate and gaseous phases of tobacco smoke: nitrogenous bases, isoprenoid compounds, tarry and phenolic substances, volatile acids, furfural and acrolein, polonium-210, nickel, and other potentially toxic substances. Because of carbon monoxide, 5–10% of circulating hemoglobin may be converted to carboxyhemoglobin as a result of continuous smoking.

Nicotine was first isolated from leaves of tobacco (*Nicotiana tabacum*) in 1828 and the actions of the drug as ganglionic stimulating drug was first described in 1889. It is a liquid alkaloid, water soluble, colorless, volatile, and strongly alkaline in reaction. On exposure to air, it turns brown and acquires the odor of tobacco. Nicotine has no known therapeutic application. The complex and often unpredictable changes that occur in the body after administration of nicotine are due not only to its actions on a variety of neuroeffector junctions, but also to the fact that the alkaloid has both stimulant and depressant phases of action. The ultimate response represents the summation of the several and opposing effects of nicotine. For example, the drug can increase the heart rate by either excitation of sympathetic or paralysis of parasympathetic cardiac ganglia. In general, small doses of nicotine stimulate the ganglion cells directly and facilitate the transmission of impulses. When larger doses of the drug are applied, the initial stimulation is followed very quickly by a blockade of transmission. In the central nervous system, appropriate doses induce tremors in both humans and laboratory animals, and larger doses can produce convulsions. Stereospecific nicotine receptors can be measured on brain membranes *(18)*. The excitation of respiration is a particularly prominent action of nicotine and at very high doses, death can result from paralysis of respiration. The acutely fatal dose of nicotine for an adult is probably about 60 mg when given parenterally: the onset of symptoms is rapid, with nausea, salivation, abdominal pain, vomiting, diarrhea, mental confusion, weakness, hypotension, breathing difficulties, and collapse. The gastric absorption of nicotine from tobacco taken by mouth is delayed, but nicotine is readily absorbed from oral and gastrointestinal mucosa, respiratory tract, and the skin. Doses given intradermally for vaccination purposes should therefore not exceed nanogram (or picogram) quantities, and must always be administered with caution.

The principle of vaccination is based on two key elements of adaptive immunity: specificity and memory *(19)*. Memory cells allow the immune system to mount a much stronger response on a second encounter with Ag. This second response is both faster and more effective than the primary response. The first introduction of immunogen, the primary stimulus, evokes the primary response in which Abs are first detectable after 1–30 d or more.

The lag period varies with dose, route of injection, the particulate or soluble nature of the immunogen, the type of adjuvant used (if any), and the sensitivity of the assay. The time required to attain maximal Ab levels and the duration of the peak titer vary with different immunogens and methods of immunization. The Abs made at various times after immunization differ in type of Ig chain (usually, IgM class are produced before the IgG class) and in affinity for the Ag (usually the affinity increases with time). After Ab values in the primary response have declined, even to the point of being no longer detectable, a subsequent encounter with the same Ag usually evokes an enhanced secondary response characterized by:

- A lower threshold dose of immunogen
- A shorter lag phase
- A higher rate and longer persistence of Ab synthesis
- Higher titers

Multiple injections of immunogen (commonly at 1- to 6-mo intervals) are usually necessary to establish the potential for a long-lasting and effective secondary response. Although current immunization practices stimulate immune responses effectively, it is still not generally possible to stimulate them selectively: for example, to elicit Ab formation without cell-mediated immunity or vice versa, or to avoid certain types of Abs, such as those of the IgE class that can cause serious allergic reactions. Furthermore, not every substance is immunogenic. Thus, it is unclear from current literature whether nicotine is immunogenic or not.

There remains a long list of serious infectious disease where no vaccine is currently available. During work in the 1920s on the production of animal sera for human therapy, it was discovered that certain substances, notably aluminum salts, added to or emulsified with an Ag, greatly enhance Ab production. It appears that the effect of adjuvants is due mainly to two activities: the concentration of Ag in a site where lymphocytes are exposed to it (depot effect) and the induction of cytokines that regulate lymphocyte function. This theory is supported by the fact that cytokines themselves have recently been shown to be effective adjuvants, particularly when coupled directly to the Ag.

Chemoprevention and Hereditary Predisposition to Cancer

In recent years, the possibility has been raised that pharmacologic agents or nutritional modification might prevent the development of human cancer, or, at least, slow down its progression. The concept of chemoprevention is gaining support, although there are still significant experimental and conceptual problems associated with it. For example, if the study population is composed of normal or nearly normal subjects (such as normal volunteers, smokers without obvious disease, or people with a history of one isolated gastrointestinal polyp), very few side effects may be acceptable. In contrast, if the subjects are at high risk of cancer (e.g., have a history of familial polyposis, hereditary predisposition to breast or colon cancer, or second tumors), considerable side effects may be acceptable.

There is also significant scientific interest in certain metabolic or detoxification phenotypes that may confer a higher cancer risk, such as aryl hydrocarbon hydroxylase (AHH) activity, debrisoquin hydroxylation, and glutathione-S-transferase (GST) activity. For example, AHH activity depends on one subfamily of cytochrome P-450 microsomal enzymes that convert polycyclic aromatic hydrocarbons into carcinogenic intermediates *(20)*. Case-control studies have yielded contradictory results regarding the association between AHH activity in lymphocytes and lung cancer risk *(21)*. The reasons why only a few heavy smokers actually develop lung cancer remain largely unknown.

Only β-carotene, the retinoids, folic acid, vitamins C and E, and tamoxifen have been used in published phase 3 clinical chemoprevention trials. The retinoids are probably the longest studied and, although their therapeutic index is somewhat narrow because of toxicities, they have achieved successful results in oral leukoplakia *(22)*, actinic keratosis *(23)*, prevention of skin cancer in xeroderma pigmentosum (XP) *(24)*, and of second primary tumors in squamous cell carcinoma of the head and neck *(25)*. More controversial is the role of other agents, such as cyclooxygenase-2 (COX-2) inhibitors in chemoprevention. COX-2, a key enzyme for the production of prostaglandins from arachidonic acid, is overexpressed in colon carcinogenesis and clinical studies with selective nontoxic inhibitors are underway.

The role of tamoxifen in chemoprevention of breast cancer has recently reached the front page of general newspapers. Estrogens have been recognized as an important promoting factor in breast cancer for several decades. Preliminary results of the Breast Cancer Prevention Trial in the United States (BCPT, NSABP-P1) indicated a 45% reduction in breast cancer incidence with prophylactic use of tamoxifen *(26,27)*, but neither of two European trials have confirmed these positive results *(28)*. Longer follow-up of completed and current trials is clearly required to clarify the relative preventive benefits and risks in different populations of women, and to confirm a possible benefit. Moreover, none of these trials have produced reliable data on mortality, which is the ultimate endpoint. The International Breast Cancer Intervention Study (IBIS) has now enrolled 5000 women, of a target of 7000, and the mature results of this trial, together with further follow-up of the BCPT, the Powles (Royal Marsden Hospital, London), and Veronesi (Istituto Europeo di Oncologia, Milan) trials will be welcomed by the scientific community and are needed to correctly advise women at risk. New agents that will function as estrogen agonists in the tissues in which estrogen is beneficial (e.g., bone and cardiovascular system), but as estrogen antagonists in tissues where estrogens may promote carcinogenesis (e.g., the endometrium) are being developed. Some are called selective estrogen-receptor modulators (SERMs), of which raloxifene is a good example.

Indeed, predictive testing might allow either long-term chemoprevention with drugs or dietary modifications, or prophylactic surgical therapy (e.g., prophylactic mastectomy in high-risk women carriers of *BRCA-1* or *-2* genes; prophylactic colectomy in young adult years in familial adenomatous polyposis), or a more intensive follow-up with relevant investigations (e.g., mammography or endoscopy). For common cancers such as breast cancer, many people will have an affected relative for reasons not related to their own susceptibility (e.g., sporadic somatic mutations). Critical to genetic counseling are the species of family history and the probability that a hereditary susceptibility is present. Computer software (e.g., Cyrillic, Cherwell Scientific, Oxford, UK) is currently available to draw family pedigrees, calculate odd ratios, and estimate individual risks. A clustering of similar tumor types within the same family (breast, breast and ovary, colon, etc.), early age at diagnosis (i.e., less than 45 yr), multifocality, or, in the case of breast cancer, bilaterality are all features that point toward an inherited predisposition to cancer. Small families may fail to fulfill all the criteria for specific syndromes because of insufficient number of cases. Epidemiological studies have demonstrated a modest (two- or threefold) increase in risk of cancer among first-degree relatives of individuals with a similar cancer. In a few cancer patients, probably some 5–10%, genetic factors may be the primary determinant, but in a second group of patients, cancer might develop because an inherited factor increases susceptibility to environmental carcinogens.

Genetic aberrations and family clustering have been described for almost every tumor type, and a comprehensive family history should be part of the assessment of all patients with cancer *(29)*. Breast cancer families and colon cancer families represent the majority of consultations at familial cancer clinics. Mutations in the *BRCA1* and *BRCA2* genes are associated with a strong predisposition to breast cancer in women; according to some estimates, a gene carrier in a high-risk family has a roughly 50% chance of developing breast cancer by the age of 50 yr, and an 80% chance by the age of 75 yr. It is likely that these risks are to some extent population dependent and are modified by both genetic background and environmental factors. In addition to female breast cancer, mutations of *BRCA1* also confer a substantially increased risk of epithelial ovarian cancer. Mutations in *BRCA2* confer, in addition to female breast cancer, a significantly increased risk of male breast cancer. The genes are very long (*BRCA1,* 5500 basepairs [bps]; *BRCA2,* 11,000 bps), and mutations can occur anywhere along their length, which makes mutation analysis very difficult, technically demanding, and expensive *(30)*. A specific region in exon 11 of the *BRCA1* gene has been associated with greater ovarian risk.

The situation is different in familial adenomatous polyposis (FAP), where current laboratory testing (Labcorp) is said to identify mutations in about 80% of individuals with the disease *(31)*. However, even in this case, the failure to identify a mutation in an individual with clinical FAP (hundreds or thousands of polyps in the late teens or early 20s) should not alter the diagnosis, nor the recommendation for surveillance and prophylactic colectomy. The adenomatous polyposis coli (APC) protein is an intracellular protein associated with catenins, which bind cell-surface cadherins and appear to regulate cellular adhesion in the crypts of the colonic mucosa (where the proliferation rate is the highest).

The Lynch syndromes, or hereditary nonpolyposis colon cancer (HNPCC), account for a greater proportion of hereditary colorectal cancer families than FAP *(32,33)*. The Amsterdam criteria for HNPCC were a bit restrictive: three individuals with colorectal cancer in a kindred, at least two in first-degree relatives, and at least one diagnosed before age 50 yr. The genes responsible are called MMR (mismatch repair) and were identified because of the observation of replication error repairs (RER) in the tumors of mutations carriers. The genes responsible are several (*hMSH2, hMLH1,hMSH6, hPMS1, hPMS2,* etc.) and usually large. Many mutations are of unclear significance and measuring the RER phenotype may be a reasonable way to begin in many families, because it is less expensive than direct genetic testing and is able to detect about 80% of HNPCC tumors. Unfortunately, RER is not widely available and RER techniques across diagnostic laboratories have not been standardized.

The so-called Li–Fraumeni syndrome requires at least three cancers for its formal definition, but the associated p53 germline mutations are not uncommon in individuals with soft tissue sarcomas and adrenal cortical carcinomas, regardless of family history. Some 50% of women with Li–Fraumeni syndrome may develop breast cancer, but this disorder probably affects fewer than 1% of all breast cancer patients.

It was thought that the same genes were involved in the genesis of both inherited and sporadic cancers, but recently it has been shown that sporadic or acquired breast and ovarian cancers have mutated *BRCA1* or *BRCA2* less than 10% of the time. Thus, lessons learned from hereditary cancer susceptibility are not necessarily relevant to sporadic cancers. It is also evident that there are more, yet unknown, breast cancer susceptibility genes in breast cancer families *(34)*.

There is some controversy about the link between ataxia telangiectasia (AT) and breast cancer. AT is a relatively rare autosomal recessive disorder characterized by a progressive cerebellar ataxia with onset in early childhood, cutaneous telangiectasia, increased sensitivity to ionizing radiation, and susceptibility to lymphoid malignancies. A gene in chromosome 11q22–23 is mutated in AT patients and has been called the ATM gene. The protein product is probably related to signaling cell death by apoptosis in response to DNA damage. Carriers (estimated at fewer than 1 in 200 in the UK population) have, according to some studies, a two- or fourfold increased risk of breast cancer *(35)*, but other studies deny a contribution to early-onset breast cancer *(36,37)*. ATM is also an important tumor suppressor in B-cell chronic lymphocytic leukemia (B-CLL) and there is some suggestion that it might share a common pathway with p53, by which damaged cells are prevented from dying through apoptosis *(38)*.

The American Society of Clinical Oncology (ASCO) has recently endorsed genetic testing as a component of a comprehensive cancer risk assessment, but not population-based genetic screening, which is unwarranted given the limitations of currently available tests *(39)*. The clinical utility of genetic testing can be determined only through adequate long-term longitudinal follow-up studies *(40)*.

Cancer Can Be Diagnosed: the Earlier the Diagnosis, the Greater the Chance of Curative Treatment

More than 90% of human cancers arise in epithelial cells (carcinomas), and most of them originate in surface epithelia (skin, respiratory tract, and gut) or secondary sexual organs (prostate and breast), suggesting some kind of interaction between carcinogenic agents that cannot penetrate very far and tissues with a high rate of cellular proliferation or hormone dependence. Less than 10% of the cancers arise in the supporting tissues of the body or the circulating cells (sarcomas and leukemias). Our diagnostic skills are, at present, better than our therapeutic skills. In particular, the advent of diagnostic techniques such as ultrasound, computed tomography (CT) scanning, flexible endoscopies, and nuclear magnetic resonance (NMR), together with cytology (fine-needle aspirates) and immunohistochemical (IHC) methods can allow the detection of comparatively small primary or secondary tumors (e.g., those measuring 1 cc in diameter) virtually anywhere in the body, and emerging molecular and cytological techniques allow the detection of precancerous lesions.

As in the case of breast cancer, improvements in prostate cancer screening methods, and particularly the introduction of PSA testing and reliable prostate ultrasound methods, have led to increased detection of early lesions. As stated by Peter Boyle recently, "It is difficult to imagine a more controversial issue in public health or oncology at present than whether widespread testing for PSA should be widely applied as a screening test for prostate cancer" *(41)*. Considering that prostate cancer is driven by androgen, the androgen receptor is an ideal target for chemoprevention of prostate cancer. The ability of the agent finasteride to prevent prostate cancer is currently being studied in the Proscar Study, a large phase 3 study that has enrolled 20,000 men. The results are expected to become available within the next 5 yr.

There are two basic biological properties of the malignant cell that have not yet been adequately explained, but that probably depend on some key regulatory pathways irreversibly altered in cancer cells: the loss of contact inhibition of cell growth, and the invasive phenotype. The former is also known as the loss of density-dependent regulation. Although contact inhibition has something to do with response to exogenous growth factors, the precise mechanisms that freeze the appetite of the cell for cell division, when a tissue culture reaches confluence, have not been determined. The latter is one of the early steps in the sequence that leads from carcinoma *in situ* to invasive cancer, allowing for the emergence of cellular clones that are able to displace their neighbors and spread through the basement membrane into the underlying tissue. Both of these behavioral changes are probably dependent on the acquisition of a new battery of genes expressed or, perhaps more likely, the loss of function of key elements in the regulatory pathways that control cell cycle checkpoints or cell position (or both). A complete molecular explanation of these phenomena is eagerly awaited, and should be seen as a priority in current cancer research.

Aging is a normal biological process that leads to senescence and eventually death. It is a process programmed in our genes that starts when we are born. From the perspective of the species, after individuals have reached the peak of their sexual maturity, they can decline in their optimal physical state to allow for the new generation. This decline in our body function (and total body water) is what we call aging and is a uniform and gradual loss of full vital fitness and faculties. For example, pinch any part of an old person's skin and it is clear that the loss of elasticity is a general and uniform phenomenon. Most people will suffer not only from this uniform type of aging, but also from a patchy tissue aging that can result in disease. For example, field cancerization (in smokers, in the oral mucosa, the bronchial tree, and the urinary bladder) and atheroma formation (in the aorta at different levels and bifurcation in patients with hypercholesterolemia) will eventually lead to cancer and cardiovascular disease. These scattered and patchy processes do not happen overnight, but can take many years (on average, more than 10 or 20) to develop into clinical pathology. Therefore, they remain subclinical over a long period, and any method or strategy to detect them might allow chemopreventive therapy. Biomarkers (e.g., loss of heterozygosity [LOH], genomic instability, DNA aneuploidy, oncogene mutations, or overexpression) can be considered signposts that significant tissue damage has already been produced, and are potential predictors for cancer occurrence. If their potential can be validated by prospective studies, biomarkers will become useful in identifying individuals at high risk of cancer who can benefit from chemoprevention therapies. Virtually all of the genetic, cellular, and circulating markers described in this book are potential intermediate endpoints of malignancy, and should be regarded as potentially relevant biomarkers.

Cancer is mainly an aging-related condition, in that almost 60% of all cancers occur in people age 65 yr or older (greater than 80% for prostate cancer, 74% for colon cancer, and 72% for pancreatic cancer).

Finally, early diagnosis is a very important objective in the follow up of individuals with an inherited predisposition to cancer.

Cancer Can Be Cured: Effects on Mortality of Present Therapies Have Been Relatively Minor

Considering that cancer usually starts as a local disease, surgical excision of the primary tumors can result in cure, or, at least, improve the quality of the patient's life.

Over the last few decades, surgeons have abandoned the most mutilating types of surgery in favor of more conservative approaches, often in addition to several other methods of treatment, such as irradiation and chemotherapy. Irradiation should also be regarded as essentially a local treatment and can reduce the extent of many cancers, bring some relief from the symptoms, and in some cases prolong the patient's life. Chemotherapy is the most widely used form of systemic therapy, though not the only one; endocrine therapies and immunological therapies should also be regarded as systemic. Despite advances in the treatment of some rare cancers (germ cell tumors, some lymphomas, HD, and some leukemias and childhood tumors), the available methods of treatment, taken as a whole, are plainly not very successful for the advanced common solid tumors: only about one-third of patients survive for more than 5 yr from the time of diagnosis. The public cannot accept defeat or death, and has been led to expect better. In 1987 the first clinical paper on the use of a recombinant human hematopoietic growth factor and cancer was published *(42)*, and in the ensuing few years the introduction of these agents to speed up bone marrow recovery after chemotherapy and the advent of peripheral blood progenitor cells (PBPCs) transplantation brought fresh hopes into the therapeutic arena (at least for chemosensitive disease) by allowing a series of clinical studies on the role of intensive and/or myeloablative chemotherapy *(43)*. Recognition that the use of dose-intensive therapies in the setting of "resistant" hematologic disease resulted in cure rates (e.g., in relapsed acute myelocytic leukemia [AML]) suggested the possibility of applying a similar strategy to some chemosensitive solid tumors. Fifteen years ago, metastatic breast cancer was invariably regarded as an incurable disease, and patients were treated only with palliative intent. Although there has been considerable controversy concerning the value of high-dose therapy in the treatment of breast cancer, most published data suggest superior outcomes for high-dose chemotherapies compared with standard therapies. Results of large, prospective, randomized, multiinstitutional studies are awaited, and newer approaches (protracted sequential chemotherapy and other dose-intensive strategies) are also being investigated. However, it seems likely that, even if the results of these studies suggest some improvement, the public will ask for more and better results.

Until recently, the main and most successful use of growth factors in cancer therapy has not been their direct or indirect antitumor effects, but their use as adjuncts to chemotherapy. Three factors have been registered for clinical application: the myeloid growth factors (granulocyte colony-stimulating factor [G-CSF] and granulocyte-macrophage colony-stimulating factor [GM-CSF]), and erythropoietin (EPO), the main regulator of erythroid growth. The genes for thrombopoietin (TPO) and megakaryocyte growth and development factor (MGDF), two agents working on platelet proliferation, were cloned, and early clinical trials (to determine safety and active dose and schedule) were reasonably encouraging, but no clinical use has been found for these recombinant products. Other growth factors are also being studied in the clinic *(44)*.

Colony-stimulating factors (CSFs) have been used to support both standard and intensified doses of chemotherapy for almost a decade. Guidelines on their optimal use have been proposed by ASCO *(45)* and a European report *(46)* among others. The main established indications in cancer medicine are the primary and, more frequently, the secondary prevention of febrile neutropenia secondary to chemotherapy for the treatment of chemosensitive solid tumors or lymphomas, and the mobilization of PBPCs in the context of high-dose chemotherapy protocols. Other uses in oncology are more developmental or controversial. Reductions in the degree, incidence, or duration of neutropenia are not considered sufficient criteria to justify the clinical use of a recombinant growth factor. Clinically relevant outcomes, such as incidence and severity of febrile neutropenic events and, particularly, improved quality of life and survival are currently the primary therapeutic endpoints of cytokine administration.

The discovery that CSF-mobilized PBPCs from the bone marrow was not expected from the early in vitro and preclinical work. These cells are now routinely harvested at most cancer centers by one or more apheresis procedures and usually cryopreserved to be infused after high-dose therapy. Indeed, many of the apheresis devices that were originally developed for plasmapheresis or for the separation of lymphokine-activated killer (LAK) cells were rapidly converted to PBPC procedures. The main advantages of these technologies are a faster trilineage recovery of hematopoiesis after myeloablation (or severe myelosuppression), and consequently a reduced requirement for platelet and red blood cell transfusions. Apheresis is a relatively simple procedure, and a general anesthetic is not required for PBPC collection as is for traditional bone marrow harvesting. Although the precise biological mechanisms that allow PBPC mobilization remain poorly understood, most patients can have their PBPCs mobilized by either CSFs alone (commonly as an outpatient procedure), or chemotherapy followed by CSFs. The latter procedure has the advantages of reducing tumor burden in vivo, as well as mobilizing PBPCs. The CD34 assay (counting labeled cells in a fluorescent-activated cell sorter) has proven to be a more reproducible and much faster assay than quantitating the number of granulocyte-macrophage colony-forming units (CFU-GM).

Cellular transfusion therapies began with mature blood cells, first with whole blood and then gradually evolving to use fractionated blood cells. The process proved to be very effective for supplementing red blood cells and platelets, but not neutrophils, primarily because of their kinetics. The second phase of cellular therapeutics began with bone marrow transplantation (BMT), and a third phase probably with the advent of recombinant human cytokines (e.g., interleukin [IL]-2) and LAK cells. A fourth exciting phase *(47)* has now begun with ex vivo stem cell expansion technologies (to allow a faster hematopoietic recovery or purging of contaminating tumor cells) and ex vivo genetic modification of blood cells (e.g., gene-marking experiments). Ex vivo expansion of tumor cells (to stimulate an antigenic response) or immune cells (to control the severity of graft-vs-host disease [GVHD] after allogeneic BMT) can be performed by inserting a suicide gene into the T lymphocytes of the donor. Gene transfection systems linked with stem cell separation devices or bioreactors, boosting the transfection efficiency of a gene transfer system, are undergoing development by several biotechnology companies, and might eventually lead to novel forms of anticancer therapy, independent of (or complementary to) traditional chemotherapy.

Abs directed against epitopes of epithelial cells are often used to detect minimal numbers of contaminating epithelial tumor cells in bone marrow of patients with solid tumors. The presence of these epithelial cells indicates systemic disease, and for several common cancers (such as breast, gastric, colorectal, and lung cancer) their presence has been reported to be a predictor for distant relapse. Novel approaches, such as RNA-based methods, are less reliable, but techniques such as sequential analysis of gene expression (SAGE) appear promising *(48)*.

Table 1
Matrix of Targets

	RP1	RP2	RP3	RP4	RP5	RP6	RP7	RP8	RP9
A	N	N	LF	N	N	LF	N	LF	N
B	N	N	N	LF	N	N	LF	N	N
C	N	N	N	N	N	N	N	N	N
D	LF	N	N	LF	N	N	GF	LF	N
E	GF	N	N	N	N	LF	N	LF	N
F	GF	LF	N	N	N	N	N	N	N

The precise aberrations of regulatory pathways involved in the control of growth, differentiation, cell death, developmental history, and invasive properties can provide a "matrix of targets" for any given cancer. This matrix represents a "molecular fingerprint" of any individual cancer at a given timepoint, and can eventually be used to select appropriate drugs and therapeutic strategies.

Abbreviations: RP, regulatory pathway; N, normal gene; LF, loss of function (mainly due to point mutation, methylation of the promoter, or deletion); GF, gain of function (mainly due to point mutation or translocation); A–F, regulatory elements in any given pathway (from upstream to downstream in each regulatory cascade); because of "crosstalk" between different pathways A–F do not necessarily imply different regulatory molecules, for the same molecule can play different roles in more than one pathway: a relatively small group of key regulatory molecules are responsible for the meaning and interpretation of multiple environmental signals; RP1–RP3, growth factor dependent pathways operating in that specific tissue; RP4, hormone-dependent pathway; RP5, invasion and metastasis pathway; RP6, DNA repair pathway; RP7, cell-cycle regulatory pathway; RP8, apoptosis pathway; RP9, angiogenesis switch pathway.

As soon as enough information on the precise molecular mechanisms involved in the regulation of cell behavior (benign or malignant) is obtained, it will be possible to classify all the players (regulatory proteins) into processes (diseased regulatory pathways). Then, not only will it be possible to tell which are the key players in each pathway, but also how each pathway is organized (from upstream to downstream), and where therapeutic intervention should be used to correct the malignant behavior of tumor cells (e.g., inhibiting angiogenesis, cell growth, or the metastatic process), to eradicate malignant cell clones (by facilitating senescence and/or apoptosis, or by stimulating the destruction of tumor cells by the immune system) (Table 1).

The number of potential therapeutic targets ranges from several hundred to perhaps only 20 or 30. Most of these processes, if not all, will have upstream regulatory elements (e.g., membrane-bound or membrane-associated), intermediate elements (cytosolic or bound to organelles, such as mitochondria), and downstream elements (transcription factors or DNA- or RNA-specific sequences). New cancer therapies will not be directed merely to hit the DNA synthetic machinery, but to hit selective targets downstream from abnormally activated catalytic functions (thereby abrogating the abnormal stimulatory signals), or upstream from inactivated or missing catalytic functions (switching on parallel or alternative regulatory pathways).

The concept of regulatory pathways involved in cell behavior is the basis of a new biochemistry. Classical biochemistry taught the basic information on how a cell obtains the energy it requires to survive. For example, in 1941 Fritz Lipmann postulated that ATP functions in a cyclic manner as a carrier of chemical energy from the degradative or catabolic reactions of metabolism, which yield chemical energy, to the cellular processes that require an energy input. The new biochemistry will tell us how a cell knows what the rest of the cells (in the same tissue or in the rest of the body) want it to do in terms of differentiating (or eventually dying) or proliferating, or moving somewhere else. Phosphate atoms are again involved in this new biochemistry, for protein phosphorylation is the common end-result of many signal pathways. In 1937 (the same year Krebs postulated the citric acid cycle), Cori and Cori began their outstanding studies of glycogen phosphorylation. However, it was not until 1988 that Tonks obtained the first partial sequence of a tyrosine phosphatase. Today, it has been suggested that the human genome might contain as many as 2000 kinase genes and up to 1000 phosphatase genes *(49)*.

A normal cell, under normal circumstances, probably decides nothing by itself (there is no cellular free will), but merely obeys orders. Normal cells can signal each other in many different ways: through pores in the membranes (gap junctions or plasmodesmata), by specific membrane receptors that recognize soluble or bound ligands (endocrine, paracrine, or autocrine mechanisms), or by synaptic transmission (special circumstances of neurons). However, a cancer cell (because of mutations, amplifications, translocations, or deletions) makes mistakes (misinterpreting the normal orders or even making them up for the wrong reasons). It cannot avoid doing so because its "software" has gone wrong, and in a progressive way. Cancer cells do not have exactly the same underlying chemistry as the normal cells of the body, which makes them vulnerable to more specific and selective drugs.

Most of these second, third, fourth, etc., intracellular messengers are binary: they are either switched on or off (by phosphorylation–dephosphorylation, for example). At any one time, a number of positive and negative signals travel from the cell membrane to the nucleus (and, perhaps, also backwards). These signals are irreversibly altered in cancer cells, and the normal balance between the on and off signals is altered.

To reestablish the normal circuits, or to kill the cells by misdirecting them into apoptosis, it will be necessary to understand these key pathways and to develop drugs to block them or to activate alternative complementary pathways. Thus, cancer is a disease process of regulatory pathways. Magic bullets to kill all cancer cells may not exist. The signal-transduction pathways involved in the proliferative response to various growth factors and mitogens are extremely complex and interactive, and they do not act as simple linear cascades. Crosstalk is an invariable feature. The new biochemistry is essentially the network of sensing and signaling in cell homeostasis.

Several key questions remain:

- How much selectivity can we expect to achieve with new drugs that will manipulate these complex signaling pathways?
- Will these new drugs be cytostatic, or cytotoxic, or both?
- How will these new drugs be obtained: serendipity, rational drug design, high-throughput screening, combinatorial chemistry, antisense technologies, gene vectors, anti-growth factors, monoclonal antibodies (mAbs)?
- Will they imply chronic or acute therapies?
- Will they have new, at times unexpected, toxicities?
- Will some malignant clones develop resistance to signal transduction therapy?

Cancer as a "malady of the genes" is an attractive model, but a large proportion of human ill health has a genetic basis. It has been estimated that at least 30%, and probably more, of pediatric admissions have a genetic component. Genetic ill health has been divided into three major types: inherited abnormal chromosomes (e.g., Down syndrome), inherited abnormal genes (e.g., cystic fibrosis), and somatic genetic diseases (e.g., cancer). Two hundred or more genes have been linked to carcinogenesis. Cancer is thought to be caused by the accumulation of two or more hits (two or more mutations affecting critical regulatory aspects such as cellular proliferation, differentiation, cell death, cellular adhesion, angiogenesis, cell contact inhibition, immune regulation, and genomic stability). The combinatorial possibilities of different mutations occurring in different genes can help to explain the extremely variable clinical and pathological features of human cancers. Moreover, clinical cancers are the result of months or years of clonal evolution and they seldom stop accumulating new mutations.

There are at least 16 ways to reduce or abolish the function of a gene product:

- Deletion of the entire gene
- Loss of the relevant chromosome
- Deletion of part of the gene
- Disruption of the gene structure (by a translocation or an inversion)
- Insertion of a sequence into the gene
- Inhibition or prevention of transcription
- Mutation of the promoter reducing mRNA levels
- Decrease in mRNA stability
- Inactivation of donor splice sites (causing read-through into the intron)
- Inactivation of donor or acceptor splice sites (causing exon to be skipped)
- Activation of cryptic splice sites
- Introduction of a frameshift in translation
- Conversion of a codon into a stop codon
- Replacement of an essential amino acid
- Prevention of posttranscriptional processing
- Prevention of correct cellular localization of product

The mutation of a gene is not the only way to abolish its function (e.g., long-range chromatin alterations, abnormal methylation, and/or imprinting). For example, in human neoplasms *p16* is silenced in at least three ways: homozygous deletion, methylation of the promoter, and point mutation. The first two represent the majority of inactivation events in most primary cancers. *p16* is a very common early event in cancer progression and is frequently seen in premalignant lesions *(50)*. The importance of *p16* is probably similar to that of *p53*. Mutations in the *p53* gene have been found in some 30% of human tumors.

Loss of function mutations usually produce recessive phenotypes, so if one allele remains normal, there are no significant phenotypic changes. For a limited number of genes, a 50% reduction in the dosage of the gene can lead to phenotypic changes (dosage effect). Certain regulatory functions are inherently dosage sensitive (e.g., gene products that compete with each other to determine a developmental or metabolic switch, or that cooperate with each other in interactions with fixed stoichiometry, or whose function depends on partial or variable occupancy of a receptor or DNA-binding site).

Less frequently, mutations can lead to a gain, rather than a loss, of function. For example, mutations can result in the ability to acquire a new substrate, overexpression of the gene product, permanently turned on receptor, inappropriately open ion channel, structurally abnormal multimers, chimeric genes, ability to bind to new DNA sequences, or the ability to trap and inactivate important regulatory molecules. If a protein has several catalytic and allosteric domains (e.g., exists at a regulatory network bottle neck), destruction or loss of function of only one of these domains can allow others to be inappropriately activated.

It is, at least theoretically, possible that some carcinogenic events may include both loss of the natural function of the gene product and gain of a function not normally associated with that particular gene product. For example, a truncated protein might be unable to perform the original function of the native protein, but could still interact functionally with other regulatory proteins by exposing the remaining protein domains.

An important issue in new drug development is whether to concentrate on abnormal oncoproteins (e.g., mutated forms of the regulatory proteins involved in carcinogenesis) or on the normal counterparts. Although some oncoproteins (e.g., Ras in pancreatic cancer) are frequently mutated at the same codon for a particular tumor type, many more derive from very large genes (e.g., *BRCA1* and *BRCA2*) or relatively large genes (*p53*) with multiple different possible mutations along the gene, which may differ according to tumor type and epidemiological reasons (e.g., different ethnic group, contact with specific carcinogens). Thus, it could prove globally more rewarding to concentrate on normal regulatory proteins (e.g., at downstream bottlenecks, or points of crosstalk) than on mutated oncoproteins. The problem here, however, is that inhibition of normal regulatory oncoproteins might prove more toxic than selective inhibition of mutated oncoproteins.

Once the relevant oncoprotein is identified and purified, gene cloning allows the production of sufficient quantities to determine its main molecular mechanisms (catalytic or regulatory) and its three-dimensional structure. Appropriate molecules (i.e., developed by empirical methods such as high-throughput screening or rational drug design) can be tested in vitro and in preclinical models to determine activity, toxicity, pharmacokinetics, and pharmacodynamics. More hospital oncology units will be devoted to clinical testing of new drugs, and cancer research is likely to undergo rapid growth, provided enough resources are made available.

The pattern of tissue-specific expression of a gene is often a poor predictor of the clinical effects of mutations. Although tissues where the gene is normally not expressed are unlikely to suffer primary pathology, the converse is not true: ectopic production of adrenocorticotrophic hormone (ACTH) by lung cancer can lead to Cushing's syndrome, whereas the *Rb* gene is ubiquitously expressed but only the retina is affected by inherited mutations. Simple correlations between a genotype at a locus and the phenotype of an individual are the exception, not the rule.

Cancer is more complex than originally thought. Simple solutions are seldom valid to solve complex problems (although, it can also be argued, a simple drug such as cisplatin can cure most germinal cell cancers), and the future will depend on finding multiple partial solutions to improve the rate of prevention and cure for this deadly disease.

A global consideration of the matrix of targets (Table 1) also helps to understand why it is so difficult to reliably and reproducibly link prognosis to changes in a single molecular marker. Many retrospective studies fail to show (by multivariate analysis) significant clinicopathological correlations between a single molecular marker and response to treatment or survival. Moreover, different studies often reach apparently contradictory results, and prospective studies fail to validate clearcut relationships. These outcomes may be because, among other possible reasons, a single marker is not truly meaningful outside the context of the full pattern or matrix of markers. Therefore, all of the relevant molecular abnormalities present in any given tumor should be taken into consideration.

The War Against Cancer Is Not Over: We Need New Therapies

If one looks at the results of cancer research from a perspective of 25 yr, one cannot help feeling satisfied with the results of this research effort in terms of progress in knowledge, although still unsatisfied in terms of therapeutic results. Twenty-five years ago, there was no knowledge of the genetic nature of malignant transformation, and almost nothing was known about growth factors, apoptosis, or regulatory pathways of cell division. Most alkylating agents, corticosteroids, antimetabolites, endocrine therapies, vinca alkaloids, and antitumor antibiotics were already used in the clinic, and platinum analogues were pending. There was no gene therapy, no mAbs, no Human Genome Project, no DNA chips, no biotechnology, no combinatorial chemistry, no high-throughput screening. People working with yeast, *Drosophila melanogaster*, or *Caenorhabditis elegans* could not have hoped that their work should become very important for oncologists. Twenty-five years ago, some prestigious scientists confessed that they could find no reproducible molecular differences between normal and malignant cells that could explain the aberrant behavior of cancer cells. Twenty-five years ago, physicians rarely told patients that they had cancer, and if specifically questioned, they routinely lied to protect the patient. Yet, 25 yr ago there was hope (irrational but comforting) that one day someone, working with exotic plants or fungi or experimenting in the vaccine world, would by chance discover a magic bullet against cancer that would be effective against most common tumor types.

Today, we know so much about cancer that, in Socratic terms, "we know almost nothing." We know that cancer is a more complex problem than most of us expected, and that, most probably, there will be no magic bullet. No two cancers are likely to be identical. Even if two cancers arise from the same tissue type and share similar regulatory pathways, they probably have different point mutations, deletions, chromosomal translocations, and genetic instability. We are using, more or less, the same drugs used 25 yr ago (except, perhaps, for taxanes, liposomal formulations, topoisomerase 1 inhibitors, some mAbs, and variants of the old antimitotic agents). We rely on the same prognostic factors: performance status, TNM stage, age/sex of the patient, histological tumor type, and differentiation. However, this book is good evidence for the imminent arrival of a new therapeutic world. The next 25 yr will be crucial in the fight against cancer.

This research effort will be unparalleled in the history of pharmacology. Hundreds of thousands of new drugs will require clinical testing (phase 1 and 2). New drug development will need to integrate molecular knowledge on specific tumors, because each cancer could prove to be different. The molecular changes induced by the test drug will need to be monitored *in situ*, to confirm that the drug produces the changes in cellular signaling that were predicted before testing. Each cancer will be screened for RNA expression, and automatic PCR devices (and sequencing devices) will provide the clinician with a matrix of targets for that particular cancer in that particular patient. Thus, primary chemotherapy (also known as neo-adjuvant therapy) will probably be more commonly used. Even with cytotoxic drugs currently available, primary chemotherapy has already been shown in several important tumor models (e.g., breast cancer, bladder cancer, head and neck cancers, and some lung cancers) to have a potentially better therapeutic index than adjuvant chemotherapies *(51)*. Neo-adjuvant therapy provides locoregional control and disease-free and overall survival rates similar to those obtained using current adjuvant therapies, has the advantage of assessing in vivo the response to specific chemotherapy agents or regimens, and improves the possibility of nonmutilating surgeries (e.g., breast-conserving surgery).

The activity of many of the cytotoxic agents used in today's practice was first detected in the traditional screening methods such as the murine leukemias (L1210 and P388) and murine solid tumors. Noncytotoxic approaches to cancer therapeutics (e.g., signal-transduction inhibitors or antiangiogenic agents) have already entered the drug development scene *(52,53)*. There are already several antiangiogenic drugs in clinical trials and the variability already seen in their activity suggests that their mechanisms in patients might be more complex and unpredictable than in inbred mice. One, at least theoretical, advantage of antiangiogenic drugs is that endothelial cells are less likely than tumor cells to become drug resistant, as they develop from normal tissue, which is genetically more stable than cancer tissue *(54)*. The crystal structure of the angiogenesis inhibitor endostatin might allow a better understanding of this important agent and provide insights into which parts of the molecule are therapeutically important *(55)*. Integration of clinically relevant inhibitors of angiogenesis into cytotoxic programs (e.g., as adjuvant long-term therapy after primary surgery or induction chemotherapy) is expected to result in improved outcomes.

New methods to overcome drug resistance or to increase the cytotoxic effect of some chemotherapy agents are already being exploited in the clinic. For example, the combination of Herceptin™ (a humanized anti-HER2 mAb, also known as trastuzumab) and paclitaxel can enhance response rates in women with breast cancer and reduce toxicity *(56)*. The exact mechanisms of this effect are still incompletely understood. In a similar manner, a humanized (chimeric) mAb (C225) has been developed that binds to the extracellular domain of epidermal growth factor receptor (EGFR) with higher affinity than the normal ligands, but upon binding does not stimulate the tyrosine kinase activity of the receptor and may enhance the therapeutic index of radiation therapy in patients with advanced head and neck cancer *(57)*.

Considering that many of the noncytotoxic anticancer agents will produce a cytostatic effect, rather than frank tumor regression, clinical trial design and endpoints will need to differ from conventional ones *(58)*.

In 1913, Paul Ehrlich wrote: "Parasites possess a whole series of chemoreceptors which differ specifically from each other. Now, if we were to succeed in discovering among these a receptor which was not represented in the organs of the host, we would have the possibility of constructing an ideal medicament by selecting a 'haptophore' (which brings about the anchoring and fixation) group which fits exclusively this particular receptor of the parasite. A medicament provided with such a chemical group would be entirely innocuous, because it is not anchored by the organs, it would, however, strike the parasites with full force and, in this sense, correspond to the immune substances ('antibodies') which, in the manner of magic bullets, seek out the enemy" (P. Ehrlich, Seventeenth International Congress of Medicine, 1913–14). Ehrlich's observations with vital stains led him to understand that different tissues display different and specific binding abilities and to the belief that it should be possible to exploit these differences in terms of selective toxic action. He began with the arsenicals and toxic dyestuffs, which led to the sulfonamides and the first clear enunciation of a principle of inhibition at a molecular level: an enzyme catalyzing the metabolism of *p*-aminobenzoic acid.

The development of sulfonamides led to the principle of metabolite analogy (i.e., an analogue of a metabolite can inhibit a relevant enzyme in a selective and therapeutically relevant manner) and to the hope that the full molecular understanding of the action of a drug leads to accurate and predictable activity of a given structure based on physical and chemical parameters. Classical biochemical targets for drug action have included:

- Inhibition at the active center (e.g., by substrate competition or cofactor inhibition)
- Allosteric inhibition and false feedback inhibitors
- Other inhibitors acting outside the active center (exo-inhibitors)
- Double blockade (pairs of compounds used together to block a single biosynthetic pathway)

Then, in a rather unpredictable way, came the discovery of penicillin (causing impairment of function or synthesis of bacterial cell wall components) and the development of screening techniques that led to the empirical discovery of most antibiotics— "toxic ones by the hundred, selectively toxic ones rarely but significantly" *(59)*. In sequential systems, such as biosynthetic pathways, the product of one enzyme is the substrate of the next and precise cytological organization must be important to secure the working of the production line. Regulatory mechanisms must apply not only to the machinery itself (enzymes in general) but also to the concentration of substrates and metabolites protecting them from dilution, contamination, ionic changes, or pH changes (membrane pumps, lipidic structures, buffer systems). The search for antibiotics rapidly provided hundreds of new toxic substances, none of which had a known mode of action at the time of their isolation. In a matter of two decades, the growth of most pathogenic bacteria could be inhibited by appropriate and clinically relevant drugs. Some of these substances were bactericidal and some were bacteriostatic. In fact, there are probably no compounds that cause instant and complete cessation of bacterial metabolism, although in some cases the effect on growth may be extremely rapid. Thus, antibiotics (even if bactericidal) do not have to kill to be effective, and they usually need some support from the host to achieve a valuable therapeutic effect. There has been endless argument as to the point at which a bacterial cell is truly dead. Some investigators regard failure to divide as death, while others think this point is reached only when all metabolism has ceased. At one extreme, bacterial spores are alive even when their metabolism is undetectable.

Cancer cells, of course, pose more formidable problems than bacterial cells. Their complexity is several orders of magnitude higher, and they are not foreign cells (such as bacteria or fungi), but daughters or granddaughters of normal body cells. However, progress in knowledge will inevitably translate into rapid new therapeutic developments. Perhaps within a decade, we shall witness a therapeutic revolution similar to that experienced in the fight against microbial infection after World War II. Scientific discoveries and progress do not follow a continuous or uniform pace, but are frequently exposed to bouts of more rapid, discontinuous development. At present, the prospects for this to happen in the fight against cancer seem rather high. For those of us who see cancer patients dying almost every day, and feel the pain associated with such premature loss of life, the intensification and coordination of cancer research is an ethical must. Because the kinds of ethics we are doing at the beginning of the third millennium must be based on logic, it follows that we must use the methods of logic. As Kant said (in his book *The Foundations of the Metaphysics of Morals),* "To help others because one has kindly feelings towards them is of no moral worth; an act has moral worth only in so far as it is done out of a sense of duty." Politicians and managers of the pharmaceutical industry should also feel this sense of duty to the public, devote more resources, and intensify cancer research efforts, without dysfunctions or duplications.

References

1. Cairns J. *Cancer: Science and Society.* WH Freeman, San Francisco, 1978.
2. Bailar JC III, Gornik HL. Cancer undefeated. *N Engl J Med.* 1997; 336:1569–74.
3. Doll R, Peto R. The causes of cancer: quantitative estimates of avoidable risks of cancer in the United States today. *J Natl Cancer Inst.* 1981; 66:1191–98.
4. Wang XD, Liu C, Bronson RT, et al. Beta-carotenes and squamous metaplasia in ferrets. *J Natl Cancer Inst.* 1999; 91:60–64.
5. Tuyns AJ. Alcohol. In: *Cancer Epidemiology and Prevention* (Schottenfeld D and Fraumeni JF Jr, eds.), WB Saunders, Philadelphia, 1982, pp. 293–304.
6. Langenfeld J, Kiyokawa H, Sekula D, Boyle J, Dmitrovsky E. Posttranslational regulation of cyclin D1 by retinoic acid: a chemoprevention mechanism. *Proc Natl Acad Sci USA.* 1997; 94:12070–4.
7. Hong WK, Sporn MB. Recent advances in chemoprevention of cancer. *Science.* 1997; 278:1073–7.
8. Buiatti E, Palli D, Decarli A, et al. A case-control study of gastric cancer and diet in Italy. II. Association with nutrients. *Int J Cancer.* 1990; 45:896–901.
9. Greenwald P, Lanza E. Dietary fiber and colon cancer. *Bol Asoc Med PR.* 1986; 78:311–3.
10. Fraumeni JF Jr. Epidemiology of cancer. In: *Origins of Human Cancer: A Comprehensive Review* (Brugge J, Curran T, Harlow E, McCormick F, eds.), Cold Spring Harbor Laboratory Press, Cold Spring Harbor, New York, 1991, pp. 171–81.
11. De Caprio JA, Ludlow JW, Lynch D, et al. The product of the retinoblastoma susceptibility gene has properties of a cell cycle regulatory element. *Cell.* 1989; 58:1085–9.
12. Heslop HE, Rooney CM. Adoptive cellular immunotherapy for EBV lymphoproliferative disease. *Immunol Rev.* 1997; 157:217–222.
13. Rickinson AB, Moss DJ. Human cytotoxic T lymphocyte responses to Epstein–Barr virus infection. *Annu Rev Immunol.* 1997; 15:405–31.
14. Bayerdörffer E, Neubauer A, Rudolph B, et al. Regression of primary gastric lymphoma of mucosa-associated lymphoid tissue type after cure of *Helicobacter pylori* infection. *Lancet.* 1995; 345:1591–4.
15. Thiede C, Alpen B, Morgner A, et al. Ongoing somatic mutations and clonal expansions after cure of *Helicobacter pylori* infection in gastric mucosa-associated lymphoid tissue B-cell lymphoma. *J Clin Oncol.* 1998; 16:3822–31.
16. Russell MAH. Cigarette smoking: a natural history of a dependence disorder. *Br J Med Psychol.* 1971; 44:1–16.

17. Patrick E, Maibach HI. Dermatotoxicology. In: *Principles and Methods of Toxicology,* 2nd edit. (Hayes AW, ed.), Raven Press, New York, 1989, pp. 383–406.

18. Romano C, Goldstein A. Stereospecific nicotine receptors on rat brain membranes. *Science.* 1980; 210:647–50.

19. Roitt I, Brostoff J, Male D. *Immunology,* 5th edit., Mosby, London, 1998.

20. Gonzalez FJ, Jaiswal AK, Nebert DW. P-450 genes: evolution, regulation, and relationship to human cancer and pharmacogenetics. *Cold Spring Harb Symp Quant Biol.* 1986; 51:879–90.

21. Law MR. Genetic predisposition to lung cancer. *Br J Cancer.* 1990; 61:195–206.

22. Hong WK, Endicott J, Itri LM, et al. 13-*cis*-retinoic acid in the treatment of oral leukoplakia. *N Engl J Med.* 1986; 315:1501–5.

23. Moriarty M, Dunn J, Darragh A, et al. Etretinate in the treatment of actinic keratosis. A double-blind crossover study. *Lancet.* 1982; 1:364–5.

24. Moshell AN. Prevention of skin cancer in xeroderma pigmentosum with oral isotretinoin. *Cutis.* 1989; 43:485–90.

25. Hong WK, Lippman SM, Itri LM, et al. Prevention of secondary primary tumors with isotretinoin in squamous-cell carcinoma of the head and neck. *N Engl J Med.* 1990; 323:795–801.

26. Margolese RG. How do we interpret the results of the Breast Cancer Prevention Trial? *CMAJ.* 1998; 158:1613–14.

27. Goel V. Tamoxifen and breast cancer prevention: what should you tell your patients? *CMAJ.* 1998; 158:1615–17.

28. Pritchard KI. Is tamoxifen effective in prevention of breast cancer? *Lancet.* 1998; 352:80–1.

29. Hodgson SV, Maher ER. *A Practical Guide to Human Cancer Genetics.* Cambridge University Press, 1993.

30. Collins FS. *BRCA1*—lots of mutations, lots of dilemmas. *N Engl J Med.* 1996; 334:186–8.

31. Giardiello FM, Brensinger JD, Petersen GM, et al. The use and interpretation of commercial APC gene testing for familial adenomatous polyposis. *N Engl J Med.* 1997; 336:823–7.

32. Kinzler KW, Vogelstein B. Lessons from hereditary colorectal cancer. *Cell.* 1996; 87:159–70.

33. Lynch HT, Smyrk T, Lynch J. An update of HNPCC (Lynch syndrome). *Cancer Genet Cytogenet.* 1997; 93:84–99.

34. Serova OM, Mazoyer S, Puget N, et al. Mutations in *BRCA1* and *BRCA2* in breast cancer families: are there more breast-cancer susceptibility genes? *Am J Hum Genet.* 1997; 60:486–95.

35. Athma P, Rappaport R, Swift M. Molecular genotyping shows that ataxia-telangiectasia heterozygotes are predisposed to breast cancer. *Cancer Genet Cytogenet.* 1996; 92:130–4.

36. Fitzgerald MG, Bean JM, Hedge SR, et al. Heterozygous ATM mutations do not contribute to early onset breast cancer. *Cancer Genet Cytogenet.* 1996; 92:130–4.

37. Swift M. Ataxia telangiectasia and risk of breast cancer. *Lancet.* 1997; 350:740.

38. Reis A. Genetics and B-cell leukemia. *Lancet.* 1999; 353:3.

39. American Society of Clinical Oncology (ASCO): Statement of the American Society of Clinical Oncology: Genetic testing for cancer susceptibility. *J Clin Oncol.* 1996; 14:1730–6.

40. Kodish E, Wiesner GL, Mehlman M, et al. Genetic testing for cancer risk: how to reconcile the conflicts. *JAMA.* 1998; 279:179–81.

41. Boyle P. Prostate specific antigen (PSA) testing as screening for prostate cancer: the current controversy. *Ann Oncol.* 1998; 9:1263–4.

42. Bronchud MH, Scarffe JH, Thatcher N, et al. Phase I/II study of recombinant human granulocyte colony-stimulating factor in patients receiving intensive chemotherapy for small cell lung cancer. *Br J Cancer.* 1987; 56:809–13.

43. Bronchud MH, Dexter TM. Clinical use of growth factors. *Br Med Bull.* 1989; 45:590–9.
44. Hernández-Bronchud M. Growth factors and cancer. *Br J Hosp Med.* 1995; 53:20–6.
45. ASCO (American Society of Clinical Oncology). Recommendations for the use of hemato-poietic colony-stimulating factors: evidence-based, clinical practice guidelines. *J Clin Oncol.* 1994; 12:2471–2508.
46. Croockewit AJ, Bronchud MH, Aapro MS, et al. A European perspective on haematopoietic growth factors in haemato-oncology: report of an expert meeting of the EORTC. *Eur J Cancer.* 1997; 33:1732–46.
47. Emerson SG. Ex vivo expansion of hematopoietic precursors, progenitors, and stem cells: the next generation of cellular therapeutics. *Blood.* 1996; 8:3082–8.
48. Lambrechts AC, van't Veer LJ, Rodenhuis S. The detection of minimal numbers of contami-nating epithelial tumor cells in blood or bone marrow: use, limitations and future of RNA-based methods. *Ann Oncol.* 1998; 9:1269–76.
49. Hancock JT. *Cell Signaling.* Addison Wesley Longman, UK, 1997.
50. Liggett WH, Sidransky D. Role of the *p16* tumor suppressor gene in cancer. *J Clin Oncol.* 1998; 16:1197–1206.
51. Valero V, Hortobagyi GN. Primary chemotherapy: a better overall therapeutic option for patients with breast cancer. *Ann Oncol.* 1998; 9:1151–4.
52. Harris AL. Are angiostatin and endostatin cures for cancer? *Lancet.* 1998; 351:1598–9.
53. Brunn GJ, Hudson CC, Sekulic A, et al. Phosphorylation of the translational repressor PHAS-1 by the mammalian target of rapamycin. *Science.* 1997; 277:99–101.
54. Boehm T, Folkman J, Browder T, O'Reilly MS. Antiangiogenic therapy of experimental cancer does not induce drug resistance. *Nature.* 1997; 390:404–7.
55. Hohenester E, Sasaki T, Olsen BR, Timpl R. Crystal structure of the angiogenesis inhibitor endostatin at 1.5 Å resolution. *EMBO J.* 1998; 17:1656–64.
56. Slamon D, Leyland-Jones B, Shak S, et al. Addition of Herceptin (humanized anti-HER2 antibody) to first line chemotherapy for HER2 overexpressing metastatic breast cancer (HER2+/MBC) markedly increases anticancer activity: a randomized, multinational con-trolled phase III trial. *Proc Am Soc Clin Oncol.* 1998; 17:98a (abstr 377).
57. Ezequiel MP, Robert F, et al. Phase I study of anti-epidermal growth factor receptor (EGFR) antibody C225 in combination with irradiation in patients with advanced squamous cell carcinoma of the head and neck (SCCHN). *Proc Am Soc Clin Oncol.* 1998; 17:395a (abstr 1522).
58. Von Hoff DD. There are no bad anticancer agents, only bad clinical trial designs—Twenty-first Richard and Hinda Rosenthal Foundation Award Lecture. *Clin Cancer Res.* 1998; 4:1079–86.
59. Gale EF, Cundliffe E, Reynolds PE, Richmond MH, Waring MJ. *The Molecular Basis of Antibiotic Action,* John Wiley & Sons, London, 1972.

2

Clinical Importance of Prognostic Factors

Moving from Scientifically Interesting to Clinically Useful

Daniel F. Hayes

Introduction

The term "prognostic factor," when used to describe patients with malignancies, has taken on several meanings. In general, a prognostic factor is considered to be useful because its results serve to separate a large heterogeneous population into smaller populations with more concisely predictable outcomes. In theory, if this separation is both reliable and disparate, one can apply therapy more efficiently to the population by exposing those most likely to need and benefit from the therapy while ensuring that the other group avoids needless toxicities.

In essence, the term "tumor markers" has come to describe a variety of molecules or processes that differ from the norm in either malignant cells or tissues, or in patients with malignancies. Assessing these alterations from normal can be used to place patients into categories that are distinguished by different outcomes, either in the absence of specific therapy or after various treatments are applied.

Tumor markers can include changes at the genetic level (e.g., mutations, deletions, or amplifications), at the transcriptional level (e.g., overexpression or underexpression), at the translational or posttranslational level (e.g., increased or decreased quantities of protein, or abnormal glycosylation of proteins), and/or at the functional level (e.g., histologic description of cellular grade or presence of neovascularization). Each of these changes can be assessed by one or more assays, which can be performed using one or more methods with differing reagents. This enormous heterogeneity of approaches is the root of considerable confusion regarding the value, in clinical terms, of a given tumor marker.

The molecular revolution is now well into its fourth decade. Despite impressive advances in the understanding of the biology of human malignancy and in the technology of investigating molecular processes, the number of clinically useful products from these advances is disappointing. For example, in 1995, the American Society of Clinical Oncology (ASCO) convened a panel of experts to establish guidelines for the use of tumor markers in colon and breast carcinoma. Although the Expert Panel reviewed many putative markers (including both tissue-based and circulating markers), their

From: *Principles of Molecular Oncology*
Edited by: M. H. Bronchud, M. A. Foote, W. P. Peters, and M. O. Robinson © Humana Press Inc., Totowa, NJ

Table 1
ASCO Practice Guidelines for Colorectal and Breast Cancer

Colorectal Cancer
- CEA
  - Not recommended for screening
  - May be used to assist staging and surgical planning, but insufficient data to use as independent prognostic variable
  - May be used to detect potentially resectable liver metastases during followup
  - May be used to monitor response to therapy in metastatic disease in association with other tests

- Other Markers
  - Insufficient data to recommend circulating LASA or CA19-9 for clinical use
  - Insufficient data to recommend DNA flow cytometry, *p53* expression or mutation, or *ras* for screening, diagnosis, staging, surveillance or monitoring.

Breast Cancer
- CA-15-3, CA27.29, CEA
  - Insufficient data to use for screening, diagnosis, prognosis, or surveillance following primary treatment
  - May be used to monitor treatment to detect progression in metastatic disease for selected patients

- ER, PR
  - Should be used to identify patients most likely to benefit from hormone therapy
  - Data insufficient to use for prognosis independent of therapy

- Other Markers
  - Insufficient data to recommend DNA flow cytometry (ploidy, S-phase fraction), c-*erbB2*, *p53*, or cathepsin D for any aspect of patient management

Modified from ASCO Expert Panel. *J Clin Oncol.* 1998; 16:793–95.
CEA = carcinoembryonic antigen; ER = estrogen receptor; PR = progesterone receptor; LASA = lipid-associated sialic acid.

ultimate recommendations were surprisingly sparse (Table 1) *(1,2)*. After careful deliberation, the Panel felt that very few of the new molecular markers (e.g., *erbB-2*, *p53*, cathepsin D) had actually been established in a scientifically rigorous fashion to be reliable and definitive.

Why were the guidelines so conservative? In reviewing the available literature, it became increasingly clear that the science of tumor-marker investigation has been haphazard and chaotic. Too often, studies of tumor markers are more inclined to fishing expeditions with the hope that something interesting will be detected with statistical significance, rather than being prospective, hypothesis-driven investigations. In light of this confusion, several authors of the Guidelines separately developed a proposal for a framework in which previously published tumor-marker studies might be critically evaluated. The authors also suggested that this framework might be used by investigators to plan future studies that lead to more rapid acceptance, or refutation, of a given marker in the clinical arena. This system, designated the Tumor Marker Utility Grading System (TMUGS), has been published elsewhere, as has a follow-up extension of TMUGS (designated TMUGS-plus) *(3,4)*. In this chapter, the systems are briefly reviewed and how they might be used to evaluate some of the more exciting markers that are currently under investigation is discussed. A detailed discussion of the role of specific tumor markers for all malignancies is beyond the scope of this review. Rather, the discussion will principally relate to examples of evaluations of tumor markers in solid tumors, although these systems are certainly applicable to other malignancies in general.

Prognosis vs Prediction

Estimating a patient's prognosis requires a complicated set of evaluations, which includes the propensity of a malignancy to expand in volume (proliferative capacity), its ability to escape its natural site of origin and establish growth in a foreign tissue (metastatic potential), and its relative sensitivity or resistance to therapy. Therapies for most solid tumors include surgery, radiation, and/or systemic therapies, such as hormone therapies or chemotherapies. In this regard, the terms "prognostic" and "predictive" have taken on separate meanings *(5,6)*. A prognostic factor is usually reserved for those markers that specifically provide an estimate of the odds of a given cancer's recurrence after local therapy only. It is usually a measure of both proliferation and metastatic potential, and it usually implies the odds of systemic recurrence and/or death in a patient who does not receive systemic therapy. Therefore, a prognostic factor is most helpful in determining if a patient is likely to be cured by local therapy alone (surgery and/or radiation therapy), or whether he or she is more likely to have a subsequent recurrence. If so, and if therapy is available that has demonstrated efficacy in that setting, knowledge of an individual's prognosis permits reasonable decision-making regarding whether or not application of further therapy is indicated. The best examples of prognostic factors for most solid tumors are the tumor, node, metastases (TNM) staging systems.

A predictive factor is a tumor marker that helps select therapies most likely to work against that patient's tumor. A predictive factor may actually be the target of the therapy, or may be an associated molecule or pathway that modifies the effectiveness of the therapy. For example, it is now clearly established that the level of estrogen receptor (ER) content in breast cancer tissue is directly related to the odds of response and benefit from antiestrogen hormonal therapy, such as ovarian ablation, tamoxifen, or aromatase inhibitors, because the ER plays a fundamental role in estrogen-dependent tumor growth and biology *(7)*. In contrast, p-glycoprotein content is a predictive factor for response to certain drugs, since this protein modulates multidrug resistance (MDR) by increasing efflux of the antineoplastic agent from the cancer cell *(8)*.

Many factors may be both prognostic and predictive. For example, in addition to serving as a predictive factor, ER is also a prognostic factor. Breast cancers with high ER content have generally slower growth potentials, and patients with ER-"positive" tumors have a better prognosis, even if they receive no treatment *(9,10)*.

Some markers may be associated with a poor prognosis independent of therapy, but they may predict for an improved outcome related to specific treatment modalities.

One such marker may be the *erbB-2* (*HER-2*, c-*neu*) proto-oncogene. Since 1987, several studies have been published that have reported conflicting results regarding whether *erbB-2* amplification and/or overexpression is a marker of poor prognosis or not *(11)*. Recent analyses have begun to suggest that *erbB-2* is independently prognostic *(12)*. However, *erbB-2* may also be predictive of resistance to hormone therapy and to alkylating agents, but predictive of sensitivity to anthracyclines, such as doxorubicin *(13–20)*.

These considerations are often ignored in many prognostic factor studies. Often, a population of patients is studied with a new, putative prognostic factor simply because the samples to be assayed are available and the outcome for the patients is known. It is not surprising that studies of a marker that might have both prognostic and predictive capabilities, especially if these effects are in opposition (as may be the case with *erbB-2*), will provide relatively random and conflicting results if not carefully planned.

Why Use Tumor Markers?

Ideally, a specific therapy will benefit all to whom it is administered, and no patient will be exposed to toxicity needlessly. However, in an imperfect world, only a fraction of patients who receive a given treatment will benefit, while all are at risk for the side effects. For example, application of adjuvant systemic therapy, designed to prevent future recurrence after local eradication of a newly diagnosed tumor to patients with a very low risk of subsequent relapse, can benefit only those few whose tumors are destined to recur. In this case, pretreatment identification of that subgroup with prognostic factors will allow the other patients to avoid being treated unnecessarily. However, simply having a poor prognosis is not justification for treatment. Many patients will have tumors that are already resistant to specific treatments. In this case, predictive factors will permit selection of those patients who will benefit from the specific therapy. Unfortunately, treatment for the other patients may not be available or as effective, but there is still no reason to expose them to toxicity with no benefit.

Do prognostic and predictive factors exist that permit such elegant selection of patients for treatment? Sadly, in most solid tumors, the answer is no. For patients with newly diagnosed solid malignancies, there is no example of a prognostic factor that predicts subsequent recurrence and death with absolute certainty. For example, most clinicians are taught that metastatic breast cancer is universally fatal, with median survival times of 18–36 mo *(21)*. However, an interesting experience published by Bloom and his colleagues *(22)* illustrates the uncertainty of predicting patient outcomes even with this disease. In this study, Bloom et al. reviewed the long-term survival of more than 200 patients who presented to the Middlesex Hospital Cancer Charity Ward from the late 18th century to the early 1900s. All patients had advanced local (and probably metastatic) breast cancer and were admitted to the ward for nursing care only, as, of course, no therapies for cancer were available at that time. Remarkably, a small group of these patients survived for 10 or more years from the time they presented, illustrating the diverse natural history of this disease.

The point of the previous illustration is that no prognostic, or predictive, marker has 100% accuracy. Therefore, when they are applied in the clinic, both physician and patient must accept some margin of error. Almost no patient with a newly diagnosed solid malignancy, no matter how favorable the prognosis, does not have some risk of recurrence and death during the succeeding decade. If effective therapy is available that reduces this risk, then not applying that therapy to all patients means that an occasional patient will relapse, and perhaps die, who would have benefited from treatment. However, if the treatment has any risks and associated costs (and all do), application of this treatment to a large group of patients with such a favorable prognosis may harm more patients than it helps.

Therefore, part of the art, and science, of medicine is to determine which markers are most reliable in separating patients into those who will do well from those who will not, and into those who will benefit from therapy from those who will not. If performed appropriately, tumor-marker analysis should permit delivery of therapy as efficiently as possible, providing benefit to the greatest number of patients while avoiding exposure to toxicities as much as possible.

TMUGS: An Overview

Clinical investigations of new cancer agents are carefully planned, using criteria and terminology that are generally agreed upon by most clinical scientists. For example, new drugs are sequentially passed through phase 1, 2, and 3 studies, in which toxicity and dose, efficacy, and definitive utility are determined, respectively. In these studies, scales have been developed to describe toxicities, responses, and overall outcomes. Such trials are prospectively planned, with detailed descriptions of the number and types of patients to be studied, how they will be treated, and how the statistical analysis will be performed. Indeed, these rules have been established so that the results of clinical studies approach the same veracity as those from laboratory investigations, in which variables and proper controls can be rigorously defined. Clinical studies that are not so rigorously defined, such as retrospective reviews of clinical experiences, may help generate hypotheses, but are rarely accepted as definitive.

In the past, no such consensus system has existed to study tumor markers. More commonly, marker studies are performed using retrospectively available samples from patients treated in a nonuniform manner. Hypotheses are often generated after the data are analyzed, and then presented as fact. Even when multiple studies of the same hypothesis are performed, the populations studied are often heterogeneous and the methods often vary from one investigator to the next. Furthermore, negative results are usually not submitted for publication (unless to refute the results of a competing laboratory). It is no wonder that most tumor markers proceed through a typical life cycle before the utility is accepted or discarded (Fig. 1). In fact, progression through such a life cycle is also common for new therapeutic ideas as well. Because the rules are better established, the time required to reach consensus may be considerably shorter.

TMUGS was proposed to similarly shorten the life cycle of tumor-marker analysis. A more detailed analysis of the TMUGS system is published elsewhere *(3)*. One component of TMUGS is the importance of a precise description of the tumor marker and the assays used to detect it. The authors also proposed a semiquantitative scale, which ranges from 0 to 3+, to grade the clinical utility of a tumor marker for any specific use (Table 2). For example, to assess whether a marker should be used to determine prognosis, the user is urged to assign a score based on his or her interpretation of the available published data. A grade of 0 implies that sufficient data exist to conclude that the marker has no utility for that use, while a grade of 2+ or 3+ implies that the

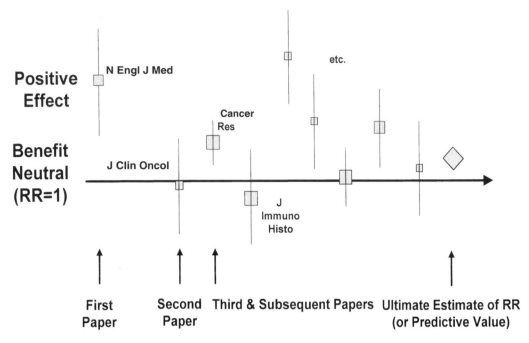

Fig. 1. Life cycle of a tumor marker.

marker should either be considered or that it absolutely should be used, respectively, in routine clinical practice. In TMUGS, the user is encouraged to support his/her evaluation by determining the level of evidence (LOE) on which his or her decision is based (Table 3). LOE I data are generated from either a prospective, highly powered study that specifically addresses the issue of tumor-marker utility or from an overview or meta-analysis of studies, each of which provides lower levels of evidence. LOE II data are derived from companion studies in which specimens are collected prospectively as part of a therapeutic clinical trial, with preestablished endpoints and statistical evaluation for the marker as well as for the therapeutic intervention. Unfortunately, most tumor-marker studies are LOE III, in which specimens happen to have been collected for a variety of reasons and are available for testing a given assay. In general, the authors of TMUGS implied that results from LOE I studies are preferred to assign clinical utility to a marker. However, they did not specifically address the strength required for a marker to be useful, nor how one might determine that strength.

TMUGS Plus

A major question left unanswered by TMUGS regards the relative strength required for a tumor marker to be clinically useful. Even if the marker divides the population into two distinct groups based on predicted outcomes (independent or dependent on therapy), do those groups differ sufficiently that the clinician will be comfortable treating them differently? This consideration begs the question of how much benefit a given patient is willing to forego to avoid toxicities. Of course, this depends on three factors: the size of the benefit, the degree of potential toxicity, and the overall attitude of the

Table 2
TMUGS Grading Scale for Clinical Utility of Tumor Marker

Utility scale	Explanation of scale
0	Marker has been adequately evaluated for a specific use and the data definitively demonstrate it has *no utility*. The marker should not be ordered for that clinical use.
NA	Data are not available for the marker for that use because marker has not been studied for that clinical use.
+/–	Data are suggestive that the marker may correlate with biological process and/or endpoint, and preliminary data suggest that use of the marker *may* contribute to favorable clinical outcome, but more definitive studies are required. Thus, the marker is still considered highly investigational and should not be used for standard clinical practice.
+	Sufficient data are available to demonstrate that the marker correlates with the biological process and/or endpoint related to the use, and that the marker results might effect favorable clinical outcome for that use. However, the marker is still considered investigational and should not be used for standard clinical practice, for one of three reasons: <ol><li>The marker correlates with another marker or test that has been established to have clinical utility, but the new marker has not been shown to clearly provide any advantage.</li><li>The marker may contribute independent information, but it is unclear whether that information provides clinical utility because treatment options have not been shown to change outcome.</li><li>Preliminary data for the marker are quite encouraging, but the level of evidence (*see below*) is lacking to document clinical utility.</li></ol>
++	Marker supplies information not otherwise available from other measures that is helpful to the clinician in decision making for that use, but the marker cannot be used as sole criterion for decision-making. Thus, marker has clinical utility for that use, and it should be considered standard practice in *selected* situations.
+++	Marker can be used as the sole criterion for clinical decision making in that use. Thus, marker has clinical utility for that use, and it should be considered standard practice.

From Hayes et al. *J Nat Cancer Inst.* 1996; 88:1456 66.

patient. Let us consider a highly life-threatening disease that can be cured only by very toxic therapy. To make the example more illustrative, let us assume that 2–3% of patients who are treated with this therapy suffer lethal toxicities. Some patients might be willing to accept the therapy if it improves their odds of survival by only 1–2% because they fear the disease worse than the treatment. Other patients would only be treated with this therapy if their odds of benefiting were substantially higher.

Table 3
Levels of Evidence for Grading Clinical Utility of Tumor Markers

Level	Type of evidence
I	Evidence from a single high-powered prospective study that is specifically designed to test marker or evidence from meta-analysis and/or overview of Level II or III studies. In the former case, the study must be designed so that therapy and followup are dictated by protocol. Ideally, the study is a prospective randomized trial in which diagnostic and/or therapeutic clinical decisions in one arm are determined based at least in part on marker results, and diagnostic and/or therapeutic clinical decisions in control arm are made independently of marker results. However, may also include prospective but not randomized trials with marker data and clinical outcome as primary objectives.
II	Evidence from study in which marker data are determined in relationship to prospective therapeutic trial that is performed to test therapeutic hypothesis but not specifically designed to test marker utility (i.e., marker study is secondary objective of protocol). However, specimen collection for marker study and statistical analysis are prospectively determined in protocol as secondary objectives.
III	Evidence from large but retrospective studies from which variable numbers of samples are available or selected. Therapeutic aspects and followup of patient population may or may not have been prospectively dictated. Statistical analysis for tumor marker was not dictated prospectively at time of therapeutic trial design.
IV	Evidence from small retrospective studies that do not have prospectively dictated therapy, followup, specimen selection, or statistical analysis. May be matched case controls, etc.
V	Evidence from small pilot studies designed to determine or estimate distribution of marker levels in sample population. May include "correlation" with other known or investigational markers of outcome, but not designed to determine clinical utility.

From Hayes et al. *J Nat Cancer Inst.* 1996; 88:1456–66

A treatment with less toxicity may be more acceptable to more patients even if the odds of benefiting are very small or do not involve survival. For example, hormonal treatment of patients with metastatic breast cancer is unlikely to cure patients or substantially prolong their survival *(23)*. However, because it has such a favorable toxicity profile, many patients may be willing to try a course of hormone therapy even if the ER profile of their tumor is unfavorable, since even an occasional patient who is deemed to be ER negative will respond *(7)*. However, if such patients have terribly symptomatic disease, or rapidly progressive (and therefore rapidly lethal) visceral metastases, they are better treated with more toxic, but potentially more effective, chemotherapy.

To return to the issue of how widely apart a tumor marker separates two populations, a weak marker may reliably separate two groups in statistical terms, but be too small to be clinically meaningful. It is now established, with a high degree of statistical significance, that patients with ER-negative breast cancer have a worse prognosis than those patients with ER-positive tumors *(24)*. However, the relative difference in outcomes between these two groups of patients is not so great that one might absolutely recommend against any adjuvant systemic therapy for ER-positive patients while strongly recommending therapy for those who are ER negative, independent of other known prognostic factors. Such a consideration raises two issues: the relative strength of given marker, and its independence from other, established factors.

How Can the Relative Strength of a Prognostic Factor Be Determined?

Prognostic and predictive factors can be placed into categories, based on their abilities to divide a single population into two or more subgroups that have distinct outcomes. Three categories have been proposed: weak, moderate, and strong. In each case, the factor may reliably distinguish two or more subgroups, but weak factors do not do so to such an extent that the patients would be treated differently. In contrast, a strong prognostic factor permits delineation between the two subgroups (e.g., those who are positive and those who are negative) with such a magnitude that one group might be observed while the other is treated.

A more detailed description of determination of the relative strengths of prognostic and predictive factors is provided elsewhere *(4)*. However, in general, factors that divide the population into subgroups that differ in outcomes by greater than twofold are considered weak, those that divide into subgroups that differ by two- to fourfold are considered moderate, and those that divide into subgroups with outcomes that differ by greater than or equal to fourfold are considered strong. The strengths of prognostic factors can be determined only by examining a population of patients who are untreated, unless the factor is a pure prognostic factor that has no interaction with treatment.

In contrast, the strength of a predictive factor is best determined in the context of a prospective clinical trial in which patients are randomly assigned to the treatment of interest or not. The ratio of the likelihood that a factor-positive patient will benefit from treatment compared with a factor-negative patient has been designated the "Benefit Ratio" *(4)*.

In the original TMUGS proposal *(3)*, determination of relative strengths is only as good as the studies in which they are analyzed. In this regard, the relative quality of the studies is essential in coming to consensus about the strength of the marker. Commonly, an early, LOE III study will report an extraordinary difference between two groups delineated by a given tumor-marker analysis. Results from subsequent studies are often more inconsistent. Therefore, it has been proposed that the relative strength of a marker should be determined only within the context of a LOE I (or at worse II) study, in which either the marker is the primary objective of a well-designed, highly powered, hypothesis-driven prospective clinical trial, or it is the objective of a statistically rigorous overview of LOE II and/or III studies. Furthermore, the strength of new prognostic or predictive factors can only be estimated by multivariate analytical methods, including preexisting, accepted factors such as TNM staging and histopathology. It is possible that a marker may be quite prognostic or predictive when considered in a univariate fashion, but that it is only reflecting information already achieved through other, established methods. In this case, acceptance of the new marker would occur only if it can be performed more easily or reliably, or less expensively.

How Can the Relative Strengths of Prognostic and Predictive Factors Be Applied Clinically?

The following discussion regarding tumor marker utility is important only in the context of currently effective therapies. For example, outside of a clinical trial, there is little value in determining that a patient has a poor prognosis unless therapy is available to change that prognosis, other than for the patient's own information. Moreover, if the patient or physician is unwilling to give up any benefit, regardless of how small and regardless of the risks, application of tumor markers is unnecessary unless the results are 100% accurate. Likewise, if the patient is unwilling to accept any therapy regardless of how large the benefit or how well tolerated the treatment, then, again, there is no point in applying tumor-marker data.

However, if the patient and physician wish to apply the therapy relatively efficiently, with some error, a matrix can be constructed in which the marker might be used in some situations but not in others (4). This matrix can be illustrated by the example of application of adjuvant systemic therapy to patients with newly diagnosed breast cancer (Table 4). In this example, it has been assumed that patients can be divided into three prognostic categories based on the odds of systemic recurrence and death during the subsequent 10 yr after diagnosis and local treatment in the absence of systemic therapy: very good (<10% chance recurrence/death), moderate (10–50%), and poor (>50%). It will be assumed, also, if no predictive factors are used, all patients will experience a proportional reduction in risk of dying of approx 30% if they receive tamoxifen or chemotherapy, and slightly higher if they receive both chemotherapy and hormone therapy (25,26).

It will also be assumed that there are four categories of absolute benefit for which physicians and patients can reach consensus regarding benefits/risks. If therapy prevents death due to breast cancer at 10 yr in 10% or more of the patients, then therapy is *absolutely* indicated (recommendation to treat is certain). If the potential absolute benefit is 6–9%, then therapy is *probably* indicated. Adjuvant systemic therapy (AST) might be *considered* but is not strongly recommended for those patients with a potential absolute benefit of 4–5%. Treatment would *not* be indicated for patients for whom the absolute benefit is 3% or less. These categories will differ based on the individual preferences of patient and physician. For example, patients might be willing to accept tamoxifen treatment for less absolute benefit, since the toxicities are less, and they might require more absolute benefit before they would consider chemotherapy.

Table 4 illustrates the decision-making process using this model, combining prognostic and predictive factors of relative strengths. In this case, a hypothetical predictive factor that is evenly distributed in the population (50% positive, 50% negative) has been chosen. In fact, ER is not substantially different than this. In Table 4, the four categories of recommendations for AST are represented by different shading. Cells that represent absolute benefits for which treatment is certain (>10%) are indicated with dark shading. Cells that represent probable treatment (6–9%) are indicated by medium shading; those that represent absolute benefit (4–5%), light shading; and those that represent benefits that do not justify AST (1–3%), no shading. As no marker has

Table 4
Absolute Benefits from Adjuvant Systemic Therapy in Context of Prognostic Factors and Predictive Factor Profiles

| Prognostic categories | Absolute probability of mortality in absence of systemic therapy (worse case) | RX | Percentage of pts who benefit from Rx if no predictive factor (assume proportional reduction = 30%) | Predictive Factors *Absolute reduction in mortality due to systemic therapy in patients for whom marker is negative compared with those for whom marker is positive* | | | | | |
| | | | | Weak (BR 1.5) | | Moderate (BR3) | | Strong (BR | |
				Neg	Pos	Neg	Pos	Neg	Pos
Very good	10%	Helps	3	1	2	<1	2	<1	3
		(Does not help)	(97)	(99)	(98)	(99)	(98)	(99)	(97)
Moderate	50%	Helps	15	6	9	4	11	2	13
		(Does not help)	(85)	(94)	(91)	(96)	(89)	(98)	(87)
Very Poor	75%	Helps	23	9	13	6	17	3	19
		(Does not help)	(77)	(91)	(87)	(94)	(83)	(97)	(81)

From Hayes Trock. Harris *Breast Cancer Res Treat.*, in press.
BR = benefit ratio.

39

100% accuracy, and because patients cannot be divided into less than 1, all cells contain at least one patient and all are rounded to the nearest integer.

For patients in a very good prognostic category, only 10% are destined to have the disease recur and die of their disease in the absence of AST. If we assume a 30% proportional reduction in death with either tamoxifen or chemotherapy, either type of AST will prevent recurrence and death due to breast cancer in only 3% (0.3 × 0.10) at most. If no predictive marker is applied to this model, 97% of patients are treated for no apparent benefit: 90% will not recur even if not treated, and 7% of those who are treated will recur anyway (Table 4). Therefore, no matter how powerful the predictive factor used, there is no subgroup in which the potential absolute benefit for one or the other type of therapy exceeds 3% (Table 4). In this case, application of a predictive factor would be of little benefit, as it would have no clinical utility within the assumptions of the model. Of course, a more effective therapy (e.g., one that reduces mortality by 50%) makes a recommendation for the use of a predictive factor more compelling, even in patients with a very good prognosis.

In contrast, up to 15% (0.30 × 50) of patients with a moderate prognosis might be helped with either type of AST. In the absence of a predictive model, 85% of patients are treated for no apparent benefit. Of the 50% in whom disease will recur, 25% will be marker positive, and 25% will be marker negative. In this case, a weak predictive factor does not sufficiently distinguish one group that might be more likely to benefit from another group that is unlikely to benefit to make different treatment recommendations (absolute benefit: 9% vs 6%; both are in the "probably treat" category). On the other hand, a moderately strong predictive factor divides these patients into a factor-negative group in which only 4% would benefit, and 96% would be treated unnecessarily. In this group, it is reasonable to consider no therapy, and certainly therapy would not be strongly recommended. In the factor-positive group, the absolute potential for benefit is sufficient that therapy is clearly indicated (factor positive: 11% benefit; 89% do not). A strong predictive factor is even more useful, dividing patients into those in whom therapy is not indicated (factor negative: 2% benefit; 98% do not) and those in whom it is absolutely indicated (factor positive: 13% benefit; 87% do not). Thus, in Table 4, there is a sharp contrast between factor-negative and factor-positive patients when a strong predictive factor is considered, only a minimal contrast between the groups when a moderate predictive factor is considered, and no contrast between the groups for a weak factor.

For patients with a very poor prognosis, weak and moderate predictive factors divide the patients into those for whom therapy is possibly indicated (6–9% absolute benefit) vs those for whom therapy is clearly indicated (>10% absolute benefit). Because most clinicians and patients would accept treatment in either category, these predictive factors are not very helpful in this situation. However, once again, a strong predictive factor is very useful, dividing patients into those for whom treatment is not indicated (factor negative: 3% benefit; 97% do not) vs those for whom treatment is very likely to be beneficial (factor positive: 19% benefit; 81% do not). Again, the strong predictive factor also minimizes the percentage of patients treated who are unlikely to benefit. In summary, prognostic and predictive factors are most helpful if they result in stark contrast between two cells in a given category, as illustrated in Table 4.

One final set of assumptions must be made to complete the proposed model. Predictive factors are helpful only if they provide an estimate of the attributable benefit within the population. The attributable benefit rests on the relative cutoff to divide the population into positive vs negative subgroups. For example, one might use a very stringent cutoff that identifies a small population (e.g., 10%) that might be very likely to benefit but that leaves the remaining population with a moderate chance of benefit. In this case, treating only the positive patients results in a substantial loss of benefit for many of the other 90%. Therefore, cutoff points must be chosen carefully and prospectively confirmed to reliably distinguish favorable from poor subgroups of patients.

The best example of a model in which the factor is roughly evenly distributed (50/50) involves the application of ER data to patients in either moderate or very bad prognostic categories. From the Early Breast Cancer Trialists Group Overview of adjuvant systemic therapy, the overall reduction in death due to tamoxifen after 10 yr of therapy is 26% *(25)*. However, the proportional reduction in mortality for those patients with ER-positive tumor approaches 50%, but it is only 6% for ER negative patients. Therefore, the benefit ratio (BR) of ER as a predictive factor is 50/6 = 8. In other words, a patient is roughly eight times more likely to benefit from tamoxifen if she is ER rich (positive) than if she is ER poor (negative). Thus, according to Table 3, ER would be assigned as a strong predictive factor. When applied to patients with a moderate or poor prognosis, ER determination clearly separates patients into those who should be treated with adjuvant tamoxifen and those who should not. In this example, it would not be recommended to treat populations of ER-negative patients, regardless of prognosis, with tamoxifen. Likewise, because 3% or fewer patients would be expected to benefit, routine use of tamoxifen would not be recommended in patients with a very good prognosis, regardless of ER status. Of course, these recommendations are for populations, and individual patients and physicians may ignore them for any of a number of reasons.

Are There Solid Tumor Markers That Fulfill the TMUGS Criteria for Routine Clinical Use?

This is a difficult question to answer in a general review such as this. For example, markers might be used in one of several different situations (determination of risk, screening, differential diagnosis, prognosis, prediction, monitoring disease course) *(3)*. Different markers may perform differently in each situation for each different disease (e.g., colon vs breast vs lung cancer). In general, the TNM-staging system has been well accepted for prognosis for most, if not all, solid tumors *(27)*. For breast and colon cancer, the ASCO Guidelines Panel has made specific recommendations based on data they felt met criteria consistent with TMUGS (Table 1) *(1)*. These guidelines have been updated once since their original publication *(2)*. However, especially in regards to *erbB-2* analysis and breast cancer, substantially more data have become available in the 2 yr since the Panel last met. These guidelines will need to be reconsidered, in regards to whether this marker can or should be used to determine prognosis, or to determine the best form of adjuvant systemic therapy for those patients for whom a relatively poor prognosis has already been determined. In this regard, *erbB-2* amplification and/or overexpression may be helpful in choosing between hormone therapy and chemotherapy, and/or in choosing between regimens that contain doxorubicin or not *(13–20)*. Moreover, recent reports have confirmed the activity of a humanized monoclonal antibody (mAb) directed against *erbB-2* in patients with metastatic breast cancer, and it must be assumed that, like ER for hormone therapy, the level of tissue expression of *erbB-2* will be critical in selecting which patients are most likely to benefit from this novel therapy *(28–31)*.

Few if any prognostic or predictive factors have been accepted for the other common solid malignancies, such as prostate, lung, and ovarian cancers *(32–34)*. For each, the TNM and grading scales are reliably prognostic. Serial circulating prostate specific antigen (PSA) values and CA125 concentrations are helpful in monitoring patients with prostate and ovarian cancers, respectively *(33,35)*.

Summary

In summary, the phrase "many are called, few are chosen" seems to reflect the current state-of-the-art in regard to tumor-marker analysis and solid tumors. However, the field is evolving rapidly, with a convergence of molecular biology and technology and understanding of clinical trial design and analysis. Several of the large cooperative trialists groups have not established separate correlative/biologic committees that are charged with designing hypothesis-driven LOE I and II studies, based on results from pilot studies. The emergence of *erbB-2* in breast cancer as a predictive factor, in a manner similar to ER, may serve as a model of directed studies that lead to determination of the relative strength of the marker, and assignment of a TMUGS score that indicates whether or not it should be used clinically.

Acknowledgments

This work was supported in part by NIH Grant CA64057 and by the Fashion Footwear Association of New York (FFANY)/QVC/Shoes on Sale.

References

1. ASCO Expert Panel. Clinical Practice Guidelines for the Use of Tumor Markers in Breast and Colorectal Cancer: Report of the American Society of Clinical Oncology Expert Panel. *J Clin Oncol.* 1996; 14:2843–77.
2. ASCO Expert Panel. 1997 update of recommendations for the use of tumor markers in breast and colorectal cancer: *J Clin Oncol.* 1998; 16:793–5.
3. Hayes DF, Bast R, Desch CE, et al. A tumor marker utility grading system (TMUGS): a framework to evaluate clinical utility of tumor markers. *J Natl Cancer Inst.* 1996; 88:1456–66.
4. Hayes DF, Trock B, Harris AL. Assessing the clinical impact of prognostic factors: When is "statistically significant" clinically useful? *Breast Cancer Res Treat.*, 1998; 52:305–19.
5. McGuire WL, Clark GM. Prognostic factors and treatment decisions in axillary-node-negative breast cancer. *N Engl J Med.* 1992; 326:1756–61.
6. Gasparini G, Pozza F, Harris AL. Evaluating the potential usefulness of new prognostic and predictive indicators in node-negative breast cancer patients. *J Natl Cancer Inst.* 1993; 85:1206–19.
7. Osborne CK. Receptors. In: *Breast Diseases,* 2nd edit. (Harris J, Hellman S, Henderson I, et al., eds.), JB Lippincott, Philadelphia, 1991, pp. 301–25.

8. Trock B, Leonessa F, Clarke R. Multidrug resistance in breast cancer: a meta-analysis of MDR1/gp170 expression and its possible functional significance. *J Natl Cancer Inst.* 1997; 89:917–31.

9. Fisher B, Costantino J, Redmond C, et al. A randomized clinical trial evaluating tamoxifen in the treatment of patients with node-negative breast cancer who have estrogen-receptor-positive tumors. *N Engl J Med.* 1989; 320:479–84.

10. Fisher B, Redmond C, Dimitrov N, et al. A randomized clinical trial evaluating sequential methotrexate and fluorouracil in the treatment of patients with node-negative breast cancer who have estrogen-receptor-negative tumors. *N Engl J Med.* 1989; 320:473–8.

11. Hayes DF. Tumor markers for breast cancer. *Ann Oncol.* 1993; 4:807–19.

12. Press MF, Bernstein L, Thomas PA, et al. *HER-2/neu* gene amplification characterized by fluorescence in situ hybridization: poor prognosis in node-negative breast carcinomas. *J Clin Oncol.* 1997; 15:2894–904.

13. Carlomagno C, Perrone F, Gallo C, et al. c-*erbB2* overexpression decreases the benefit of adjuvant tamoxifen in early-stage breast cancer without axillary lymph node metastases. *J Clin Oncol.* 1996; 14:2702–8.

14. Leitzel K, Teramoto Y, Konrad K, et al. Elevated serum c-*erbB-2* antigen levels and decreased response to hormone therapy of breast cancer. *J Clin Oncol.* 1995; 13:1129–35.

15. Yamauchi H, O'Neill A, Gelman R, et al. Prediction of response to antiestrogen therapy in advanced breast cancer patients by pretreatment circulating levels of extracellular domain of the HER-2/c-neu protein. *J Clin Oncol.* 1997; 15:2518–25.

16. Ravdin P, Green S, Albain K, et al. Initial report of the SWOG biological correlative study of c-*erbB-2* expression as a predictor of outcome in a trial comparing adjuvant CAF T with tamoxifen (T) alone. *Proc Am Soc Clin Oncol.* 1998; 97a (abstract 374).

17. Allred DC, Clark G, Tandon A, et al. *HER-2/neu* in node-negative breast cancer: prognostic significance of overexpression influenced by the presence of in situ carcinoma. *J Clin Oncol.* 1992; 10:599–605.

18. Gusterson BA, Gelber RD, Goldhirsch A, et al. Prognostic importance of c-*erbB-2* expression in breast cancer. *J Clin Oncol.* 1992; 10:1049–56.

19. Thor A, Berry D, Budman D, et al. *erbB-2*, *p53*, and adjuvant therapy interactions in node positive breast cancer. *J Natl Cancer Inst.* 1998; 16:1346–60.

20. Paik S, Bryant J, Park C, et al. *erbB-2* and response to doxorubicin in patients with axillary lymph node-positive, hormone receptor-negative breast cancer. *J Natl Cancer Inst.* 1998; 90:1361.

21. Harris J, Morrow M, Norton L. Malignant tumors of the breast. In: *Cancer: Principles and Practice of Oncology,* 5th edit. (DeVita V, Hellman S, Rosenburg S, eds.), Lippincott-Raven, Philadelphia, 1997, pp. 1557–616.

22. Bloom H, Richardson W, Harrier EJ. Natural history of untreated breast cancer. *Br Med J.* 1962; 2:213–21.

23. Hayes DF, Henderson IC, Shapiro CL. Treatment of metastatic breast cancer: present and future prospects. *Semin Oncol.* 1995; 22:5–21.

24. Fuqua S. Estrogen and progesterone receptors in breast cancer. In: *Diseases of the Breast,* (Harris J, Lippman M, Morrow M, et al., eds.), Lippincott-Raven, Philadelphia, 1996, pp. 261–72.

25. Early Breast Cancer Trialists' Collaborative Group. Tamoxifen for early breast cancer: Overview of the randomised trials. *Lancet.* 1998; 351:1451–67.

26. Early Breast Cancer Trialists' Collaborative Group. Polychemotherapy for early breast cancer: an overview of the randomised trials. *Lancet.* 1998; 352:930–42.

27. American Joint Committee on Cancer: Breast. In: *AJCC Cancer Staging Manual,* 5th

edit. Fleming I, Cooper J, Henson D, et al., eds.), Lippincott-Raven, Philadelphia, 1997, pp. 171–80.

28. Baselga J, Tripathy D, Mendelsohn J, et al. Phase II study of weekly intravenous recombinant humanized anti-*p185HER2* monoclonal antibody in patients with *HER2/neu*-overexpressing metastatic breast cancer. *J Clin Oncol.* 1996; 14:737–44.

29. Cobleigh M, Vogel C, Tripathy D, et al. Efficacy and safety of Herceptin™ (humanized anti-*HER-2* antibody) as a single agent in 222 women with *HER-2* overexpression who relapsed following chemotherapy for metastatic breast cancer. *Proc Am Soc Clin Oncol.* 1998; 17:97a (abstract 376).

30. Pegram M, Lipton A, Hayes DF, et al. Phase II study of receptor-enhanced chemosensitivity using recombinant humanized anti-*p185HER2/neu* monoclonal antibody plus cisplatin in patients with *HER2/neu*-overexpressing metastatic breast cancer refractory to chemotherapy treatment. *J Clin Oncol.* 1998; 16:2659–71.

31. Slamon D, Leyland-Jones B, Shak S, et al. Addition of Herceptin™ (humanized anti-HER2 antibody) to first line chemotherapy for HR2 overexpressing metastatic breast cancer (HER2+/MBC) markedly increases anticancer activity: a randomized multinational controlled phase III trial. *Proc Am Soc Clin Oncol.* 1998; 17:98a (abstract 377).

32. Strauss GM, Skarin AT. Use of tumor markers in lung cancer. In: *Hematology/Oncology Clinics of North America: Tumor Markers in Adult Solid Malignancies* (Hayes DF, ed.), WB Saunders, Philadelphia, 1994, pp. 507–32.

33. Kantoff PW, Talcott JA. The prostate specific antigen: its use as a tumor marker for prostate cancer. In: *Hematology/Oncology Clinics of North America: Tumor Markers in Adult Solid Malignancies* (Hayes DF, ed.), WB Saunders, Philadelphia, 1994, pp. 555–72.

34. Ozols R, Schwartz P, Eifel P. Ovarian cancer, fallopian tube carcinoma, and peritoneal carcinoma. In: *Cancer: Principles and Practice of Oncology,* 5th edit. (DeVita V, Hellman S, Rosenburg S, eds.), Lippincott-Raven, Philadelphia, 1997, pp. 1502–39.

35. Fritsche HA, Bast RC. CA 125 in ovarian cancer: advances and controversy. *Clin Chem.* 1998; 44:1379–80.

3

Genetic Markers in Sporadic Tumors

S. Birindelli, A. Aiello, C. Lavarino, G. Sozzi, Silvana Pilotti, and
Marco A. Pierotti

Introduction

Progress in understanding the molecular basis of neoplastic transformation has strengthened the concept that cancer is a genetic disease. This concept, however, lumps together two types of genetic diseases with the same outcome: the first linked to an entirely somatic cell-gene deregulation and the second one dealing with a genetic susceptibility. At the somatic cell level, deregulation of cancer genes that control the careful balance between increase in cell number and withdrawal from the cell cycle promotes neoplastic growth by disrupting this balance. This occurs as a result of circumvention of the apoptotic machinery, promotion of cell division and cell proliferation, loss of cell differentiation pathways, and disruption of cell–cell communication and interaction. Thus, cancer represents the endpoint of a multistep process involving cancer genes and stimulatory and inhibitory signals provided by and controlled by products of the cancer genes.

In the first type of genetic disease, alterations in cancer genes can involve either dominant, gain-of-function mutations within proto-oncogenes that result in abnormal positive signals for cell proliferation or recessive, loss-of-function mutations within the tumor suppressor genes (TSGs) that interfere with the negative regulation of cell growth. Mutations within TSGs also may have a dominant-negative effect, one in which an altered protein is produced that competes with its wild-type counterpart and prevents its activity. Mutant versions of TSG *TP53* provide a paradigmatic example of such a mechanism. A third type of cancer gene recently has been identified in colorectal tumors associated with hereditary nonpolyposis colorectal cancer (HNPCC). These genes control mismatch repair (MMR), a process associated with the fidelity of DNA replication, and have been designated mutator genes. Their alterations cause microsatellite instability (MSI), characterized by random contractions or expansions in the length of simple sequence repeats (SSRs) or microsatellites, and may have important prognostic implications.

The second type of genetic disease is based on the recognition of a genetic susceptibility in about 8–10% of cancer patients. This latter disease results from the inheritance of altered alleles of genes, which are almost always of the tumor-suppressor type.

From: *Principles of Molecular Oncology*
Edited by: M. H. Bronchud, M. A. Foote, W. P. Peters, and M. O. Robinson © Humana Press Inc., Totowa, NJ

Along with different penetrance, this tumor-suppressor type determines the genetic risk of cancer, which can be almost 100% during a lifetime.

In these cases, including genes that predispose to a genetic risk of cancer *(1),* alterations of cancer-associated genes provide molecular markers. These markers are useful for novel diagnostic approaches and for genetic profiling of the tumor cell, with the aim of providing better prognostic evaluation and prediction of therapeutic drug response.

To provide a more rational view of the problems, this chapter organizes the subject by genetic markers from cancer-associated genes that were altered by point mutation, deletion, or inappropriate expression. The classes of genetic markers derived from chromosomal instability and from nonrandom chromosomal abnormalities are discussed, and genetic markers useful for the determination of clonality illustrated.

Genetic Markers Derived from Cancer-Associated Genes

TP53

The *TP53* gene, located on chromosome 17p13.1 and encompassing 20 kb of DNA, comprises 11 exons, the first of which is noncoding. In a cross-species comparison, the p53 proteins show five highly (>90%) conserved regions within the amino-acid residues that are considered essential to the functional activity of p53 *(2).*

This gene encodes a 393-amino-acid nuclear phosphoprotein, which contains phosphorylation sites at the amino (N) and carboxy (C) termini, a central zinc-binding core domain that interacts with DNA, and a nuclear localization and tetramerization domain at the C-terminus. It is classified as a TSG because the wild-type p53 protein restrains inappropriate cellular proliferation that regulates the transition from G_1 to S phase (as a checkpoint control factor) of the cell cycle and determines cell death through apoptosis. These regulatory functions are mediated by the interaction of p53 protein with specific DNA sequences, which may allow regulation at the transcriptional level of important genes in the p53-mediated growth suppression (e.g., *GADD45, MDM2,* and *WAF1–Cip1*).

When DNA is damaged, p53 protein accumulates and promotes cell cycle arrest before DNA synthesis by inducing the expression of a downstream gene, *WAF1–Cip1,* whose protein product (p21) binds to cyclin/cyclin-dependent kinases (CDK) complex and inhibits retinoblastoma (Rb) phosphorylation. This process allows the cell to repair DNA damage. The p53 protein also can block DNA synthesis by upregulating the transcription of *GADD45* (product: growth arrest DNA damage protein), which binds to proliferating cell nuclear antigen (PCNA) and inhibits DNA synthesis *(2).*

In response to DNA damage, p53 can induce apoptosis by increasing *bax* gene transcription, which inhibits *BCL-2* activity and drives the cell toward apoptosis *(3).*

TP53 mutations are involved in almost all tumor types, especially carcinomas of the colorectum, breast, lung, esophagus, stomach, liver, and bladder, but the frequency and type of mutation differ substantially among cancers.

More than 80% of the *TP53* mutations reported in human cancers are clustered between exons 5 and 8 within the evolutionary conserved regions of the gene (codons 110 to 307) *(4,5).* The mutations are usually missense and produce altered proteins. Sites in which mutations are detected at high frequency are called hot-spot mutations. They include codons 175, 248, 273, and 282 *(6).* Growing evidence suggests that mutation of *TP53* may involve not only a loss of function of wild-type *p53* activity but also a gain of function phenotype contributed by the mutant p53 protein.

Recent results suggest that *TP53* mutations may be one of the most important predictors for poor prognosis, increased risk of relapse *(7)*, and cancer-death risk *(8–10)*. Unfortunately, the clinical application of *TP53* mutation status as a prognostic tool remains controversial.

TP53 alterations can be detected though single-strand conformation polymorphism (SSCP), constant denaturant gel electrophoresis (CDGE), denaturing gradient gel electrophoresis (DGGE), or sequencing analysis.

TP53 has potential clinical applications in early-detection strategies. Detection of *TP53* mutations in the sputum of patients with lung cancer, combined with K-*ras* mutation analysis, may be a suitable target for early detection strategies *(11)*. This method has a limitation: the percentage of tumor cells identified is very low.

The potential clinical application for prognosis with *TP53* has been studied. In patients with breast cancer, analysis of *TP53* mutations in fine-needle aspirates *(12)* or core biopsy may be useful for prognostic assessment and prediction of response to adjuvant chemotherapy before radical surgery. In patients with node-positive breast cancer, detection of *p53* mutations (combined with the detection of *HER-2/neu* gene amplification) *(10)* in surgical specimens can be used as a molecular tool for prognostic assessment *(7,13,14)* and therapy planning.

The most important subgroup of breast cancer patients needing reliable prognostic factors is women without axillary lymph node involvement. Introduction of routine *TP53* mutation screening may assist in the selection of patients with node-negative breast cancer who can be considered for postoperative adjuvant treatment *(15–17)*.

In colorectal cancer, detection of *TP53* point mutations, particularly mutations in the conserved domains (e.g., Arg-175) *(7,18)*, may be a valuable prognostic adjunct in defining more aggressive tumors.

TP53 mutations are frequent in late-stage ovarian cancer (50% of stage III and IV epithelial ovarian cancers) *(19)* and have been associated with reduced overall survival rates *(19,20)*.

Righetti et al. *(21)* reported a significant correlation between presence of *TP53* missense mutations and resistance to cisplatin-based therapy in ovarian cancer. Moreover, Wahl et al. *(22)* and Lavarino et al. *(23)* suggest that inactivation of wild-type *p53* may confer increased sensitization to the chemotherapeutic agent paclitaxel and thus help overcome resistance in tumors that do not respond to platinum drug alone. These results could make the detection of *TP53* mutations a useful marker for therapy planning. However, as described by Sørensen et al. *(19)*, conflicting findings imply the need for further studies to elucidate the role of p53 in the response to chemotherapy.

RAS

The *ras* genes, one of the first oncogenes identified, constitute a multigene family that is highly conserved among eukaryotes, which suggests that they may play a fundamental role in cellular proliferation. They are named H-*ras* (homologous to Harvey murine sarcoma virus oncogene), K-*ras* (homologous to Kirsten murine sarcoma virus oncogene), and N-*RAS* (initially isolated from a neuroblastoma cell line) *(24)*. The human *RAS* genes encode for similar membrane-bound 21-kDa proteins (189 amino acids) involved in signal transduction, with a guanine nucleotide-binding activity and an intrinsic guanosine triphosphatase (GTP) activity *(25)*. Normally, these proteins (p21ras) exist in equilibrium between active and inactive states. The p21ras proteins remain inactive, characterized by a conformation that allows binding to guanosine diphosphate (GDP), until they receive a stimulus from another protein upstream of the pathway of transduction. This stimulus results in the exchange of GDP for GTP followed by conformational change of p21ras to its active state. These activated proteins transduce the signal by linking tyrosine kinases to downstream serine/threonine kinases, such as raf, and mitogen-activated protein kinases (MAPK) *(24)*. They subsequently become inactivated by their intrinsic GTPase activity, which catalyzes the hydrolysis of GTP and permits the return to the inactive GDP-bound state *(26)*.

Stabilization of ras proteins in their active state causes a continuous flow of signal transduction, which results in malignant transformation. The p21ras proteins can acquire transforming potential secondary to a point mutation at codon 12, 13, or 61 in the coding gene. Transformation can occur with mutations at or near the GTP-binding domain of p21ras protein, which prevents the inactivation of GTP and results in continuous p21ras activity *(24)*. Normal *RAS* genes can induce malignant transformation if highly overexpressed *(26)*.

Activated *RAS* genes are the most frequently found oncogenes in a variety of human cancers *(27)*, including adenocarcinomas of the pancreas (90%), colon cancer (50%), and lung cancer (30%). Adenocarcinomas show mutations in K-*RAS* oncogene, predominantly in codon 12 with a G-T transversion *(27)*.

Methods for detecting *RAS* alterations include SSCP, CDGE, DGGE, restriction fragment length polymorphism (RFLP) analysis, allele-specific oligodeoxynucleotide (ASO) hybridization, and sequencing analysis.

RAS has potential clinical applications in the early detection of pancreatic tumors. Because 80% of pancreatic carcinomas contain *K-RAS* mutations *(28)*, the detection of *K-RAS* mutations in pancreatic juice *(29–31)* combined with other somatic mutations common to this cancer (e.g., *TP53*) might be a valuable tool for the detection of pancreatic carcinoma. This method appears to be useful mainly for differentiating pancreatic cancer from chronic pancreatitis *(32)*. This method has limitations: a recent report demonstrated that *RAS* gene mutations are found in hyperplasia in pancreatic tissue of patients with chronic pancreatitis *(31)*. Further studies are required to completely determine the specificity of *K-RAS* mutations in the carcinogenesis of pancreatic tumors.

Detection of *K-RAS* mutations in stool specimens could be a noninvasive presymptomatic indicator of colonic adenomas (mostly adenomas >1 cm) *(33,34)* or colorectal tumors, but this method is limited by difficulties in DNA isolation from colonic cells within stool specimens. Furthermore, *K-RAS* mutations are present only in 50% of colorectal tumors. The detection of other mutant genes (e.g., *APC* and *TP53*) in stool specimens would increase the potential sensitivity of this strategy *(33)*.

Detection of *K-RAS* mutations in sputum or bronchoalveolar lavage fluid from patients with lung cancer may serve as an important adjunct to cytology in the diagnosis of lung cancer *(11,35)*. However, the percentage of tumor cells identified is much lower than those identified in urine and stool specimens *(11)*.

As a prognostic tool, evidence in colorectal cancer increasingly suggests a link between poor outcome and specific types of *K-RAS* mutations (codon 12 G-T transversions) *(24,36)*. Demonstration of such a prognostic effect may allow appropriate targeting of intensive follow-up and adjuvant therapy, especially for intermediate-stage tumors in which outcome could be more closely related to the genetically determined aggressiveness. However, a relationship between *K-RAS* status and prognosis in colorectal cancer has not yet been firmly established *(36)* and the usefulness of its determination is unclear. In patients with non-small-cell lung cancer (NSCLC), presence of *K-RAS* mutations has been related to an unfavorable prognosis *(24,27,37)*.

HER-2/neu

The *HER-2/neu* gene, part of the tyrosine kinase oncogene family, is located on chromosome 17q21 and encodes for a transmembrane receptor-like phosphoglycoprotein (185 kDa) that is closely related in structure but biologically distinct from the epidermal growth factor receptor (EGFR) *(38)*.

The EGF and HER-2/neu receptors have a glycosylated extracellular N-terminus where the ligand binds, a hydrophobic transmembrane region, and a kinase domain contained within the intracytoplasmic C-terminus. The cytoplasmic domains of these receptors contain several tyrosines that can become phosphorylated upon activation and then bind to proteins that contain SH2 domains and that are part of the signal transduction pathway *(24)*.

Amplification and overexpression of the *HER-2/neu* proto-oncogene have been reported in approx 25% of breast, ovarian, endometrial, gastric, and salivary gland carcinomas and are associated with poor prognosis in patients with each of these cancers *(39)*. Data from clinical trials in breast cancer suggest an association between *HER-2/neu* overexpression and resistance to chemotherapy. Thus, overexpression of this oncogene may represent not only a prognostic but also a predictive factor for response to chemotherapy *(40)*.

Methods for detecting *HER-2/neu* amplification include fluorescence *in situ* hybridization (FISH), Southern blot analysis, slot-blot hybridization, and quantitative polymerase chain reaction (PCR).

HER-2/neu has potential prognostic clinical applications in breast cancer: detection of *HER-2/neu* amplification has utility in identifying highly aggressive node-positive breast carcinomas *(10,39,41)*. In patients with axillary node-negative breast cancer, *HER-2/neu* amplification has been reported as an independent prognostic factor for risk of recurrence *(42)*.

HER-2/neu gene expression has been reported as a new factor for predicting treatment response in breast cancer. In particular, information on expression of this oncogene may become determinant for the prediction of response to antracycline-containing chemotherapy and resistance to treatment with tamoxifen or CMF (cyclophosphamide, methotrexate, fluorouracil) *(43)*. The role of *HER-2/neu* in the response to chemotherapy has not yet been inconvertibly established; therefore these results need confirmation with further studies. In endometrial cancer, *HER-2/neu* amplification is a potential prognostic marker of poor outcome and may have clinical utility in selecting patients for adjuvant therapy *(44)*.

RET

The *RET* proto-oncogene is located on chromosome 10q11.2 and comprises 21 exons, which encode a receptor-type tyrosine kinase (RTK) that likely is involved in the control of neural crest cell proliferation, migration, survival, and/or differentiation. The Ret receptor comprises an extracellular ligand-binding domain that contains a region of cadherin homology of unknown significance, a transmembrane domain, an intracellular tyrosine kinase domain, and additional amino-acid sequences that function as regulatory domains *(45)*. This receptor is expressed in three isoforms due to alternative splicings involving the last three exons *(46)*. Ligand binding induces receptor dimerization and autophosphorylation in a *trans* fashion and functions to recruit intracellular signaling proteins. *RET* expression occurs predominantly in neural crest-derived cells *(45)*.

Germline mutations in the *RET* proto-oncogene are associated with multiple endocrine neoplasia (MEN) type 2 (2A and 2B) and familial medullary thyroid carcinoma. On the other hand, somatic point mutations of *RET* have been described in 23–69% of sporadic medullary thyroid carcinomas (MTCs) *(47)*. The most common somatic mutation occurs in the intracellular tyrosine kinase domain of *RET* at codon 918 within exon 16 and causes the substitution of a methionine by a threonine.

Methods for detecting *RET* amplification include mutation-specific restriction enzyme analysis and sequencing analysis.

Potential clinical applications include diagnosis (analysis of *RET* mutations in both peripheral blood leukocytes and tumor specimens enables discrimination between hereditary and sporadic MTC *[48]*) and prognosis (tumor-specific mutation at codon 918 has been reported to correlate with tumor recurrence and poor prognosis *[48]*).

BCL2

The *BCL2* (B-cell leukemia/lymphoma 2) gene, located on chromosome 18q21, spans more than 230 kb of DNA and consists of three exons of which exon 2 and a small part of exon 3 encode for protein. Dependent on splicing of intron 2, *BCL2* encodes for two mRNAs, BCL2α and BCL2β, of which only BCL2α seems to have biologic relevance. The BCL2α protein is a 26-kDa membrane protein located at the cytosolic site of the nuclear envelope, endoplasmic reticulum (ER), and outer mitochondrial membrane. *BCL2* inhibits apoptosis under stress conditions and prolongs cell survival. In normal tissues, BCL2 protein displays a restricted topographic distribution within mature tissues that are characterized by apoptotic cell death. In secondary follicles, *BCL2* is strongly expressed in mantle zone, which comprises long-lived recirculating cells. In the thymus, *bcl2* is present in the surviving mature thymocytes of the medulla. *BCL2* is usually expressed in hematopoietic precursor cells, but it is absent in their most differentiated and terminal progeny *(49)*. *bcl2* is present in complex differentiating epithelium, where it is restricted to stem cell and proliferating zones. Because of its antiapoptotic function, the *bcl2* gene initiated a new category of oncogenes called regulators of cell death. Recently, bcl2 homologues, some of which bind to bcl2, have been identified, suggesting that bcl2 functions at least in part through protein–protein interaction. Site-directed mutagenesis of bcl2 protein BH1 and BH2 domains showed that these two regions were important for binding of bcl2 to bax, a member of the bcl2-family that promotes cell death and whose interaction with BCL2 is necessary to regulate the apoptotic pathway *(50–52)*.

The *BCL2* gene was discovered by virtue of its involvement in t(14;18) of follicular lymphomas. Although translocation is the main mechanism of *BCL2* gene activation (discussed later), *BCL2* point mutations and amplification also have been reported.

Mutations clustering in the *BCL2* open-reading frame occur in high-grade B-cell lymphomas transformed from low-grade follicular lymphomas carrying *BCL2* gene rearrangement *(53,54)*. *BCL2* gene amplification, which leads to increased protein production, has been detected in about 30% of high-grade diffuse large cell lymphomas (DLCLs) lacking *BCL2* translocation *(55)*.

BCL2 expression has been investigated both in lymphoid and nonlymphoid tumors. In solid tumors, *BCL2* expression occurs in tumors of some hormonally responsive epithelium, such as breast and prostate *(51)*. Detection of BCL2 protein has diagnostic utility and some prognostic value.

Detection methods include Southern blot hybridization (for gene amplification) and PCR–SSCP and direct sequencing for gene mutation; BCL2 protein expression can be determined by immunocytochemistry (IHC), Western blot, or flow cytometry.

The clinical applications of *BCL2* include diagnosis of lymphomas where BCL2 protein expression is used as a marker for the differential diagnosis between reactive follicular hyperplasia and follicular lymphoma *(50,56,57)*. Prognosis of patients with leukemia and lymphomas can be helped by bcl2. Due to the occurrence of *BCL2* gene mutations in transformed high-grade B-cell lymphomas *(53,54)*, this genetic lesion may represent a predictive marker of progression in *BCL2*-rearranged tumors. Clinical correlation studies in DLCL indicated that *BCL2* amplification is associated with advanced-stage disease at presentation *(58)*.

In high-grade B-cell lymphomas, BCL2 protein expression is a strong, major predictor of overall survival, disease-free survival, and relapse-free survival either alone *(59,60)* or in association with *p53* expression *(61)*, being related to poor outcome. High *BCL2* expression is associated with low remission rate in acute myeloid leukemia (AML) *(62)* and is an indicator of poor response in acute lymphocytic leukemia (ALL) *(63)*.

Clinical utility has been shown in solid tumors. *BCL2* expression is found in tumors of some hormonally responsive epithelia, such as tumors of the breast and prostate. In neuroblastoma and carcinoma of the prostate, bcl2 positivity is a poor prognostic marker, whereas breast cancer patients with bcl2-positive tumors have better survival *(51,64)*. In the thyroid gland, *BCL2* expression is downregulated in adenomas and well-differentiated carcinomas and is frequently completely lost in anaplastic carcinoma *(65–68)*. In MTC, lack of bcl2 immunoreactivity correlated significantly with a shorter survival *(69)*; therefore, down-regulation of *BCL2* expression in MTC may identify a subset of tumors with a more aggressive clinical course. The association between immunohistochemical staining for BCL2 protein and the histological type and prognosis of NSCLC is controversial *(70,71)*.

In cancers that overexpress *BCL2*, decreasing its expression by targeting BCL2 directly or indirectly through an upstream regulator of *BCL2* may render the neoplastic cells more sensitive to chemotherapeutic agents *(51)*.

BCL1–PRAD1–CCND1

The *PRAD1* gene, which was first cloned from a parathyroid adenoma with inv(11) (p15;q13) *(72)* and subsequently identified as *BCL1 (73)*, maps on chromosome 11q13. Transcription gives rise to two major mRNAs of 4.5 and 1.5 kb through alternative polyadenylation. The *BCL1* gene encodes for a 36-kDa nuclear protein of 295 amino acids, cyclin D1, which belongs to the cyclin G1 family *(74)*. The bcl1–cyclin D1 protein binds and activates the CDK4 and CDK6 and seems to regulate the cell cycle G_1–S checkpoint through phosphorylation of Rb protein *(75)*. In normal tissue, the bcl1–cyclin D1 protein is expressed in the proliferating fraction of epithelial tissues, whereas it is absent in lymphoid tissues such as lymph node, spleen, and tonsil *(76)*.

The main mechanisms of *BCL1* gene activation include translocation and amplification, both of which result in overexpression of normal RNA of 1.5 and 4.5 kb and of intact 36 kDa cyclin D1 protein. The 11q13 region is involved in B-cell lymphomas, parathyroid adenoma, breast cancer, squamous cell cancer of the head and neck, esophagus and bladder carcinoma, and in MEN 1 *(77)*.

Detection methods include Southern blot analysis for amplification; and Northern blot, reverse transcriptase PCR (RT-PCR), RNA *in situ* hybridization (RNA-ISH), Western blot, and IHC for overexpression.

The *BCL1* gene has diagnostic applications in patients with lymphoma. bcl1 protein expression is a marker that enables a differential diagnosis of mantle cell lymphoma (MCL), being positive in more than 80% of cases *(77)*.

In solid tumors, prognosis can be determined by the *BCL1* gene. In cancers of the breast and of the head and neck region, 11q13 amplification is associated with poor clinical course of the disease *(78)*. In a study performed in esophageal carcinoma *(79)*, *BCL1* was amplified in a subset of primary tumors and lymph node metastases. Metastases tended to be more common in patients with *BCL1* amplification than in those without this abnormality. Moreover, *BCL1* amplification was associated with decreased 1-yr survival, thus providing useful prognostic information.

REL

The *REL* gene, the human homologue of the reticuloendotheliosis virus strain T (*REV-T*), which induces leukemia in chickens, was identified in a human genomic DNA library and assigned to chromosome 2. By FISH, *REL* was mapped to the 2p15;14 position *(80)*. *REL,* which consists of seven exons, belongs to the REL–NF-kB family of transcriptional activators. These molecules can heterodimerize and participate in cytoplasmic/nuclear signal transduction in response to cytokines, mitogens, physical and oxidative stress, and other pathogenic products *(81)*. In humans, high concentrations of REL mRNA are found in relatively mature lymphocytes. Its expression is depressed in immature thymocytes and may therefore play a role in lymphocytic differentiation *(82)*. The *REL* oncogene has been found amplified in a subset of DLCL *(81)*. Detection methods include Southern blot hybridization.

Potential clinical applications include diagnosis and prognosis. A 35-fold *REL* amplification has been described in about 20% of DLCL, >70% of which are primary extranodal lymphomas *(58)*. The occurrence of this abnormality in advanced stage disease, and the association with other genetic lesions, suggest that *REL* may represent a progression-associated marker of primary extranodal lymphomas.

MYC

MYC is a member of the helix–loop–helix/leucine zipper superfamily, a gene family containing at least seven closely related genes. The most studied are *C-MYC* (cellular), *N-MYC* (originally isolated from neuroblastoma cells), and *L-MYC* (originally isolated from small-cell lung cancer [SCLC] cells). The *MYC* genes encode for nuclear DNA-binding proteins that are involved in transcriptional regulation. MYC proteins form homodimers or heterodimers through their C-terminal helix–loop–helix domains. MYC can heterodimerize with proteins such as max, mad, and MX11. Max can bind Myc to repress the transcriptional activation of *MYC* genes, whereas mad and MX11 can bind max and release *MYC* to function as a transcriptional activator *(24)*. *MYC* is implicated in the control of normal cell proliferation, transformation, and differentiation. *MYC* expression in untransformed cells is growth-factor dependent and essential for progression through the cell cycle *(83)*. A recently defined biologic function of *MYC* is apoptosis control: in different cell types, *MYC* can induce apoptosis if a cell is deprived of specific growth factors.

C-MYC, the major member of the *MYC* family, is located on human chromosome 8q24 and consists of three exons, the first of which is noncoding. *N-MYC* maps on chromosome 2p24.1.

MYC abnormalities can be in the form of chromosome translocation (discussed later), gene mutation, or gene amplification. The result is usually an elevated *MYC* expression rather than a change of the protein structure. Gu et al. *(84)* suggested that tumor-associated *MYC* alteration may be related to an imbalance of the myc/max system and promotion of cell proliferation. In lymphomas, *C-MYC* gene mutation can occur in the gene transactivation domain and in the coding region after translocation into the *Ig* gene *(85)*. Mutations can occur in the noncoding gene exon 1 and at the exon 1/intron 1 boundary with or without *C-MYC* gene translocation *(85)*. This region is considered the *C-MYC* regulatory region and is responsible for mRNA stability. In Burkitt's lymphoma (BL), mutations frequently occur at sites of phosphorylation, a finding that suggests that they may have a pathogenetic role.

C-MYC deregulation is associated with its amplification in DLCL, SCLC, ovarian cancer, and breast cancer. *N-MYC* is frequently amplified in neuroblastomas, retinoblastomas, and SCLC.

Methods for detecting *MYC* include: Southern blot, FISH, and PCR for *MYC* amplification; and PCR–SSCP and direct sequencing for *MYC* mutations.

In patients with DLCL, *C-MYC* amplification, in association with other genetic lesions, occurs in about 20% of cases with advanced-stage disease, and is considered a progression marker *(58)*. In solid tumors, *C-MYC* amplification and overexpression, combined with *HER-2/neu,* have been reported to be associated with poor prognosis, including a shorter disease-free survival and reduced survival, in patients with breast carcinoma *(41)*.

In neuroblastoma, *N-MYC* amplification has been correlated with increased metastases and poor outcome *(86)*. Contradictory findings exist about the association between *N-MYC* amplification and *BCL2* expression in neuroblastoma *(86,87)*.

BCL6

The *BCL6* gene (also known as *BCL5* or *LAZ-3*) maps on chromosome 3q27 and consists of nine exons, the first two of which are noncoding. The gene is transcribed as a 3.8-kb message predominantly in normal adult skeletal muscle and in some patients with non-Hodgkin's lymphoma (NHL) carrying 3q27 chromosomal defects. *BCL6* encodes for a 79-kDa nuclear protein containing six C-terminal zinc finger domains and an N-terminal POZ domain, which mediates its sequence-specific transcriptional repressor function *(88,89)*. The BCL6 protein is predominantly expressed in the B-cell lineage, where it is found in mature B cells. In normal human lymphoid tissues, *BCL6* expression is topographically restricted to germinal centers, including all centroblasts and centrocytes. This restriction indicates that *BCL6* is specifically regulated during B-cell differentiation and suggests a role for *BCL6* in germinal-center development and function *(90,91)*.

The *BCL6* gene can be activated by chromosomal translocation (discussed later) or somatic mutations. Breakpoints and mutations cluster in the *BCL6* 5′ regulatory region, in a 3.3 kb *Eco*RI fragment that defines the major translocation cluster (MTC). *BCL6* somatic mutations are multiple and often biallelic. They are found in tumors displaying either normal or rearranged *BCL6* alleles, indicating their independence from chromosomal rearrangement and from linkage to *Ig* genes. *BCL6* gene mutations have been found in >70% of DLCL and 45% of follicular lymphomas *(92)*. Detection methods for *BCL6* somatic mutations include PCR–SSCP and direct sequencing.

Recently, *BCL6* gene mutations have been found in a high proportion of normal B cells *(93,94)* and in most germinal center derived lymphomas *(95)*, so this genetic abnormality does not seem to have a diagnostic utility. Investigation of the prognostic value of *BCL6* mutations is still at early stages. Cesarman et al. *(96)* showed that *BCL6* mutations predict shorter survival and refractoriness to reduced immunosuppression and/or surgical excision in posttransplantation lymphoproliferative disorders.

p16–INK4a–CDKN2A

Regulation of the cell cycle at the G_1–S transition point involves several genes, and the complex of *p16* [also known as *MTS1* (major tumor suppressor 1], *INK4a* [inhibitor of CDK4a], and *CDKN2A* [CDK inhibitor 2A]) is a G_1-specific negative regulator of cell proliferation. Consistent with high frequency of allelic loss (loss of heterozygosity [LOH]) detection at the 9p21 chromosomal region in many human malignancies and tumor cell lines, the human gene *p16* was isolated in 1993 and is located at the 9p21 locus.

The *p16* gene comprises three exons coding for a 15.8-kDa protein of 156 amino acids that show a four tandem repeat motif structure. The p16 protein is the prototype of a family of not functionally redundant cyclin-dependent kinase (CDK) inhibitors (i.e., p15INK4b, p18INK4c, and p19INK4d). Their function is to block the association of CDK4/6 with cyclin D and then prevent the activation of the kinase activity of the CDK4/6–cycD complex. The CDK4/6–cycD complex can phosphorylate the pRB protein which concomitantly releases E2F, a factor that permits transcription of cell-cycle regulator genes and progression into S phase. On the contrary, binding of CDK4 or 6 with p16 protein blocks the cell cycle in G_1 phase. These functional relations are known as the p16INK4a–CDK4–cycD1–Rb pathway.

The amount of p16 mRNA in nonpathologic human tissue is quite low, but accumulation of *p16* transcript and protein has been shown in response to cellular senescence, oncogenic *RAS* gene stimulus, and inactivation of the *RB* gene.

To date, three main mechanisms of genetic inactivation of the *p16* gene have been found: deletion of both alleles, deletion of one allele and mutation in the remaining allele, and deletion of one allele and methylation-mediated silencing of the remaining allele *(97)*.

A common event in tumorigenesis, affecting both hereditary (malignant melanoma) and sporadic tumors, is the deregulation of the G_1–S transition point.

Deletions, point mutations, and methylation of the 5′ CpG island are molecular abnormalities that could affect *p16* function in many human cancers. Specifically, *p16* point mutations commonly occur in pancreatic, esophageal, lung, and head and neck tumors. Deletions of *p16* have been identified in melanoma, bladder, prostate adenocarcinoma, T-cell acute lymphocytic leukemia (ALL), glioma, mesothelioma, sarcoma, ovarian, and renal cell carcinoma. Finally, methylation of the 5′ CpG island was associated with breast, colon, bladder, head and neck, lung, and brain tumors.

On the contrary, alterations of p16 protein expression do not have diagnostic or prognostic relevance. An alternative transcript to *p16,* termed *p16β,* does not seem a primary target in oncogenesis.

Intragenic mutations can be uncovered by mutation analysis (SSCP and direct sequencing); allele inactivation is detected by LOH analysis microsatellites or Southern blot. To determine LOH and the methylation state of *p16,* comparison with normal tissue is required.

Potential clinical applications include risk assessment: LOH as well as mutations of *p16* have been reported in sporadic dysplastic nevi, thereby suggesting their role in the development of malignant melanomas and offering a possible tool for risk assessment *(98)*. In diagnosis, sporadic pancreatic cancers have been affected by *p16* mutations, which seem to be useful as diagnostic markers, but their biologic meaning is undefined *(99)*. Preliminary findings suggest that *p16* inactivation through LOH and hypermethylations may be useful in predicting pituitary tumors with an aggressive behavior *(100)*. In hematopoietic tumors, *p16* gene inactivation has been frequently observed (e.g., ALL and some B- and T-cell lymphomas, and NHL). Adults with B- or T-cell lymphoma who carry such an alteration probably have a poor prognosis *(101)*. Paired sequential analyses showed that transformation from low- to high-grade B-cell lymphoma is associated with loss of *p16* activity *(102,103),* suggesting that *p16* may be involved in progression and may represent a target for new therapeutic strategies *(101)*.

Genetic Markers Derived from Chromosomal Instability

The term "chromosomal instability" refers to a wide spectrum of alterations that occur either at the DNA or chromosomal level. At the DNA level, chromosomal instability encompasses MSI and LOH, whereas at the chromosomal level, instability is restricted to LOH. MSI and LOH represent two unrelated phenomena that share a common analysis tool: microsatellite sequences.

Microsatellites, also known as "simple sequences repeat" (SSR), are short genomic sequences that usually are present in the human genome as mono- to esa-nucleotides, repeated *n* times in tandem in large clusters. Their presence has been demonstrated in all human chromosomes with a frequency proportional to their dimension. Specific localization of microsatellites is mostly extragenic, but intragenic sequences also have been described *(104,105)*. Tandem clusters tend to be highly polymorphic in terms of size: wide variations between individuals suggest their use as polymorphic markers in characterizing individual genomes. Consistent with their simple sequence and condensed structure, microsatellite DNA are not transcribed or translated.

Errors occurring in microsatellite sequences during DNA replication produce expanded or shortened repetitive sequence units within the microsatellite and lead to the appearance of additional bands in otherwise normal alleles. This phenomenon (MSI) often but not always occurs in conjunction with mutations in MMR genes that are involved in DNA repair pathways *(106)*. It has been proposed that MMR genes represent a third class of genes in addition to TSGs and oncogenes that could promote oncogenesis if altered.

Confusion surrounds the terminology used to define MSI. Acronyms such as MSI, MIN, and MI refer to instability detected within microsatellite sequences. Moreover, there is no consensus in the literature regarding the number of markers necessary to classify a specimen positive or negative for MSI or regarding an unequivocal definition of MSI and replication error repair (RER). As to the first issue, several authors proposed a minimum range of three to seven loci analyzed. For definitions of MSI and RER, it has been suggested that the presence of MSI in at least one locus may be termed MSI-positive or low-frequency MSI, while MSI detected in more loci tested, or in a generalized fashion, should be defined as RER-positive phenotype or high-frequency MSI. Biologically, RER-positive phenotype definitely contributes to the development of cancer, whereas MSI could lead to cellular death or proliferation advantage followed by selection of clones prone to malignant transformation. In addition, a cutoff of 29% has been proposed for the frequency of MSI, to discriminate between MSI and RER. Unfortunately, this cutoff cannot be applied to all types of tumors. It has been also proposed that studies of sequences contained within cancer-associated genes be preferred for their better result accuracy rather than screening of markers outside of such genes.

Another unsolved issue concerns the choice on nucleotide repeats: dinucleotide microsatellites should be preferred over trinucleotides or tetranucleotides for monitoring genomic instability.

At variance with MSI, LOH has been shown to reflect loss-of-function mutations in the retained allele of a TSG within the affected chromosomal region *(107)*. In fact, the "two-hit" hypothesis of oncogenesis postulated by Knudson *(108)* indicates a first inactivation of one allele of a TSG by mutations ranging from alteration of a single amino acid to a large gene deletion, with the second allele often inactivated by a less precise pattern. The aforementioned model was first applied to hereditary tumors, where the "first hit" represents a germline mutation and the "second hit" is the LOH that occurred at a somatic level and that affected the wild-type allele. It is possible that the "two-hit" hypothesis can be applied to sporadic tumors also, except that the two aforementioned events occurred at a somatic level. LOH detection relies heavily on cellular economy for its implication in tumor transformation and progression, and it acquires meaning as an early diagnosis marker and as a prognostic and therapeutic response marker.

The rest of this chapter summarizes the still-contrasting data reported in the published literature regarding the clinical value of such markers in early diagnosis and their usefulness in the definition of prognosis and therapeutic response in neoplastic diseases. The data show a clustering of such markers within organs/sites/systems and in particular for prognosis a correlation with several clinical–pathologic parameters (i.e., histotype, localization, timing progression, multifocality, and familiarity) which may serve to better define the disease outcome. Finally, the unresponsiveness to alkylating agents shown by MSI-positive patients makes such a marker a valid tool for chemotherapy response evaluation.

Detection of microsatellite alterations in pathologic tissue requires a comparison with normal tissue from the same patient *(109)*.

Microsatellite analysis (LOH and MSI) is an easy, fast test. The relative small size of microsatellite sequences (100–300 base pairs [bps]) allows analysis on DNA specimens extracted from fresh or frozen tissue and also from formalin-fixed and sometimes bouin-fixed specimens (in the latter case, nested PCR is required). Common methods for detecting MSI and LOH are radioactive PCR or Southern blot (LOH only) and denaturing acrylamide gel electrophoresis and fluorochrome PCR with an automatic sequencer. The last approach allows a higher grade of analysis standardization and an objective interpretation of the results that no longer depends on the expertise of operator.

Microsatellite Instability, Loss of Heterozygosity, and Cancer

MSI and LOH have been observed in sporadic tumors of the colon, stomach, pancreas, bladder, hematopoietic system, lung, ovary, breast, endometrium, prostate, brain, head and neck, and skin. Both types of alterations show loci clustering by tumor type, site, and body system. Consistent with a role in tumor initiation, such molecular alterations appear to occur early in the tumor development and occasionally may be detected at a preneoplastic stage, as well as in nonmalignant tissue. This finding suggests that, at least in some cases, such a pattern is compatible with a normal phenotype *(110)*. MSI and LOH reportedly are useful in the evaluation of prognosis and therapeutic response in different tumors. As for prognosis, a wide spectrum of positive or negative correlations of these markers with traditional clinical–pathologic parameters (i.e., histotype, localization, timing of progression, multifocality, and familiarity) has proved partly useful for better defining the disease outcome. MSI could offer a valid tool for evaluating responsiveness to chemotherapy because most cancer cells that resist alkylating agents exhibit the MSI phenotype (Table 1).

Genetic Markers Derived from Nonrandom Chromosomal Abnormalities

Recurring and highly consistent chromosomal aberrations have led to the identification of new proto-oncogenes at or spanning chromosomal breakpoints. Studies have shown that these genes are oncogenic and confirmed the pivotal role of chromosomal aberrations in tumor development. Specific translocations initially have been identified in hematologic tumors, and subsequently they also have been demonstrated in a subset of solid neoplasms. In hematopoietic tumors, chromosomal translocations have two main consequences: the juxtaposition of a proto-oncogene to the gene for a T-cell receptor or an immunoglobulin (Ig) protein, inducing oncogenic activation, and creation of a fusion gene encoding a chimeric protein. The genes involved often encode transcription factors, suggesting that disruption of transcriptional control plays a major role in oncogenesis. The main clinical application of these nonrandom chromosomal abnormalities is the diagnostic definition of several morphologically equivocal tumors followed by the assessment of minimal residual disease and therapeutic response. Because of the high number of chromosomal translocations identified in hematopoietic tumors, this chapter describes in detail only those with significant clinical relevance. Other translocations reported in hematopoietic tumors are listed in Tables 2 and 3.

Table 1
Microsatellite Instability (MSI) and Loss of Heterozygosity (LOH) in Cancer.
Evaluation of MSI and LOH in neoplastic diseases that cannot yet be considered of clinical relevance has been reported for ovarian and breast carcinomas and melanocytic lesions. A possible role of these markers in disease progression, poor outcome, and risk of malignant transformation has been suggested for these and other cancers.

- GASTRIC CANCER
  - –RER+ detection ranges from 15–30% *(111)*, without any correlation with MMR gene mutations.

  - –RER+ (scored with 3 or more loci involved) are associated with antral location, intestinal subtype, both early and advanced stages, and nodal positive cases *(112)*.

  - –RER+ (scored as more than 6 loci involved) not restricted to patients with familial disease background and is significantly associated with female sex, lower tumor stage, and tumor localization in the distal part of the stomach *(113)*.

  - –RER+ as diagnostic or prognostic marker outside the context of HNPCC cases is currently of limited clinical value *(110)*.

  - –Correlation of RER+ with tumor stage, localization, and histologic subtype seems to be a promising field.

- BLADDER CANCER (Data concerning Transitional Cell Carcinoma—TCC)
  - –The 60 tri- and tetranucleotide markers were screened for 50 TCC urine samples obtaining at least one marker alteration, namely MSI and/or LOH, in 80% of cases analyzed *(114)*.

  - –Data confirmed by using a microsatellite panel comprehensive of 20 markers *(115)*.

  - –Candidate TSGs involved in bladder cancer mapped at chromosome 9 are *p16, GAS1,* and *PTC* genes, but none showed alterations *(116)*.

  - –LOH at 8p and 10q, namely 10q24.1–q24.3 and 10q26.1–26.2 bands *(117,118)*, have been proposed as adverse prognostic markers; 8p deletion has been found to correlate with high-grade tumors *(119)*, but putative TSGs as POLB and PPP2CB, mapped at 8p region, did not reveal any mutations *(120)*.

  - –Loss of function of TSGs as DEL27, APC, DCC, TP53, and Rb have been proposed as adverse prognostic markers; LOH at DEL27 locus seems to be involved in cases showing an aggressive behavior *(121)*.

  - –Consistent with their role in the regulation of the cell cycle, LOH of TP53 and Rb have been mainly observed in high-grade and/or wide-invasive tumors *(122)*, and associated with disease progression and survival reduction, especially if both the markers are simultaneously altered.

  - –Taken individually, Rb correlates with increased mitotic index, whereas TP53 seems useful in identifying chemotherapy-unresponsive patients *(123)*.

  - –Generalized LOH and MSI may discriminate for presence or absence of tumor cells in urine cytological samples. LOH at 8p, 10q, DEL27, Rb, and TP53 loci seems to correlate with poor outcome and chemotherapy unresponsiveness. LOH on chromosome 9 appears to correlate with both early and late events and its role needs to be further investigated.

RER = replication error repair; HNPCC = hereditary nonpolyposis colon cancer; MMR = mismatch repair; MSI = microsatellite instability; Rb = retinoblastoma protein; TCC = transitional cell carcinoma; TSG = tumor-suppressor gene

continued

Table 1 (*continued*)

- HEAD AND NECK CANCER (Data concerning head and neck squamous cell carcinoma—HNSCC)

  –HNSCC develops from accumulations of genetic events sometimes specific for early or advanced stage of the disease.

  –Losses of 9p21 and 3p14 regions are frequently detected in oral premalignant lesions *(124,125),* although mutations occurring at *p16* and *VHL* genes mapped within the above mentioned regions, have never been found.

  –Correlation between generalized LOH and histology high-grade as well as advanced tumor has been reported, and evidence suggests that chromosome 18, more than others, is involved in short survival. In this view, at least three minimal deleted regions of chromosome 18, encompassing the q12, q21.1, and q21.2 bands, were frequently found lost in more aggressive cases *(126,127).*

  –Candidate TSGs on 18q are *DCC, DPC4,* and *MADR2. DCC* gene, located within one of the three minimal regions of deletion above mentioned, is frequently found in a homozygous deletion status in HNSCC cell lines but it is still controversial its involvement in cancerogenesis and progression of human HNSCC.

  –Evidence suggests that simultaneous LOH at *TP53* and *Rb* loci is associated with poor survival and that these markers may be usefully applied for prognosis *(128).*

  –LOH at 18q and 8p loci seem to correlate with the tumor aggressiveness *(129,130).*

- PROSTATE CANCER

  –Positive correlation between frequency of LOH at specific loci and both tumor high-grade and cancer death has been reported (3.6% grade I vs 12% grade II) *(131,132).*

  –LOH detection at 10q, 18q, 16q, and 11p chromosomal regions have been found associated with high histologic grade and recurrence *(133).*

  –Although frequently referenced, LOH at 18q21 region and progression of prostate carcinoma and TSGs possibly involved remain undetected *(134,135).*

  –The 16q13–q24.3 region, and in particular the 16q24.1–q24.2 band, have been frequently found associated with aggressive disease (i.e., histologic high-grade and metastasis development but no mutations have been found occurring at CDH1, HPR CBFB TSGs here located) *(136,137).*

  –High rate of LOH (70%) at 11p region, harboring the *KAI1* gene, observed in metastatic foci from human prostate cancer, but further investigation required *(138).*

  –LOH at 10q, 11p, 16q, and 18q chromosomal regions as well as the frequency of generalized LOH correlate with adverse prognostic parameters such as high tumor grade, recurrence of neoplasia, advanced stage, and cancer death; 16q LOH could be a promising marker to identify patients who do not benefit from androgen therapy.

- RENAL CELL CARCINOMA

  –Validation provided for the microsatellite markers panel useful for the differential diagnosis in RCC subtypes (i.e., nonpapillary RCC, papillary RCC, chromophobe RCC, renal oncocytoma, and collecting duct carcinoma) *(139).*

HNSCC = head and neck squamous cell carcinoma; LOH = loss of heterozygosity; RCC = renal cell carcinoma; TSG = tumor suppressor genes

continued

Table 1 (*continued*)

- RENAL CELL CARCINOMA (*continued*)
  – Nonpapillary RCC marked by LOH at chromosome 3p (98%); 8p (33%), 9 (33%), 14q (48%) and duplication of chromosome 5q (70%); papillary RCC shows trisomies of chromosome 3q (35%), 7 (80%), 8 (20%), 12 (35%), 16 (60%), 17 (90%), and 20 (30%); chromophobe RCC characterized by a combination of LOH at chromosome 1 (100%), 2 (95%), 6 (88%), 10 (88%), 13 (95%), 17 (76%), and 21 (70%).

  – A positive association has been found between trisomy 16, 12, 20, and partial loss of chromosome 14 and clinically more aggressive RCCs *(140);* 14q deletion positively associates with increased tumor grade and stage, demonstrating its validity as a marker in prognosis evaluation.

  – Microsatellite markers located at chromosome 1, 2, and 3 can be used for differential diagnosis of RCC; LOH at 14q may be usefully applied as adverse prognostic marker overall, whereas LOH at 8p and 9p correlates with high stage in a subset of RCCs.

- LUNG CANCER
  – Morphologic steps leading to lung neoplasia including, at least for SCC, hyperplasia, metaplasia, dysplasia, carcinoma *in situ,* invasive and metastatic carcinoma, reflect the typical multistep process of carcinogenesis.

  – Molecular mechanism of the lung carcinoma has focused on the role of inactivation of K-*ras (141),* TP53 *(142),* p16–CDKN2–MTS1 *(143),* and FHIT *(144).*

  – Allelotype studies showed that LOH at 3p, 13q, and 17p are involved in carcinogenesis of NSCLC, whereas deletions especially involving 2q, 9p, 18q, and 22q may play an important role in its progression *(145).*

  – Both invasive carcinomas and the corresponding preneoplastic lesions were found widely affected by LOH at 3p; such loss could be an early and crucial step in pathogenesis of NSCLC and usefully applied as marker in the risk assessment *(146).*

  – Preliminary data suggest that MSI at 2p and 3p regions (scored as 1 or more loci involved) may be detected at a high rate (69%) and may show a statistically significant correlation with poor prognosis; MSI at 2p and 3p loci may provide a useful prognostic marker in both stage I NSCLC and in relapse risk assessment of operable forms *(147,148).*

  – Frequency of MSI at 2p and 3p has provided to be an independent factor that could predict a decreased survival as well as familial clustering of malignancy, suggesting the presence of putative defects that might increase the sensitivity to a wide variety of environmental carcinogens *(149).*

  – LOH occurring at chromosome 2 was found significantly associated with brain metastases, whereas specific 2q deletion seems to occur more frequently in moderately and poorly differentiated tumors than in well-differentiated ones *(150).*

  – Recent data, focused on the carcinogenic role of the 16q 24.1–24.2 band deletion, not fitting with localization of CDH1, suggest existence of a different TSG involved in lung cancer progression *(151).*

SCC = squamous cell carcinoma; NSCLC = non-small-cell lung cancer; LOH = loss of heterozygosity; MSI = microsatellite instability; RCC = renal cell carcinoma; SCC = squamous cell carcinoma

continued

Table 1 (*continued*)

- LUNG CANCER (*continued*)
  - –LOH occurring at two bands of the long arm of chromosome 10, 10q21, and 10q23–25, never associated with *PTEN* gene mutations, has been proposed as adverse prognostic marker in SCLC cases *(152)*.

  - –The *p16* region seems to be the major target of deletion in primary NSCLC and preneoplastic lesions *(153,154)* whereas LOH at the same region has been reported to be present in a decreasing fashion in a large cell carcinomas, SCC, and adenocarcinomas.

  - –LOH at two distinct regions between D11S1758 and D11S12 and between HRAS and D11S1363, encompassing the 11p15.5 chromosomal portion, were found to be associated the former with tumor type and advanced stage, and the latter with cigarette consumption, female sex, and reduction of survival *(155)*.

  - –LOH at 1p32/LMYC significantly correlates with regional nodal involvement as well as advanced clinical stages in NSCLC *(156)*.

  - –The 3p and 9p losses seem to be related to the early stages and then useful in risk assessment; LOH spanning chromosome 2 is associated with poorly differentiation and brain metastases; MSI occurring at 2p and 3p in addition to LOH at 1p32, 10q, 11p, and 16q may be associated with adverse prognosis and cigarette consumption *(157)*.

- COLON CANCER
  - –Clinical and pathologic stage are the only available prognostic parameters in colorectal cancer patients, but in a relevant percentage of cases, they failed to predict outcome or survival.

  - –Generalized LOH frequency was found equally distributed among the three types of colon and rectum cancers investigated (i.e., sporadic RER– cancers, sporadic RER+ cancers, and cancers associated with ulcerative colitis); RER+ phenotype seems to be associated with a survival advantage *(158)*.

  - –LOH at 18q seems to correlate with adverse outcome; by contrast, RER+ phenotype seems to contribute to better survival.

SCLC = small-cell lung cancer; SCC = squamous cell cancer; LOH = loss of heterozygosity; RER = replication area repair; NSCLC = non-small-cell lung cancer

Hematopoietic Tumors: Proto-oncogene Activation

BCL2

BCL2 was one of the first oncogenes shown to be involved in nonrandom chromosomal translocations. It usually is rearranged with *Ig* heavy and light chain genes on chromosomes 14q32 (*IgH*), 2p11 (κ), and 22q11 (λ). In t(14;18)(q32;q21), approx 70% of the breakpoints on chromosome 18 cluster within a major breakpoint region (MBR) in the untranslated region of exon 3, 20% occur in the minor cluster region (MCR) 20 kb downstream of *BCL2,* and a minority cluster in the variant cluster region (VCR), 1.5 kb upstream or within the first noncoding exon *(52)*. As a consequence of the breakpoint locations, the protein coding domain is maintained during translocation.

Gene rearrangement therefore results in overexpression of intact BCL2 protein under the control of *Ig* enhancer sequences *(50)*. The role of t(14;18) and *BCL2* overexpression in tumorigenesis was demonstrated by in vivo studies. Transgenic mice bearing *BCL2–Ig* minigene harbor expanded B-cell compartments and developed follicular hyperplasia that eventually progressed to high-grade monoclonal lymphomas. When expression is directed to T cells, fully one-third of the mice develop peripheral T-cell lymphomas. Long latency and progression from polyclonal hyperplasia to monoclonal malignancy are consistent with the hypothesis that oncogenic events in addition to *BCL2* overexpression are necessary for tumor formation. Accordingly, in lymphomas arising in *BCL2–Ig* transgenic mice, a common second tumorigenic hit is translocation of the *C-MYC* oncogene *(51)*.

Detection methods include Southern blot hybridization with probes specific for the MBR, MCR, and 5′ regions of *BCL2;* PCR with primers specific for the MBR or MCR breakpoint regions; long-distance PCR (LD-PCR), and FISH *(159)*.

t(14;18) is the molecular hallmark of follicular lymphomas and is associated with 60–80% of these tumors. The translocation is found in 20% of DLCL, likely transformed from low-grade follicular lymphomas, and about 10% of Hodgkin's diseases (HD). The t(2;18) and t(18;22) variant translocations have been described in 10% of B-cell chronic lymphatic leukemias (B-CLL). Combined with morphologic and clinical observations, the finding of t(14;18) in lymph node aspirate may help define a differential diagnosis of follicular lymphoma *(160)*.

t(14;18) is not exclusively associated with tumors. Using sensitive nested PCR, rare *BCL2–JH* harboring cells have been demonstrated in up to 50% of reactive tonsil and spleen and in peripheral blood of normal individuals, in whom the translocation frequency increases with age *(161,162)*. Controversial data still surround the prognostic impact of *BCL2* translocation. Studies have demonstrated that *BCL2*-rearranged and germline tumors undergo the same clinical behavior, and a negative prognostic marker is represented by BCL2 protein overexpression *(59,61)*.

The presence of t(14;18) provides a useful genetic marker to monitor patients after therapy. The PCR persistence of residual *BCL2* rearranged cells in the peripheral blood and bone marrow of patients in clinical remission identifies a group of people at high risk of relapse.

BCL1

t(11;14) (q13;q32) translocation involves the *BCL1* locus on chromosome 11q13 and one of the joining regions of the *IgH* genes on chromosome 14q32, resulting in juxtaposition of *BCL1* with the *IgH* enhancer. Only sporadically variable (*VH*) genes or switch *IgM* (Sμ) may be involved *(163)*. t(11;14) probably reflects an error in normal variable diversity joining (VDJ) recombination during normal precursor B-cell development. More than 80% of the breakpoints on chromosome 11 cluster in a 300-bp region known as MTC, centromeric to *BCL1 (77)*. Two MTCs have been identified (*mTc1* 22 kb telomeric to *BCL1,* and *mTc2,* clustering in the 5′ flanking region of *BCL1*) that are less frequently involved in translocation.

Inv(11) (p15;q13) was found in a parathyroid adenoma and involved the parathyroid hormone locus on 11p15 and *BCL1–PRAD1* on 11q13 *(72)*. In this reciprocal translocation, the *PRAD1* gene was placed under the regulatory sequences of the *PTH* gene and resulted in mRNA overexpression.

Detection methods include conventional cytogenetics, Southern blot hybridization, PCR, FISH, and fiber FISH.

t(11;14) (q13;q32), the molecular hallmark of MCL, is detectable by Southern blotting and PCR, in up to 50% of these tumors *(164–166)*. The finding that the percentage of *BCL1*-positive cases increases by FISH analysis *(167)* and the evidence that up to 90% of MCL overexpress BCL1 protein *(168,169)* suggest that deregulation of the *BCL1* gene occurs in many more cases than originally thought. No clinical differences were observed between *BCL1*-rearranged and germline MCL, an indication that *BCL1* does not identify a clinically different MCL subset. Sporadically, t(11;14) has been found in lymphoid malignancies other than MCL, including B-CLL and multiple myeloma *(170,171)*. In some cases, however, reclassification of these t(11;14)-bearing tumors included them in the MCL histotype.

c-myc

The translocations involving the *C-MYC* gene on chromosomes 8 and one of the *Ig* loci are of three types. Approximately 80% of cases involve translocation t(8;14)(q24;q32), which occurs between *C-MYC* and the genes for the *Ig* heavy chain. The remainder involve translocation between *C-MYC* and *Ig* light chain sequences on chromosomes 2p11 and 22q11. In plasmacytomas, the breakpoints on chromosome 8 occur within the first noncoding intron of *C-MYC*, while in BLs, the translocations are more variable and occur in the 5′ or 3′ sequences flanking the gene or up to 300 kb upstream from the gene. Owing to the relocation of *C-MYC* near or within the strong transcription controls of the *Ig* gene, the translocation results in a loss of normal gene regulation and leads to constitutive *C-MYC* expression. Detection methods include Southern blot hybridization, LD-PCR, and FISH.

t(8;14)(q24;q32), and its variants t(8;22)(q24;q11) and t(2;8)(p11;q24), the molecular hallmark of BL, are observed in almost all cases of BLs/leukemias *(172)*. These translocations occasionally can be detected in 15% of other intermediate to high-grade B-cell lymphomas, and sporadically in low-grade B-cell lymphomas. In sporadic BL, translocation breakpoints cluster within the first exon or intron or immediately upstream from the gene, whereas in endemic BL, translocations with breakpoints dispersed over about 300 kb upstream from the gene are most frequent. Among other B-cell lymphomas, *C-MYC* rearrangement is observed in *BCL2*-positive follicular lymphomas undergoing high-grade transformation *(173),* and is considered a secondary genetic event involved in tumor progression.

BCL6

Chromosomal translocations with the *Ig* gene regions are among the most common rearrangements involving chromosome 3q27. The *BCL6* gene frequently can rearrange with the *IgH* loci on chromosome 14 in t(3;14)(q27;q32), but occasional rearrangement with the *IgL* loci, in t(3;22)(q27;q11) and t(2;3)(p11;q27), is also observed *(174)*. In t(2;3), the *BCL2* and *IgL* κ genes are juxtaposed in a head-to-head configuration. Rearrangements of *BCL6* with non-*Ig* genes have been described. Although many of the partner genes translocated with *BCL6* are still unknown, some have been identified, including a novel H4 histone gene located on chromosome 6p21 *(175)*, the B-cell transcriptional coactivator BOB1 OBF1 on chromosome 11q23.1 *(176,177)*, and the *TTF* gene which encodes a novel G protein on chromosome 4p11 *(178)*. Many variant rearrangements of *BCL6,* affecting chromosomes 1p32, 1p34, 3p14, 6q23, 12p13, 14q11, and 16p13, involve genes that have not been characterized *(179)*.

Detection methods include Southern blot hybridization and FISH with a cosmide spanning the 3q27 breakpoint region.

BCL6 chromosomal translocations are associated to approx 50% of cases of DLCL and 10% of follicular lymphomas *(180)*. In DLCL, *BCL6* rearrangement correlates with clinical presentation at extranodal sites, including the gastrointestinal tract. Offit et al. *(181)* showed that patients with *BCL6* gene rearrangement had a favorable overall survival and survival without disease progression. Since this finding has not been supported by Bastard et al. *(182)*, the prognostic meaning of *BCL6* rearrangement remains to be determined.

TAL1

TAL1 (T-cell acute leukemia)–*SCL* (stem cell leukemia hematopoietic transcription factor) gene is located on chromosome 1p32. The encoded gene product is homologous to a number of proteins that are involved in the control of cell growth and differentiation. The region of homology is restricted to a 56-amino-acid domain to form two amphipathic helices separated by an intervening loop. Such helix–loop–helix (HLH) proteins are proposed to function as transcriptional regulatory factors based on their ability to bind in vitro to the E-box motif of eukaryotic transcriptional enhancers. It is suggested that the TAL1 protein may function as a transcriptional regulatory factor. Studies in mice indicate that TAL1 is essential for embryonic blood formation in vivo *(183)*. In tissues, *TAL1* is expressed in developing brain, normal bone marrow and mast cells, leukemic T cells, and endothelial cells but not in normal T cells *(184)*. A recent report indicated an antiapoptotic effect of ectopic *TAL1* expression in response to cytotoxic agents *(185)*.

Tumor-specific alteration of *TAL1* arises by either of two distinct mechanisms. One mechanism is represented by t(1;14)(p32;q11), which transposes *TAL1* from its normal location on chromosome 1p32 into the T-cell receptor α/δ chain complex on chromosome 14q11. The second consists of a 90-kb deletion upstream of one allele of the *TAL1* locus, probably due to aberrant Ig recombinase activity that results in the fusion between *SCL–TAL1* and *SIL* (SCL interrupting locus, chromosome 1p33) *(186,187)*. Both mechanisms disrupt the 5′ end of the *TAL1* gene so that its expression is controlled by the regulatory elements of the *TCR*δ or *SIL* genes that are normally expressed in T-cell ontogeny. The consequence may be an ectopic TAL1 production that activates a specific set of target genes that are normally silent. Breakpoints affecting the 3′ side of *TAL1* or occurring 25 kb downstream from the gene have been recently described *(188)*.

Detection methods for t(1;14) (p32;q11) include conventional cytogenetics and Southern blot hybridization. Detection methods for deletions originating the *TAL1–SIL* fusion gene include Southern blot, DNA PCR, and RT-PCR.

Alteration of the *TAL1* gene is the most common genetic lesion known to be associated with T-cell ALL (T-ALL). Almost 25% of T-ALL patients exhibit *TAL1* deletions, and an additional 3% harbor the t(1;14) translocation. T-NHL or adult T-cell malignancies do not display *TAL1* aberrations. A recent study indicates that T-ALL patients with *TAL1* recombination had a significantly better outcome than other T-ALL patients without the recombination *(189)*.

Hematopoietic Tumors: Chimeric Proteins

NPM–ALK

The nucleolar phosphoprotein gene, nucleophosmin (*NPM*), is located on chromosome 5q35. It is highly conserved, and its protein product is involved in the late stages of ribosomal assembly. The anaplastic lymphoma kinase (*ALK*) gene, a newly characterized gene located on chromosome 2p23, codes for a novel 200-kDa transmembrane protein kinase that belongs to the insulin-receptor subfamily. Whereas NPM is expressed ubiquitously at high levels, the normal expression of *ALK* is restricted to neural tissues and is important for normal neural development and function.

t(2;5)(p23;q35) generates a fusion *NPM–ALK* gene that encodes a chimeric protein. The NPM–ALK protein consists of N-terminal sequences derived from the *NPM* gene fused to C-terminal cytoplasmic sequences from the *ALK* gene, including the consensus protein tyrosine kinase residues *(190)*. Therefore, t(2;5) results in the transcription of *ALK* driven off the strong *NPM* promoter, leading to inappropriate expression and constitutive activation of a truncated 80-kDa ALK protein. Because of the breakpoint location, the fusion protein lacks extracellular and transmembrane domain and has intracellular localization. The NPM–ALK hybrid protein is thought to play a key role in tumorigenesis by aberrant phosphorylation of intracellular substrates *(191)*.

The detection method for DNA is two-color FISH; for RNA, RT-PCR; and for protein, IHC with monoclonal antibodies (mAbs) recognizing a formalin-resistant epitope in both the 80-kDa NPM–ALK chimeric and the 200-kDa normal human ALK proteins.

The presence of t(2;5) is specifically associated with 50–60% of CD30-positive anaplastic large-cell lymphomas (ALCLs), which represent a subset of high-grade NHL. This marker identifies a subgroup of morphologically heterogeneous ALCLs with T/null phenotype that are characterized by a more favorable clinical course than *NPM–ALK*-negative ALCLs *(192)*.

BCR–ABL t(9;22)(q34;q11)

The normal cellular *BCR* gene is located on chromosome 22q11.21. It spans a 135-kb region and contains 23 exons. The *BCR* gene is expressed as mRNAs of 4.5 and 6.7 kb. It encodes a 160-kDa phosphoprotein associated with a serine/threonine kinase activity *(193)* and shows autophosphorylation activity as well as transphosphorylation activity for several protein substrates *(194)*. The c-*ABL* gene, mapping on chromosome 9q34, is 225 kb in size and is expressed as either a 6- or 7-kb mRNA transcript. The *ABL* gene codes for a 145-kDa tyrosine kinase with nuclear localization. The DNA-binding activity of the ABL protein is regulated by CDC2-mediated phosphorylation, suggesting a cell cycle function for *ABL*. The gene is also implicated in processes of cell differentiation, cell division, cell adhesion, and stress response. The tyrosine kinase activity of nuclear ABL is regulated in the cell cycle through a specific interaction with Rb protein *(195)*. *ABL* activity is negatively regulated by its SH3 domain through an unknown mechanism, and deletion of the SH3 domain turns *ABL* into an oncogene *(196)*.

t(9;22)(q34;q11) translocation, which transposes the *ABL* gene from chromosome 9 to the center of the *BCR* gene on chromosome 22, results in a head-to-tail fusion of these two genes and the formation of the Philadelphia (Ph) chromosome. The 5′ exon of the *ABL* gene lies at least 300 kb upstream from the remaining *ABL* exons, and the very long intron is the target for translocation *(197)*. Although the position of the breakpoint on chromosome 9 varies considerably, the breakpoint on chromosome 22 is clustered in an area called bcr for "breakpoint cluster region" *(198)*. The *BCR–ABL*-encoded product is a chimeric 210-kDa protein that has bcr information at its N-terminus and retains most of the normal ABL protein sequences. In some tumors, the *ABL* gene can be juxtaposed to the 5′ region of the *BCR* gene in a t(9;22) translocation cytogenetically indistinguishable from the Ph chromosome. In these cases, a unique *ABL*-derived tyrosine kinases of 180 kDa is produced *(199)*. The functional consequence of the *BCR–ABL* fusion is increased tyrosine kinase activity. Sequences within the first exon of *BCR* appear to be essential for this activation and probably work through direct physical binding to the kinase regulatory domain of *ABL*.

Detection methods include conventional cytogenetics, Southern blot hybridization, two-color FISH, and RT-PCR.

t(9;22) (Ph⁺) represents a diagnostic tumor-specific marker associated with more than 90% of chronic myelogenous leukemias (CMLs), which have an unfavorable evolution to AML or ALL. A striking correlation between the site of the breakpoint within the breakpoint cluster region on chromosome 22 and the length of time between presentation and onset of acute phase was demonstrated; the patients with 5′ breakpoint had a fourfold longer chronic phase than those with a 3′ breakpoint *(200,201)*. The optimization of RT-PCR protocols has allowed monitoring of minimal residual disease in Ph⁺ CML patients undergoing bone marrow transplantation (BMT). Several studies showed that PCR-negativity indicates complete eradication of the leukemic clone, and PCR-positivity is associated with relapse in T-depleted transplanted patients or those undergoing transplantation in the advanced phase. PCR-positive patients undergoing transplantation in the chronic phase or those receiving nonmanipulated bone marrow have a slightly higher risk of relapse than PCR-negative patients. In these cases it has been demonstrated by competitive PCR that a low number of *BCR–ABL* transcript molecules is associated with prolonged complete remission, and patients with an increasing number of transcript molecules are subject to relapse *(202,203)*.

The variant t(9;22), a translocation cytogenetically undistinguishable from that of CML but with a different breakpoint in the *BCR* gene, is found in about 10% of patients with *de novo* ALL *(204)*.

PML–RARA (t15;17)(q22;q12)

The *PML* (promyelocytic leukemia) gene maps on chromosome 15q22. It codes for a DNA-binding zinc finger protein with a potential leucine zipper motif. Its physiological role is unknown, but a putative transcription-factor function is suggested. The PML protein is expressed at significant high levels in G_1 phase of the cell cycle and at a lower level in S, G_2, and M phases *(205)*. In mice, *PML* regulates hematopoietic differentiation and controls cell growth and tumorigenesis *(206)*. *PML* function is essential for the tumor-growth-suppressive activity of retinoic acid (RA) and for its ability to induce terminal myeloid differentiation of precursor cells. *PML* is needed for the RA-dependent transactivation of the p21 (*WAF1–Cip1*) gene, which regulates cell-cycle progression and cellular differentiation *(206)*.

The *RARA* gene maps on chromosome 17q12. It is homologous to the receptors for steroid and thyroid hormones *(207)* and codes for a nuclear receptor protein that binds the RA ligand and DNA through a zinc finger region, thereby presumably activating a set of target genes.

t(15;17)(q22;q12) is an important example of a transcription fusion factor, in which the *PML* gene on chromosome 17 is fused with the *RARA* gene on chromosome 15. In the chimeric gene, the promoter and first exon of the *RARA* gene are replaced by part of the *PML* gene *(208)*. The *PML* breakpoints are clustered in two regions on either side of an alternative spliced exon *(209)*. The translocation chromosome generates a *PML–RARA* chimeric transcript. Alternative splicing of *PML* exons produces multiple isoforms of the *PML–RARA* mRNAs, even within a single patient. The *PML–RARA* fusion RNA encodes a predicted 106-kDa chimeric protein that contains most of the *PML* sequences fused to a large part of the *RARA* gene, including its DNA- and hormone-binding domains *(208)*. The ability of the chimeric *NPM–RARA* gene to initiate tumorigenesis was demonstrated in transgenic mice, which exhibited a partial block of differentiation in the neutrophil lineage and eventually progressed to overt myeloid leukemia *(210)*. It is speculated that the PML–RARA fusion protein may functionally interfere with the *PML* and *RXR–RAR* pathways at multiple levels, leading to proliferative advantage and block of hematopoietic differentiation *(206)*.

Detection methods include conventional cytogenetics, Southern blot hybridization, FISH, and RT-PCR.

t(15;17)(q22;q21) is associated with almost 100% of cases of acute promyelocytic leukemia (APL) (AML3 or M3 in the FAB classification). The molecular characterization of *PML–RARA* has clinical prognostic impact. This genetic aberration represents a tumor-specific marker for a correct diagnosis of APL and because its presence is related to a good response to all-*trans* retinoic acid (ATRA), it permits the use of a specific therapy based on the use of this retinoid. It has been observed that the persistence of residual transcript during clinical remission allows identification of patients with high risk of relapse for whom further therapeutic treatment might be required *(211)*.

AML–ETO t(8;21)(q22;q22)

The *AML* gene, located on chromosome 21q22, is the human homologue of *Runt,* an important gene in *Drosophila* that regulates segmentation. The structure analysis of the *AML* gene showed that the 5′ portion of the gene contains the *Runt* homologous sequences, a DNA-binding domain, and dimerization sequences, whereas the 3′ portion contains gene transactivation sequences *(212)*. In adults, the *AML* gene is ubiquitously expressed in several tissues, particularly in bone marrow cells. Because *AML* knockout mice die during embryonic development, secondary to the complete absence of fetal liver-derived hematopoiesis, it is suggested that *AML*-regulated target genes are essential for definitive hematopoiesis of all lineages *(213)*. The *ETO* gene maps on chromosome 8q22. It comprises 13 exons distributed over 87 kb of genomic DNA *(214)*. *ETO* structurally belongs to the zinc finger transcription factor genes. By Western blot analysis, the ETO product was identified as a 70-kDa protein associated with the nuclear matrix *(215)*. Its biologic function is still unknown. *ETO* is expressed in several tissues, mainly during fetal life, with the highest mRNA levels occurring in brain and heart. Recent data show that *ETO* is also specifically expressed in CD34[+] hematopoietic stem cells *(216).*

t(8;21)(q22;q22) leads to the fusion of the *AML* and *ETO* genes. The resulting fusion gene transcribes a hybrid mRNA and is translated into a 94-kDa AML–ETO chimeric protein. The *AML–ETO* chimeric gene contains in 5′ *Runt* but not transactivation sequences of *AML*; in 3′, the gene contains the whole coding sequence of *ETO,* whose expression is regulated by the *AML* promoter *(212).* In vitro transfection experiments suggest that the AML–ETO fusion protein can suppress the normal AML protein function by inhibiting myeloid differentiation *(217).* Thus, the neoplastic transformation may result either by a dominant negative effect of the AML–ETO hybrid protein, which blocks the transcription of specific genes involved in myeloid differentiation, such as granulocyte-macrophage colony-stimulating factor (GM-CSF) or alternatively may be promoted by aberrant ETO transcription under the effect of AML promoter. Detection methods include two-color FISH, RT-PCR, and Western blot.

t(8;21), the most frequent cytogenetic alteration observed in AML, is associated with 20% of AML M2 and is found in about 5% of AML M1 by RT-PCR analysis *(218).* Except in rare pediatric cases, patients carrying this genetic abnormality usually have a favorable clinical course *(219).* In patients with complete clinical remission after conventional chemotherapy, and autologous or allogenic BMT, the *AML–ETO* transcript is frequently found by RT-PCR *(220,221).* The biological meaning of this finding is unknown. It is speculated that rare t(8;21)-positive cells persistent in the bone marrow of patients in clinical remission represent a clonal population only partially transformed and are not able to develop into overt leukemia. Owing to the constant persistence of genetically aberrant cells during remission, the minimal residual disease monitoring by RT-PCR does not seem to provide useful clinical and therapeutic information.

Other Translocations

A number of other chromosomal translocations have been described in hematopoietic tumors, which either juxtapose proto-oncogenes to Ag-receptor genes or lead to the formation of fusion genes *(222–224).* These specific translocations are listed in Tables 2 and 3.

Solid Tumors

Investigation of solid-tumor translocations has concentrated on sarcomas, whose cytogenetics have been well studied *(222).* In sarcomas, specific chromosomal translocations have been associated with distinct tumor histotypes, thus providing a clinical application in the differential diagnosis of sarcomas with difficult morphological diagnosis assessment (e.g., primitive neuroectodermal tumors [PNET], synovial sarcoma, rhabdomyosarcoma) and in some cases, a prognostic assessment. Moreover, these markers can be potentially used for monitoring minimal residual disease. One gene more frequently involved in these specific chromosomal translocations is *EWS*. Molecularly, the oncogenic conversion of *EWS* follows a common scheme of activation that exchanges its putative RNA binding domain with the DNA-binding domains of ETS-family transcription factor genes *(FLI1, ERG, ETV1, E1AF, FEV)* or other transcription

Table 2
Nonfusion Genes in Hematopoietic Tumors

Type	Translocation	Affected gene	Rearranged gene	Disease
Basic helix-loop-helix	t(7;19)(q35;p13)	*LYL1*	*TCR*β	T-ALL
	t(7;9)(q35;q34)	*TAL2*	*TCR*β	T-ALL
Cysteine-rich (LIM) proteins	t(11;14)(p15;q11)	*LMO1*	*TCR-δ*	T-ALL
	t(11;14)(p13;q11)	*LMO2*	*TCR-δ/α/β*	T-ALL
	t(7;11)(q35;p1 31)	*LMO2*	*TCR-δ/α/β*	T-ALL
Homeobox protein	t(10;14)(q24;q11)	*HOX11*	*TCR-α/β*	T-ALL
	t(7;10)(q35;q24)	*HOX11*	*TCR-α/β*	T-ALL
Others	t(10;14)(q24;q32)	*lyt-10*	*IgH*	B-NHL
	t(14;19)(q32;q13)	*BCL-3*	*IgH*	B-CLL
	t(5;14)(q31;q32)	*IL-3*	*IgH*	Pre-B ALL
	t(7;9)(q34;q34)	*TAN1*	*TCR*β	T-ALL
	t(1;17)(p34;q34)	*LCK*	*TCR*β	T-ALL
	t(X;14)(q28;q11)	*C6.1B*	*TCR-α*	T-PLL
	t(9;14)(p13;q32)	*PAX-5*	*IgH*	LPL B-NHL

Abbreviations: TCR, T-cell receptor; IgH, immunoglobulin heavy chain; ALL, acute lymphoblastic leukemia (T, B, or pre-B cell); B-NHL, B non-Hodgkin's lymphoma; B-CLL, B chronic lymphocytic leukemia; T-PLL, T prolymphocytic leukemia; LPL, lymphoplasmacytoid lymphoma.

factor genes (*ATF1, WT1*). This fusion may be necessary for *EWS*-associated oncogenesis, and the transcription factor partner in the chimeric proteins may determine the specific tumor type. In fact the fusion of a member of the ETS-family of DNA-binding proteins (FL1, ERG, ETV1, E1AF, FEV) with EWS gives rise to pPNET, ATF1 with EWS to clear-cell sarcoma, and WT1 with EWS to intraabdominal desmoplastic small-round-cell tumor. On the other hand FUS and EWS protein may functionally act as equivalents when fused with the transcription factor CHOP in myxoid liposarcomas (Table 4). These apparently opposite findings lead to the hypothesis that EWS and FUS proteins also may be interchangeable in the EWS-associated tumors.

Detection of these chimeric transcripts can be performed by conventional cytogenetics, molecular cytogenetics (FISH with painting probes or gene-specific probes), and at the transcriptional level by RT-PCR, and has formed the basis of a sensitive and specific diagnostic assay for these tumors (225).

Soft Tissues

EWS–FLI1 t(11;22)(q24;q12)

Karyotype analyses have revealed a tumor-specific chromosomal translocation t(11;22)(q24;q12) in 86% of both Ewing sarcoma (ES) and PNET. The (11;22) translocation results in the fusion of the N-terminal region of the *EWS* gene rich in glutamine,

Table 3
Fusion Genes in Hematopoietic Tumors

Translocation	Affected gene	Disease
t(1;19)(q23;p13)	*PBX1-E2A*	Pre-B ALL
t(17;19)(q22;p13)	*HLF-E2A*	Pro-B ALL
t(11;17)(q23;q21)	*PLZF-RARA*	APL
t(4;11)(q21;q23)	*AF4-MLL*	ALL/Pre-B ALL/ANLL
t(9;11)(q21;q23)	*AF9-MLL*	ALL/Pre-B ALL/ANLL
t(11;19)(q23;p13)	*MLL-ENL*	Pre-B ALL/T-ALL/ANLL
t(x;11)(q13;q23)	*AFX1-MLL*	T-ALL
t(1;11)(p32;q23)	*AF1P-MLL*	ALL
t(6;11) (q27;q23)	*AF6-MLL*	ALL
t(11;17)(q23;q21)	*MLL-AF17*	AML
t(3;21)(q26;q22)	*EVI-1-AML1*	CML
t(3;21)(q26;q22)	*EAP-AML1*	MDS
t(16;21)(p11;q22)	*FUS-ERG*	AML
t(6;9)(p23;q34)	*DEK-CAN*	AML
t(5;12)(q33;p13)	*PDGFβ-TEL*	CMML

Abbreviations: ALL, acute lymphoblastic leukemia (T or B cell); AML, acute myelogenous leukemia; ANLL, acute non-lymphoblastic leukemia; APL, acute promyelocytic leukemia; CMML, chronic myelomonocytic leukemia; MDS, myelodysplastic syndromes.

serine, and tyrosine residues to the *ETS*-like DNA-binding domain of the *FLI1* (Friend leukemia integration site 1) gene *(222)*. *EWS* is an ubiquitously expressed gene located on chromosome 22 that encodes for a RNA-binding protein, whereas FLI1, located on chromosome 11, is a member of the ETS family of transcription factors. The oncogenic effect of t(11;22) is caused by the formation of a chimeric protein. The protein has the potential to promote tumorigenesis by acting as an aberrant transcription factor *(226)* that is functionally distinct from the normal *FLI1 (225)*. Several EWS–FLI1 fusion types have been observed: the two main types, fusion of *EWS* exon 7 to FLI1 exon 6 (type 1) and fusion of *EWS* exon 7 to *FLI1* exon 5 (type 2), account for about 85% of EWS–FLI fusions *(227)*. Type 1 EWS–FLI1 fusion has been shown to be a significant positive predictor of overall survival *(227)*. Thus, molecular detection of the t(11;22) translocation is valuable in the differential diagnosis of small-round-cell tumors and provides important information for the staging and prognosis of ES *(228)*. EWS–FLI1-positive cells were amplified by RT-PCR in bone marrow and peripheral blood of a subset of patients with both nonmetastatic and metastatic ES or PNET, a finding that suggests a possible application of RT-PCR in the early identification of patients who may benefit from alternative therapy or who may be spared overtreatment *(229)*.

EWS–ERG *t(21;22)(q22;q12)*

t(21;22) is a variant translocation of *EWS* gene present in 5% of patients with ES. This translocation gives origin to the fusion of *EWS* to a different *ETS* family member, the *ERG* gene located on chromosome 21. After this translocation, identical EWS nucleotide sequences found in the EWS–FLI1 fusion transcripts are fused to portions

Table 4
Fusion Genes in Sarcomas

Tumor	Translocation	5'/3' Fusion Gene	Type
Ewing/PNET	t(11;22)(q24;q12)	*EWS/FLI-1*	*RNA binding/ETS TF*
	t(21;22)(q22;q12)	EWS/ERG	RNA binding/ETS TF
	t(7;22)(p22;q12)	*EWS/ETV1*	RNA binding/ETS TF
	t(2;22)(q33;q12)	*EWS/FEV*	*RNA binding/ETS TF*
Melanoma of soft parts	t(12;22)(q13;q12)	EWS/ATF1	RNA binding/bZIP TF
Intra-abdominal desmoplastic small round cell tumours	t(11;22)(p13;q12)	EWS/WT1	RNA binding/Zn finger TF
Myxoid chondrosarcoma	t(9;22)(q22-31;q11-12)	*EWS/CHN*	RNA binding/Steroid thyroid receptor gene
Undifferentiated sarcoma of infancy	t(17;22)(q12;q12)	EWS/EIAF	RNA binding/TF
Liposarcoma (myxoid & round cell)	t(12;16)(q13;p11)	TLS(FUS)/CHOP	RNA binding/bZIP
	t(12;22)(q13;q12)	EWS/CHOP	RNA binding/bZIP
Alveolar RMS	t(2;13)(q35;q14)	PAX3/FKHR	PB&HD/FD
	t(1;13)(p36;q14)	PAX7/FKHR	
Synovial sarcoma	t(X;18)(p11.2;q11.2)	SYT/SSX1	?/?
		SYT/SSX2	
Dermatofibrosarcoma protuberans	t(17;22)(q22;q13)	PDGFB/COL1A1	Platelet growth factor/collagene type 1α1

of ERG encoding an ETS DNA-binding domain, resulting in the expression of a hybrid EWS/ERG protein *(225).*

EWS–ETV1 *t(7;22)(p22;q12)*

This rare variant chromosomal translocation, recently identified in two pPNET cases *(230,231),* fuses *EWS* to the *ETV1* (for ETS translocation variant 1) gene, a member of the ETS family of transcription factors located on chromosome 7p22. Identical *EWS* nucleotide sequences found in most *EWS–FLI1* and *EWS–ERG* chimeric transcripts are fused to a region of *ETV1* encoding an *ETS* domain with sequence-specific DNA-binding activity *(231).*

EWS–fev *t(2;22)(q33;q12)*

EWS can be fused to *fev* in the chromosomal translocation t(2;22) in a subset of ES. The *fev* gene is located on chromosome 2 and consists of three exons. It is a new member of the *ETS* family that encodes a 238-amino-acid protein containing an *ETS* DNA-binding domain closely related to that of *FLI1* and *ERG*. However, compared with *FLI1* and *ERG, FEV* lacks transcription regulatory domains in its N-terminal part. The C-terminal part of fev is alanine rich, suggesting a potential transcription repressor activity. *FEV* expression is detected in adult prostate and small intestine, but not in other adult or in fetal tissues *(232).*

EWS–E1AF *t(17;22)(q12;q12)*

The t(17;22) chromosomal translocation, leading to the fusion of *EWS* with *E1AF,* was described in an undifferentiated sarcoma of infancy *(233). E1AF* is a newly isolated member of *ETS* family of genes that is located on chromosome 17q21 and that encodes for the adenovirus E1A enhancer-binding protein. The breakpoint on chromosome 17 lies in the region upstream to the *ETS* domain of the *E1AF* gene. As in other fusion proteins previously characterized in ES and Ewing family sarcoma, it is assumed that the RNA-binding domain of *EWS* may be replaced by the DNA-binding domain of *E1AF.*

EWS–ATF1 *t(12;22)(q13;q12)*

This translocation is frequently and specifically found in malignant melanoma of soft tissues (clear-cell sarcoma) and causes the fusion of *EWS* to the transcription factor *ATF1.* The chimeric EWS–ATF1 protein consists of the N-terminal domain of EWS linked to the βZIP DNA-binding domain of *ATF1,* and possibly results in the activation of *ATF1* target genes *(234).*

EWS–WT1 *t(11;22)(p13;q12)*

This translocation, recurrently associated with desmoplastic small-round-cell sarcoma, juxtaposes *EWS* to the Wilms' tumor gene *WT1* on chromosome 11p13. *WT1* encodes a zinc finger transcription factor that may play a crucial role in normal genitourinary development *(235).* It is expressed in the developing kidney, gonads, spleen, mesothelium, and brain. *WT1* is an oncosuppressor gene specifically inactivated in a subset of Wilms' tumors, and mutations have been found in the germline of susceptible individuals *(236).* In the *EWS–WT1* rearrangement, the breakpoints involve the intron between *EWS* exons 7 and 8 and the intron between *WT1* exons 7 and 8, producing an in-frame fusion of the functional domains of the two genes. The chimeric protein consists of the N-terminal domain of *EWS* and the DNA-binding zinc finger domain of *WT1* and is predicted to modulate transcription at *WT1* target sites *(237).*

EWS–CHN *t(9;22)(q22–31;q11–12)*

A recurrent translocation, t(9;22) (q22;q12), has been recognized in myxoid chondrosarcoma (MCS), specifically the extraskeletal subtype *(238).* In this specific translocation, the *EWS* gene becomes fused to CHN, a novel orphan nuclear receptor with a zinc finger DNA-binding domain located at 9q22–31 *(238).* CHN may be the human homologue of the rat gene *NOR1,* which was recently identified as a sequence overexpressed in brain cells undergoing apoptosis. The chimeric *EWS–CHN* gene encodes a EWS–CHN fusion protein in which the C-terminal RNA-binding domain of *EWS* is replaced by the entire CHN protein, including a large N-terminal domain, a central DNA-binding domain, and a C-terminal ligand-binding/dimerization domain *(239).* An alternative splicing of the 3′ end of the fusion transcript has been described *(238).*

EWS–CHOP *t(12;22)(q13;q12)*

t(12;22) was described in myxoid/round cell liposarcomas, the most common subtype of liposarcoma *(240–242).* This chromosomal translocation leads to the fusion between the N-terminal part of *EWS* and the *CHOP* gene, creating an *EWS–CHOP* chimeric gene. *CHOP* maps on chromosome 12q13 and was previously demonstrated to be consistently involved in rearrangements with the *FUS* gene in the t(12;16) in myxoid/ round cell liposarcomas. At molecular level, the breakpoints on *EWS* occurred within intron 7, close to an A L U sequence, and similarly, the breaks on *CHOP* were observed to cluster in intron 1 near A L U sequences *(242).* The presence of the *EWS–CHOP* chimeric gene in myxoid/round cell liposarcomas indicates that the N-terminal part of *FUS* may be replaced by the N-terminal portion of *EWS* in a Chop fusion oncoprotein and that the two N-terminal parts, when fused to certain transcription factors, have a common or very similar oncogenic potential.

Comparing the clinicopathologic features of the t(12;22)-carrying myxoid/round cell liposarcomas cases with those of cases harboring the more usual t(12;16), no clinical or pathologic differences were identified *(240).*

FUS–CHOP *t(12;16)(q13;p11)*

t(12;16)(q13;p11) is characteristic of the human myxoid/round cell liposarcomas *(240,243).* This chromosomal abnormality results from the fusion of a gene on chromosome 16 called *FUS* or *TLS* and a gene on chromosome 12 that encodes for a dominant inhibitor of transcription, *CHOP.* The FUS product contains a Q S Y-rich segment and an RNA-binding domain, as in the EWS protein. After the rearrangement, the putative RNA-binding domain of *FUS* is replaced by the entire *CHOP* coding region, which contains a basic leucine zipper domain. As in the *EWS* fusion, the *FUS* domain provides a transcriptional activation domain to a presumptive DNA-binding activity of *CHOP* *(222).*

PAX3–FKHR *t(2;13)(q35;q14)* and PAX7–FKHR *t(1;13)(p36;q14)*

Pediatric solid tumor alveolar rhabdomyosarcoma often harbors specific translocations that result in the fusion of a forkhead-domain gene *FKHR* at 13p14 with either the *PAX3* or *PAX7* developmental control genes at 2p35 and 13q14, respectively *(244).*

PAX3 and *PAX7* encode a transcription factor with DNA-binding domains (paired box and homeodomain) that control development by activating specific target genes. After translocation, the resulting chimeric transcription factor contains the DNA-binding domain, a truncated *FKHR* DNA-binding domain, and the C-terminal region of *FKHR (222)*.

SYT–SSX *t(X;18)(p11.2;q11.2)*

A characteristic *SYT–SSX* fusion gene that results from the chromosomal translocation t(X;18)(p11;q11) is detectable in almost all (>80%) synovial sarcomas (SSs). As a result of this translocation, the *SYT* gene from chromosome 18 fuses to either of two highly homologous genes, *SSX1* or *SSX2*, at Xp11.2. *SYT–SSX1* and *SYT–SSX2* express fusion proteins in which the C-terminal amino acids of Syt are replaced by amino acids from the C-terminus of the SSX proteins *(245)*. The fusion proteins function as aberrant transcriptional regulators *(246)*. A significant relationship between histologic SS subtype (monophasic vs biphasic) and *SSX1* or *SSX2* involvement was found: all *SYT–SSX1*-positive SSs were biphasic, and all *SYT–SSX2*-positive were SS monophasic. Moreover, the patients with *SYT–SSX2* had considerably better metastasis-free survival than those with *SYT–SSX1 (246)*.

PDGFB–COL1A1 *t(17;22)(q22;q13)*

This chromosomal translocation was identified in dermatofibrosarcoma protuberans (DP), an infiltrative skin tumor of intermediate malignancy. This tumor, and its juvenile form, giant cell fibroblastoma (GCF), are cytogenetically characterized by the presence of supernumerary ring(s) derived from t(17;22) *(247,248)*. The breakpoints from translocations and rings in DP and GCF contain the fusion of *PDGFβ* chain and collagen type 1α1 (*COL1A1*) genes *(249)*. PDGFβ (c-*sis* proto-oncogene) has transforming activity and is a potent mitogen for several cell types. COL1A1 is a major constituent of the connective tissue matrix. The gene fusion leads to the deletion of exon 1 of *PDGFβ* which results in the release of growth factor from its normal regulation *(249)*. DP DNA transfection onto NIH3T3 fibroblast cells provided direct evidence of the transforming activity of *COL1A1/PDGFβ* chimeric sequence *(250)*. Because the *PDGFβ* pathway is well known and several chemical compounds for blocking PDGFβ signaling are available, therapies specific for DP could reasonably be expected.

Epithelial Tissue

Cytogenetic and molecular analyses of thyroid tumors have indicated these neoplasms as a good model for analyzing human epithelial cell multistep carcinogenesis *(251)*. Thyroid gland manifests a wide spectrum of malignant neoplasms, including MTC, which develop from the neural crest-derived C cells, and tumors arising from the epithelial follicular cells. The latter comprise several tumor types with different phenotypic characteristics and variable biologic and clinical behavior.

Molecular studies have identified specific genetic alterations in these different tumor types. In particular, the well-differentiated carcinomas of the papillary type are characterized by the activation of the RTKs *RET* and *NTRK1* proto-oncogenes. Somatic rearrangements of both *ret* and *NTRK1* produce several forms of oncogenes *(251)*. In all cases, *ret* or *NTRK1* TK domains are fused to the N-terminus of different genes (Table 4).

Detection methods include Southern blot, extra-long PCR, and RT-PCR.

RET

The *RET–PTC1* oncogene, a chimeric transforming sequence, is generated by the fusion of the TK domain of *RET* to the 5′-terminal region of the gene *H4–D10S170*. Both genes have been localized to chromosome 10q. *H4–D10S170* contains a coiled-coil sequence that confers to the oncoprotein the ability to form dimers, resulting in a constitutive activation of the TK function.

In the case of the *RET–PTC2* oncogene, the rearrangement involves the TK domain of *RET* and the gene of the regulatory subunit RIα of protein kinase A (PKA), which maps to chromosome 17q23 *(253,254)*. Cytogenetic analysis has revealed that this oncogene arises from a t(10;17)(q11.2;q23) reciprocal translocation *(255)*. RIα, like the *H4* gene, contains a dimerization domain involved in the activity of the oncogene.

The *RET–PTC3* oncogene is generated by the fusion of the TK domain of *RET* and a gene named *ELE1* (also known as *RFG*) *(256,257)* located in the same region, 10q11.2. In this case, a paracentric inversion of the long arm of chromosome 10 was identified.

NTRK1

NTRK1, located on chromosome 1q22 *(258)*, encodes one of the receptors for nerve growth factor (NGF). *NTRK1*, originally detected in a human colon carcinoma as an oncogene *(TRK)*, was generated from the chromosomal rearrangement by fusing the *NTRK1* TK domain to sequences of a tropomyosin gene, *TPM3*.

The extracellular region of NTRK1 protein contains three leucine-rich motifs (LRMs) flanked by conserved cysteine residues. This extracellular domain also contains two C2 Ig-like loops similar to those present in neural cell adhesion molecules and in receptors for fibroblast growth factors (FGF), platelet-derived growth factor (PDGF), and colony-stimulating factor (CSF)-1.

NTRK1 is expressed primarily in the nervous system and appears essential for the development of both the peripheral and central nervous systems *(251)*.

The *TRK* oncogene is generated by a 1q intrachromosomal rearrangement involving an isoform of the nonmuscle tropomyosin *(TPM3)* mapped to chromosome 1q31 and *NTRK1 (259)*. Molecular analysis revealed the presence not only of the product of the oncogenic rearrangement (5′ TPM3-3′ NTRK1), but also of that related to the reciprocal event (5′ NTRK1-3′ TPM3).

The *TRK–T1* (T2; T4) oncogene, formed by the fusion of *NTRK1* TK domain to sequences of the *TPR* (Translocated Promoter Region) gene localized on chromosome 1q25 *(260)*, generates three chimeric transforming sequences. *TRK–T1* is encoded by a hybrid mRNA that contains 598 nucleotides of *TRP* and 1148 nucleotides of *NTRK1*. An inversion of 1q is responsible for formation of *TRK*. *TRK-T2* and *TRK-T4* rearrangements involve different genomic regions of the two partner genes, *TPR* and *NTRK1*, but occur in the same intron of both these genes. As a consequence, the same mRNA and oncoprotein are produced in both cases. The molecular characterization of these rearrangements indicates that the chromosomal mechanism leads to oncogenic activation as an inv(1q) *(261)*.

The *TRK–T3* oncogene contains 1412 nucleotides of NTRK1 preceded by 598 nucleotides belonging to a novel gene, *TGF* (TRK-fused gene) located on chromosome 3. The latter gene displays a coiled-coil region that could confer to the oncoprotein the ability to form complexes *(251)*.

Table 5
Somatic Rearrangements of Both *ret* and *NTRK1*.

Tyrosine kinase	Activating gene	Oncogene
ret	*H4(D10 5170)*	*ret/PTC1*
	R1α	*ret/PTC2*
	ELE1	*ret/PTC3*
NTRK1	*Tropomyosin*	*TRK*
	TPR	*TRK/T1 (T2; T4)*
	TFG	*TRK/T3*

The most significant clinical relevance of *RET* rearrangements are the correlation with radiation exposure. In fact, a significant proportion of papillary thyroid carcinomas (PTCs) from children exposed to the consequences of the Chernobyl nuclear accident contain a rearranged form of *RET (262,263)*.

In addition, a correlation between the combination of *RET* and *NTRK1* positivity and young age of patients at diagnosis and a significant association between *RET7–NTRK1* positivity and locally advanced stage of disease at onset (pT4: $p < 0.015$) was reported *(264)*. A multivariate analysis confirmed that *RET–NTRK1* activation parallels an unfavorable disease presentation, which may correlate with less favorable disease outcome, and also showed that within these tumors, the frequency of *RET–NTRK1* positivity occurs irrespective of subtypes and degree of differentiation *(265)* (Table 5).

Genetic Markers for Determination of Clonality

It is widely accepted that most tumors are of unicellular origin and result from the progeny of a single cell that has acquired one or more genetic lesions. Therefore, monoclonality is generally considered the hallmark of tumors, although situations exist in which clonality is not unequivocally associated to malignancy. Clonal markers have significance both for the diagnosis and for subsequent studies of disease progression of both solid and hematologic tumors. The methods of clonality determination can be categorized by X-chromosome inactivation and by immunoglobulin and T-cell receptor (TCR) gene rearrangement analysis. All methods depend on the demonstration that a cell population is homogeneous with respect to a particular marker.

X-Chromosome Inactivation

In females, inactivation of one X chromosome occurs in each somatic cell during early embryonic development and is passed to the progeny of the cell in a stable fashion. Evidence relates X-chromosome inactivation to differential methylation of cytosine in the DNA of X-chromosome genes *(266)*. The inactivation or methylation patterns of X-chromosome genes can be used for detecting the clonality of tumors in females heterozygous for a particular X-linked polymorphism. The paternal and maternal X chromosomes can be distinguished by identification of polymorphism at certain alleles, and differences in methylation of DNA sequences within these alleles can be detected by digestion of the DNA with methylation-sensitive restriction enzymes. Polymorphisms have been identified in the hypoxanthine phosphoribosyl transferase (HPRT) and phosphoglycerate kinase (PGK) genes which are near sites that show differential methylation *(267,268)*. Both genes, which are located on the long arm of the X chromosome at Xq26.1-q26.2 and Xq13.3, are constitutively active and therefore amenable to study in various cell types. The limiting factor in the application of this method is the relatively low frequency of polymorphism (20–40%). Recently, the androgen receptor (AR) *(268)* and monoamine oxidase type A (MAOA) *(270)* have been reported to have a very high heterozygosity rate (AR 90%, MAOA 75%), thus increasing the number of tumors that can be analyzed by X-linked RFLP analysis.

For detection, both normal and tumor DNA are first digested with the appropriate restriction endonuclease to distinguish the maternal and paternal copies of the gene through an X-linked RFLP. A second endonuclease that is sensitive to methylation of cytosine residues distinguishes active from inactive copies of the gene through changes of the DNA methylation pattern. In a polyclonal cell population, where X-chromosome inactivation occurs randomly, the paternal and maternal alleles are cleaved by this enzyme so that two fragments of reduced intensity remain visible. In DNA extracted from a tumor with monoclonal composition, one of the two allelic fragments is completely digested, while the other remains unaltered *(271)*. Most methods for X-linked clonality analysis are based on these principles and performed by Southern blot hybridization. The polymorphic and methylation sites of some X-linked genes (such as *PGK, AR,* and *AOA*) are closely clustered within a short region, which allows clonality analysis by PCR amplification after methylation-sensitive enzyme digestion and nonradioactive detection *(272)*. The human AR assay (HUMARA) is an example of PCR-based technique for X-linked clonality analysis *(273)* that also allows detection of clonal cells in selected areas of tissue section both from fresh and archival specimens *(274)*.

X-linked polymorphism can be a useful tumor marker for all tumors that lack specific genetic lesions (e.g., chromosomal translocations), such as myeloproliferative disorders, some ALLs, and many solid tumors. Neoplasms determined to be clonal by X-linked DNA polymorphism include acute and chronic leukemias *(275)*, benign solid tumors (e.g., uterine leiomyomas and parathyroid adenomas), locally aggressive tumors (e.g., sporadic basal cell carcinoma) *(276)*, malignant tumors (Wilms' tumors and gastrointestinal carcinoma), and desmoid tumor *(277)*.

Immunoglobulin Heavy Chain and T-cell Receptor Gene Rearrangement

The genes encoding for human IgH are located on chromosome 14q32. The locus comprises many nonidentical gene segment repeats, which rearrange into a functional unit before transcription and production of the Ig protein. The *IgH* chain gene consists of clusters of more than 100 variable (V), 20 diversity (D), and 6 joining (J) regions. Rearrangement of the gene involves exclsion of DNA between the D and J clusters. The result is DJ joining, which is followed by a second excision between the D and V clusters, and results in VDJ joining. The VDJ unit becomes the coding sequence for the variable part of the Ig protein, which is expressed in conjunction with constant region (C) exons. Variable numbers of untemplated nucleotides (N regions) are inserted at the junctions between the V, D, and J segments. Therefore, each B cell has a unique *IgH* gene rearrangement.

As with B cells, the ability of a particular clonal line of T cells to recognize a given Ag is fixed. The receptors on T cells (*TCR* genes) contain two polypeptide subunits, α and β, in more than 95% of T lymphocytes and γ and δ in a few cells. The genes encoding for each subunit are located on chromosomes 14q11.2 (α), 7q35 (β), 7p15-p14 (γ), and 14q11.2, near the α chain genes (δ). The *TCR* γ and δ regions are rearranged early during T-cell ontogeny before either the α or β chain genes. When subsequent rearrangement of the α chain gene occurs, the *TCR* δ region is deleted, and the rearranged γ region is conserved. As for *Ig* genes, the variable portions of TCR subunits are assembled from VJ or VDJ gene segments, and random N nucleotides are inserted at the junction sites *(278)*.

The unity of the VDJ and VJ assembly in *IgH* and *TCR* genes can be exploited to analyze clonality in tumors of B- and T-cell origin, respectively. By detecting VDJ rearrangement, tissues originating from a single cell display unique *IgH* or *TCR* rearrangement pattern, while tissues originated from multiple B- or T-cell populations display multiple different rearrangements.

The analysis of *IgH* and *TCR* gene rearrangement can be performed by Southern blotting. PCR approaches have recently been defined to identify B- and T-cell mono-clonal proliferations based on the use of 5′ primers complementary to V sequences in conjunction with 3′ primers complementary to the consensus J sequence of the genes. Based on the length of the rearranged fragment, the monoclonal population produces single-size PCR products, and the polyclonal population originates a wide range of product sizes *(279–281)*. Because of the great complexity of the *TCRα* genes and the frequent deletion of the δ gene, PCR analysis of *TCR* rearrangement is usually performed on *TCRβ* and/or γ genes *(282)*.

The use of gas chromatography (GC)-clamp primers and DGGE can be helpful in isolating a clonal *IgH*- or *TCR*-amplified band in the presence of a strong polyclonal background *(283)*. Another reported method for *IgH* and *TCR* clonality is heteroduplex analysis, which is based on denaturation and renaturation of PCR products at low temperature followed by separation on nondenaturating polyacrylamide according to their conformation *(284)*.

PCR analysis of *IgH* and *TCR* gene rearrangement can be easily and rapidly performed on paraffin-embedded archived tissues or in small samples such as lymph node fine-needle aspiration and endoscopic biopsies *(160,285)*. By this analysis, the lineage of proliferation and the differential diagnosis between reactive and neoplastic B- and T-cell proliferation can be assessed with morphologic and clinical information. Notably, detection of *IgH* and *TCR* genes rearrangement gives information about clonality, not malignancy per se. Benign conditions (e.g., benign monoclonal gammopathy) and so-called premalignant conditions (e.g., lymphomatoid granulomatosis, lymphomatoid papulosis, Langerhans cell histiocytosis, lymphoepithelial salivary gland lesion of Sjö-gren) may show monoclonal rearrangement without necessarily developing malignancy after prolonged follow-up *(286)*. Moreover, in PCR-based tests, well-defined mono-clonal bands can be observed when the lymphoid DNA template is present in trace amounts. On the other hand, false-negative results can be achieved when the presence of DNA is below the sensitivity level (1%) or when the target genes undergo somatic mutation that prevents primer binding, as in germinal center-derived B-cell lympho-mas *(279)*.

Clinically, the unity of the VDJ and VJ *IgH* and *TCR* gene rearrangement has been widely exploited to design tumor-specific primers and monitor minimal residual disease in B- and T-cell-derived malignancies.

Conclusions

In this chapter, we have reviewed the main representatives of the different classes of cancer genes that have already found tentative clinical applications. Much work has been done in this area, but it is evident from our review that much more work remains. Hopefully, this research will have direct benefits for patients with cancer.

References

1. Lindor NM, Green MH, Mayo Familial Cancer Program. The concise handbook of Family Cancer Syndromes. *J Natl Cancer Inst.* 1998; 90:1039–71.
2. Chang F, Syrjänen S, Syrjänen K. Implications of the *p53* tumor-suppressor gene in clinical oncology. *J Clin Oncol.* 1995; 13:1009–22.
3. Selvakurrmaran M, Lin H-K, Toshiyuki M, et al. Immediate early up-regulation of *bax* expression by *p53* but not TGFβ1: a paradigm for distinct apoptotic pathways. *Oncogene.* 1994; 9:1791–8.
4. Hollstein M, Sidransky D, Vogelstein B. et al. *p53* mutations in human cancers. *Science.* 1991; 253:49–53.
5. deFromentel CC, Soussi T. *TP53* tumor suppressor gene: a model for investigating human mutagenesis. *Genes Chrom Cancer.* 1992; 4:1–15.
6. Greenblat MS, Bennet WP, Hollstein M, Harris CC. Mutations in p53 tumor suppressor gene: clues to cancer etiology. *Cancer Res.* 1994; 54:4855–4878.
7. Berns EM, van Staveren IL, Look MP, et al. Mutations in residues of *TP53* that directly contact DNA predict poor outcome in human primary breast cancer. *Br J Cancer.* 1998; 77:1130–6.
8. Thorlacius S, Thorgilsson B, Björnsson J, et al. *TP53* mutations and abnormal p53 protein staining in breast carcinomas related to prognosis. *Eur J Cancer.* 1995; 31A:1856–61.
9. Kovach JS, Hartmann A, Blaszyk H, et al. Mutation detection by highly sensitive methods indicates that *p53* gene mutations in breast cancer can have important prognostic value. *Proc Natl Acad Sci USA.* 1996; 93:1093–6.
10. Tsuda H, Sakamaki C, Tsugane S, et al. A prospectuve study of the significance of gene and chromosome alterations as prognostic indicators of breast cancer patients with lymph node metastases. *Breast Cancer Treat.* 1998; 48:21–32.
11. Mao L, Hruban H, Boyle JO, et al. Detection of oncogene mutations in sputum precedes diagnosis of lung cancer. *Cancer Res.* 1994; 54:1634–7.
12. Lavarino C, Corletto V, Mezzelani A, et al. Detection of *TP53* mutation, loss of heterozygosity and DNA content in fine-needle aspirates of breast carcinoma. *Br J Cancer.* 1998; 77:125–30.
13. Bergh J, Norberg T, Sjögren S, et al. Complete sequencing of the *p53* gene provides prognostic information in breast cancer patients, particularly in relation to adjuvant systemic therapy and radiotherapy. *Nat Med.* 1995; 1:1029–34.
14. Børrensen AL, Andersen TI, Eyfjörd JE, et al. *TP53* mutations and breast cancer prognosis: particularly poor survival rates for cases with mutations in the zinc-binding domains. *Genes Chrom Cancer.* 1995; 14:71–5.
15. Iacopetta B, Grieu F, Powell B, et al. Analysis of *p53* gene mutation by polymerase

chain reaction-single strand conformation polymorphism provides independent prognostic information in node-negative breast cancer. *Clin Cancer Res.* 1998; 4:1597–602.

16. Hartmann A, Blaszyk H, Kovach JS, et al. The molecular epidemiology of *p53* gene mutations in human breast cancer. *Trends Genet.* 1997; 13:27–33.

17. Falette N, Paperin MP, Treilleux I, et al. A. Prognostic value of *P53* gene mutations in a large series of node-negative breast cancer patients. *Cancer Res.* 1998; 58:1451–5.

18. Goh HS, Yao J, Smith DR. *p53* point mutation and survival in colorectal cancer patients. *Cancer Res.* 1995; 55:5217–21.

19. Sørensen BS, Kærn J, Holm R, et al. Therapy effect of either paclitaxel or cyclophosphamide combination treatment in patients with epithelial ovarian cancer and relation to *TP53* gene status. *Br J Cancer.* 1998; 78:375–1.

20. Auersperg N, Edelson MI, Mok SC, et al. The biology of ovarian cancer. *Semin Oncol.* 1998; 25:281–304.

21. Righetti S, Della Torre G, Pilotti S, et al. A comparative study of *p53* gene mutations, protein accumulation, and response to cisplatin-based chemotherapy in advanced ovarian carcinoma. *Cancer Res.* 1996; 56:689–93.

22. Wahl AF, Donaldson KL, Fairchild C, et al. Loss of normal *p53* function confers sensitization to taxol by increasing G2/M arrest and apoptosis. *Nat Med.* 1996; 2:72–9.

23. Lavarino C, Delia D, Di Palma S, et al. *p53* in drug resistance in ovarian cancer. *Lancet.* 1997; 349:1556.

24. Salgia R, Skarin AT. Molecular abnormalities in lung cancer. *J Clin Oncol.* 1998; 16:1207–17.

25. Siegfried JM, Gillespie AT, Mera R, et al. Prognostic value of specific K*RAS* mutations in lung adenocarcinoma. *Cancer Epidemiol Biom Prev.* 1997; 6:841–7.

26. Barbacid M. *Ras* genes. *Annu Rev Biochem.* 1987; 56:779–827.

27. Cho JY, Kim JH, Lee YH, et al. Correlation between K-*ras* gene mutation and prognosis of patients with nonsmall cell lung carcinoma. *Cancer.* 1997; 79:462–7.

28. Wilentz RE, Chung CH, Sturm PD, et al. K-*ras* mutations in the duodenal fluid of patients with pancreatic carcinoma. *Cancer.* 1998; 82:96–103.

29. Tada M, Omata M, Kawai S, et al. Detection of *ras* gene mutations in pancreatic juice and peripheral blood of patients with pancreatic adenocarcinoma. *Cancer Res.* 1993; 53:2472–74.

30. Kondo H, Sugano K, Fukayama N, et al. Detection of point mutations in the K-*ras* oncogene at codon 12 in pure pancreatic juice for diagnosis of pancreatic carcinoma. *Cancer.* 1994; 73:1589–94.

31. Kondo H, Sugano K, Fukayama N, et al. Detection of K-*ras* gene mutations at codon 12 in the pancreatic juice of patients with intraductal papillary mucinous tumors of the pancreas. *Cancer.* 1997; 79:900–5.

32. Howe JR, Conlon KC. The molecular genetics of pancreatic cancer. *Surg Oncol.* 1997; 6:1–18.

33. Sidransky D, Tokino T, Hamilton SR, et al. Identification of *ras* oncogene mutations in the stool of patients with curable colorectal tumors. *Science.* 1992; 256:102–5.

34. Tomlinson I, Ilyas M, Novelli M. Molecular genetics of colon cancer. *Cancer Metas Rev.* 1997; 16:67–79.

35. Mills NE, Fishman CL, Scholes J, Anderson SE, Rom WN, Jacobson DR. Detection of K-ras oncogene mutations in bronchoalveolar lavage fluid for lung cancer diagnosis. *J Natl Cancer Inst.* 1995; 87:1056–1060.

36. Cerottini JP, Caplin S, Saraga E, et al. The type of K-*ras* mutation determines prognosis in colorectal cancer. *Am J Surg.* 1998; 175:198–202.

37. Fukuyama Y, Mitsudomi T, Sugio K, et al. K-*ras* and *p53* mutations are an independent unfavourable prognostic indicator in patients with non-small-cell lung cancer. *Br J Cancer.* 1997; 75:1125–30.

38. Quénel N, Wafflart J, Bonichon F, et al. The prognostic value of c-*erbB2* in primary breast carcinomas: a study on 942 cases. *Breast Cancer Res Treat.* 1995; 35:283–329.

39. Press MF, Bernstein L, Thomas PA, et al. *HER-2/neu* gene amplification characterized by fluorescence in situ hybridization: poor prognosis in node-negative breast carcinomas. *J Clin Oncol.* 1997; 15:2894–904.

40. Anan K, Morisaki T, Katano M, et al. Assessment of c-*erbB2* and vascular endothelial growth factor mRNA expression in fine-needle aspirates from early breast carcinomas: pre-operative determination of malignant potential. *Eur J Surg Oncol.* 1998; 24:28–33.

41. Persons DL, Borelli KA, Hsu PH. Quantitation of *HER-2/neu* and c-*myc* gene amplification in breast carcinoma using fluorescence in situ hybridization. *Mod Pathol.* 1997; 10:720–7.

42. Andrulis IL, Bull SB, Blackstein ME, et al. *neu/erbB-2* amplification identifies a poor-prognosis group of women with node-negative breast cancer. *J Clin Oncol.* 1998; 16:1340–9.

43. Goldhirsh A, Wood WC, Senn HJ, et al. Meeting highlights: international consensus panel on the treatment of primary breast cancer. *J Natl Cancer Inst.* 1995; 87:1441–5.

44. Saffari B, Jones LA, El-Naggar A, et al. Amplification and overexpression of *HER-2/neu* (c-*erbB2*) in endometrial cancers: correlation with overall survival. *Cancer Res.* 1995; 55:5693–8.

45. Porter AC, Vaillancourt RR. Tyrosine kinase receptor-activated signal transduction pathways which lead to oncogenesis. *Oncogene.* 1998; 16:1343.

46. Pasini B, Ceccherini I, Romeo G. *RET* mutations in human disease. *Trends Genet.* 1996; 12:138–44.

47. Bugalho MJ, Frade JP, Santos JR, et al. Molecular analysis of the *RET* proto-oncogene in patients with sporadic medullary thyroid carcinoma: a novel point mutation in the extracellular cysteine-rich domain. *Eur J Endocrinol.* 1997; 136:423–6.

48. Uchino S, Noguchi S, Adachi M, et al. Novel point mutations and allele loss at the *RET* locus in sporadic medullary thyroid carcinomas. *Jpn J Cancer Res.* 1998; 89:411–8.

49. Delia D, Aiello A, Soligo D, et al. *bcl-2* proto-oncogene expression in normal and neplastic human myeloid cells. *Blood.* 1992; 79:1291–8.

50. Korsmeyer SJ. *Bcl-2* initiates a new category of oncogenes: regulators of cell death. *Blood.* 1992; 80:879–86.

51. Yang E, Korsmeyer ST. Molecular thanatopsis: a discourse on the *BCL2* family and cell death. *Blood.* 1996; 88:386–401.

52. Meijerink JPP. t(14;18), a journey to eternity. *Leukemia.* 1997; 11:2175–87.

53. Reed JC, Tanaka S. Somatic point mutations in the translocated *bcl-2* genes of non-Hodgkin's lymphomas and lymphocytic leukemias: implications for mechanisms of tumor progression. *Leuk Lymphoma.* 1993; 10:157–63.

54. Matolcsy A, Casali P, Warnke RA, et al. Morphologic transformation of follicular lymphoma is associated with somatic mutation of the translocated *Bcl-2* gene. *Blood.* 1996; 88:3937–44.

55. Monni O, Joensuu H, Franssila K, et al. *BCL2* overexpression associated with chromosomal amplification in diffuse large B cell lymphoma. *Blood.* 1997; 3:1168–74.

56. Aiello A, Delia D, Borrello MG, et al. Flow cytometric detection of the mitochondrial BCL-2 protein in normal and neoplastic human lymphoid cells. *Cytometry.* 1992; 13:502–9.

57. Ashton-Key M, Diss TC, Isaacson PG, Smith ME. A comparative study of the value of

immunohistochemistry and the polymerase chain reaction in the diagnosis of follicular lymphoma. *Histopathology.* 1995; 27:501–8.

58. Rao PH, Houldsworth J, Dyomina K, et al. Chromosomal and gene amplification in diffuse large B cell lymphoma. *Blood.* 1998; 92:234–40.

59. Gascoyne RD, Adomat SA, Krajewski S, et al. Prognostic significance of Bcl-2 protein expression and *Bcl-2* gene rearrangement in diffuse aggressive non-Hodgkin's lymphoma. *Blood.* 1997; 90:244–51.

60. Hill ME, Maclennan A, Cunningham DC, et al. Prognostic significance of *BCL-2* expression and *bcl-2* major breakpoint region rearrangement in diffuse large cell non-Hodgkin's lymphoma: a British National Lymphoma Investigation Study. *Blood.* 1996; 88:1046–51.

61. Piris MA, Pezzella F, Martinez-Montero JC, et al. *p53* and *bcl-2* expression in high-grade B-cell lymphomas: correlation with survival time. *Br J Cancer.* 1994; 69:337–41.

62. Campos L, Rouault JP, Sabido O, et al. High expression of bcl-2 protein in acute myeloid leukemia. *Blood.* 1993; 81:3091–7.

63. Maung ZT, MacLean FR, Reid MM, et al. The relationship between *bcl-2* expression and response to chemotherapy in acute leukaemia. *Br J Haematol.* 1994; 88:105–9.

64. Castle VP, Heidelberger KP, Bromberg J, et al. Expression of the apoptosis-suppressing protein Bcl-2 in neuroblastoma is associated with poor stage disease, unfavorable histology and N-*myc* amplification. *Am J Pathol.* 1993; 143:1543–50.

65. Pilotti S, Collini P, Del Bo R, et al. A novel panel of antibodies that segregates immunocyto-chemically poorly differentiated carcinoma from undifferentiated carcinoma of the thyroid gland. *Am J Surg Pathol.* 1994; 18:1054–64.

66. Pilotti S, Collini P, Rilke F, et al. Bcl-2 protein expression in carcinomas originating from the follicular epithelium of the thyroid gland. *J Pathol.* 1994; 172:337–42.

67. Pollina L, Pacini F, Fontanini G, et al. *bcl-2, p53* and proliferating cell nuclear antigen expression is related to the degree of differentiation in thyroid carcinomas. *Br J Cancer.* 1996; 73:139–43.

68. Kanthan R, Radhi JM. Immunohistochemical analysis of thyroid adenomas with Hurthle cells. *Pathology.* 1998; 30:4–6.

69. Viale G, Roncalli M, Grimelius L, et al. Prognostic value of bcl-2 immunoreactivity in medullary thyroid carcinoma. *Hum Pathol.* 1995; 26:945–50.

70. Pezzella F, Turley H, Kuzu I, et al. bcl-2 protein in non-small-cell lung carcinoma. *N Engl J Med.* 1993; 329:690–4.

71. Fleming MV, Guinee DG, Chu WS, et al. Bcl-2 immunohistochemistry in a surgical series of non-small cell lung cancer patients. *Hum Pathol.* 1998; 29:60–4.

72. Arnold A, Kim HG, Gaz RD, et al. Molecular cloning and chromosomal mapping of DNA rearranged with the parathyroid hormone gene in a parathyroid adenoma. *J Clin Invest.* 1989; 83:2034–40.

73. Komatsu H, Iida S, Yamamoto K, et al. A variant chromosome translocation at 11q13 identifying *PRAD1/cyclin D1* as the *BCL-1* gene. *Blood.* 1994; 84:1226–31.

74. Motokura T, Bloom T, Kim HG, et al. A novel cyclin encoded by a *bcl1*-linked candidate oncogene. *Nature.* 1991; 350:512–5.

75. Muller H, Lukas J, Schneider A, et al. *Cyclin D1* expression is regulated by the retinoblas-toma protein. *Proc Natl Acad Sci USA.* 1994; 91:2945–49.

76. Bartkova J, Lukas J, Strauss M, et al. Cell cycle-related variation and tissue restricted expression of human cyclin D1 protein. *J Pathol.* 1994; 172:237–45.

77. De Boer J, Van Krieken JH, Schuuring E, et al. *Bcl-1–cyclin D1* in malignant lymphoma. *Ann Oncol.* 1997; 8:S109–17.

78. Schuuring E. The involvement of the chromosome 11q13 region in human malignancies: *cyclin D1* and *EMS1* are two new candidates oncogenes. A review. *Gene.* 1995; 159:83–96.
79. Gramlich TL, Fritsch CR, Maurer D. et al. Differential polymerase chain reaction assay of *cyclin D1* gene amplification in esophageal carcinoma. *Diagn Mol Pathol.* 1994; 3:255–9.
80. Mathew S, Murty VV, Dalla-Favera R, et al. Chromosomal localization of genes encoding for transcription factors, c-*rel, NF-κ-Bp50, NF-κ-Bp65,* and *lyt*-10 by fluorescence in situ hybridization. *Oncogene.* 1993; 8:191–3.
81. Houldsworth J, Mathew S, Rao PH, et al. *REL* proto-oncogene is frequently amplified in extranodal diffuse large cell lymphoma. *Blood.* 1996; 87:25–9.
82. Brownell E, Mathieson B, Young HA, et al. Detection of c-*rel*-related transcripts in mouse hematopoietic tissues, fractionated lymphocyte populations, and cell lines. *Mol Cell Biol.* 1987; 7:1304–9.
83. Seth A, Gupta S, Davis RJ. Cell cycle regulation of the c-*Myc* transcriptional activation domain. *Mol Cell Biol.* 1993; 13:4125–36.
84. Gu W, Checova K, Tassi V, et al. Opposite regulation of gene transcription and cell proliferation by c-Myc and Max. *Proc Natl Acad Sci USA.* 1993; 90:2935–39.
85. Johnston JM, Carroll WL. c-*myc* hypermutation in Burkitt's lymphoma. *Leuk Lymphoma.* 1992; 8:431–9.
86. Ikegaki N, Katsumata M, Tsujimoto Y, et al. Relationship between *bcl-2* and *myc* gene expression in human neuroblastoma. *Cancer Lett.* 1995; 91:161–8.
87. Mejia MC, Navarro S, Pellin A, et al. Study of bcl-2 protein expression and the apoptosis phenomenon in neuroblastoma. *Anticancer Res.* 1998; 18:801–6.
88. Kerkaert JP, Deweindt C, Tilly H, et al. LAZ3, a novel zinc finger encoding gene, is disrupted by recurring chromosome 3q27 translocations in human lymphomas. *Nat Genet.* 1993; 5:66–70.
89. Chang CC, Ye BH, Chaganti RS, et al. BCL-6, a POZ/zinc-finger protein, is a sequence-specific transcriptional repressor. *Proc Natl Acad Sci USA.* 1996; 93:6947–52.
90. Cattoretti G, Chang CC, Cechova K, et al. BCL-6 protein is expressed in germinal-center B cells. *Blood.* 1995; 86:45–53.
91. Ye BH, Cattoretti G, Shen Q, et al. The *BCL-6* proto-oncogene controls germinal-center formation and Th2-type inflammation. *Nat Genet.* 1997; 16:161–70.
92. Migliazza A, Martinotti S, Chen W, et al. Frequent somatic hypermutations of the 5′ noncoding region of the *BCL6* gene in B-cell lymphoma. *Proc Natl Acad Sci USA.* 1995; 92:12520–4.
93. Shen HM, Peters A, Baron B, et al. Mutation of *BCL-6* gene in normal B cells by the process of somatic hypermutation of *Ig* genes. *Science.* 1998; 280:1750–2.
94. Pasqualucci L, Migliazza A, Fracchiolla N, et al. *BCL-6* mutations in normal germinal center B-cells: evidence of somatic hypermutation acting outside Ig loci. *Proc Natl Acad Sci USA.* 1998; 95:11816–21.
95. Peng HZ, Du MQ, Koulis A, et al. Non-immunoglobulin gene hypermutation in germinal center B cells. *Blood.* 1999; 93:2167–72.
96. Cesarman E, Chadburn A, Liu YF, et al. *BCL-6* gene mutations in posttransplantation lymphoproliferative disorders predict response to therapy and clinical outcome. *Blood.* 1998; 92:2294–302.
97. Liggett WH, Sidransky D. Role of *p16* tumor suppressor gene in cancer. *J Clin Oncol.* 1998; 16:1197–206.
98. Lee JY, Dong SM, Shin MS, et al. Genetic alterations of *p16INK4a* and *p53* genes in sporadic dysplastic nevus. *Biochem Biophys Res Commun.* 1997; 237:667–72.

99. Sirivatanauksorn V, Sirivatanauksorn Y, Lemoine NR. Molecular pattern of ductal pancreatic cancer. *Arch Surg.* 1998; 383:105–15.

100. Farrel WE, Clayton RN. Molecular biology of human pituitary adenomas. *Ann Med.* 1998; 30:192–8.

101. Drexler HG. Review of alterations of the cyclin-dependent kinase inhibitor INK4 family genes *p15, p16, p18,* and *p19* in human leukemia-lymphoma cells. *Leukemia.* 1998; 12:845–59.

102. Elenitoba-Johnson KE, Gascoyne RD, Lim MS, et al. Homozygous deletions at chromosome 9p21 involving *p16* and *p15* are associated with histologic progression in follicle center lymphoma. *Blood.* 1998; 12:4677–85.

103. Villuendas R, Sanchez-Beato M, Martinez JC, et al. Loss of p16/INK4A protein expression in non-Hodgkin's lymphomas is a frequent finding associated with tumor progression. *Am J Pathol.* 1998; 153:887–97.

104. Levinson G, Gutman GA. Slipped-strand mispairing: a major mechanism for DNA sequence evolution. *Mol Biol Evol.* 1987; 4:203–21.

105. Csink AK, Henikoff S. Something from nothing: the evolution and utility of satellite repeats. *Trends Genet.* 1998; 14:200–4.

106. Levin B. *Genes VI.* Oxford University Press, 1997.

107. Croce CM. Genetic approaches to the study of the molecular basis of human cancer. *Cancer Res.* 1991; 51:5015–8.

108. Knudson AG. Mutation and cancer. Statistical study of retinoblastoma. *Proc Natl Acad Sci USA.* 1971; 68:820–3.

109. Weber JL, May PE. Abundant class of human DNA polymorphisms which can be typed using polymerase chain reaction. *Am J Hum Genet.* 1989; 44:338–96.

110. Arzimanoglou II, Gilbert F, Barger HR. Microsatellite instability in human solid tumors. *Cancer.* 1998; 82:1808–20.

111. Hayden JD, Martin IG, Cawkwell L, et al. The role of microsatellite instability in gastric carcinoma. *Gut.* 1998; 42:300–3.

112. Wu MS, Lee CW, Shun CT, et al. Clinicopathological significance of altered loci of replication error and microsatellite instability-associated mutations in gastric cancers. *Cancer Res.* 1998; 58:1494–7.

113. Keller G, Rudelius M, Vogelsang H, et al. Microsatellite instability and loss of heterozygosity in gastric carcinoma in comparison to family history. *Am J Pathol.* 1998; 152:1281–9.

114. Mao L, Schoenberg MP, Scicchitano M, et al. Molecular detection of primary bladder cancer by microsatellite analysis. *Science.* 1996; 271:659–62.

115. Steiner G, Schoenberg MP, Linn JF, et al. Detection of bladder cancer recurrence by microsatellite analysis of urine. *Nat Med.* 1997; 3:621–4.

116. Habuchi T, Devlin J, Elder PA, et al. Detailed deletion mapping of chromosome 9q in bladder cancer: evidence of two tumor suppressor loci. *Oncogene.* 1995; 11:1671–4.

117. Cappellen D, Gil Diez de Medina S, Chopin D, et al. Frequent loss of heterozygosity on chromosome 10q in muscle-invasive transitional cell carcinomas of the bladder. *Oncogene.* 1997; 14:3059–66.

118. Kagan J, Liu J, Stein JD, et al. Cluster of allele losses within a 2.5 cM region of chromosome 10 in high-grade invasive bladder cancer. *Oncogene.* 1998; 16:909–13.

119. Takle LA, Knowles MA. Deletion mapping implicates two tumor suppressor genes on chromosome 8p in the development of bladder cancer. *Oncogene.* 1996; 12:1083–7.

120. Eydmann ME, Knowles MA. Mutation analysis of 8p genes *POLB* and *PPP2CB* in bladder cancer. *Cancer Genet Cytogenet.* 1997; 93:167–71.

121. Bohm M, Kirch H, Otto T, et al. Deletion analysis at the DEL-27, APC and MTS1 loci in bladder cancer: LOH at the DEL-27 locus on 5p13–12 is a prognostic marker of tumor progression. *Int J Cancer.* 1997; 74:291–5.

122. Miyamoto H, Shuin T, Ikeda I, et al. Loss of heterozygosity at the p53, RB, DCC and APC tumor suppressor gene loci in human bladder cancer. *J Urol.* 1996; 155:1444–7.

123. Ozer H. Bladder cancer. *Curr Opin Oncol.* 1998; 10:273–8.

124. Waber P, Dlugosz S, Cheng QC, et al. Genetic alterations of chromosome band 9p21–22 in head and neck cancer are not restricted to *p16INK4a. Oncogene.* 1997; 15:1699–704.

125. Mao L, Lee JS, Fan YH, et al. Frequent microsatellite alterations at chromosomes 9p21 and 3p14 in oral premalignant lesions and their value in cancer risk assessment. *Nat Med.* 1996; 2:682–5.

126. Papadimitrakopoulou VA, Oh Y, El-Naggar A, Izzo J, Clayman G, Mao L. Presence of multiple incontiguous deleted regions at the long arm of chromosome 18 in head and neck cancer. *Clin Cancer Res.* 1998; 4:539–44.

127. Frank CJ, McClatchey KD, Devaney KO, et al. Evidence that loss of 18q is associated with tumor progression. *Cancer Res.* 1997; 57:824–7.

128. Gleich LL, Li YQ, Biddinger PW, et al. The loss of heterozygosity in retinoblastoma and *p53* suppressor genes as a prognostic indicator for head and neck cancer. *Laryngoscope.* 1996; 106:1378–81.

129. El-Naggar AK, Hurr K, Batsakis JG, et al. Sequential loss of heterozygosity at microsatellite motifs in preinvasive and invasive head and neck squamous carcinoma. *Cancer Res.* 1995; 55:2656–9.

130. Erber R, Conradt C, Homann N, et al. *TP53* DNA contact mutations are selectively associated with allelic loss and have a strong clinical impact in head and neck cancer. *Oncogene.* 1998; 16:1671–9.

131. Suzuki H, Komiya A, Emi M, et al. Three distinct commonly deleted regions of chromosome arm 16q in human primary and metastatic prostate cancers. *Genes Chrom Cancer.* 1996; 17:225–33.

132. Wernert N, Bieroff E, Hugel A. Pathological aspects of prostate cancer and benign nodular hyperplasia. *Anticancer Res.* 1997; 17:2907–10.

133. Wang SI, Parsons R, Ittman M. Homozygous deletion of the *PTEN* tumor suppressor gene in a subset of prostate adenocarcinomas. *Clin Cancer Res.* 1998; 4:811–5.

134. Crundwell MC, Chughatai S, Knowles M, et al. Allelic loss on chromosomes 8p, 22q and 18q (DCC) in human prostate cancer. *Int J Cancer.* 1996; 69:295–300.

135. Ueda T, Komiya A, Emi M, et al. Allelic losses on 18q21 are associated with progression and metastasis in human prostate cancer. *Genes Chrom Cancer.* 1997; 20:140–7.

136. Latil A, Cussenot O, Fournier G, et al. Loss of heterozygosity at chromosome 16q in prostate adenocarcinoma: identification of three independent regions. *Cancer Res.* 1997; 57:1058–62.

137. Elo JP, Harkonen P, Kyllonen AP, et al. Loss of heterozygosity at 16q24.1–q24.2 is significantly associated with metastatic and aggressive behaviour of prostate cancer. *Cancer Res.* 1997; 57:3356–9.

138. Kawana Y, Komiya A, Ueda T, et al. Location of *KAI1* on the short arm of human chromosome 11 and frequency of allelic loss in advanced human prostate cancer. *Prostate* 1997; 32:205–13.

139. Bugert P, Kovacs G. Molecular differential diagnosis of renal cell carcinomas by microsatellite analysis. *Am J Pathol.* 1996; 149:2081–8.

140. Herbers J, Schullerus D, Muller H, Kenck C, Chudek J, Weimer J, Bugert P, Kovacs G.

Significance of chromosome arm 14q loss in nonpapillary renal cell carcinomas. *Genes Chrom Cancer.* 1997; 19:29–35.

141. Rodhenius S, Slebos RJ. Clinical significance of *ras* oncogene activation in human lung cancer. *Cancer Res.* 1992; 52:2665–9.

142. Takahashi T, Nau M, Chiba I, et al. *p53:* a frequent target for genetic abnormalities in lung cancer. *Science.* 1989; 246:491–4.

143. Hayashi N, Sugimoto Y, Tsuchiya E, et al. Somatic mutation of the *MTS* (multiple tumor suppressor) *1/CDK41* (cyclin-dependent kinase 4 inhibitor) gene in human primary non-small cell lung carcinoma. *Biochem Biophys Res Commun.* 1994; 15:1426–30.

144. Sozzi G, Veronese ML, Negrini M, et al. The *FHIT* gene at 3p14.2 is abnormal in lung cancer. *Cell.* 1996; 85:7–26.

145. Shiseki M, Kohno T, Adachi J, et al. Comparative allelotype of early and advanced stage non-small cell lung carcinomas. *Gene Chrom Cancer.* 1996; 17:71–7.

146. Hung J, Kishimoto Y, Sugio K, et al. Allele-specific chromosome 3p deletions occur at an early stage in the pathogenesis of lung carcinoma. *JAMA.* 1995; 273:558–63.

147. Rosell R, Pifarre A, Monzo M, et al. Reduced survival in patients with stage-I non-small cell lung cancer associated with DNA-replication errors. *Int J Cancer.* 1997; 74:330–4.

148. Pifarre A, Rossel R, Monzo M, et al. Prognostic value of replication errors on chromosomes 2p and 3p in non-small-cell lung cancer. *Br J Cancer.* 1997; 75:184–9.

149. Suzuki K, Ogura T, Yokose T, et al. Microsatellite instability in female non-small-cell lung cancer patients with familial clustering of malignancy. *Br J Cancer.* 1998; 77:1003–8.

150. Otsuka T, Kohno T, Mori M, et al. Deletion mapping of chromosome 2 in human lung carcinoma. *Genes Chrom Cancer.* 1996; 16:113–9.

151. Sato M, Mori Y, Sakurada A, et al. Identification of a 910-Kb region of common allelic loss in chromosome bands 16q24.1–q24.2 in human lung cancer. *Genes Chrom Cancer.* 1998; 22:1–8.

152. Petersen S, Wolf G, Bockmuhl U, et al. Allelic loss on chromosome 10q in human lung cancer: association with tumour progression and metastatic phenotype. *Br J Cancer.* 1998; 77:270–6.

153. Kishimoto Y, Sugio K, Hung JY, et al. Allele-specific loss in chromosome 9p loci in preneoplastic lesions accompanying non-small-cell lung cancers. *J Natl Cancer Inst.* 1995; 86:1224–9.

154. Okami K, Cairns P, Westra WH, et al. Detailed deletion mapping at chromosome 9p21 in non-small cell lung cancer by microsatellite analysis and fluorescence in situ hybridization. *Int J Cancer.* 1997; 74:588–92.

155. O'Briant KC, Bepler G. Delineation of the centromeric and telomeric chromosome segment 11p15.5 lung cancer suppressor regions LOH11A and LOH11B. *Genes Chrom Cancer.* 1997; 18:111–4.

156. Fong KM, Kida Y, Zimmerman PV, et al. MYCL genotypes and loss of heterozygosity in non-small cell lung cancer. *Br J Cancer.* 1996; 74:1975–8.

157. Sozzi G, Sard L, De Gregorio L, et al. Association between cigarette smoking and *FHIT* gene alterations in lung cancer. *Cancer Res.* 1997; 57:2121–23.

158. Tomlinson I, Ilyas M, Johnson V, et al. A comparison of the genetic pathways involved in the pathogenesis of three types of colorectal cancer. *J Pathol.* 1998; 184:148–52.

159. Poetsch M, Weber-Matthiesen K, Plendl HJ, et al. Detection of the t(14;18) chromosomal translocation by interphase cytogenetics with yeast-artificial-chromosome probes in follicular lymphoma and nonneoplastic lymphoproliferations. *J Clin Oncol.* 1996; 14:963–9.

160. Aiello A, Delia D, Giardini R, et al. PCR analysis of *IgH* and *BCL2* gene rearrangement in the diagnosis of follicular lymphoma in lymph node fine-needle aspiration. *Diagn Mol Pathol.* 1997; 6:154–60.

161. Limpens J, de Jong D, van Krieken JH, et al. *Bcl-2/JH* rearrangements in benign lymphoid tissues with follicular hyperplasia. *Oncogene.* 1991; 6:2271–6.

162. Limpens J, Stad R, Vos C, et al. Lymphoma-associated translocation t(14;18) in blood B cells of normal individuals. *Blood.* 1995; 85:2528–36.

163. Koduru PRK, Offit K, Filippa DA. Molecular analysis of breaks in *BCL-1* proto-oncogene in B-cell lymphomas with abnormalities of 11q13. *Oncogene.* 1989; 4:929–34.

164. Ott MM, Helbing A, Ott G, et al. *bcl-1* rearrangement and cyclin D1 protein expression in mantle cell lymphoma. *J Pathol.* 1996; 179:238–42.

165. Molot RJ, Meeker TC, Wittwer CT, et al. Antigen expression and polymerase chain reaction amplification of mantle cell lymphomas. *Blood.* 1994; 83:1626–31.

166. Pott C, Tiemann M, Linke B, et al. Structure of *Bcl-1* and *IgH-CDR3* rearrangements as clonal markers in mantle cell lymphomas. *Leukemia.* 1998; 12:1630–7.

167. Vaandrager JW, Zwikstra E, De Boer CJ, et al. Direct visualization of dispersed 11q13 chromosomal translocation in mantle cell lymphoma by multi-color DNA fiber FISH. *Blood.* 1996; 88:1177–82.

168. Bosch F, Jarers P, Campo E, et al. *PRAD1/cyclin D1* gene overexpression in chronic lymphoproliferative disorders: a highly specific marker of mantle cell lymphoma. *Blood.* 1994; 84:2726–32.

169. Ott MM, Bartkova J, Bartek J, Durr A, Fischer L, Ott G, Muller-Hermelink HK, Kreipe H. Cyclin D1 expression in mantle cell lymphoma is accompanied by downregulation of cyclin D3 and is not related to the proliferative activity. *Blood.* 1997; 90:3154–9.

170. Raffeld M, Jaffe ES. BCL-1, t(11;14) and mantle cell-derived lymphomas. *Blood.* 1991; 78:259–63.

171. Shivdasani RA, Hess JL, Skarin AT, et al. Intermediate lymphocytic lymphoma: clinical and pathological features of a recently characterized subtype of non-Hodgkin's lymphoma. *J Clin Oncol.* 1993; 11:802–11.

172. Ambinder RF, Griffin CA. Biology of the lymphoma: cytogenetics, molecular biology, and virology. *Curr Opin Oncol.* 1991; 3:806–12.

173. Takimoto Y, Takafuta T, Imanaka F, et al. Histological progression of follicular lymphoma associated with *p53* mutation and rearrangement of the *C-MYC* gene. *Hiroshima J Med Sci.* 1996; 85:902–7.

174. Suzuki K, Miki T, Kawamata, et al. Variant translocation of the *BCL6* gene to immunoglobulin kappa light chain gene in B-cell lymphoma. *Jpn J Cancer Res.* 1994; 85:911–7.

175. Akasaka T, Miura I, Takahashi N, et al. A recurring translocation, t(3;6) (q27;p21), in non-Hodgkin's lymphoma results in replacement of the 5′ regulatory region of *BCL6* with a novel *H4* histone gene. *Cancer Res.* 1997; 57:7–12.

176. Galieguezouitina S, Quief S, Hildebrand MP, et al. The B-cell transcriptional coactivator *BOB1/OBF1* gene fuses to the *LAZ3/BCL6* gene by t(3-11) (q27 q23.1) chromosomal translocation in a B-cell leukemia line (Karpas-231). *Leukemia.* 1996; 10:579–87.

177. Yuille MAR, Galieguezouitina S, Hiorns LR, et al. Heterogeneity of breakpoints at the transcriptional coactivator gene, *BOB-1,* in lymphoproliferative disease. *Leukemia.* 1996; 10:1492–96.

178. Dallery E, Galieguezouitina S, Collyndhooghe M, et al. *TTF,* a gene encoding a novel small G-protein, fuses to the lymphoma-associated *LAZ3* gene by t(3;4) chromosomal translocation. *Oncogene.* 1995; 10:2171–8.

179. Wlodarska I, Mecucci C, Stul M, et al. FISH identifies new chromosomal changes involving 3q27 in non-Hodgkin's lymphomas with *BCL6/LAZ3* rearrangement. *Genes Chrom Cancer.* 1995; 14:1–7

180. Bastard C, Tilly H, Lenormand B, et al. Translocations involving band 3q27 and Ig gene regions in non-Hodgkin's lymphoma. *Blood.* 1992; 79:2527–31.

181. Offit K, Lo Coco F, Luoie D, et al. Rearrangement of the *bcl-6* gene as a prognostic marker in diffuse large cell lymphoma. *N Engl J Med.* 1994; 331:74–80.

182. Bastard C, Deweindt C, Kerkaert JP, et al. LAZ3 rearrangements in non-Hodgkin's lymphoma: correlation with histology, immunophenotype, karyotype, and clinical outcome in 217 patients. *Blood.* 1994; 83:2423–27.

183. Shivdasani RA, Mayer EL, Orkin SH. Absence of blood formation in mice lacking the T-cell leukemia oncoprotein tal-1/SCL. *Nature.* 1995; 373:432–4.

184. Hall W, Hall E. The *SCL/TAL1* gene: roles in normal and malignant hematopoiesis. *Bioessays.* 1997; 19:607–13.

185. Bernard M, Delabesse E, Novault S, et al. Antiapoptotic effect of ectopic *TAL1/SCL* expression in a human leukemic T-cell line. *Cancer Res.* 1998; 58:2680–7.

186. Aplan PD, Lombardi DP, Reaman GH, et al. Involvement of the putative hematopoietic transcription factor SCL in T-cell acute lymphoblastic leukemia. *Blood.* 1992; 79: 1327–33.

187. Delabesse E, Bernard M, Landman-Parker J, et al. Simultaneous SIL-TAL1 RT-PCR detection of all tal(d) deletions and identification of novel tal(d) variants. *Br J Haematol.* 1997; 99:901–7.

188. Xia Y, Brown L, Tsan JT, et al. The translocation (1;14)(p34;q11) in human T-cell leukemia: chromosome breakage 25 kilobase pairs downstream of the *TAL1* protooncogene. *Genes Chrom Cancer.* 1992; 4:211–16.

189. Kikuchi A, Kobayashi S, Hanada R, et al. *TAL1* gene analysis in T-cell malignancies. *Jpn J Clin Hematol.* 1998; 39:259–66.

190. Morris SW, Kirstein MN, Valentine MB, et al. Fusion of a kinase gene, *ALK,* to a nucleolar protein gene, *NPM,* in non-Hodgkin's lymphoma. *Science.* 1994; 263:1281–84.

191. Bischof D, Pulford K, Mason DY, et al. Role of nucleophosmin (NPM) portion of the non-Hodgkin's lymphoma-associated NPM-anaplastic kinase fusion protein in oncogenesis. *Mol Cell Biol.* 1997; 17:2312–35.

192. Falini B, Bigerna B, Fizzotti M, et al. ALK expression defines a distinct group of T/null lymphomas ("ALK lymphomas") with a wide morphological spectrum. *Am J Pathol.* 1998; 153:875–86.

193. Stam K, Heisterkamp N, Reynolds FH, et al. Evidence that the *phl* gene encodes a 160,000-dalton phosphoprotein with associated kinase activity. *Mol Cell Biol.* 1987; 7:1955–60.

194. Maru Y, Witte ON. The *BCR* gene encodes a novel serine/threonine kinase activity within a single exon. *Cell.* 1991; 67:459–68.

195. Welch PJ, Wang JYJ. A C-terminal protein-binding domain in the retinoblastoma protein regulates nuclear c-*abl* tyrosine kinase in the cell cycle. *Cell.* 1993; 75:779–90.

196. Shore SK, Bogart SL, Reddy EP. Activation of murine c-*abl* protooncogene: effect of a point mutation on oncogenic activation. *Proc Natl Acad Sci USA.* 1990; 87:6502–6.

197. Bernards A, Rubin CM, Westbrook CA, et al. The first intron in the human c-*abl* gene is at least 200 kb long and is a target for translocations in chronic myelogenous leukemia. *Mol Cell Biol.* 1987; 7:3231–36.

198. Prakash O, Yunis JJ. High resolution chromosomes of the t(9;22) positive leukemias. *Cancer Genet Cytogenet.* 1984; 11:361–7.

199. Fainstein E, Marcelle C, Rosner A, et al. A new fused transcript in Philadelphia chromosome positive acute lymphocytic leukemia. *Nature.* 1987; 330:386–8.

200. Mills KI, Hynds SA, Burnett AK, et al. Further evidence that the site of the breakpoint in the major breakpoint cluster region (M-bcr) may be a prognostic indicator. *Leukemia.* 1989; 3:837–40.

201. Mills KI, MacKenzie ED, Birnie GD. The site of the breakpoint within the bcr is a prognostic factor in Philadelphia-positive CML patients. *Blood.* 1988; 72:1237–41.

202. Gaiger A, Henn T, Horth E, et al. Increase of BCR–ABL chimeric mRNA expression in tumor cells of patients with chronic myeloid leukemia precedes disease progression. *Blood.* 1995; 86:2371–8.

203. Lin F, van Rhee F, Goldman JN, et al. Kinetics of increasing *BCR–ABL* transcript numbers in chronic myeloid leukemia patients who relapse after bone marrow transplantation. *Blood.* 1996; 87:4473–8.

204. Hermans A, Heisterkamp N, von Lindern M, et al. Unique fusion of *bcr* and c-*abl* genes in Philadelphia chromosome positive acute lymphoblastic leukemia. *Cell.* 1987; 51:33–40.

205. Chang KS, Fan YH, Andreeff M, et al. The *PML* gene encodes a phosphoprotein associated with the nuclear matrix. *Blood.* 1995; 85:3646–53.

206. Wang Z, Delva L, Gaboli M, et al. Role of *PML* in cell growth and the retinoic acid pathway. *Science.* 1998; 279:1547–51.

207. Petkovich M, Brand NJ, Krust A, et al. A human retinoic acid receptor which belongs to the family of nuclear receptors. *Nature.* 1987; 330:444–50.

208. de The H, Chomienne C, Lanotte M, et al. The t(15;17) translocation of acute promyelocytic leukemia fuses the retinoic acid receptor alpha gene to a novel transcribed locus. *Nature.* 1990; 347:558–61.

209. Goddard AD, Borrow J, Freemont PS, et al. Characterization of a zinc finger gene disrupted by the t(15;17) in acute promyelocytic leukemia. *Science.* 1991; 254:1371–4.

210. Brown D, Kogan S, Lagasse E, et al. A *PMLRAR-alpha* transgene initiates murine acute promyelocytic leukemia. *Proc Natl Acad Sci USA.* 1997; 94:2551–56.

211. Frassoni F, Martinelli G, Saglio G, et al. *BCR/ABL* chimeric transcript in patients in remission after marrow transplantation for chronic myeloid leukemia: higher frequency of detection and slower clearance in patients grafted in advanced disease as compared to patients grafted in chronic phase. *Bone Marrow Transplant.* 1995; 16:595–601.

212. Erickson, P, Gao J, Chang KS, et al. Identification of breakpoints in t(8;21) acute myelogenous leukemia and isolation of a fusion transcript, *AML1/ETO,* with similarity to *Drosophila* segmentation gene, runt. *Blood.* 1992; 80:1825–31.

213. Okuda T, van Deursen J, Hiebert SW, et al. *AML1,* the target of multiple chromosomal translocations in human leukemia, is essential for normal fetal liver hematopoiesis. *Cell.* 1996; 84:321–30.

214. Wolford JK, Prochazka M. Structure and expression of the human *MTG8/ETO* gene. *Gene.* 1998; 212:103–9.

215. Le XF, Claxton D, Kornblau S, et al. Characterization of the ETO and AML1/ETO proteins involved in 8;21 translocation in acute myelogenous leukaemia. *Eur J Haematol.* 1998; 60:217–25.

216. Erickson P, Dessev G, Lasher RS, et al. ETO and AML1 phosphoproteins are expressed in CD34+ hematopoietic progenitors: implication for t(8;21) leukemogenesis and monitoring residual disease. *Blood.* 1996; 88:1813–23.

217. Meyers S, Lenny N, Hiebert SW. The t(8;21) fusion protein interferes with AML1b-dependent transcriptional activation. *Mol Cell Biol.* 1995; 15:1974–82.

218. Andrieu V, Radford Weiss I, Toussard X, et al. Molecular detection of t(8;21) *AML–ETO* in M1/M2: correlation with cytogenetics, morphology and immunophenotype. *Br J Haematol.* 1996; 92:855–65.

219. Nucifora G, Rowley J. *AML1* and 8;21 and 3;21 translocations in acute and chronic myeloid leukemia. *Blood.* 1996; 86:1–14.

220. Chang KS, Fan YH, Stass SA, et al. Expression of *AML1–ETO* transcripts and detection of minimal residual disease in t(8;21)-positive acute myeloid leukemia. *Oncogene.* 1993; 8:983–8.

221. Guerrasio A, Rosso C, Martinelli G, et al. Polyclonal hematopoiesis associated with long-term persistence of the *AML–ETO* transcript in patients with FAB M2 acute myeloid leukemia in continuous clinical remission. *Br J Haematol.* 1995; 90:364–8.

222. Rabbits TH. Chromosomal translocations in human cancer. *Nature.* 1994; 372:143–9.

223. Iida S, Rao P, Nallasivam P, et al. The t(9;14)(p13;q32) chromosomal translocation associated with lymphoplasmacytoid lymphoma involves the *PAX-5* gene. *Blood.* 1996; 88:4110–7.

224. Rubnitz JE, Look AT. Molecular basis of leukemogenesis. *Curr Opin Hematol.* 1998; 5:264–70.

225. Söensen PHB, Lessnick SL, Lopez-Terrada, D, et al. A second Ewing's sarcoma transloca-tion, t(21;22), fuses the *EWS* gene to another ETS-family transcription factor, ERG. *Nat Genet.* 1994; 6:146–51.

226. May WA, Gishizky ML, Lessinck SL, et al. Ewing sarcoma 11;22 translocation produces a chimeric transcription factor that requires the DNA-binding domain encoded by *FLI1* for transformation. *Proc Natl Acad Sci USA.* 1993; 90:5752–56.

227. de Valva E, Kawai A, Healey JH, et al. *EWS–FLI1* fusion transcript structure is an independent determinant of prognosis in Ewing's sarcoma. *J Clin Oncol.* 1998; 16:1248–55.

228. Dockhorn-Dworniczak B, Schafer KL, Dantcheva R, et al. Diagnostic value of the molecu-lar genetic detection of the t(11;22) translocation in Ewing's tumours. *Virchows Arch.* 1994; 425:107–12.

229. West DC, Grier HE, Michelle MS, et al. Detection of circulating tumor cells in patients with Ewing's sarcoma and peripheral primitive neuroectodermal tumor. *J Clin Oncol.* 1997; 15:583–8.

230. Squire J, Zielenska M, Thorner P, et al. Variant translocations of chromosome 22 in Ewing's sarcoma. *Genes Chrom Cancer.* 1993; 8:190–4.

231. Jeon IS, Davis JN, Braun BS, et al. A variant Ewing's sarcoma translocation (7;22) fuses the *EWS* gene to the *ETS* gene *ETV1. Oncogene.* 1995; 10:1229–34.

232. Peter M, Couturier J, Pacquement H, et al. A new member of the *ETS* family fused to *EWS* in Ewing tumor. *Oncogene.* 1997; 14:1159–64.

233. Kaneko Y, Yoshida K, Handa M, et al. Fusion of an *ETS*-family gene, *E1AF,* to *EWS* by t(17;22)(q12;q12) chromosomal translocation in an undifferentiated sarcoma of infancy. *Genes Chrom Cancer.* 1996; 15:115–21.

234. Zucman J, Delattre O, Desmaze C. *EWS* and *ATF-1* gene fusion induced by t(12;22) translocation in malignant melanoma of soft parts. *Nat Genet.* 1993; 4:341–5.

235. Call KM, Glaser T, Ito CY, et al. Isolation and characterization of a zinc finger polypeptide gene at the human chromosome 11 Wilms' tumor locus. *Cell.* 1990; 60:509–20.

236. Haber DA, Housman DE. Role of the *WT1* gene in Wilms' tumor. *Cancer Surv.* 1992; 12:105–17.

237. Gerald WL, Rosai J, Ladanyi M. Characterization of the genomic breakpoint and chimeric

transcripts in the *EWS–WT1* gene fusion of desmoplastic small round cell tumor. *Proc Natl Acad Sci USA.* 1995; 92:1028–32.

238. Brody RI, Ueda T, Hamelin A, et al. Molecular analysis of the fusion of *EWS* to an orphan nuclear receptor gene in extraskeletal myxoid chondrosarcoma. *Am J Pathol.* 1997; 150:1049–58.

239. Clark J, Benjamin H, Gill S. et al. Fusion of the *EWS* gene to CHN, a member of the steroid/thyroid receptor gene superfamily, in a human myxoid chondrosarcoma. *Oncogene.* 1996; 12:229–35.

240. Dal Cin P, Sciot R, Panagopoulos I, et al. Additional evidence of a variant translocation t(12;22) with *EWS/CHOP* fusion in myxoid liposarcoma: clinicopathological features. *J Pathol.* 1997; 182:437–41.

241. Panagopoulos I, Aman P, Mertens F, et al. Genomic PCR detects tumor cells in peripheral blood from patients with myxoid liposarcoma. *Genes Chrom Cancer.* 1996; 17:102–7.

242. Panagopoulos I, Lassen C, Isakkson M, et al. Characteristic sequence motifs at the breakpoints of the hybrid genes *FUS/CHOP, EWS/CHOP* and *FUS/ERG* in myxoid liposarcoma and acute myeloid leukemia. *Oncogene.* 1997; 15:1357–62.

243. Sanchez-Garcia I, Rabbitts TH. Transcriptional activation by TAL1 and FUS-CHOP proteins expressed in acute malignancies as a result of chromosomal abnormalities. *Proc Natl acad Sci USA.* 1994; 91:7869–73.

244. Weber-Hall S, McManus A, Anderson J, et al. Novel formation and amplification of the PAX7-FKHR fusion gene in a case of alveolar rhabdomyosarcoma. *Genes Chrom. Cancer.* 1996; 17:7–13.

245. Brett D, Whitehouse S, Antonson P, et al. The SYT protein involved in the t(X;18) synovial sarcoma translocation is a transcriptional activator localised in nuclear bodies. *Hum Mol Genet.* 1997; 6:1559–64.

246. Kawai A, Woodruff J, Healey JH, et al. *SYT–SSX* gene fusion as a determinant of morphology and prognosis in synovial sarcoma. *N Engl J Med.* 1998; 338:153–60.

247. Minoletti F, Miozzo M, Pedeutour F, et al. Involvement of chromosomes 17 and 22 in dermatofibrosarcoma protuberans. *Genes Chrom Cancer.* 1995; 13:62–5.

248. Pedeutour F, Simon MP, Minoletti F, et al. Translocation, t(17;22) (q22;q13), in dermatofibrosarcoma protuberans: a new tumor-associated chromosome rearrangement. *Cytogen Cell Genet.* 1996; 72:171–4.

249. Simon MP, Pedeutour F, Sirvent N, et al. Deregulation of the platelet-derived growth factor B-chain gene via fusion with collagen gene *COL1A1* in dermatofibrosarcoma protuberans and giant-cell fibrosarcoma. *Nat Genet.* 1997; 15:95–8.

250. Greco A, Fusetti L, Villa R, et al. Transforming activity of the chimeric sequence formed by the fusion of collagen gene *COL1A1* and the platelet derived growth factor b-chain gene in dermatofibrosarcoma protuberans. *Oncogene.* 1998; 17:1313–9.

251. Pierotti MA, Bongarzone I, Borrello MG, et al. Cytogenetics and molecular genetics of carcinomas arising from thyroid epithelial follicular cells. *Gene Chrom Cancer.* 1996; 16:1–14.

252. Grieco M, Santoro M, Berlingieri MT, Melillo RM, Donghi R, Bongarzone I, Pierotti MA, Della Porta G, Fusco A, Vecchio G. PTC is a novel rearranged form of the ret proto-oncogene and is frequently detected in vivo in human thyroid papillary carcinomas. *Cell.* 1990; 60:557–563.

253. Bongarzone I, Monzini N, Borrello MG, et al. Molecular characterization of a tumor-specific transforming sequence formed by fusion of *ret* tyrosine kinase and the regulatory subunit RI of cyclic AMP-dependent protein kinase A. *Mol Cell Biol.* 1993; 13:358–66.

254. Sozzi G, Bongarzone I, Miozzo M, et al. A t(10;17) translocation creates the *RET/ptc2* chimeric transforming sequence in papillary thyroid carcinoma. *Genes Chrom Cancer.* 1994; 9:244–50.

255. Minoletti M, Butti MG, Coronelli S, et al. The two genes generating *RET/PTC3* are localized in chromosomal band 10q11.2. *Genes Chrom Cancer.* 1994; 11:51–7.

256. Bongarzone I, Butti MG, Coronelli S, Borrello MG, Santoro M, Mondellini P, Pilotti S, Fusco A, Della Porta G, Pierotti MA. Frequent activation of ret protooncogene by fusion with a new activating gene in papillary thyroid carcinomas. *Cancer Res.* 1994; 54:2979–85.

257. Santoro M, Dathan NA, Berlingieri MT, Bongarzone I, Paulin C, Grieco M, Pierotti MA, Vecchio G, Fusco A. Molecular characterization of RET/PTC3; a novel rearranged version of the RETproto-oncogene in a human thyroid papillary carcinoma. *Oncogene.* 1994; 9:509–16.

258. Weier HUG, Rhein A P, Shadravan F, Collins C, Polikoff D. Rapid physical mapping of the human trk protooncogene (NTRK1) to human chromosome 1q21–22 by P1 clone selection, fluorescence *in situ* hybridization (FISH), and computer-assisted microscopy. *Genomics.* 1995; 26:390–393.

259. Martin-Zanca D, Hughes SH, Baracid M. A human oncogene formed by the fusion of truncated tropomyosin and protein tyrosine kinase sequences. *Nature* 1994; 319:748.

260. Miranda C, Minoletti M, Greco A, et al. Refined localization of the human *TPR* gene to chromosome 1q25 by in situ hybridization. *Genomics.* 1994; 23:714–5.

261. Greco A, Mariani C, Miranda C, et al. Characterization of the *NTRK1* genomic region involved in chromosomal rearrangements generating *TRK* oncogenes. *Genomics.* 1993; 18:397–400.

262. Fugazzola L, Pilotti S, Pinchera A, et al. Oncogenic rearrangements of the *RET* proto-oncogene in papillary thyroid carcinomas from children exposed to Chernobyl nuclear accident. *Cancer Res.* 1995; 55:5617–20.

263. Klugbauer S, Lengfelder E, Demidchik EP, et al. High prevalence of RET rearrangement in thyroid tumors of children from Belarus after the Chernobyl reactor accident. *Oncogene.* 1995; 11:2459–67.

264. Bongarzone I, Fugazzola L, Vigneri P, et al. Age-related activation of the tyrosine kinase receptor protooncogenes *RET* and *NTRK1* in papillary thyroid carcinoma. *J Clin Endocrinol Metab.* 1996; 81:2006–9.

265. Bongarzone I, Vigneri P, Mariani L, et al. *RET/NTRK1* rearrangements in thyroid gland tumors of the papillary carcinoma family: correlation with clinicopathological features. *Clin Cancer Res.* 1998; 4:223–8.

266. Holliday R. Ageing: X-chromosome reactivation. *Nature.* 1987; 327:661–2.

267. Vogelstein B, Fearon ER, Hamilton SR, et al. Clonal analysis using recombinant DNA probes from the X-chromosome. *Cancer Res.* 1987; 47:4806–13.

268. Vogelstein B, Fearon ER, Hamilton SR, et al. Use of restriction fragment length polymorphisms to determine the clonal origin of human tumors. *Science.* 1985; 227:642–5.

269. Allen RC, Zoghbi HY, Moseley AB, et al. Methylation of *Hpa*II and *Hha*I sites near the polymorphic CAG repeat in the human androgen receptor gene correlates with X-chromosome inactivation. *Am J Hum Genet.* 1992; 51:1229–39.

270. Hendricks RW, Chen ZY, Hinds H, et al. An X chromosome inactivation assay based on differential methylation of a CpG island coupled to a VNTR polymorphism at the 1385′ end of the monoamine oxidase A gene. *Hum Mol Genet.* 1992, 1:87–94.

271. Wainscoat JS, Fey MF. Assessment of clonality in human tumors: a review. *Cancer Res.* 1990; 50:1355–60.

272. Kopp P, Jaggi R, Tobler A, et al. Clonal X-inactivation analysis of human tumours using the

human androgen receptor gene (HUMARA) polymorphism: a non-radioactive and semiquantitative strategy applicable to fresh and archival tissue. *Mol Cell Probes.* 1997; 11:217–28.

273. Gale RE, Mein CA, Linch DC. Quantification of X-chromosome inactivation patterns in hematological samples using the DNA PCR-based HUMARA assay. *Leukemia.* 1996; 10:362–7.

274. Peng H, Du M, Diss TC, et al. Clonality analysis in tumors of women by PCR amplification of X-linked genes. *J Pathol.* 1997; 181:223–7.

275. Gale RE, Linch DC. Clonality studies in acute myeloid leukemia. *Leukemia.* 1998; 12:117–20.

276. Walsh DS, Peacocke M, Harrington A, et al. Patterns of X-chromosome inactivation in sporadic basal cell carcinoma: evidence for clonality. *J Am Acad Dermatol.* 1998; 38:49–55.

277. Lucas DR, Shroyer KR, McCarthy PJ, et al. Desmoid tumor is a clonal cellular proliferation: PCR amplification of HUMARA for analysis of patterns of X-chromosome inactivation. *Am J Surg Pathol.* 1997; 21:306–11.

278. Hannum C, Freed JH, Tarr G, et al. Biochemistry and distribution of the T cell receptor. *Immunol Rev.* 1984; 81:161–76.

279. Diaz-Ciano S. PCR-based alternative for diagnosis of immunoglobulin heavy chain gene rearrangement. Principles, practice and polemics. *Diagn Mol Pathol.* 1996; 5:3–9.

280. Achille A, Scarpa A, Montresor M, et al. Routine application of polymerase chain reaction in the diagnosis of monoclonality of B cell lymphoid proliferations. *Diagn Mol Pathol.* 1995 4:14–24.

281. Tbakhi A, Tubbs R. Utility of polymerase chain reaction in detecting B cell clonality in lymphoid neoplasms. *Cancer.* 1996; 77:1223–5.

282. Diss TC, Watts M, Pan LX, et al. The polymerase chain reaction in the demonstration of monoclonality in T cell lymphomas. *J Clin Pathol.* 1995; 48:1045–50.

283. Lozano MD, Tierens A, Greiner TC, et al. Clonality analysis of B-lymphoid proliferations using the polymerase chain reaction. *Cancer.* 1996; 77:1349–55.

284. Szczepanski T, Langerak AW, Wolvers-Tettero IL, et al. Immunoglobulin and T cell receptor gene rearrangement patterns in acute lymphoblastic leukemia are less mature in adults than in children: implications for selection of PCR targets for detection of minimal residual disease. *Leukemia.* 1998; 12:1081–8.

285. Aiello A, Giardini R, Tondini C, et al. PCR-based clonality analysis: a reliable method for the diagnosis and follow-up monitoring of conservatively treated gastric B cell MALT lymphomas. *Histopathology.* 1999; 34:326–30.

286. Collins RD. Is clonality equivalent to malignancy: specifically, is immunoglobulin gene rearrangement diagnostic of malignant lymphoma? *Hum Pathol.* 1997; 28:757–9.

4

Cellular and Tissue Markers in Solid Tumors

Thomas Lindahl, Torbjön Norberg, Gunnar Åström,
Sigrid Sjögren, and C. Jonas Bergh

Introduction

The preceding two chapters have provided the groundwork discussion on the prognostic value and potential clinical utility of markers.

This chapter broadly discusses the present and potential future use of cellular and tissue markers for the management of patients with solid malignant tumors, and attempts to highlight potential developments within this area, with some focus on breast cancer (as this tumor type has served as a model for studies on prognostic and predictive factors).

Preclinical Medicine and Clinical Oncology

During the last two decades, we have experienced remarkable advances in understanding basic cell and molecular biology. Cornerstones in this development were the discovery of oncogenes in human cancer, followed by the identification of the tumor-suppressor genes (TSGs) (reviewed in ref. *1*). The detailed characterization of the different cyclines and cycline-dependent kinases (CDKs), responsible for the immediate regulation of the different phases of the cell cycle, were also major achievements (reviewed in refs. *2,3*). The factors involved in cell-cycle regulation are presently being studied in human cancers to investigate their potential as diagnostic markers and possible targets for antiproliferative drugs. The diagnostic tools used in cancer medicine have been remarkably improved *(4)*. For example, the use of population-based screening mammography programs for early diagnosis of breast cancer have resulted in a statistically improved breast cancer survival *(5)*. Early (adjuvant) therapy of systemic micrometastases has statistically significantly improved the survival of patients with breast and colorectal carcinoma *(6–9)*. Despite these latter achievements, there is a need to avoid undertreatment and to diminish overtreatment. A better use of cellular and tissue markers may be helpful to obtain these goals. To diminish overtreatment, it may be necessary to explore the techniques aimed at identifying micrometastases. The microscopic identification of epithelial, breast cancerlike cells in the bone marrow has been done for decades *(10,11)*. The prognostic value of micrometastases in relation to the nodal status has been demonstrated in one study, which definitely must be confirmed in prospective studies *(12)*. With more advanced techniques, it may be possible to monitor the effect

From: *Principles of Molecular Oncology*
Edited by: M. H. Bronchud, M. A. Foote, W. P. Peters, and M. O. Robinson © Humana Press Inc., Totowa, NJ

of adjuvant chemotherapy by analyzing epithelial marrow cells before and after chemo-therapy, thus giving these cells a potential predictive value. Despite these achievements using adjuvant therapy for breast and colorectal carcinoma, these malignant tumors and other common solid tumors are still major causes of death. In the macrometastatic situation, the effects of the present conventional therapy modalities (i.e., surgery, radiotherapy, chemotherapy, and hormonal manipulations) are limited or even absent.

Potential Obstacles

The transition to potentially more complicated diagnostic procedures will most likely require more resources compared with the present strategies. This change may be complicated, as some clinicians and scientists tend to be very cautious, sometimes too conservative, in accepting and integrating new routines for the management of cancer patients. As an example, one may mention the late acceptance of adjuvant polychemo-therapy for breast cancer patients with poor prognosis *(13)*. The positive effects of this type of early therapy were first described in a randomized study published in 1977 *(14)*. Although a number of studies could repeat these data, and the first overview was performed in 1985 *(15)*, it was not until the early 1990s that this therapy principle was generally accepted in some regions and countries. This circumspective attitude among physicians and scientists, combined with the economic strain on the healthcare sector in many western European countries, will thus be complicating factors *(13)*. Another example of conservatism and skepticism is the reluctance to accept and the slow introduction over decades of fine-needle cytology in the United States for the diagnostic management of cancer patients *(16)*. In this case, the economic factors regulating the management of the patients may influence the selection of method. These are the environments in which new principles will be launched for diagnosis using cellular and tissue-marker therapy selection.

The Identification of New Human Genes

All human genes will be sequenced within the coming few years *(17,18)*. The next important step will be to identify the protein structures and functions of the translated genes. These new genes and proteins may be used for the improved diagnoses of different diseases, including malignant tumors. For cancers, it is very likely in the coming years that new factors with prognostic and predictive potential will be identified in solid malignant tumors.

Prognostic and Predictive Factors for the Management of Cancer Patients: Present Standards and the Future

We have a long list of established prognostic factors based on clinical variables, the tumor, node, metastasis (TNM) staging; different morphological parameters; proteolytic enzymes; mutant oncogenes; and TSGs with loss of function. The present arsenal allows us to give rather accurate prognostic information for groups of patients, but not for individual patients. The use of new prognostic factors aimed at an individual fingerprint-ing of each tumor has the potential to improve prognostic information on an individual level. Although important, it would be better if the identification of new *predictive* factors applicable on the individual level (e.g., a factor with high sensitivity and specificity correlating with the therapeutic effects by a certain oncologic therapeutic modality) could be done. Estrogen and progesterone receptor status is a good example of useful predictive factors for the selection of hormonal therapy in patients with breast cancer; a receptor-positive cancer has a 60–70% chance of responding to hormonal therapy, whereas a receptor-negative cancer has only a 5–10% chance of responding to the same hormonal agents *(19)*. New predictive factors should aim to produce better results than these.

Morphological Tumor Diagnosis and the Future Integration of Molecular Biological Diagnostic Tools

The classic diagnoses of malignant tumors have almost exclusively been based on microscopic examination of the morphology of representative portions of the tumor. Pathologists have developed a marked skill in the diagnoses of malignant vs benign tumors and other pathological conditions. The histopathologic description of a malignant tumor is primarily based on visual comparison between tumor tissue in relation to normal tissue. In general, this is also the major basis for the malignancy grading of the tumors. The histopathologic classification, grading, and staging systems have been shown to be largely reproducible and highly useful for the clinical management of patients with cancer. However, it is not certain that this type of morphological classification will be used in the future for all tumor types. Future methods should try to better reflect the tumor heterogeneity and variability seen during tumor progression. It is possible that within 10 yr, the histopathological classification and grading systems will be supplemented with additional information based on different genotypic and phenotypic factors. A not far-fetched view is that in the future these factors may decide the individual therapy selections rather than the formal histopathological diagnosis. However, these new phenotypic and genotypic markers must have demonstrated their value in repeated, large-scale clinical studies, ideally prospective ones. The use of microchips, the microarray technique, and other molecular biological techniques will most likely create a revolution when properly applied to large, population-based clinical materials in the detailed knowledge of the molecular changes during the different tumor stages from early atypia by invasive carcinoma to widespread metastases *(20–23)*. These techniques will create an enormous amount of data, which must be analyzed in a systematic way, in collaboration with biostatistical expertise, using prospectively designed protocols with predefined primary and secondary endpoints.

Primary Tumors vs Metastases: Biopsy and Noninvasive Techniques

A potential shortcoming with the diagnostic procedures outlined earlier is that almost all studies are focused on analyses of the primary tumors, despite the fact that many studies relate to the metastatic situation. This situation occurs because morphological material is rarely taken from the metastases. Except for scientific purposes, this oversight may be important from a clinical point of view to verify that the patient truly has a relapsing malignant disease, or benign lesions, or metastases from another primary malignant tumor. The biopsy techniques for investigations of metastatic lesion should be safe to perform and ideally should be applicable for repeated sampling of tumor lesions to monitor dynamic changes over time in both the primary tumor and in the metastases. Biopsy techniques, not requiring open surgery, have developed markedly during the last few years. It is now possible in the outpatient setting to safely perform ultrasound and computed tomography (CT)-guided biopsies from the primary disease, metastases in visceral organs, and suspected skeletal lesions *(24–33)*. These biopsies could then be analyzed for different genotypic and phenotypic markers in comparison with the primary tumor (Lindahl et al., *manuscript in preparation*). The information could then be used for tailor-made therapy selections. Parallel with this is a rapid development of noninvasive diagnostic procedures aimed at mirroring the effect by certain oncologic therapeutic modalities in relation to baseline status. An example of the latter is the positron emission tomography (PET) technique *(34,35)*. This technique could be used to visualize different major metabolic steps and processes in the tumors and the surrounding normal tissues. The PET technique could also be used for dynamic studies of metabolic marker changes in tumors in relation to a certain oncologic therapy, for receptor occupancy and pharmacokinetic studies, and in the search for potential tumor-specific markers aimed at increasing the selectivity of the different oncologic therapeutic modalities, and thus increasing the therapeutic ratio. However, the outlined biopsy and PET techniques will most likely not completely mirror each other nor will they have the resolution to appreciate the marked tumor-cell heterogeneity almost always present in all solid malignant human tumors. In the future, biopsy and noninvasive techniques must be further refined to be able to identify heterogeneity and to identify even minute changes during tumor progression.

Tailoring of Therapy: Pharmacokinetics

Individual tailoring of chemotherapy should be based on the relevant predictive tumor biological factors outlined earlier. Adding to the complexity, with the present arsenal of cytostatics, we have an interpatient (up to 10-fold) variability in clearance/systemic exposure in patients with normal liver and hepatic function *(36–39)*. This variation in clearance is due to genetic and functional factors. The pharmacokinetic variability may, of course, potentially influence the outcome for individual patients. This means that the pharmacokinetic variability also must be taken into account when designing tailor-made approaches based on the tumor's biological factors *(36,40,41)*.

c-*erbB-2* and *p53*

The oncogene c-*erbB-2* and the TSG *p53* are used as examples of potentially interesting cellular markers for prognosis and prediction. These factors are also discussed in the context of how to quantify and measure them to obtain optimal results. The advantages and disadvantages of these analyses should be restudied when new potential markers (to be used in the coming decade) are developed to better fingerprint the individual tumor, resulting in improved prognosis, prediction, and therapy selections at the individual patient level.

c-erbB-2

Background

c-*erbB-2* (HER2–neu) is an oncogene that is homologous to epidermal growth factor receptor (EGFR). Other members of this family are c-*erbB-3* and c-*erbB-4*. The c-

erbB-2 oncogene encodes a 185-kDa transmembrane glycoprotein from the gene located at 17q21 (reviewed in ref. *42* and chapter 3 of this book).

Methods for c-erbB-2 Determination

c-*erbB-2* status has been studied by many techniques (reviewed in ref. *42*). Southern blots and polymerase chain reactions (PCRs) have been used for studies of gene amplification (reviewed in ref. *42*). Overexpression has been investigated with RNA- and protein-based methods, Northern blots, fluorescent *in situ* hybridization (FISH), Western blots, and immunohistochemistry (IHC) (reviewed in ref. *42*). For the last technique, 17 different polyclonal and monoclonal antibodies (mAbs) were used (reviewed in ref. *42*). Other authors have previously demonstrated a marked variability by the c-*erbB-2* Abs to detect antigen (Ag) overexpression on archival biopsies *(43)*. The PCR-based method revealed positivity in 30.6% of the tested biopsies, while the other methods demonstrated mean values in the same range, 22.7–29.7% (reviewed in ref. *42*). We have used the CB11 mAb for IHC on a population-based breast cancer cohort of 315 patients with a similar result of 19% positivity *(44)*. No direct comparative studies between the different techniques have been presented on large and population-based material, with reference to the prognostic and predictive value for c-*erbB-2*. It would be interesting to investigate, on a larger amount of patient material, those potential discrepancies between protein expression and gene amplification in relation to prognosis and prediction.

c-erbB-2-Correlations with Other Markers

An increased protein expression or gene amplification of c-*erbB-2* has been shown to correlate with estrogen receptor (ER) negativity *(44–53)*. c-*erbB-2* positivity has also been shown to correlate with worse histopathological and nuclear grades, high S-phase, and aneuploidy (reviewed in ref. *42*).

c-erbB-2 and Tamoxifen

c-*erbB-2* positivity is known to be associated with a worse response to endocrine therapy in patients with breast cancer, both for metastatic breast cancer and in the adjuvant setting *(44,47,54–57)*. Conversely, in one study with 205 patients with advanced breast cancer, the effect of tamoxifen was not related to the c-*erbB-2* status *(58)*.

c-erbB-2 and Cytostatics

The receptor-positive human breast carcinoma cell line MCF-7 was transfected with c-*erbB-2* which resulted in resistance to tamoxifen and a low level of resistance to cisplatin, but retained sensitivity to doxorubicin and 5-fluorouracil (5-FU) *(59)*.

In a retrospective study, poor survival was demonstrated for adjuvant polychemotherapy with cyclophosphamide, methotrexate, and 5-FU in breast cancer patients with tumors overexpressing c-*erbB-2 (48)*. In the National Surgical Adjuvant Breast Program (NSABP) B11 study with 638 patients, patients with tumors overexpressing c-*erbB-2* had a significant benefit with the addition of doxorubicin to the melphalan- and 5-FU-based regimen *(60)*. Furthermore, a statistically significantly improved relapse-free survival was demonstrated in a group of patients receiving standard doses of 5-FU, doxorubicin, and cyclophosphamide compared with two groups receiving a lower dose intensity *(61)*. Clahsen and co-workers *(62)* demonstrated a trend for improved disease-free survival ($p = 0.17$) in patients with overexpression of c-*erbB-2* receiving one course of perioperative 5-FU, doxorubicin, and cyclophosphamide. A borderline, disease-free survival benefit was demonstrated for the c-*erbB-2*-negative patients receiving therapy compared with those receiving no adjuvant therapy ($p = 0.05$) *(62)*. However, contradictory results have also been presented in a study with 103 patients with metastatic breast cancer and a study with neo-adjuvant chemotherapy; in these studies, the patients received epirubicin-based polychemotherapy and doxorubicin-based chemotherapy together with radiotherapy, respectively *(63,64)*.

c-erbB-2 *and Trastuzumab*

The trastuzumab mAb directed against c-*erbB-2* has recently been explored in patients with breast cancer with tumors with c-*erbB-2* overexpression. The c-*erbB-2* mAb trastuzumab (Herceptin™) has, alone or in combination with chemotherapy, demonstrated objective responses, in the range of 16% using the Ab alone or 48% in combination with paclitaxel *(65,66)*. Only patients with markedly c-*erbB-2*-positive tumors were included in these studies after IHC-based selection. Therapy with trastuzumab is being explored in the adjuvant setting in patients with micrometastases. The likelihood that the therapy will function better in the micrometastatic situation is most likely higher.

p53

Background

The p53 protein is encoded from a gene locus on the short arm of chromosome 17, p13.1. *p53* is responsible for the control of essential cellular functions such as apoptosis, cell-cycle control, chromosomal segregation, gene transcription, and genomic stability (reviewed in ref. *67*). p53 is a nuclear phosphoprotein with 393 amino acids. The *p53* gene can be activated by the telangiectasia gene (ATM) by ultraviolet (UV) light, carcinogens, cytostatics, and radiation. The activated wild-type protein can either activate p53-dependent apoptotic machinery or downstream, by p21, inhibit CDKs. *p53* can be inactivated by somatic or germline mutations or by binding to certain viral oncoproteins (human papilloma virus [HPV] protein E6, SV-40 large T-Ag, hepatitis B viral X protein, and adenovirus protein E1A; or binding to the oncogene *MDM2*). *MDM2* has been demonstrated to bind to the N-terminal of the p53 protein *(68)*.

Methods for p53 Determination

IHC using different monoclonal and polyclonal Abs is the most frequently used method for detecting p53 in clinical samples. The basis for IHC determination of p53 is related to the fact that the mutant protein has a markedly prolonged half-life of 4–20 h *(69–72)*, while the wild-type p53 protein has a half-life of only 15–20 min *(73)*. A major problem with the commonly used mAbs is their inability to discriminate between mutant p53 and enhanced levels of normal wild-type p53 *(74)*. The p53 protein is normally localized to the nucleus and IHC techniques will, of course, provide information on the subcellular localization of the Ag, the tissue distribution in malignant cells vs stroma cells, and the heterogeneity within the tumor. The degree of immunohistochemical positivity has been quite variable in the different studies.

This potential discrepancy could be related to the Abs used for the p53 determinations. Furthermore, the fixative and fixation time have also been demonstrated to be of importance *(75,76)*. In a comparative study between the p53 Abs Pab 1801, p53–BP-12, D07, and CM1, Pab 1801 and D07 were demonstrated, after microwave Ag retrieval, to give the best localization of p53 Ag *(77)*. The authors claimed that the mAb Pab 1801 was most useful with reference to prognostic information *(77)*. The same Abs, together with Pab 240 and signet, were investigated in another study using biopsies from patients with colorectal carcinoma; the Ab D07 was considered to be best *(78)*. Flow cytometry has also recently been explored for determination of the p53 status *(79)*.

We have compared immunohistochemical determination of the p53 protein using Pab 1801 with cDNA sequencing of the same breast cancer material consisting of more than 300 primary breast cancer biopsies *(74)*. IHC with this Ab could detect only 2 of 13 deletions, none of 6 stop codons, and only 2 of 3 insertions, but almost all point mutations, 40 of 45 *(74)*. In our study, immunohistochemical detection of p53 resulted in a 30% false-positive rate and 9% false-negative rate *(74,80)*.

We also have studied the luminometric immunoassay for p53 determination using Pab 1801 and D01 compared with above-mentioned immunohistochemical technique and cDNA sequencing *(74,81)*. The luminometric method gave very similar result as the immunohistochemical study, and both these techniques were inferior compared with cDNA sequencing *(81)*.

The cDNA sequencing of p53 on homogenized breast cancer biopsy material has been compared with genomic sequencing of microdissected tumors from the same material (total, 100 biopsies) *(82)*. The cDNA technique detected 22 of 23 mutations in the exons; 1 stop codon was missed *(82)*. Three further mutations in the intron and splice regions were detected with genomic sequencing of microdissected tumor material. The potential clinical relevance for these mutations is unknown. We have also performed a comparative study using genomic sequencing without microdissection compared with cDNA sequencing on the same homogenized material from 16 breast cancer biopsies with known p53 mutations. All 16 mutations were detected with the cDNA technique, but 2 were missed with the genomic sequencing technique when the microdissection step was omitted *(82)*. Sequencing is a laborious and expensive technique, and thus other molecular biological techniques are frequently used for screening for mutations. The most commonly used technique is the combination of PCR with single-strand conformation polymorphism (SSCP). The sensitivity for the SSCP technique has been described as varying from 58% to 100% in samples with p53 mutation *(83,84)*. For optimal SSCP results, different temperatures and glycerol concentrations must be tested. Furthermore, the technique has a higher sensitivity for smaller segments compared with larger segments. However, a negative SSCP result will not exclude the possibility of a p53 mutation.

Denaturing gradient gel electrophoresis (DGGE) has been shown to be a useful screening method for mutations *(85,86)*. The major advances with this technique is that this method has been able to detect 1% mutated cells surrounded by cells without mutations *(87)*. This finding may be of importance for detailed studies of tumor heterogeneity and this type of information may be particularly interesting in studies of early molecular biological events in the tumor development. Studies of loss of heterozygosity (LOH) are aimed at identifying a potential difference in the expression of the paternal and maternal allele. In our study of 26 p53 mutations, we demonstrated that 21 tumors had LOH, 4 samples were not informative, and 1 sample had retention of 1 allele *(82)*.

p53 Mutations Are Common

p53 mutation is the most common genetic abnormality described to date for human cancer *(75,88–104)*. Fifty percent of patients with colon and lung carcinoma have been demonstrated to have *p53* mutations. *p53* mutations are rare in patients with nephroblastomas (Wilms' tumors) or testicular teratomas *(105,106)*. *p53* abnormalities can be demonstrated in dysplastic lesion in the skin, in esophagus, in the bronchus, and in *in situ* carcinoma (ISC) of the breast *(107–110,* Norberg et al., *unpublished data)*. *p53* mutations have also been shown to occur in relation to tumor progression or as a late event in the tumor development. The latter statement is valid for cervical, colon, and thyroid carcinoma; the blast crises in chronic myeloid leukemia; and the progression of low-grade astrocytomas *(111–120)*.

p53 and Prognoses

Patients with somatic *p53* mutations or increased p53 protein expression have been shown to have worse prognosis for a long list of malignant tumors compared with those patients with normal, wild-type p53 *(75,88–104)*.

Breast cancer patients with mutations in the evolutionary regions II and V or mutations in the zinc finger binding regions L2 and L3 have been demonstrated to have a particularly poor prognosis *(89,92)*. Interestingly, in colorectal carcinoma, mutations outside the evolutionarily conserved regions were associated with statistically significantly worse survival *(121)*.

p53 as Predictive Factor

p53 has also been extensively investigated in relation to its possible predictive potential. Tamoxifen therapy has been shown to work less well both in the adjuvant setting and in patients with metastatic disease if the tumors contain mutant *p53* or increased p53 protein levels *(89,122)*. However, a negative study on 92 patients has also been published with reference to *p53* and tamoxifen *(123)*. The effect of chemotherapy in relation to p53 status has been investigated in at least 15 breast cancer studies (reviewed in ref. *124)*. In five of these studies, the patients with increased p53 protein levels or with mutant *p53* had poor relapse-free and disease-free survival and overall survival *(61,62,125–127)*. Furthermore, patients with a mutant *p53* status and acute myeloid leukemia, chronic lymphocytic leukemia, myelodysplastic syndromes, T-cell leukemia, malignant lymphoma, and ovarian carcinoma have been reported to have resistance/poorer response to conventional chemotherapy *(125–132)*.

Conclusions

The discovery of new genes and their corresponding proteins as part of the HUGO project may be useful for the detailed fingerprinting of individual tumors and a better use of the present arsenal of cellular and tissue markers aimed at better prediction and therapy selection at the individual level based on these markers. The aim should be to tailor the therapy for each patient to diminish both over- and undertreatment.

Acknowledgments

Our work has been supported by the Swedish Cancer Society and the Nordic Cancer Union. The excellent secretarial assistance of Marléne Forslund is greatly appreciated.

References

1. Perkins A, Stern D. Molecular biology of cancer. Oncogenes. In: *Cancer: Principles & Practice of Oncology,* 5th edit. (DeVita V, Heilman S, Rosenberg S, eds.), Lippincott-Raven, Philadelphia, 1997, pp. 79–102.

2. Kastan M. Molecular biology of cancer: the cell cycle. In: *Cancer: Principles & Practice of Oncology,* 5th edit. (DeVita V, Heilman S, Rosenberg S, eds.), Lippincott-Raven, Philadelphia, 1997, pp. 121–34.

3. Landberg G, Roos G. The cell cycle in breast cancer. *APMIS.* 1197; 105:575–89.

4. Catellino R. Imaging techniques in cancer management. Section 1, overview. In: *Cancer: Principles & Practice of Oncology,* 5th edit. (DeVita V, Hellman S, Rosenberg S, eds.), Lippincott-Raven, Philadelphia, 1997, pp. 633–43.

5. Nystrom L, Rutqvist LE, Wall S, et al. Breast cancer screening with mammography: overview of Swedish randomised trials. *Lancet.* 1993; 341:973–8.

6. Early Breast Cancer Trialists' Collaborative Group. Systemic treatment of early breast cancer by hormonal, cytotoxic, or immune therapy. *Lancet.* 1992; 339:1–15.

7. Early Breast Cancer Trialists' Collaborative Group. Polychemotherapy for early breast cancer: an overview of the randomised trials. *Lancet.* 1998; 352:930–42.

8. Early Breast Cancer Trialists' Collaborative Group. Tamoxifen for early breast cancer: an overview of the randomised trials. *Lancet.* 1998; 351:1451–67.

9. NIH consensus conference. Adjuvant therapy for patients with colon and rectal cancer. *JAMA.* 1990; 264:1444–55.

10. Redding W, Coombes R, Monaghan P, et al. Detection of micrometastases in patients with primary breast cancer. *Lancet.* 1983; 2:1271–4.

11. Ridell B, Landys K. Incidence and histopathology of metastases of mammary carcinoma in biopsies from the posterior iliac crest. *Cancer.* 1979; 44:1872–8.

12. Diel I, Kaufmann M, Costa S, et al. Micrometastatic breast cancer cells in bone marrow at primary surgery: prognostic value in comparison with nodal status. *J Natl Cancer Inst.* 1996; 88:1652–68.

13. Bergh J. Determination and use of p53 in the management of cancer patients with special focus on breast cancer—a review. In: *Prognostic and Predictive value of p53.* (Klijn J, ed.), Elsevier, Amsterdam, 1997, pp. 35–50.

14. Bonadonna G, Rossi A, Valagussa P, et al. The CMF program for operable breast cancer with positive axillary nodes. *Cancer.* 1977; 39:2904–15.

15. Early Breast Cancer Trialists' Collaborative Group. Effects of adjuvant tamoxifen and of cytotoxic therapy on mortality in early breast cancer. An overview of 61 randomized trials among 28,896 women. *N Engl J Med.* 1988; 319; 1681–92.

16. Eisenhut CL, King DE, Nelson WA, Olson LC, Wall RW, Glant MD. Fine-needle biopsy of pediatric lesions: a three-year study in an outpatient biopsy clinic. *Diagn Cytopathol.* 1996; 14:43–50.

17. Collins F, Patrinos A, Jordan E, et al. New goals for the US Human Genome Project: 1998–2003. *Science.* 1998; 282:682–9.

18. van Ommen G. The human genome project and the role of genetics in health care. *Clin. Chem Lab Med.* 1998; 36:515–7.

19. Roodi N, Bailey L, Kao W, et al. Estrogen receptor gene analysis in estrogen receptor-positive and receptor-negative primary breast cancer. *J Natl Cancer Inst.* 1995; 87:446–51.

20. Cole K, Krizman DB, Emmert-Buck MR. The genetics of cancer—a 3D model. *Nat Genet.* 1999; 21:38–41.

21. Debouck C, Goodfellow P. DNA microarrays in drug discovery and development. *Nat Genet.* 1999; 21:48–50.

22. Forozan F, Karhu R, Kononen J, Kallioniemi A, Kallioniemi OP. Genome screening by comparative genomic hybridization. *Trends Genet.* 1997; 13:405–9.

23. Hacia J. Resequencing and mutational analysis using oligonucleotide microarrays. *Nat Genet.* 1999; 21:42–7.

24. Bernardino M. Automated biopsy devices: significance and safety. *Radiology.* 1990; 176:615–6.

25. Burbank F, Kaye K, Belville J, et al. Image-guided automated core biopsies of the breast, chest, abdomen, and pelvis. *Radiology.* 1994; 191:165–71.

26. Ciray I, Aström G, Sundström C, Hagberg H, Ahlstrom H. Assessment of suspected bone metastases. CT with and without clinical information compared to CT-guided bone biopsy. *Acta Radiol.* 1997; 38:890–5.

27. Elvin A, Andersson T, Jaremko G, et al. Significance of operator experience in diagnostic accuracy of biopsy gun biopsies. *Eur Radiol.* 1994; 4:430–3.

28. Fraser-Hill MA, Renfrew DL, Hilsenrath PE. Percutaneous needle biopsy of musculoskeletal lesions. 1. Effective accuracy and diagnostic utility. *Am J Roentgenol.* 1992; 158:809–12.

29. Moulton JS, Moore PT. Coaxial percutaneous biopsy technique with automated biopsy devices. Value in improving accuracy and negative predictive value. *Radiology* 1993; 186:515–22.

30. Parker S, Hopper K, Yakes W, et al. Image-directed percutaneous biopsies with a biopsy gun. *Radiology.* 1989; 171:663–9.

31. Tikkakoski T, Paivansalo M, Siniluoto T, et al. Percutaneous ultrasound-guided biopsy. Fine needle biopsy, cutting needle biopsy, or both? *Acta Radiol.* 1993; 34:30–4.

32. Welch T, Sheedy P, Johnson C, et al. CT-guided biopsy: prospective analysis of 1,000 procedures. *Radiology.* 1989; 171:493–6.

33. Aström KG, Sundström JC, Lindgren PG, Ahlstrom KH. Automatic biopsy instruments used through a coaxial bone biopsy system with an eccentric drill Eip. *Acta Radiol.* 1995; 36:237–42.

34. Brock CS, Meikle SR, Price MP. Does fluorine-18 fluorodeoxyglucose metabolic imaging of tumours benefit oncology? *Eur J Nucl Med.* 1997; 24:691–705.

35. Timothy AR, Cook GJ. PET scanning in clinical oncology. *Ann Oncol.* 1998; 9:353–5.

36. Gurney H. Dose calculation of anticancer drugs: a review of the current practice and introduction of an alternative. *J Clin Oncol.* 1996; 14:2590–611.

37. Gurney H, Ackland S, Gebski V, et al. Factors affecting epirubicin pharmacokinetics and toxicity: evidence against using body-surface area for dose calculation. *J Clin Oncol.* 1998; 16:2299–304.

38. Karlsson MO, Molnar V, Bergh J, Freijs A, Larsson R. A general model for time-dissociated pharmacokinetic-pharmacodynamic relationship exemplified by paclitaxel myelosuppression. *Clin Pharmacol Ther.* 1998; 63:11–25.

39. Sandström M, Freijs A, Larsson R, et al. Lack of relationship between systemic exposure for the component drugs of the fluorouracil, epirubicin, and 4-hydroxycyclophosphamide regimen in breast cancer patients. *J Clin Oncol.* 1996; 14:1581–8.

40. Bergh J. Tailored chemotherapy to equal toxicity—is it possible? In: *Adjuvant Therapy of Primary Breast Cancer.* (Senn HJ, Gelber R, Goldhirsch A, Thurlimann B, eds.), Springer-Verlag, Berlin, 1998, pp. 328–40.

41. Bergh J, Wikllund T, Erikstein B, et al. Dosage of adjuvant G-CSF (filgrastim)-supported FEC polychemotherapy based on equivalent haematological toxicity to high-risk breast cancer patients. *Ann Oncol.* 1998; 9:403–11.

42. Revillion F, Bonneterre J, Peyrat J. *ERBB2* oncogene in human breast cancer and its clinical significance. *Eur J Cancer.* 1998; 34:791–808.

43. Press MF, Hung G, Godolphin W, Slamon DJ. Sensitivity of HER-2/neu antibodies in archival tissue samples. Potential source of error in immunohistochemical studies of oncogene expression. *Cancer Res.* 1994; 54:2771–7.

44. Sjögren S, Inganas M, Lindgren A, Holmberg L, Bergh J. The prognostic and predictive value of c-*erbB*-2 overexpression in primary breast cancer, alone and in combination with other prognostic markers. *J Clin Oncol.* 1998; 16:462–9.

45. Barbareschi M, Leonardi E, Mauri FA, Sergio G, Dalla Palma P. p53 and c-erbB-2 protein expression in breast carcinoma. An immunohistochemical study including correlations with receptor status, proliferation markers, and clinical stage in human breast cancer. *Am J Clin Pathol.* 1992; 98:408–18.

46. Berns EM, Klijn JG, van Staveren IL, Portengen H, Noordegraaf E, Foekens JA. Prevalence of amplification of the oncogenes *c-myc, HER2/neu,* and *int-2* in one thousand human breast tumours: correlation with steroid receptors. *Eur J Cancer.* 1992; 28:697–700.

47. Carlomagno C, Perrone F, Gallo C, et al. c-*erbB2* overexpression decreases the benefit of adjuvant tamoxifen in early-stage breast cancer without axillary lymph node metastases. *J Clin Oncol.* 1996; 14:2702–8.

48. Gusterson BA, Gelber RD, Goldhirsch A, et al. Prognostic importance of c-*erbB-2* expression in breast cancer. *J Clin Oncol.* 1992; 10:1049–56.

49. Hartmann LC, Ingle JN, Wold LE, et al. Prognostic value of c-*erbB2* overexpression in axillary lymph node positive breast cancer. Results from a randomized adjuvant treatment protocol. *Cancer.* 1994; 74:2956–63.

50. Lipponen HJ, Aaltomaa S, Syrjanen S, Syrjanen K. c-*erbB*-2 oncogene related to p53 expression, cell proliferation and prognosis in breast cancer. *Anticancer Res.* 1993; 13:1147–52.

51. Marx D, Schauer A, Reiche C, et al. c-*erbB2* expression in correlation to other biological parameters of breast cancer. *J Cancer Res Clin Oncol.* 1990; 116:15–20.

52. Takahashi S, Narimatsu E, Asanuma H, et al. Immunohistochemical detection of estrogen receptor in invasive human breast cancer: correlation with heat shock proteins, pS2 and oncogene products. *Oncology.* 1995; 52:371–5.

53. Tang R, Kacinski B, Validire P, et al. Oncogene amplification correlates with dense lymphocyte infiltration in human breast cancers: a role for hematopoietic growth factor release by tumor cells? *J Cell Biochem.* 1990; 44:189–98.

54. Borg A, Baldetorp B, Fernö M, et al. *ERBB2* amplification is associated with tamoxifen resistance in steroid-receptor positive breast cancer. *Cancer Lett.* 1994; 81:137–44.

55. Leitzel K, Teramoto Y, Konrad K, et al. Elevated serum c-erbB-2 antigen levels and decreased response to hormone therapy of breast cancer. *J Clin Oncol.* 1995; 13:1129–35.

56. Wright C, Nicholson S, Angus B, et al. Relationship between c-erbB-2 protein product expression and response to endocrine therapy in advanced breast cancer. *Br J Cancer.* 1992; 65:118–21.

57. Yamauchi H, O'Neill A, Gelman R, et al. Prediction of response to antiestrogen therapy in advanced breast cancer patients by pretreatment circulating levels of extracellular domain of the HER-2/c-neu protein. *J Clin Oncol.* 1997; 15.2518–25.

58. Elledge R, Green S, Ciocca D, et al. HER-2 expression and response to tamoxifen in estrogen receptor-positive breast cancer: a Southwest Oncology Group Study. *Clin Cancer Res.* 1998; 4:7–12.

59. Benz CC, Scott GK, Sarup JC, et al. Estrogen-dependent, tamoxifen-resistant tumorigenic growth of MCF-7 cells transfected with HER2/neu. *Breast Cancer Res Treat.* 1993; 24:85–95.

60. Paik S, Bryant J, Park C, et al. *erbB-2* and response to doxorubicin in patients with axillary lymph node-positive, hormone receptor-negative breast cancer. *J Natl Cancer Inst.* 1998; 90:1361–70.

61. Thor AD, Berry DA, Budman DR, et al. *erbB-2, p53,* and efficacy of adjuvant therapy in lymph node-positive breast cancer. *J Natl Cancer Inst.* 1998; 90:1346–60.

62. Clahsen PC, van de Velde CJ, Duval C, et al. p53 protein accumulation and response to adjuvant chemotherapy in premenopausal women with node-negative early breast cancer. *J Clin Oncol.* 1998; 16:470–9.

63. Niskanen E, Blomqvist C, Franssila K, Hietanen P, Wasenius VM. Predictive value of *c-erbB-2,* p53, cathepsin-D and histology of the primary tumour in metastatic breast cancer. *Br J Cancer.* 1997; 76:917–22.

64. Rozan S, Vincent-Salomon A, Zafrani B, et al. No significant predictive value of c-*erbB-*2 or p53 expression regarding sensitivity to primary chemotherapy or radiotherapy in breast cancer. *Int J Cancer.* 1998; 79:27–33.

65. Cobleigh M, Vogel C, Tripathy D, et al. Efficacy and safety of Herceptin™ (humanized anti-HER2 antibody) as a single agent in 222 women with *HER2* overexpression who relapsed following chemotherapy for metastatic breast cancer. *Proc Am Soc Clin Oncol.* 1998; 17:97a (abstr 376).

66. Slamon D, Leyland-Jones B, Shak S, et al. Addition of Herceptin™ (humanized anti*HER2* antibody) to first line chemotherapy for *HER2* overexpressing metastatic breast cancer (HER2[+]MBC) markedly increases anticancer activity: a randomized, multinational controlled phase III trial. *Proc Am Soc Clin Oncol.* 1998; 17:98a (abstr 377).

67. Harris C. Structure and function of the *p53* tumor suppressor gene: clues for rational cancer therapeutic strategies. *J Natl Cancer Inst.* 1996; 88:1442–55.

68. Kussie PH, Gorina S, Marechal V, et al. Structure of the MDM2 oncoprotein bound to the p53 tumor suppressor transactivation domain. *Science.* 1996; 274:948–53.

69. Finlay C, Hinds P, Tan TH, et al. Activating mutations for transformation by *p53* produce a gene product that forms an *hsc70–p53* complex with an altered half-life. *Mol Cell Biol.* 1988; 8:531–9.

70. Hinds PW, Finlay CA, Quartin RS, et al. Mutant *p53* cDNAs from human colorectal carcinomas can cooperate with *ras* in transformation of primary rat cells: a comparison of the "hot spot" mutant phenotypes. *Cell Growth Different.* 1990; 1:571–80.

71. Iggo R, Gatter K, Bartek J, Lane D, Harris AL. Increased expression of mutant forms of *p53* oncogene in primary lung cancer. *Lancet.* 1990; 335:675–9.

72. Reich N, Levine A. Growth regulation of a cellular tumour antigen, p53, in nontransformed cells. *Nature* 1984; 308:199–201.

73. Gronostajski R, Goldberg A, Pardee A. Energy requirement for degradation of tumor-associated protein p53. *Mol Cell Biol.* 1984; 4:442–8.

74. Sjögren S, Inganas M, Norberg T, et al. The *p53* gene in breast cancer: prognostic value

of complementary DNA sequencing versus immunohistochemistry. *J Natl Cancer Inst.* 1996; 88:173–82.

75. Silvestrini R, Benini E, Daidone MC, et al. p53 as an independent prognostic marker in lymph node-negative breast cancer patients. *J Natl Cancer Inst.* 1993; 85:965–70.

76. Silvestrini R, Rao S, Benini E, Daidone MG, Pilotti S. Immunohistochemical detection of p53 in clinical breast cancers: a look at methodologic approaches. *J Natl Cancer Inst.* 1995; 87:1020.

77. Horne GM, Anderson JJ, Tiniakos DG, et al. p53 protein as a prognostic indicator in breast carcinoma: a comparison of four antibodies for immunohistochemistry. *Br J Cancer.* 1996; 73:29 35.

78. Baas IO, Mulder JW, Offerhaus GJ, Vogelstein B, Hamilton SR. An evaluation of six antibodies for immunohistochemistry of mutant *p53* gene product in archival colorectal neoplasmas. *J Pathol.* 1994; 172:5–12.

79. Kraggerud SM, Jacobsen KD, Berner A, et al. A comparison of different modes for the detection of p53 protein accumulation. *Pathol Res Pract.* 1997; 193:471–8.

80. Sjögren S. Prognostic factors with predictive potential in breast cancer. Special focus on the tumour suppressor p53. Acta Universitatis Upsahensis, Uppsala. Comprehensive Summaries of Uppsala Dissertations from the Faculty of Medicine, No 722, 1997.

81. Norberg T, Lennerstrand J, Inganas M, Bergh J. Comparison between p53 protein measurement using the luminometric immunoassay and immunohistochemistry 24 with detection of *p53* gene mutations using cDNA sequencing in human breast tumours. *Int J Cancer.* 1998; 79:376–83.

82. Williams C, Norberg T, Ahmadian A, et al. Assessment of sequence-based *p53* gene analysis in human breast cancer: messenger RNA in comparison with genomic DNA targets. *Clin Chem.* 1998; 44:455–62.

83. Hayashi K, Yandell DW. How sensitive is PCR-SSCP? *Hum Mutat.* 1993; 2:338–46.

84. Sarkar G, Yoon HS, Sommer SS. Dideoxy fingerprinting (ddF): a rapid and efficient screen for the presence of mutations. *Genomics.* 1992; 13:441–3.

85. Borresen AL, Hovig E, Smith-Sorensen B, et al. Constant denaturant gel electrophoresis as a rapid screening technique for *p53* mutations. *Proc Natl Acad Sci USA.* 1991; 88: 8405–9.

86. Fischer S, Lerman L, DNA fragments differing by single base-pair substitutions are separated in denaturing gradient gels: correspondence with melting theory. *Proc Natl Acad Sci USA.* 1983: 80:1579–83.

87. Borresen-Dale A. Subgroups of *p53* mutations may predict the clinical behaviour of cancers in the breast and colon and contribute to therapy response. In: *Prognostic and Predictive Value of p53.* (Klijn J, ed.), Elsevier, Amsterdam, 1997, pp. 23–33.

88. Andersen TI, Holm R, Nesland JM, Heimdal KR, Ottestad L, Borresen AL. Prognostic significance of TP53 alterations in breast carcinoma. *Br J Cancer.* 1993; 68:540–8.

89. Bergh J, Norberg T, Sjögren S, Lindgren A, Holmberg L. Complete sequencing of the *p53* gene provides prognostic information in breast cancer patients, particularly in relation to adjuvant systemic therapy and radiotherapy. *Nat Med.* 1995; 1:1029–34.

90. Borg A, Lennerstrand J, Stenmark-Askmalm M, et al. Prognostic significance of *p53* overexpression in primary breast cancer; a novel luminometric immunoassay applicable on steroid receptor cytosols. *Br J Cancer.* 1995; 71:1013–17.

91. Bosari S, Viale G, Radaelli U, Bossi P, Bonoldi E, Coggi G. *p53* accumulation in ovarian carcinomas and its prognostic implications. *Hum Pathol.* 1993; 24:1175–79.

92. Borresen AL, Andersen TI, Eyfjörd JE, et al. *TP53* mutations and breast cancer prognosis:

particularly poor survival rates for cases with mutations in the zinc-binding domains. *Genes Chromosom Cancer.* 1995; 14:71–5.

93. Chang F, Syrjanen S, Syrjanen K. Implications of the *p53* tumor suppressor gene in clinical oncology. *J Clin Oncol.* 1995; 13:1009–22.

94. Drobnjak M, Latres E, Pollack D, et al. Prognostic implications of *p53* nuclear overexpression and high proliferation index of Ki-67 and adult soft-tissue sarcomas. *J Natl Cancer Inst.* 1994; 86:549–54.

95. Elledge RM, Clark GM, Fuqua SA, Yu YY, Allred DC. p53 protein accumulation detected by five different antibodies: relationship to prognosis and heat shock protein 70 in breast cancer. *Cancer Res.* 1994; 54:3752–57.

96. Ellege RM, Fuqua SA, Clark GM, Pujol P, Allred DC, McGuire WL. Prognostic significance of *p53* gene alterations in node-negative breast cancer. *Br Cancer Res Treat.* 1993; 26:225–35.

97. Martin HM, Filipe MI, Morris RW, Lane DP, Silvestre F. *p53* expression and prognosis in gastric carcinoma. *Int J Cancer.* 1992; 50:859–62.

98. Mitsudomi T, Oyama T, Kusano T, et al. Mutations of the *p53* gene as a predictor of poor prognosis in patients with non-small-cell lung cancer. *J Natl Cancer Inst.* 1993; 85:2018–23.

99. Remvikos Y, Tominaga O, Hammel P, et al. Increased p53 protein content of colorectal tumours correlates with poor survival. *Br J Cancer.* 1992; 66:758–64.

100. Sarkis AS, Dalbagni G, Cordon-Cardo C, et al. Nuclear overexpression of p53 protein in transitional cell bladder carcinoma: a marker for disease progression. *J Natl Cancer Inst.* 1993; 85:53–9.

101. Starzynska T, Bromley M, Ghosh A, Stern PL. Prognostic significance of *p53* overexpression in gastric and colorectal carcinoma. *Br J Cancer.* 1992; 66:558–62.

102. Thor A, Moore DH, Edgerton SM, et al. Accumulation of *p53* tumor suppressor gene protein: an independent marker of prognosis in breast cancers. *J Natl Cancer Inst.* 1992; 84:845–55.

103. Thorlacius S, Borresen A, Eyfjörd J. Somatic *p53* mutations in human breast carcinomas in an Icelandic population: a prognostic factor. *Cancer Res.* 1993; 53:1637–41.

104. Visakorpi T, Kallioniemi OP, Heikkinen A, Koivula T, Isola J. Small subgroup of aggressive, highly proliferative prostatic carcinomas defined by p53 accumulation. *J Natl Cancer Inst.* 1992; 84:883–7.

105. Greenblatt MS, Bennett WP, Hollstein M, Harris CC. Mutations in the *p53* tumor suppressor gene: clues to cancer etiology and molecular pathogenesis. *Cancer Res.* 1994; 54:4855–78.

106. Velculescu VE, El-Deiry WS. Biological and clinical importance of the *p53* tumor suppressor gene. *Clin Chem.* 1996; 42:858–68.

107. Jones DR, Davidson AG, Summers CL, Murray GF, Quinlan DC. Potential application of p53 as an intermediate biomarker in Barrett's esophagus. *Ann Thorac Surg.* 1994; 57:598–603.

108. Nuorva K, Soini Y, Kamel D, et al. Concurrent *p53* expression in bronchial dysplasias and squamous cell lung carcinomas. *Am J Pathol.* 1993; 142:725–32.

109. Sozzi G, Miozzo M, Donghi R, et al. Deletions of *17p* and *p53* mutations in preneoplastic lesions of the lung. *Cancer Res.* 1992; 52:6079–82.

110. Wang LD, Hong JY, Qiu S, Gao H, Yang CS. Accumulation of p53 protein in human esophageal precancerous lesions: a possible early biomarker for carcinogenesis. *Cancer Res.* 1993; 53:1873–77.

111. Ahuja H, Bar-Eli M, Arlin Z, et al. The spectrum of molecular alterations in the evolution of chronic myelocytic leukemia. *J Clin Invest.* 1991; 87:2042–47.

112. Crook T, Vousden KH. Properties of *p53* mutations detected in primary and secondary cervical cancers suggest mechanisms of metastasis and involvement of environmental carcinogens. *EMBO J.* 1992; 11:3935–40.

113. Crook T, Wrede D, Tidy J, et al. Clonal *p53* mutation in primary cervical cancer: association with human-papillomavirus-negative tumours. *Lancet.* 1992; 339:1070–3.

114. Donghi R, Longoni A, Pilotti S, Michieli P, Della Porta G, Pierotti MA. Gene *p53* mutations are restricted to poorly differentiated and undifferentiated carcinomas of the thyroid gland. *J Clin Invest.* 1993; 91:1753–60.

115. Foti A, Ahuja HG, Allen SL, et al. Correlation between molecular and clinical events in the evolution of chronic myelocytic leukemia to blast crisis. *Blood.* 1991; 77: 2441–44.

116. Haapasalo H, Isola J, Sallinen P, Kalimo H, Helin H, Rantala I. Aberrant *p53* expression in astrocytic neoplasms of the brain: association with proliferation. *Am J Pathol.* 1993; 142:1347–51.

117. Ito T, Seyama T, Mizuno T, et al. Unique association of *p53* mutations with undifferentiated but not with differentiated carcinomas of the thyroid gland. *Cancer Res.* 1992; 52:1369–71.

118. Kakeji Y, Korenaga D, Tsujitani S, et al. Gastric cancer with *p53* overexpression has high potential for metastasising to lymph nodes. *Br J Cancer.* 1993; 67:589–93.

119. Sidransky D, Mikkelsen T, Schwachheirner K, Rosenblum ML, Cavanee W, Vogelstein B. Clonal expansion of *p53* mutant cells associated with brain tumour progression. *Nature.* 1992; 355:846–7.

120. Wada H, Asada M, Nakazawa S, et al. Clonal expansion of *p53* mutant cells in leukemia progression in vitro. *Leukemia.* 1994; 8:53–9.

121. Kresser U, Inganas M, Byding S, et al. Prognostic value of *p53* genetic changes in colorectal cancer. *J Clin Oncol.* 1999; 17:593–9.

122. Berns EM, Klijn JG, van Putten WL, et al. p53 protein accumulation predicts poor response to tamoxifen therapy of patients with recurrent breast cancer. *J Clin Oncol.* 1998; 16:121–7.

123. Archer SG, Eliopoulos A, Spandidos D, et al. Expression of *ras, p21, p53* and c-*erbB*-2 in advanced breast cancer and response to first line hormonal therapy. *Br J Cancer.* 1995; 72:1259–66.

124. Bergh J. Clinical studies of p53 in treatment and benefit of breast cancer patients. 1999, in press.

125. Aas T, Borresen AL, Geisler S, et al. Specific *p53* mutations are associated with de novo resistance to doxorubicin in breast cancer patients. *Nat Med.* 1996; 2:811–14.

126. Larsson L, Carlsson G, Sjögren S, et al. Mutations in the *p53* gene predict the outcome of adjuvant therapy in node-positive patients with breast cancer. *Proc Am Soc Clin Oncol.* 1999, 18:610a (abstract 2356).

127. Linn SC, Pinedo HM, van Ark-Otte J, et al. Expression of drug resistance proteins in breast cancer, in relation to chemotherapy. *Int J Cancer.* 1997; 71:787–95

128. Al-Azraqi A, Chapman C, Challen C, et al. *p53* mutations in primary human ovarian cancer as a determinant of resistance to carboplatin. *Proc Am Assoc Cancer Res.* 1995; 36:228 (abstr 1356).

129. Diccianni MB, Yu J, Hsiao M, Mukherjee S, Shao LE, Yu AL. Clinical significance of *p53* mutations in relapsed T cell acute lymphoblastic leukemia. *Blood.* 1994; 84:3105–12.

130. Ichikawa A, Kinoshita T, Watanabe T, et al. Mutations of the *p53* gene as a prognostic factor in aggressive B-cell lymphoma. *N Engl J Med.* 1997; 337:529–34.

131. Smith-Sorensen B, Kaern J, Holm R, et al. Therapy effect of either paclitaxel or cyclophos-

phamide combination treatment in patients with epithelial ovarian cancer and relation to *TP53* gene status. *Br J Cancer.* 1998; 78:375–81.

132. Wattel E, Preudhomme C, Hacquet B, et al. *p53* mutations are associated with resistance to chemotherapy and short survival in hematologic malignancies. *Blood.* 1994; 84:3148–57.

5

Circulating Tumor Markers

Alan Horwich and Gill Ross

Introduction

The concept of a circulating tumor marker applies to a secreted chemical product of a tumor cell such that the concentration of the chemical in the blood may in some way represent a quantifiable assessment of the tumor burden at that time. Probably the earliest examples were the proteins produced from myeloma cells discovered by Bence Jones in the mid-19th century. Currently the range of possible tumor markers is broad; however, relatively few have been incorporated in routine oncologic practice (Table 1). The clinical roles of circulating markers might include screening; diagnosis; staging; assessment of prognosis; and monitoring of response, remission, and relapse. Additionally, as relatively specific tumor products, marker substances may confer tissue specificity for immunohistochemistry (IHC) and antibody (Ab)-based techniques for imaging and therapy.

To be useful in clinical practice, an ideal marker should be both sensitive and specific. Furthermore, the marker test should reliably indicate the situation to which there is an appropriate therapeutic response.

The sensitivity of a test is the probability of the test being positive in patients with the disease. Based on the symbols in Table 2, sensitivity equals $A/(A+C)$. The specificity of the test is the probability of a normal test result in patients without the cancer. From Table 2, specificity equals $D/(B+D)$. A further concept of value in judging markers is the positive predictive value, which is the probability of a patient having the cancer when the test is positive [i.e., the number of true positive results divided by the total number of positive results: $A/(A+B)$].

These relatively simple concepts become more complex for marker tests where there is no clear cutoff between a normal and abnormal result, for example, with a measure of prostate-specific antigen (PSA) as a diagnostic test for prostate cancer (discussed later). In this setting, higher values of the marker represent a greater probability of the presence of prostate cancer and the appropriate choice of cutoff level for finding cancer may depend upon patient-related factors such as age *(1)*.

From: *Principles of Molecular Oncology*
Edited by: M. H. Bronchud, M. A. Foote, W. P. Peters, and M. O. Robinson © Humana Press Inc., Totowa, NJ

Table 1
Circulating Markers in Oncology

Marker	Abbreviation	Tumor(s)
Human chorionic gonadotrophin	hcG	Gestational trophoblastic Germ cell Urothelial Gastrointestinal
α-Fetoprotein	AFP	Germ-cell hepatocellular
Lactate dehydrogenase	LDH	Germ cell
Placental alkaline phosphatase	PLAP	Germ cell Lymphoma
Prostate-specific antigen	PSA	Prostate
Carcinoembryonic antigen	CEA	Gastrointestinal, esp. colorectal; Breast
Neuron specific enolase	NSE	Small cell lung cancer Neuroendocrine
CA125	—	Ovarian
CA19.9	—	Pancreas Gastrointestinal Ovarian

Table 2
Evaluation of a Marker Test[a]

	Marker positive	Marker negative
Cancer present	A	B
Cancer absent	C	D

[a]Sensitivity, A/(A+B); specificity, D/(C+D); predictive value, A/(A+C).

Use of Markers for Particular Cancers

Testicular Cancer

The serum tumor markers α-fetoprotein (AFP) and human chorionic gonadotropin (hCG) are in widespread clinical use to aid in the diagnosis and management of patients with nonseminomatous tumors, one or both of these markers being increased in approx 75% of patients with metastatic disease *(2–4)*. More recently, lactate dehydrogenase (LDH) has proven useful in assessment of prognosis *(5)*. (These markers are discussed in greater detail.) There has been some assessment of the use of placental-like alkaline phosphatase (PLAP) as a tumor marker for seminoma; however, the level of sensitivity and specificity of assays developed to date have not encouraged widespread use of PLAP as a serum marker *(6,7)*.

α-*Fetoprotein*

AFP is an embryonic protein produced by the yolk sac and subsequently by the fetal liver. It has a molecular mass of 70,000 Da, is structurally similar to albumin, and probably serves a similarly diverse number of functions in the fetus. Serum levels decrease around the time of birth; when found in the serum of adults, it is indicative of hepatocellular carcinoma *(8,9)*. AFP has also been found in a proportion of patients with testicular nonseminoma and occasionally other tumors *(10)*. In nonseminoma, AFP is usually associated with yolk sac differentiation. The general view is that AFP is not produced by pure seminoma despite a small number of case reports of the association.

Human Chorionic Gonadotropin

hCG production is mainly from syncytiotrophoblastic cells. It is a hormone of molecular weight 45,000 Da and is produced normally by the placenta. It comprises two dissimilar subunits, α and β. The amino-acid sequence of the α-subunit is similar to that of some other human hormones including luteinizing hormone (LH), follicle-stimulating hormone (FSH), and thyroid-stimulating hormone (TSH). The β-subunit is unique, although it shares some amino-acid sequence with the LH subunit. The usual Ab-based assays for hCG are directed at the β-subunit but measure both intact hCG and the β fragments. Normal values, except during pregnancy, are generally <2 international units per liter (IU/L) with normal urinary values <30 IU/L.

Staging of Testicular Cancer

One or both of the tumor markers AFP and hCG are increased in the serum of about 75% of patients with metastatic nonseminoma. Moderate increases of hCG are found in 33–50% of patients with seminoma. In most cases, the diagnosis of a testicular germ-cell tumor is not difficult on clinical grounds, although the presence of a palpably abnormal testis may indicate a tumor or a possible diagnosis of local granulomatous infection. When the tumor is painful, there may be confusion with epididymoorchitis or torsion. The presence of an increased marker can complement further investigations such as local ultrasound. Furthermore, in approx 5% of germ-cell tumors, the primary site remains occult, possibly because it is extragonadal, or alternatively because the primary tumor has remained microscopic or infarcted. In these cases, the presentation may be with lymphadenopathy; retroperitoneal or mediastinal mass; or, rarely, a pineal or pelvic tumor.

Additionally, tumor markers can help in staging assessments including prognosis. Typically, staging occurs after orchidectomy and comprises assessment of tumor markers and a computed tomography (CT) scan of thorax and abdomen. The presence of an elevated AFP or hCG after orchidectomy does not automatically indicate the presence of metastatic disease because of the time needed for clearing of these markers from the serum. The physiological half-life of hCG as determined by a standard immunoassay is approx 36 h; half-life for AFP, 5–7 d. Thus, particularly for AFP, patients whose tumor has been completely resected by orchidectomy may have abnormal AFP levels in the serum for some weeks. Therefore, staging assessments after orchidectomy require a sequence of markers for accurate interpretation.

AFP, hCG, and LDH are tumor products that have contributed considerably to accurate assessment of prognosis and appropriate management of patients with metastatic nonseminoma *(11)*. An International Germ Cell Cancer Collaborative Group (IGCCCG) produced a database containing more than 5000 patients with advanced

Table 3
International Germ Cell Cancer Collaborative Group Prognosis Schedule

Prognosis	Definition
Good (5- yr survival 92%)	Testis/retroperitoneal primary and No nonpulmonary visceral metastases and Low serum markers (AFP <1000 ng/mL, hCG <5000 U/L, and LDH <1.5 × NUL)
Intermediate (5-yr survival 80%)	As for good prognosis but with Intermediate serum markers (AFP = 1000–10,000 ng/mL, hCG 5000–50,000 U/L, or LDH 1.5–10 × NUL)
Poor (5-yr survival 48%)	Mediastinal primary or Nonpulmonary visceral metastases or High markers (AFP > 10,000 ng/mL, or hCG 50,000 U/L, or LDH>10 × NUL)

Abbreviations: AFP, α-fetoprotein; hCG, human chorionic gonadotropin; LDH, lactate dehydrogenase; NUL, normal upper limit.

nonseminoma who had been treated with platinum-based chemotherapy schedules. This work led to publication of a consensus stratification of germ-cell cancer prognosis (Table 3). Apart from a somewhat uncommon situation of primary mediastinal germ-cell cancer or the presence of nonpulmonary visceral metastases (usually liver, bone, or brain), the division of patients into three prognostic groups is based entirely on marker concentrations; these allow categorization of prognosis ranging from a group with an identified 48% 5-yr survival to a group with a 92% 5-yr survival with the presumption in this particular tumor that 5-yr survivals equate to cure rates.

In this study, prognosis of patients with metastatic seminoma was dominated by the rare adverse subgroup with nonpulmonary visceral metastases. However, a more detailed analysis of 286 of these patients (12) and a series of patients from the Memorial Sloan-Kettering Cancer Center *(13)* demonstrated that an increased serum LDH was also an independent adverse indicator.

Monitoring of Response in Testicular Cancer

Because AFP, hCG, and LDH represent tumor products, it is anticipated that a decline in the number of marker-producing tumor cells would lead to a decline in the serum concentration of the marker. It should also be recognized that a change in marker concentration could follow alteration in the rate of production of marker per cell and that the concentration of marker in the serum represents a balance between production and metabolism/excretion. Thus, although a decline in serum marker is encouraging evidence of response, occasionally the pattern of decline can be complex *(14).* Aspects that have been investigated include:

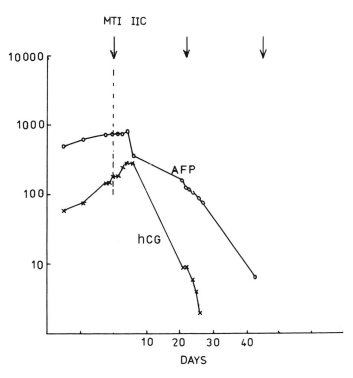

Fig. 1. Marker surge phenomenon after chemotherapy for germ cell tumor. *Arrows* indicate start of chemotherapy cycle. AFP, α-fetoprotein; hCG, human chorionic gonadotropin.

- The surge phenomenon refers to a transient initial increase in marker after initiation of chemotherapy (Fig. 1) which has been thought to be due either to release of stored marker or to an impact of chemotherapy on tumor differentiation *(15,16)*.
- The rate of serum marker decline after start of chemotherapies: Horwich and Peckham *(14)* found that this was not a precise prognostic factor based on a simple comparison of marker level on d 21 of chemotherapy compared with the value before chemotherapy on d 1 with the result expressed as an apparent half-life in days. It was found that the hCG half-life in 22 patients who subsequently remained relapse-free ranged from 2.5 to 9 d (mean, 4.4 d). Of the 7 patients who relapsed after chemotherapy, hCG half-life was within the same range in 6. One patient with very extensive disease had a prolonged half-life of 34 d; this patient never achieved clinical or marker remission. There was a narrow range of AFP half-life for patients remaining disease-free (5–9 d); for 11 patients who relapsed, the range of AFP half-life was 6–14 d. However, all 3 patients with half-life >9 d relapsed.

It seems that for most patients the initial marker pattern was determined by tumor cells that were sensitive to chemotherapy such that even those who relapsed after chemotherapy had a dramatic initial response. The possible exception is the population of patients with drug-resistant disease and AFP-producing tumors. de Wit et al. *(17)* studied 669 patients treated with cisplatin combination chemotherapy. Sixty-three percent had abnormal AFP values at the start of chemotherapy and 58% had abnormal hCG. In the half-time analysis confined to those patients with abnormal marker concentration 3 wk after the start of chemotherapy, it was found that prolongation either of hCG or AFP half-lives did not accurately predict treatment failure. However, studies at the

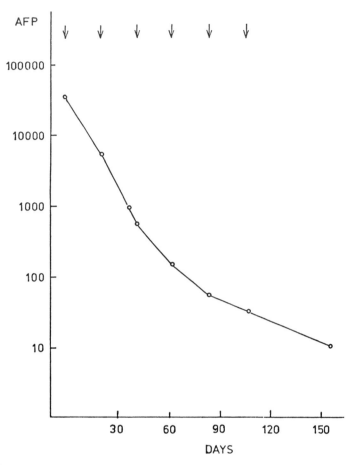

Fig. 2. Late changes in marker regression rate. *Arrows* indicate start of chemotherapy cycle.

Memorial Sloan-Kettering Cancer Center have identified marker regression rate as a useful predictor of outcome after chemotherapy. These studies were based on the rate of regression after two cycles of therapy as prolonged half-life defined for hCG as >3 d and for AFP >7 d. Marker regression was deemed satisfactory either if less than these values or if the marker decreased to within normal limits (complete marker response). Satisfactory decline was associated with a median event-free survival of 20.7 mo *(18)*.

- Late change in marker regression rate (Fig. 2) has unclear significance. In general, continued regression is seen as equivalent to continued response although clearly a change in slope may be a harbinger of overt marker increase and relapse. For patients presenting with high serum hCG levels, a slowing in the rate of decline of marker concentration in the serum is common even in patients who are cured by their initial chemotherapy *(19)*.
- More than half of patients treated with chemotherapy for bulky germ-cell tumors have evidence of a residual mass at the site of their previous disease when assessed by CT scanning after completion of the course of chemotherapy. For nonseminomas, these masses

may represent fully differentiated or mature teratoma, areas of extensive necrosis, undifferentiated persisting germ-cell tumors, or a combination. For seminoma, the masses may be entirely fibrotic although a proportion contain residual viable seminoma. Tumor markers can have a valuable role in diagnosis of the presence of persisting undifferentiated tumor in these settings, and can offer a useful guide to appropriate management.

Monitoring of Remission in Testicular Cancer

Serum markers can help in the continued monitoring of patients after completion of their initial treatment. From 5% to 10% of patients who have had a satisfactory response to initial treatment will nonetheless relapse. The expression of markers at the time of relapse is approximately equivalent in frequency to expression of markers at presentation. However, change in pattern of marker expression in the individual patient can be noted, and thus sensitive monitoring requires an analysis of markers even in those patients whose original tumors were not apparently marker positive.

Tumor Markers in Prostate Cancer

Introduction

The first marker used for prostate cancer was prostatic acid phosphatase (PAP). The acid phosphatases are found in a variety of tissues and their isozymes have different properties and substrate specificities. PAP is predominantly composed of two of the isozymes which are also found in granulocytes and pancreas and may be abnormal in concentration in the serum in a range of conditions including polycythemia rubra vera, granulocytic leukemia, Gaucher's disease, and pancreatic cancer. PAP has a molecular mass of 100,000 Da and is produced by the epithelial cells lining the prostatic acini. It is found in high concentration in prostatic fluid and elevated amounts are found in the serum of more than 75% of patients with metastatic prostate cancer. To avoid false-positive results, it is important that a blood sample is not taken immediately after rectal examination. Currently, serum PAP measurements have a limited role in view of the relatively low sensitivity and specificity of this marker. In practice, it has been replaced by serum PSA.

PSA is an important marker for prostate cancer with relevance for population screening for diagnosis, for prognosis, and for monitoring of treatment effects, and as a possible target mechanism in research on gene therapy. PSA is a glycoprotein of molecular mass 34,000 Da and is produced by prostatic epithelium. It is a serine protease whose function is thought to be to liquefy seminal coagulum by proteolysis. The gene encoding PSA is on chromosome 19 and occupies approx 6 kb.

PSA is measured in the serum by radioimmunoassay and the test kits may vary slightly in their normal range. Elevated amounts are found both in patients with benign prostatic conditions and those with prostate cancer. As discussed, there have been attempts to increase the sensitivity and specificity in PSA diagnosis of prostate cancer by refining the concentration using parameters such as PSA density (relating to size of the prostate gland), PSA velocity (rate of change with time), PSA relating to age, PSA fractionation (free vs bound), and measurement of cells in the circulation expressing PSA mRNA.

PSA in Diagnosis

As with PAP, PSA values can be increased by prior digital rectal examination, although it is rare for this examination to elevate the value beyond the normal range *(20)*. The incidence of an elevated PSA increases with the stage of the tumor from approx 40% in patients with occult presentations to 70% in those with tumors penetrating the capsule to almost 100% in patients with extension of the primary tumor to seminal vesicles or involvement of local lymph nodes *(21,22)*.

There have been a number of large studies designed to evaluate PSA in the screening of prostate cancer. For example, in more than 1200 men over 50 yr of age, serum PSA was found to be increased in 187 (15%), 32 of whom had cancer detected by biopsy (detection rate, 2–6%) *(23)*. In a similar study based on 1653 patients, PSA was between 4 and 9.9 ng/mL in 107 (6.5%) and >10 ng/mL in 30 (1.8%) men. Cancer was eventually diagnosed in 22% of the former and in 66% of the latter, with an overall detection rate of cancer in the study of 2.2% *(24)*. However, not all screen-detected cancers are associated with an abnormal PSA and in a typical series, 20% of such tumors are associated with a normal value *(25,26)*.

Though PSA offers a relatively inexpensive and highly acceptable screening test for prostate cancer, the rationale of this technology must be based on its specificity and on a demonstration that early treatment of the disease improves the prognosis. A formal screening trial in prostate cancer has not yet been completed, and therefore PSA screening has not been adopted in all countries.

PSA and Staging

As discussed, the incidence of an abnormal PSA value increases with advancing stage of the cancer. There is an increase in the mean PSA with advancing stage. This is likely to be a consequence of the relationship between serum PSA and the volume of the prostate tumor *(27)*.

The study by Partin et al. *(28)* demonstrated that the mean serum PSA was 5–6 ng/mL in patients with organ-confined cancers, 7.7 ng/mL in those with localized cancers but capsular penetration, 23.2 ng/mL in those with seminal vesicle involvement, and 26.2 ng/mL in those with involved lymph nodes. The level of PSA may also be useful in the prediction of bone scan findings. A study in 521 patients with newly diagnosed prostate cancer revealed that of those with a PSA of 20 ng/mL or less (*n* = 306) only 1 had a positive bone scan and no patient with a PSA of <10 ng/mL had a positive bone scan *(29)*.

PSA as a Marker of Response to Treatment

As may be predicted, a decrease in PSA to undetectable levels after radical prostatectomy defines a subset of patients with a good prognosis *(30)*. This finding has been confirmed by biopsy studies after prostatectomy which are more frequently positive in patients with an increased PSA *(31)*. This assay can provide a key indication for post-prostatectomy irradiation. In this setting, the rate of increase of PSA can be helpful in distinguishing those patients with locoregional disease from those with advanced metastatic disease, as the latter tend to have a doubling time of <6 mo.

After radiotherapy for localized prostate cancer, the serum PSA has been found to decrease with a half-life of between 1 and 3 mo *(32,33)*. This slow regression reflects the known slow disappearance of malignancy after radiotherapy, thought to be a consequence of tumor cell death occurring only on attempted cell division. However, a longitudinal study has suggested that PSA values regress very predominantly in the first year after treatment; continued regression after 1 yr appeared in only 8% of patients *(27)*. In a different study based on 143 patients followed for a median of 27 mo after radiotherapy, 94% of those patients whose PSA normalized within 6 mo remained relapse-free compared with only 8% of those whose serum PSA remained increased after 6 mo.

PSA after Hormonal Therapy

There is a clear correlation between PSA response and clinical response to hormone therapy *(21)*. The degree of decrease of PSA is an indicator of remission duration *(34)*. An increase in serum PSA after hormone therapy is a predictor of clinical progression with a mean lead time of approx 7 mo. Although the value of this is much less established, there also appears to be a relationship between decrease in serum PSA and patient benefit *(35,36)*.

Gastrointestinal Tumors

Carcinoembryonic Antigen

Carcinoembryonic antigen (CEA), a 200,000 Da glycoprotein, was isolated in 1965 by Gold and Freemen using an Ab raised by injection of an extract derived from human colonic carcinoma into rabbits. Immunochemical electron microscopy techniques can demonstrate the presence of this protein in normal colonic columnar cells.

Assays are now available using both polyclonal and monoclonal antibodies (mAbs). Serum CEA values are increased in carcinomas of the gastrointestinal tract (GI), but can also be raised in a variety of nonmalignant conditions, reducing the specificity of the test. These nonmalignant conditions include GI inflammation, collagen disorders, infection, trauma, infarction, renal impairment, and smoking. Generally, however, values achieved in these conditions do not reach those documented in colonic malignancy. The low sensitivity and specificity of serum CEA precludes its routine use in screening general populations for colorectal cancer; hence interest has turned to evaluating its use in assessing prognosis or monitoring therapy in established disease.

The value of preoperative CEA level as an independent prognostic marker is not clear, although values broadly reflect tumor burden, and increase and decrease with response to therapy *(37)*. Serum CEA values should decrease to normal within 6 wk of complete tumor resection. Fewer than 5% of patients with Dukes A colorectal carcinoma will have increased serum CEA, increasing to 25% of Dukes B cases, 44% of Dukes C cases, and 65% of patients with metastatic disease. A number of authors have reported that increased amounts of CEA predict increased risk of recurrence *(38–40)*, but others have reported its prognostic value to be limited *(41,42)*. In a large modern series of 377 patients with advanced colorectal cancer, serum CEA was an independent predictor of survival *(43)*.

Monitoring for recurrent disease status by serum CEA is of limited value *(44)*. Up to 30% of patients with recurring disease will have normal levels.

Increased amounts of serum CEA can be found in patients with advanced noncolorectal tumors, including breast, lung, cervical, endometrial, and ovarian cancer, and may be useful in monitoring response to therapy.

Ca19.9

This antigen (Ag) was derived from a human colonic adenocarcinoma cell line, and several commercial kits are now available for its clinical measurement. Levels of the Ag are increased in up to 75% of patients with advanced colorectal malignancy. The primary value of this maker currently lies in its greater sensitivity than CEA in monitoring gastric, pancreatic, and biliary tumors *(45)*. Recent research suggests serial analysis of amounts of 19.9 can be used to predict response to radiotherapy in inoperable cases of pancreatic cancer *(46)*, where conventional imaging may have limited clinical sensitivity.

Ovarian Cancer

The Ag CA125 was first reported in 1983 after a murine mAb was raised to a human ovarian cystadenocarcinoma. CA125 is produced by tissues derived from coelomic epithelium, which includes the peritoneum, fallopian tube, endometrium, endocervix, pleura, and pericardium, but not the normal ovary. It is present as a cell-surface glycoprotein in approx 80% of epithelial ovarian tumors, with a serum half-life of 4 d. While levels >35 IU/mL are seen during the first trimester of pregnancy, in a range of benign conditions (cirrhosis, endometriosis), and in advanced intraabdominal malignancies, 99% of normal blood bank donors will have values lower than this. Increases above 35 IU/mL is seen preoperatively in >90% of women with stage III or IV ovarian carcinoma, but only 50% of those with stage I disease. Unfortunately the low specificity of CA125 precludes its use in screening general populations, and its sensitivity is too low to use alone in the screening of high-risk women *(47)*. However, combined with ultrasound and knowledge of menopausal status, CA125 levels provided 85% sensitivity and 98% specificity for the diagnosis of pelvic malignancy in a cohort of 143 women investigated for a pelvic mass *(48)*.

Serial CA125 levels are currently accepted to be the best method of monitoring response to therapy. A decrease of >50% maintained for more than 28 d is highly predictive of response, and conversely, a serial increase of 50% indicates progression. In a detailed study by Mogensen *(49)*, CA125 was measured during early chemotherapy in 121 patients with FIGO stage III or IV ovarian cancer to investigate if the Ag could be used as a prognostic parameter. CA125 was determined before the start of chemotherapy and 1 mo after the first, second, and third courses. The Ag level before the start of chemotherapy held no prognostic information. CA125 was a significant prognostic parameter in all three courses, but its correlation with survival improved with the number of courses. Patients with high marker levels (greater than 100 U/mL) 1 mo after the third course had a median survival of 7 mo. This should be compared with a 50% 5-yr survival in patients who had 10 U/mL or less and a median survival of 22 mo among patients with intermediate CA125 levels. Cox regression analysis of the covariation between survival, CA125, and five variables (age, FIGO stage, histopathology, tumor grade, and bulk of residual tumor) showed that the CA125 value was the most significant prognostic parameter. As a consequence of this study, the authors suggested that chemotherapy of patients with high CA125 values 1 mo after the third course could be discontinued and treated with palliative therapy if other curative regimens are not available. Similar conclusions were reached in a large Medical Research Council (MRC) study involving 573 cases confirming that serum CA125 levels after three cycles of chemotherapy are predictive for the probability of achieving complete remission.

Breast Cancer Related Markers

A number of mAbs have been raised to mucins, high-molecular-weight glycoproteins produced by epithelial cells of the breast. The most heavily investigated mucin marker is known as CA15.3, which is increased in about 11% of women with operable breast cancer, and 60% of women with metastatic disease. It is also increased in 10% of women with benign breast disease. The lack of specificity and low sensitivity preclude the use of CA15.3 in screening or diagnosis of symptomatic breast disease, but serial estimations may be of value in monitoring response of metastatic disease. A prospective study was undertaken to define the optimal combination of bone scan and tumor marker assays in staging a breast cancer cohort of 157 consecutive cases. The results suggest that in asymptomatic patients, a CA15.3 level of < 25 U/mL (upper normal value chosen as the threshold) is strongly predictive of a negative bone scan; by contrast, high tumor marker levels are predictive of neoplastic bone involvement. When a doubtful bone scan is obtained in a patient with breast cancer, a normal marker value makes it highly probable that bone scan abnormalities are not related to malignancy *(50)*.

Summary

Tumor markers are substances that often can be detected in higher-than-normal amounts in serum or tissues of patients with certain forms of cancer. Although measurements of tumor marker levels can be useful when used in conjunction with other clinical tests in the detection and diagnosis of some forms of cancer, measurements of tumor marker values alone are not sufficient to diagnose cancer. The reason is that tumor markers can be increased in patients with benign conditions, but are not increased in every patient with cancer, especially in the early stages of the disease. Many tumor markers are not specific to a particular type of cancer, and the amount of a tumor marker may be increased by more than one type of cancer. Possibly the best use of tumor markers is to assess a patient's response to treatment and to check for recurrence of disease. It is hoped that further research will refine the properties of tumor markers, giving them more clinical utility.

Acknowledgments

This work was undertaken by The Royal Marsden NHS Trust who received a proportion of its funding from the NHS Executive; the views expressed in this publication are those of the authors and not necessarily those of the NHS Executive. This work was also supported by the Institute of Cancer Research and the Bob Champion Trust and the Cancer Research Campaign.

References

1. Brawer MK. How to use prostate-specific antigen in the early detection or screening for prostatic carcinoma. *CA Cancer J Clin.* 1995; 45:148–64.
2. Perlin E, Engeler J, Edson M, Karp D, McIntire KR, Waldman TA. The value of serial measurement of both HCG and AFP for monitoring germ cell tumours. *Cancer.* 1976; 37:215–9.
3. Norgaard-Pedersen B, Albrechtsen R, Bagshawe KD, et al. Clinical use of AFP and HCT in testicular tumours, of germ, cell origin. *Lancet.* 1978, ii:1042.
4. Thompson DK, Haddow JE. Serial monitoring of serum alpha-fetoprotein and chorionic gonadotropin in males with germ cell tumors. *Cancer.* 1979; 43:1820–9.
5. International Germ Cell Cancer Group. International germ cell consensus classification: a prognostic factor-based staging system for metastatic germ cell cancers. *J Clin Oncol.* 1997; 15:594–603.
6. Tucker DF, Oliver RT, Travers P, Bodiner WF. Serum marker potential of placental alkaline phosphatase-like activity in germ cell tumours evaluated by H17 E2 monoclonal antibody assay. *Br J Cancer.* 1985; 51:631–9.
7. Horwich A, Tucker DF, Peckham MJ. Placental alkaline phosphatase as a tumour marker in seminoma using the H17 E2 monoclonal antibody assay. *Br J Cancer.* 1985; 51:625–9.
8. Tatarinov Y. Detection of embryo-specific alpha globulin in the blood sera of patients with primary liver tumour. *Vopr Med Khim.* 1964; 10:90–1.
9. Kohn J, Weaver P. Serum-alpha-1-fetoprotein in hepatocellular carcinoma. *Lancet.* 1974; 2:344–6.
10. Waldmann TA, McIntire KR. The use of a radioimmunoassay for alpha-fetoprotein in the diagnosis of malignancy. *Cancer.* 1974; 34:1510–5.
11. Horwich A, Huddart R, Dearnaley D. Markers and management of germ-cell tumours of the testes. *Lancet.* 1998; 352:1535–8.
12. Wanderas EH, Fossa SD, Tretli S. Risk of a second germ cell cancer after treatment of a primary germ cell cancer in 2201 Norwegian male patients. *Br J Cancer.* 1997; 33:244–52.
13. Mencel PJ, Motzer RJ, Mazumdar M, Vlarnis V, Bajorin DF, Bosl GJ. Advanced seminoma: treatment results, survival, and prognostic factors in 142 patients. *J Clin Oncol.* 1994; 12:120–6.
14. Horwich A, Peckham MJ. Serum tumour marker regression rate following chemotherapy for malignant teratoma. *Eur J Cancer Clin Oncol.* 1984; 20:1463–70.
15. Speeg KV, Azizkhan JC, Stromberg K. The stimulation by methotrexate of human chorionic gonadotrophin and placental alkaline phosphatase in cultured choriocarcinoma cells. *Cancer Res.* 1976; 36:4570–6.
16. Browne P, Bagshawe KD. Enhancement of human chorionic gonadotrophin production by antimetabolites. *Br J Cancer.* 1982; 46:22–9.
17. de Wit R, Sylvester R, Tsitsa C, et al. Tumour marker concentration at the start of chemotherapy is a stronger predictor of treatment failure than marker half-life: a study in patients with disseminated non-seminomatous testicular cancer. *Br J Cancer.* 1997; 75:432–5.
18. Murphy BA, Motzer RJ, Mazumdar M, et al. Serum tumor marker decline is an early predictor of treatment outcome in germ cell tumor patients treated with cisplatin and ifosfamide salvage chemotherapy. *Cancer.* 1994; 73:2520–6.
19. Andreyev HM, Dearnaley DP, Horwich A. Testicular non-seminoma with high serum human chorionic gonadotrophin: the trophoblastic teratoma syndrome. *Diagn Oncol.* 1993; 3:67–71.

20. Chybowski FM, Bergstralh EJ, Oesterling JE. The effect of digital rectal examination on the serum prostate specific antigen concentration: results of a randomized study. *J Urol.* 1992; 148:83–6.
21. Ercole CJ, Lange PH, Mathisen M, Chiou RK, Reddy PK, Vessella RL. Prostatic specific antigen and prostatic acid phosphatase in the monitoring and staging of patients with prostatic cancer. *J Urol.* 1987; 138:1181–4.
22. Oesterling JE, Chan DW, Epstein JI, et al. Prostate specific antigen in the preoperative and postoperative evaluation of localized prostatic cancer treated with radical prostatectomy. *J Urol.* 1988; 139:766–72.
23. Brawer MK, Chetner M, Beatie J, Buchner DM, Bessella RL, Lange PH. Screening for prostatic carcinoma with prostate specific antigen, *J Urol.* 1992; 137:841–5.
24. Catalona WJ, Smith DS, Ratliff TL, et al. Measurement of prostate-specific antigen in serum as a screening test for prostate cancer. *N Engl J Med.* 1991; 324:1156–61.
25. Cooner WH, Mosley BR, Rutherford CJ, Jr, et al. Prostate cancer detection in a clinical urological practice by ultrasonography, digital rectal examination and prostate specific antigen. *J Urol.* 1990; 143:1146–52.
26. Labrie F, Dupont A, Suburu R, et al. Serum prostate specific antigen as pre-screening test for prostate cancer. *J Urol.* 1992; 147:846–851.
27. Stamey TA, Kabalin JN, Ferrari M, Yang N. Prostate specific antigen in the diagnosis and treatment of adenocarcinoma of the prostate. IV. Anti-androgen treated patients, *J. Urol.* 1989; 141:1088–90.
28. Partin AW, Carter HB, Chan DW, et al. Prostate specific antigen in the staging of localized prostate cancer: influence of tumor differentiation, tumor volume and benign hyperplasia. *J Urol.* 1990; 143:747–52.
29. Chybowski FM, Keller JJ, Bergstralh EJ, et al. Predicting radionuclide bone scan findings in patients with newly diagnosed untreated prostate cancer. Prostate specific antigen is superior to all other clinical parameters. *J Urol.* 1991; 145:313–8.
30. Lange PH, Ercole CJ, Lightner DJ, et al. The value of serum prostate specific antigen determination before and after radical prostatectomy. *J Urol.* 1991; 141:313–8.
31. Lightner DJ, Lange PH, Reddy PK, Moore L. Prostate specific antigen and local recurrence after radical prostatectomy. *J Urol.* 1990; 144:921–6.
32. Meek AG, Park TL, Oberman E, Wielopolski L. A prospective study of prostate specific antigen levels in patients receiving radiotherapy for localized carcinoma of the prostate. *Int J Radiat Oncol Biol Phys.* 1990; 19:733–41.
33. Ritter MA, Messing EM, Shanahan TG, Potts S, Chappell RJ, Kinsella TJ. Prostate-specific antigen as a predictor of radiotherapy response and patterns of failure in localized prostate cancer. *J Clin Oncol.* 1992; 10:1208–17.
34. Miller PD, Eardley I, Kirby RS. Prostate specific antigen and bone scan correlation in the staging and monitoring of patients with prostatic cancer. *Br J Urol.* 1992; 70:295–8.
35. Kelly WK, Scher HI, Mazumdar M, Vlamis V, Schwartz M, Fossa SD. Prostate-specific antigen as a measure of disease outcome in metastatic hormone-refractory prostate cancer. *J Clin Oncol.* 1993; 11:607–15.
36. Tannock IF, Osoba D, Stockler MR, et al. Chemotherapy with mitroxantrone plus Prednisone or Prednisone along for symptomatic hormone-resistant prostate cancer: a Canadian randomised trial with palliative end points. *J Clin Oncol.* 1996; 14:1756–64.
37. Primrose JN, Bleiberg H, Daniel F, et al. Marimasat in recurrent colorectal cancer-. exploratory evaluation of biological activity by measurement of carcinoembryonic antigen. *Br J Cancer.* 1999; 79:509–14.

38. Aabo K, Pedersen H, Kjaer M. Carcinoembryonic antigen (CEA) and alkaline phosphatase in progressive colorectal cancer with special reference to patient survival. *Eur J Cancer Clin Oncol.* 1986; 22:211–7.

39. Staab HJ, Anderer FA, Biummendorf T, Stumpf E, Fischer R. Prognostic value of preoperative serum CEA level compared to clinical staging. *Br J Cancer.* 1981; 44:652–62.

40. Wanebo HJ, Rao B, Pinskey C. Preoperative carcinoembryonic antigen level as a prognostic indicator in colorectal cancer. *N Engl J Med.* 1978; 299:448–51.

41. Lewi H, Blumgart LH, Carter DC. Pre-operative carcino-embryonic antigen and survival in patients with colorectal cancer. *Br J Surg.* 1984; 71:206–8.

42. Goslin R, Steele G, MacIntyre J. The use of preoperative plasma CEA levels for the stratification of patients after curative resection of colorectal cancer. *Ann Surg.* 1980; 192:747–9.

43. Webb A, Scott-Mackie P, Cunningham D. The prognostic value of CEA, beta HCG, AFP, CA125, CA19-9 and C-erb B- 2, beta HCG immunohistochemistry in advanced colorectal cancer. *Ann Oncol.* 1995; 6:581–7.

44. Weiss NS, Cook LS. Evaluating the efficacy of screening for recurrence of cancer. *J Natl Cancer Inst.* 1998; 90:1870–2.

45. Safi F, Schlosser W, Kolb G, Beger HG. Diagnostic value of CA 19-9 in patients with pancreatic cancer and non specific gastrointestinal symptoms. *J Gastrointest Surg.* 1997; 1:106–12.

46. Okusaka T, Okada S, Sato T, et al. Tumor markers in evaluating the response to radiotherapy in unresectable pancreatic cancer. *Hepatogastroenterology.* 1998; 45:867–72.

47. Jacobs I, Davies AP, Bridges J. Prevalence screening for ovarian cancer in postmenopausal women by CA 125 measurement and ultrasonography. *Br Med J.* 1993; 306:1030–4.

48. Jacobs I, Oram D, Fairbanks J, Turner J, Frost C, Grudzinskas JG. A risk of malignancy index incorporating CA 125, ultrasound and menopausal status for the accurate preoperative, diagnosis of ovarian cancer. *Br J Obstet Gynaecol.* 1990; 97:922–9.

49. Mogensen O. Prognostic value of CA 125 in advanced ovarian cancer. *Gynecol Oncol.* 1992; 44:207–212.

50. Buffaz PD, Gauchez AS, Caravel JP. Can tumour marker assays be a guide in the prescription of bone scan for breast and lung cancers? *Eur J Nucl Med.* 1999; 26:8–11.

II

Diseased Regulatory Pathways

6

Growth Factor-Signaling Pathways in Cancer

Daniel Kalderon

Introduction

Growth factor-signaling pathways were first directly implicated in cancer by the discovery that retroviruses induce cancer in animals by using activated or overexpressed versions of normal genes (proto-oncogenes). These oncogenes encode for membrane-associated receptors (e.g., *erb2* and epidermal growth factor receptor [EGFR]), their extracellular ligands (e.g., v-*sis* and platelet-derived growth factor [PDGF]), cytoplasmic signal transduction molecules (e.g., *src, ras,* and *raf*), or nuclear mitogen-inducible transcription factors (e.g., *jun, fos,* and *myc*). In some cases these same proto-oncogenes were mutationally activated in human tumors (especially constitutively active *ras* and overexpressed *myc*). Other genes were later revealed as tumor suppressors by studies linking gene inactivation with cancer. Again, some tumor suppressors were implicated in growth factor-signaling pathways (e.g., APC–Wnt signaling and Smad4–TGFβ [transforming growth factor] signaling). Others were found to be regulators of the cell cycle (e.g., retinoblastoma protein [Rb] and p16INK4a) or components of checkpoint controls that monitor DNA damage, e.g., *p53,* and respond by inducing cell-cycle arrest or cell death by apoptosis. Further studies of how oncogenes and tumor suppressors fit into signal-transduction pathways, cell-cycle regulation, and regulation of apoptosis have provided a substantial framework for understanding how each genetic change might contribute to cancer and why multiple mutations generally are required for tumorigenesis.

The emerging picture is of a cell that focuses multiple environmental impacts onto the activity of a small group of key regulatory molecules. These molecules collaborate to select one of a few mutually exclusive programs: temporary quiescence, cell division, terminal differentiation, senescence, or apoptosis. These key regulatory molecules (or close relatives) are widely expressed, suggesting a core of regulatory interactions that are common to all cell types. As an example, a number of growth factors lead to activation of Ras, which consequently results in increases in cyclin-dependent kinase (CDK) activities, inhibition of Rb, and progress through the cell cycle. Hence, in most cell types, mutagenic activation of Ras or loss of Rb can contribute to proliferation that is independent of environmental signals.

From: *Principles of Molecular Oncology*
Edited by: M. H. Bronchud, M. A. Foote, W. P. Peters, and M. O. Robinson © Humana Press Inc., Totowa, NJ

The molecular links between members of a signal-transduction pathway and the key regulators of specific cellular programs have been studied primarily in a synthetic tissue culture environment. Animal studies sometimes reveal unexpected outcomes or tissue-specific differences. Similar variability occurs in different tissue culture cell types, particularly when comparing primary and established cells. Moreover, in several instances, particular proto-oncogenes or tumor-suppressor mutations (e.g., *ras*) are associated with specific tumor types in humans. Mutagenic activation of *ras* can promote cell proliferation, differentiation, senescence, or apoptosis depending on the cellular context *(1–3)*. Activated *ras* occurs in many late-stage colorectal adenomas but expression of activated *ras* alone does not promote colonic tumor formation *(4)*.

To understand why various cells respond differently to the same mutagenic event despite a shared core of key regulatory interactions, it is necessary to understand how cells use signaling pathways to control growth and development. This chapter summarizes the principles used by a complex organism to direct development through cell communications. The chapter also describes the molecular details of some major signaling pathways and how they most commonly are subverted by mutations in cancer. Finally, this chapter discusses how these signaling pathways affect the cell cycle, senescence, differentiation, and apoptotic programs and how choices are made among these programs.

Signaling Pathways Were Designed for Development and Homeostasis

During the development of multicellular organisms, including humans, many signals pass between cells to coordinate a variety of temporally and spatially appropriate cellular decisions. The secreted or cell surface-associated molecules that act as signals fall into several traditional families, including hormones, neurotransmitters, growth factors, and adhesion molecules. This classification is based largely on how the signals are dispersed, which ranges from the general circulation of hormones to the synapse-specific release of neurotransmitters. Molecules from each class interact with a recipient cell in much the same way and can elicit responses that include restriction or specification of developmental fate, arrest or initiation of proliferation, and survival or cell death. These cell communication systems are designed so that a limited number of molecules can mediate a large number of decisions without confusion.

The expression of signals and receptors is highly regulated temporally and spatially during development, ensuring specificity of cell communication. To avoid confusion in tissues undergoing several simultaneous signaling events, a moderately large number of different signaling molecules (ligands) and a roughly corresponding number of receptors are involved. Nevertheless, a specific ligand or receptor often appears in more than one place and at more than one time in development *(5)*.

A much more dramatic molecular economy occurs within signal-transduction pathways. The specific message of a particular signal could theoretically be preserved by a signal-transduction pathway that is unique to each receptor; however, this is not the case. Very few entirely distinct signal-transduction pathways exist, so, inevitably, each one can be activated by a wide variety of receptor–ligand pairs. For example, many ligand families, including PDGF, EGF, nerve growth factor (NGF), and fibroblast growth factor (FGF) activate receptor tyrosine kinases (RTKs) and the Ras–MAP kinase (MAPK) pathway, and each depends on this pathway to elicit an appropriate response.

Different signals at different times and sites elicit characteristic responses. Several strategies might be used to achieve different responses. First, the signals and receptors could be the source of specificity. Ligands of the PDGF, EGF, and NGF families activate the Ras–MAPK pathway, but they also activate other signaling pathways. Different ligands might therefore produce qualitative and quantitative differences in the spectrum of respondent signal-transduction pathways, which could be instrumental in conferring an appropriate, unique response. Second, the status of the responding cell also may dictate the appropriate response by altering the concentrations or activities of cytoplasmic signal-transduction components. This could, in turn, alter the responsiveness of specific pathways, again generating a relatively complex signaling code that the cell may be able to translate into a specific action. Third, differences in nuclear targets of signal-transduction pathways and their collaborators may underlie cell-specific responses. These key targets include transcription factors that dictate developmental fate, differentiation, and the expression of regulators of apoptosis and the cell cycle. Based on results from a limited number of relevant developmental studies, cell-specific expression of transcription factors is probably the most common mechanism responsible for producing a unique response to a generic signaling pathway.

In some special situations, ligand concentration is critical. Hedgehog (Hh), Wnts, and TGFβ family members can each dictate cell fate in a concentration-dependent manner *(6–8)*. In some situations, a specific branch of an RTK-signaling pathway is critical in one cell type but not in another *(9)*. More commonly, the nature of the response depends on a cell's developmental history.

In the *Drosophila* leg imaginal disc (an epithelial monolayer that develops into the cuticle of the adult leg), for example, Hh protein induces transcription of the TGFβ family member, *dpp,* in dorsal anterior cells and simultaneously induces the Wnt-family member, *wg,* in ventral anterior cells *(10)*. Neither *dpp* nor *wg* can be induced by activating the Hh signaling pathway in posterior cells because the prior expression of the transcription factor, Engrailed, represses expression of a protein (Ci) that is the key transcriptional effector of the Hh signal-transduction pathway *(11)*. Furthermore, failure to induce *wg* in dorsal anterior cells results from the prior and continued expression of *dpp* in these cells that signals to repress *wg* even in the face of an activating Hh signal *(12)*. Similarly, prior *wg* expression in ventral cells prevents ventral induction of *dpp* by Hh.

A second example of cell status affecting the response to a signal is provided by EGFR in *Drosophila* eye development. Stimulation of EGFR is required for many aspects of eye development, including cell proliferation before differentiation, initiation of neural differentiation that results in an "R8" precursor, successive recruitment and specification of each of the seven photoreceptor types that join the founder R8 cell to form a unit eye, and prevention of subsequent apoptosis of photoreceptor and accessory cells *(13,14)*. A single cell can undergo three different responses to EGFR stimulation within a single day. At least one of these responses is sensitive to the strength of RTK signaling *(15)*, but almost certainly these temporally distinct responses to EGFR stimulation are dictated primarily by successive changes in the status of expression of transcription factors in the responding cells *(16)*.

Based on these and similar observations, a theory emerges that precise orchestration of successive changes (developmental history) in gene expression is the major mechanism used during development to accommodate necessary economies in the number of molecules dedicated to cell communications. Thus, a cell receives a signal to which it is responsive and alters various properties, including induction and repression of specific genes. All or part of the new transcription program then stabilizes through intrinsic mechanisms that involve stable chromatin changes, positive autoregulation, or more complex circuitry among transcription factors. As a result, the cell's new status becomes independent of the initial signal. Negative feedback mechanisms sometimes make the cell refractory to the initial signal during this stabilization period, thereby defining a signaling episode. The cell now has a modified response to a second signal. In some cases, a cell may only now produce receptors only for the second signal, become the source of a second signal to which other cells respond, or move to a new environment in response to the first signal.

Repeated use of this strategy produces a complex choreography of patterns of gene expression that is preprogrammed to provide the organism's basic developmental framework. Continual reciprocal interactions between different developing cell types also ensure a regulative quality, whereby cell types are maintained in appropriate proportions and locations. Generally, signaling errors are automatically corrected because they lead to an inappropriate signaling environment for a cell that either directs the cell to adopt a different fate or leads to apoptosis, because it cannot support proliferation or differentiation of the misplaced cell.

The above scenario emphasizes the overwhelming importance of a cell's developmental history and implies that a specific signal or activated signal-transduction pathway has no intrinsic meaning. A signal can be interpreted as a differentiation, growth, or apoptotic signal, depending on cell status. Hence, potential responses to signaling pathways can be explored in various cell types, but the relevant response can be ascertained only by studying the cell of interest in its normal context.

The formation of a tumor is progressive; it generally involves successive mutation of genes. These genes are involved in signaling, regulation of the cell cycle, and apoptosis. The consequences of these mutations resemble normal cellular signals and are interpreted by the same context-dependent logic that is used in normal development. The order of these changes and the changing environment of the tumor cell precursor must therefore be known to understand how each mutagenic change alters cell behavior.

Activation of certain signaling pathways and inhibition of others frequently induce cell proliferation and, most importantly, is causally implicated in the development of tumors. Some pathways originally were defined by their growth-stimulatory behavior in tissue culture cells and are considered the classic growth-factor pathways, instigated by EGF, PDGF, TGFα, TGFβ, insulin-like growth factors (IGF-I, -II), and various hematopoietic cell growth factors (cytokines/interleukins [ILs]). These same growth factors also can stimulate cell migration; act as survival factors, particularly in the nervous system (neurotrophic actions); and direct developmental programs. Conversely, several ligands were first studied in the context of their developmental roles (i.e., Wnt family, bone morphogenetic protein [BMP] branch of the TGFβ family, Hh) or according to their neurotrophic activities (i.e., NGF) and were subsequently implicated in growth control. Discussion of the major growth factor-signaling pathways implicated in early stages of tumorigenesis follows.

Growth Factor-Signaling Pathways

Signaling pathways are complex and incompletely understood. For clarity, many details are omitted and important new connections probably will emerge even before publication of this chapter.

Tyrosine Kinase-Receptor Pathways

Numerous growth factors (e.g., PDGF, EGF, fibroblast growth factor [FGF], NGF, and TGFα) signal by inducing dimerization and activation of receptors that are protein tyrosine kinases *(17)* (Fig. 1). The proximity of two receptors in a ligand-complexed dimer allows intermolecular receptor autophosphorylation at multiple sites. These phosphorylations stimulate additional tyrosine kinase activity and create binding sites for signaling molecules that contain SH2 (Src-Homology 2) or PTB (phosphotyrosine-binding) domains *(18,19)*. Each SH2 domain recognizes phosphotyrosine and a short amino acid sequence carboxy (C)-terminal to the tyrosine that determines the specificity of SH2-phosphotyrosine binding (PTB) *(20)*.

RTKs have variable numbers and contexts of tyrosine residues phosphorylated upon activation, and therefore can recruit different subsets of SH2 or PTB domain molecules. PDGFR has 12 sites and can bind many SH2-domain-containing proteins, including phospholipase Cγ (PLCγ); cytoplasmic tyrosine kinases of the Src family; p85 regulatory subunit of phosphatidyl inositol 3′ kinase (PI3K); protein tyrosine phosphatase, SHP-2; adapter proteins Grb2, Shc, Hck, and Grb7; Ras GTPase activating-protein GAP; and transcription factors of the STAT family *(21)*. In each case, binding to the receptor can produce activation of the recruited signaling molecule. Activation can be induced by an allosteric change, tyrosine phosphorylation, apposition to binding partners or substrates at the membrane, or a combination of these effects. Thus, ligand binding to a single type of RTK can activate many types of molecules at the plasma membrane, and produce numerous diverse responses; however, many of these receptor-bound signaling molecules feed into common pathways *(22)*. The major activated pathways are described.

Ras–MAP Kinase Pathway

The most prominent RTK signaling pathway is the Ras–MAPK pathway. Ras is associated with the plasma membrane and is activated by binding GTP (guanosine triphosphate), a process catalyzed by the GTP/GDP (guanosine diphosphate) exchange factor, son-of-sevenless (Sos). Sos is brought to its substrate by association with the adapter protein Grb2, which binds specific phosphotyrosines of activated RTKs (e.g., PDGFR and EGFR) *(23)*. The adapter protein, Shc, also can stimulate this process, but less directly *(24)*. Shc can bind a different subset of receptor phosphotyrosines and then be phosphorylated by RTKs or by associated Src-family tyrosine kinases. Phosphorylated Shc provides binding sites for the SH2 domain of Grb2 and recruits Sos to the membrane. EGFR and PDGFR recruit Sos through both Shc and direct Grb2 binding. RTKs for insulin, IGF-I, and IGF-II, do not have activation-dependent binding sites for Grb2, but they can bind and phosphorylate insulin receptor substrates (IRS-1 and IRS-2), thereby providing PTB sites for several molecules, including Grb2 and Shc *(25)*. Similarly, FGFR and NGFR can phosphorylate a membrane-associated substrate, FRS2, that subsequently recruits Grb2–Sos and activates Ras *(26)*. All RTKs can activate Ras by at least one of these pathways.

GTP bound Ras recruits the serine/threonine protein kinase Raf to the plasma membrane, where it is phosphorylated and activated *(27,28)*. Although Ras can bind directly to Raf, the activation of Raf involves many additional proteins and is not completely understood *(29,30)*. Raf, in turn, activates another protein kinase, MAP/ERK kinase (MEK) by serine phosphorylation. MEKs then activate the MAPKs, extracellular signal-regulated kinase (ERK1) and ERK2, by dual phosphorylation of threonine and tyrosine residues *(2)*. The Raf–MEK-ERK phosphorylation cascade is one of several MAPK phosphorylation cascades in mammalian cells *(31,32)*. The first two components have very restricted substrate specificity, which may be limited further by association with scaffold proteins *(33)*. The terminal MAPK component, on the other hand, generally is considered the final effector of the signaling pathway. ERKs can phosphorylate membrane-associated and cytoplasmic components and, especially during sustained activation, translocate to the nucleus and phosphorylate transcription factors of the ternary complex factor (TCF) and Ets families. This step leads to activation of immediate-early genes, including *fos, jun,* and *myc,* which encode transcription factors *(34)*. Transcriptional changes are important mediators of the mitogenic actions of Ras and are described below in more detail.

Activation of the c-*fos* promoter depends in part on a binding site recognized by a complex of serum response factor (SRF) and a TCF that has an Ets-family DNA-binding domain. Phosphorylation of TCFs at multiple sites by ERKs stimulates transcriptional activation *(34)*. Induction of c-*fos* by mitogens through the SRF–TCF binding site (SRE) also can be mediated by activation of SRF via an ERK-independent pathway that involves the small GTPase, Rac. Mitogen stimulation of the c-*fos* promoter is enhanced further by the action of the transcription factor CREB (cAMP-responsive binding protein) at its cognate site. CREB can be activated by a number of protein kinases, including RSK2, which can itself be activated by ERKs *(35)*. Hence, mitogens act in various ways, including activation of Ras and ERKs, to induce c-*fos*.

Other promoters have not been studied as intensively as c-*fos,* but c-*jun* is induced partly through a site for a CREB-related activating transcription factor (ATF) protein and is therefore responsive to ERK and RSK2 activation. The c-*myc* promoter is not well understood, but it includes an E2F–Ets site. In some cases activation by Raf (and hence ERK) is sufficient for c-*myc* induction and is necessary for induction by serum *(36,37)*. In other cases, however, Raf activation suffices for *fos,* but not *myc* induction, and *myc* induction relies partly on poorly defined inputs from Src-family tyrosine kinases *(38)*. Proteins outside the TCF family (Ets-1, -2) can associate with transcription factors other than SRF and can be phosphorylated by ERKs to stimulate activation or abrogate repression at a variety of promoter elements *(34)*. Hence, the immediate effects of ERK activation are not limited to SRE and CRE sites or to induction of *fos, jun,* and *myc*.

c-fos protein associates with c-jun protein to form the transcription factor, AP-1 *(34)*. c-myc protein associates with Max protein to form a transcriptional activator that binds to E-box sites *(37)*. Activation of immediate-early genes by the Ras–ERK pathway is generally mediated by binding sites for Ets proteins and CREB, whereas delayed immediate-early genes (which respond later and require new protein synthesis for

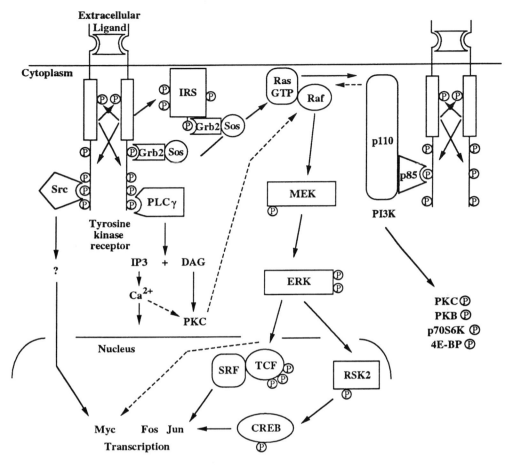

Fig. 1. Tyrosine kinase signaling pathways. Ligand binding induces receptor dimerization and autophosphorylation and generates many binding sites for molecules with SH2 domains of appropriate specificity. In some cases, a receptor substrate, such as IRS, contributes some of these binding sites. Recruitment of a Grb2–Sos complex to the membrane activates Ras. Ras recruits Raf, leading to successive activation of members of the MAPK cascade, Raf, MEK, and ERK. Activated ERK moves to the nucleus and phosphorylates transcription factors that activate immediate-early genes, including *fos* and *jun*. *myc* also responds to Src and related tyrosine kinases through an ill-defined pathway. PI3K is activated by recruitment of the p85 regulatory subunit to the membrane and by Ras. PI3K can activate Ras and the ERK pathway in addition to several other effectors, as shown in Fig. 2. PLCγ binds activated receptor and is activated by phosphorylation. PLCγ generates activators of PKC, which can activate the Ras–ERK pathway. *Dashed arrows* indicate less robust or widespread activations than *solid arrows*.

induction) might additionally respond to Myc–Max heterodimers and transcription factors of the AP-1 family through E-boxes and AP-1 sites, respectively. Tracing the effects of Ras–ERK stimulation beyond immediate-early gene expression is very difficult because of complex interactions among transcription factors and because other signaling pathways are sometimes triggered in conjunction with Ras–ERK. For example, the *jun* family includes several members that can form complexes that bind to AP-1 sites. Some Jun proteins can be activated through phosphorylation by MAPKs related to ERKs, especially by the Jun N-terminal kinase (JNK) that responds to stress stimuli *(39)*. The consequences of c-*fos* and c-*jun* induction on AP-1 activity are therefore quite variable.

Although transcriptional responses to Ras–ERK are very important, the Ras–ERK pathway also can affect the translation of mRNAs. The phosphorylation of eIF–4E by MNK1 (MAPK signal-integrating kinase), which itself is activated by ERK phosphorylation, increases its binding affinity for the 5'-cap structure of mRNAs and increases the efficiency of translation initiation *(40)*.

PI3 Kinase Pathways

Activation of PI3K initiates a second major branch of RTK signaling. Recruitment of the PI3K p110 catalytic subunit by receptor association of the p85 regulatory subunit stimulates activity, perhaps largely by plasma membrane apposition, close to a source of phospholipid substrates *(41)*. PI3K phosphorylates the 3' position of the inositol residue in phosphatidyl inositol (PtdIns), phosphatidyl inositol 4-phosphate (PtdIns 4-P), and phosphatidyl inositol 4,5-diphosphate (PtdIns[4,5]P2) (Figure 2).

The PtdIns(3,4,5)P3 (PIP3) product in particular stimulates the activation of a number of serine/threonine protein kinases, including protein kinase B (PKB) and p70 ribosomal protein S6 kinase (p70^{S6K}) *(42,43)*. Activation of these kinases requires threonine phosphorylation in the kinase domain and a second specific serine or threonine phosphorylation C-terminal to the kinase domain. In each case the kinase-domain phosphorylation requires a priming step to make the substrate accessible to the PIP3-stimulated protein kinase, PDK1 *(42,44,45)*. For PKB, the requisite conformational change follows binding of PIP3 to the pleckstrin homology (PH) domain of PKB. For p70^{S6K}, conformational priming requires phosphorylation of multiple C-terminal residues that are MAPK consensus sites and also phosphorylation of a "FRAP–mTOR" site (discussed later). For PKB, the second critical phosphorylation event is triggered by a PIP3-dependent kinase activity, termed PDK2. PDK2 has not been identified molecularly.

PDK1 can also bind and phosphorylate the kinase domain of all protein kinase C (PKC) isozymes tested, thereby activating atypical PKC *(46)*. An additional event, such as diacylglycerol (DAG) binding for the conventional isozymes PKCα and β, is required for activation of allosterically regulated PKC isozymes. PDK1 has a PH domain that is required for PIP3 to stimulate the phosphorylation of PKC and PKB by PDK1 in vitro. PH-domain binding to PIP3 probably stimulates PDK1 actions by ensuring membrane localization.

PI3K can lead to activation of small GTPases of the Rac, Rho, and Cdc42 families, perhaps by altering the activity of PH-domain-containing GTP/GDP exchange factors, such as Vav and Sos *(47–50)*. Rac, Rho, and Cdc42, like Ras, are membrane associated, activated by catalyzing GTP loading, and inactivated by catalyzing GTP hydrolysis. The downstream effectors of the different Ras superfamily members are quite varied. However, two major actions of Rac, Rho, and Cdc42 proteins are regulation of the actin cytoskeleton and transcription through the JNK MAPK cascade *(51)*. PI3K does not activate the transcriptional branch of Rho family actions but does induce cytoskeletal changes *(52)*. Furthermore, PI3K-activated Rac1 and Cdc42 can bind to p70^{S6K} and contribute to its activation, perhaps by targeting to a lipid environment where PDK1

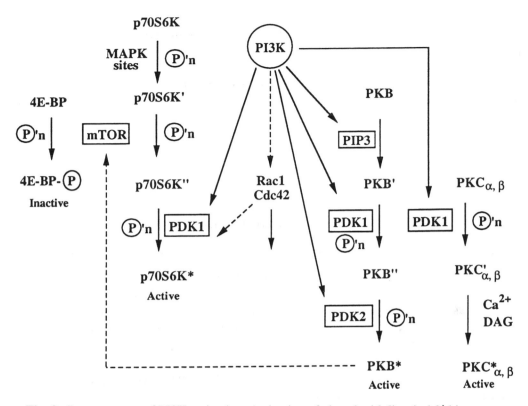

Fig. 2. Consequences of PI3K activation. Activation of phosphatidylinositol 3′-kinase generates phosphoinositides phosphorylated at the 3′ position, including PIP3. PIP3 can bind various PH domains to bring molecules together at membrane locations, including PKB as a substrate and PDK1 and PDK2 as kinases. PDK phosphorylations activate PKB and p70S6K, and prime conventional PKC isozymes for activation. The p70S6K activation requires prior phosphorylation at consensus MAPK sites and at a site that is phosphorylated by mTOR (or an associated kinase). The mTOR activation depends on PI3K and PKB, but the mechanism is unclear (*dashed arrow*). The mTOR also phosphorylates and inactivates the eIF–4E binding protein (4E–BP). The p70S6K activation can be facilitated by Rac1 and Cdc42, perhaps via membrane targeting, and PI3K can induce activation of Rac and in some cases Cdc42.

can act *(53)*. Thus, generation of PIP3 by PI3K catalysis contributes through several mechanisms, including PKB conformational changes, PDK1 activation, PDK2 activation, Rho family GTPase activation, and membrane association to the activation of at least three serine/threonine kinases: PKB, p70^{S6K}, and PKCs.

Several effects of PI3K alteration lead to changes in translation of mRNAs. These changes are mediated by PKC *(54)*, p70^{S6K}, and 4E–BPs (eIF–4E binding proteins), a family of proteins that bind to the initiation factor, eIF–4E. Phosphorylation of ribosomal protein S6 by P70^{S6K} leads to a modest general increase in protein translation but a very large stimulation for a subset of mRNAs (including those for ribosomal proteins) that include a polypyrimidine stretch in their 5′ untranslated region (UTR) *(55)*. eIF–4E binds to the 5′ terminal cap structure of mRNAs and to eIF–4G. The scaffolding protein eIF–4G binds to the 40S ribosome and to eIF–4A, which works together with eIF–4B to unwind secondary RNA structure. The binding of eIF–4E to eIF–4G is important for association of mRNAs with the ribosome; it also facilitates scanning for the translation initiation codon by reducing the secondary structure. 4E–BPs compete with eIF–4G for binding to eIF–4E, and therefore inhibit translation; however, 4E–BPs are inactivated by phosphorylation *(40)*. Phosphorylation of 4E–BP1 stimulates general translation about twofold but can stimulate translation more than 20-fold for specific mRNAs (e.g., c-*myc*) that contain highly structured 5′-UTRs *(56)*. Thus, PI3K activation can increase translation generally and more dramatically for a subset of mRNAs that affects growth and cell cycle regulation.

The mechanisms of growth factor or PI3K-induced phosphorylation of p70^{S6K} and 4E-BP are not completely understood but appear linked by a member of the PI3 kinase family that was initially identified in yeast as the target of (the immunosuppressant) rapamycin (TOR). TOR and the mammalian homolog (mTOR–FRAP1–RAFT-1) are inhibited by binding to a complex of rapamycin and the FKB12 (another immunosuppressant)-binding protein. Rapamycin inhibits phosphorylation of 4E–BP1 and one of the key activating phosphorylations of p70^{S6K} *(40)*. mTOR from cell extracts can phosphorylate p70^{S6K} and 4E–BP1 on the appropriate critical functional residues *(57)*. Because 4E–BP1 phosphorylation by mTOR is relatively inefficient in vitro, an intermediate kinase may be involved. mTOR probably also reduces the activity of phosphatases that affect the target phosphorylation sites in 4E–BP and p70^{S6K} *(40,58)*. How mTOR is activated is unknown, but phosphorylation of 4E–BP1 requires PI3K and PKB activity.

Thus, activation of p70^{S6K} is an extremely complex process. The process involves several steps that are sensitive to PI3K activity, including mTOR and PDK1 activation and possibly membrane targeting by Rac and Cdc42 activation. The Ras–ERK pathway is not required for activation of p70^{S6K}, although in theory ERKs could phosphorylate the primary C-terminal p70^{S6K} sites that permit subsequent activation by mTOR and PDK1. Activation of p70^{S6K} is probably an important consequence of mitogen stimulation, as antibodies (Abs) to p70^{S6K} can arrest cell proliferation *(55)*.

Phospholipase C Pathway

PLCγ bound to an activated RTK can be phosphorylated on tyrosine and activated to catalyze cleavage of phospholipids into DAG and inositol triphosphates (IP3) *(22)*. Binding of IP3 to specific receptors on internal membranes leads to Ca^{2+} release from intracellular pools. DAG and Ca^{2+} together activate conventional PKC isozymes. PKC can activate Raf and ERK kinases in a Ras-dependent manner *(59)*.

STATs

Tyrosine phosphorylation of receptor-bound STATs leads to dimerization and translocation to the nucleus, where they act as direct activators of transcription *(60)*. STAT activation is not a universal property of RTKs, and its importance has not been thoroughly assessed; however, STATs are essential mediators of tyrosine kinase signaling that results from the action of a large family of cytokines.

Summation of RTK-Activated Pathways

The above pathways exhibit collaborative effects that involve both common effectors and cross-regulation. PI3K is at the heart of several such interactions. PI3K stimulation of PIP3 synthesis provides adequate local substrate for PLCγ activation to produce sustained calcium signals *(61)*. Both PI3K and PLCγ contribute to activation of PKC isozymes, which can in turn contribute to Ras–ERK pathway activation. p70[S6K] activation depends on two PI3K-activated phosphorylations (i.e., mediated by mTOR and PDK1) activated by PI3K and another set of phosphorylations that may be ERK dependent. Most importantly, Ras can bind and activate PI3K *(62)*, and in some cell types, PI3K activation requires Ras activity *(47,63)*. Conversely, PI3K stimulates Ras activity *(64)* and also may contribute to Raf activation through phosphorylation by the Rac or Cdc42-regulated kinase Pak3 *(65)*.

Initiation of several molecular changes at an activated RTK, followed by considerable convergence and cross-regulation of the consequent signaling pathways, has a number of consequences. First, RTK signaling can activate several terminal protein kinase effectors (i.e., ERKs, p70[S6K], mTOR, PKB, and PKC), allowing a complex response. Second, all of these effectors are likely to be activated to some degree regardless of the specific RTK activated, but the magnitude of activation of each effector will depend on the specific receptor and the level of expression of a variety of signaling molecules. The combination of cell status and specific receptors activated can produce a variety of distinguishable responses, albeit based on a common theme.

An important question is whether the different terminal effectors of RTK signaling have an independent influence on the cellular response or whether their convergent action is normally required to elicit a specific cellular program, such as proliferation or differentiation. This question has been investigated by using mutations affecting specific phosphorylated tyrosine residues of the receptor, by delivering inhibitors of specific downstream effectors, or by creating artificially activated forms of single or multiple effectors. The results of such manipulations are cell type-dependent and can overestimate the normal contribution of a specific effector, if artificially activated proteins are overexpressed beyond physiologically attainable levels of activity. Nevertheless, some generalizations have emerged. Stimulation of cell proliferation by growth factors generally requires activation of the ERK pathway and sometimes additionally requires PI3 kinase activity *(2,47,66)*. Ras activation is sufficient for ERK activation. In some cases Ras also is sufficient to activate PI3 kinase and is required for mitogens to activate PI3K effectively *(47,63)*. In other situations, Ras is neither sufficient nor necessary for PI3K activation. PKB activation is very important in countering apoptosis. The relevant targets of these protein kinases are discussed later in the context of the cell cycle, senescence, and apoptosis.

Mutational Alteration of Tyrosine Kinase Receptor Pathways

Developmentally regulated presentation of ligands is an important mechanism for restricting the activity of signaling pathways, so it follows that inappropriate production of ligand could stimulate inappropriate growth, as recognized years ago in the autocrine growth factor hypothesis *(67)*. During development, the temporally and spatially restricted production of ligands is generally itself a response to activation of a signaling pathway by another ligand (as outlined at the beginning of this chapter). The frequent association of growth factor production with tumors is probably, therefore, secondary to internal disruption of a different growth factor-signaling pathway rather than to mutational alteration of the promoter for the autocrine factor. Inappropriate production of growth factors is nevertheless common in tumors and may contribute to the oncogenic process by reinforcing the effects of a primary aberration in a tyrosine kinase-signaling pathway *(68)*.

Specific mutations affecting receptors can produce ligand-independent dimerization and activation. Such changes include loss of the extracellular region and changes in the transmembrane domain, or even expression of the normal protein at high levels *(68,69)*. Inappropriate receptor activation has the virtue of activating all downstream pathways but may not always be effective because of down-regulation mechanisms. Feedback inhibition frequently occurs at multiple sites along a signaling pathway, but the receptor is invariably a prime target. Ligand binding can promote binding of a phosphatase (SHP2) that can dephosphorylate receptor phosphotyrosines. It can also stimulate receptor serine/threonine phosphorylation by downstream protein kinases (e.g., PKC for the EGFR) that reduce ligand affinity and tyrosine kinase activity, or ligand can induce receptor internalization and degradation *(21,70)*. Also, several activated receptors recruit and activate Ras–GAP, and in doing so, limit the extent of Ras activation.

The EGFR family (ErbB1–4) illustrates some of these principles *(68)*. There are several ligands for ErbB1 (i.e., EGF, TGFα, amphiregulin, heparin-binding EGF, β-cellulin, and epiregulin), and erbB3 and 4 (two families of alternatively spliced neuregulins), but none for ErbB2. Nevertheless, *erbB2* can be activated in response to ligands by forming heterodimers with other family members. Such heterodimers are the most potent activators of downstream pathways and of cell proliferation in tissue culture. Only *erbB2* overexpression suffices to transform established tissue culture cell lines, and although *erbB1* amplification also is seen in cancers, a particularly strong link exists between *erbB2* overexpression and rapid tumor growth. Furthermore, an activating mutation affecting the transmembrane region of ErbB2 is associated with tumors in rats and Abs to erbB2 have been successful in reducing tumor growth in animal studies and clinical trials *(68)*.

ErbB2 is particularly potent at stimulating growth for at least two reasons. First, monomeric EGF family ligands have a high-affinity binding site that dictates specificity for ErbB1 or for ErbB3/4 and a low-affinity site that binds better to ErbB2 than to the other receptors. Hence ErbB2 is preferentially incorporated into an activated heterodimer and produces the most stable, persistent signaling complex *(71)*. Second, a homodimeric ErbB1 complex with EGF is internalized and degraded, whereas an activated ErbB1–ErbB2 complex is recycled to the membrane after internalization *(70)*. Thus, ErbB2 overexpression enhances the response of other EGFR family members to normal low levels of ligand, in part because it is relatively insensitive to negative feedback. By contrast, ectopic production of TGFα, found in several tumors, is presumably at sufficiently high level that it can activate tyrosine kinase signaling despite negative feedback controls.

The most common and effective method of synthetically activating tyrosine kinase-proliferation pathways may be through activating mutations of *ras*. This can be attributed to the design of Ras as an on/off switch, whereby specific mutations that compromise GTPase activity leave Ras in a permanent "on" state that is inert to negative feedback mechanisms (e.g., Ras–GAP activity). On the other hand, Ras also occupies a focal point that is sufficient to activate the ERK pathway and sometimes also the PI3K pathway, as well as associated activation of Rho family GTPases.

Individual activation of downstream cytoplasmic targets in the Raf–MAPK and PI3K–PKB pathways also can contribute to oncogenesis in animals, as shown by the transforming retroviruses-harboring activated *raf* and PKB(*Akt*) genes. However, such mutations are not frequently found in human tumors. The Ras–ERK pathway can suffice for transcriptional induction of c-*jun* and c-*fos (38)*. Regulation of c-*myc* expression is complex and strong activation requires more than just the Ras–ERK pathway *(37)*. *fos, jun,* and *myc* genes have corresponding retroviral oncogenes, but only genetic alterations of *myc* (generally amplification) are commonly found associated with human tumors.

The prevalence in human tumors of *ras* mutations, which activate several downstream pathways, and of increased *myc* expression, which normally requires more than one upstream signaling pathway, suggests that more than one branch of a RTK signaling pathway generally is required to alter the regulation of cell proliferation significantly.

Cytokine and Antigen-Receptor Pathways

Hematopietic growth factors, termed cytokines, contribute to lineage, differentiation, and proliferation decisions during the maturation of specific blood cell types from a pluripotent stem cell. Proliferation and activation of mature peripheral T and B cells in response to immune challenge are triggered by binding to antigen (Ag) receptor complexes but additionally depend on signals elicited by cytokines (Figure 3). Some cytokine receptors, such as those for colony-stimulating factor (CSF)-1 and stem cell factor (SCF), are tyrosine kinases, whereas another large class of cytokine receptors triggers tyrosine kinase phosphorylation events indirectly. This latter class of cytokine receptors includes four main families (erythroid [EpoR], IL-2R, IL-3R, and IL-6R) that are activated by hetero- or homodimeric ligands, most likely through dimerization *(72)*. In each case, a signaling subunit has a sequence motif, known as Box1 and 2, close to the plasma membrane and C-terminal tyrosine residues that become phosphorylated in response to activation. The tyrosine kinases responsible for phosphorylation are members of the Janus kinase (JAK) and Src-families. The JAKs bind to the Box1,2 region. As with RTKs, receptor dimerization allows initial *trans*-phosphorylation between JAKs in a receptor complex. This phosphorylation activates the JAKs further and stimulates phosphorylation of tyrosine residues in the receptor and on substrates that become associated with the receptor. At least one receptor phosphotyrosine forms a binding site for a specific member of the STAT family of proteins, which is subsequently phosphorylated by JAK on a single tyrosine residue *(60)*. This phosphorylation triggers STAT dissociation from the receptor and homo- or heterodimerization through mutual interaction of phosphotyrosine regions and SH2 domains. Only STAT dimers can accumulate in the nucleus, bind DNA, and activate transcription.

Although STATS are important effectors for cytokines, JAK activity also leads to recruitment and activation of other signaling molecules, often including Shc, p85, and IRS1 or 2, and hence subsequent activation of Ras and PI3K pathways *(73)*. Members of the Src tyrosine kinase family, including Lck, Fyn, Lyn, Hck, and Syk, also associate with cytokine receptors and initiate tyrosine kinase signaling pathways, but their role is minor compared with that of the JAK kinases *(74)*.

Stimulation of Ag receptors of T cells and B cells leads initially to the sequential activation of two families of tyrosine kinases *(74–76)*. The exact events that lead to

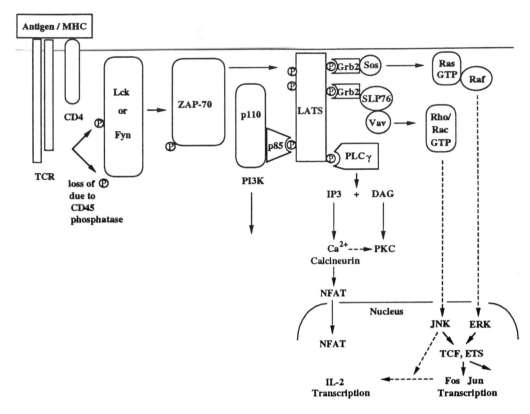

Fig. 3. T-cell receptor signaling. Antigen–MHC stimulation of the T-cell receptor (TCR) and associated CD4 receptor elicits two events that activate the tyrosine kinases, Lck and Fyn: phosphorylation and dephosphorylation of an inhibitory tyrosine by CD45 phosphatase. Zap-70 is then activated by phosphorylation, and it phosphorylates LATS, which acts as a scaffold for SH2-domain-containing proteins. This leads to activation of Ras and the ERK pathway, PI3K, and PLCγ, as for RTKs (Fig. 1). However, Rho and Rac GTPases also are strongly activated via the exchange factor Vav, leading to activation of the JNK MAPK cascade. An important response to intracellular calcium release is translocation of activated NF-AT transcription factors to the nucleus, where they contribute to IL-2 induction.

activation of Src-family kinases (Lck and Fyn in T cells; Lyn, Fyn, BIh, and Fgr in B cells) are unclear but are thought to involve both intermolecular autophosphorylation and dephosphorylation of an inhibitory C-terminal phosphotyrosine by the phosphatase CD45, in each case triggered by receptor clustering. A characteristic motif (ITAM; immunoreceptor tyrosine-based activation motif) on the T-cell or B-cell receptor is then phosphorylated on two tyrosines by the activated Src-family kinase to form a binding site for a Syk-family kinase (Syk in B cells; ZAP-70 and Syk in T cells). Recruitment leads to activation of Syk (by autophosphorylation) and ZAP-70 (involving phosphorylation by a Src-family kinase). Syk and ZAP-70 are the major instigators of downstream signaling events.

In T cells, an integral membrane protein, linker for activation of T cells (LAT), is a key substrate for ZAP70 that can provide binding sites for the SH2 domains of phospholipase Cγ (PLCγ), p85 of PI3K, and Grb2 *(77)*. Such an adapter also must act in B cells, as both T-cell and B-cell Ag receptor engagement leads to activation of the Ras/ERK pathway (through Grb2 and Sos), PI3K activity (by p85), PKC activation (by PLCγ and DAG), and calcineurin phosphatase activity (by PLCγ, IP3, and Ca^{2+}). Calcineurin controls the activity of NF-AT transcription factors that, together with immediate-early gene products *(fos, jun)* induced by MAPK pathways, activate transcription of the cytokine IL-2 in T cells.

Another adapter protein, SLP-76, becomes phosphorylated in T cells and recruits Vav, which becomes tyrosine phosphorylated and activated. Vav is a guanine nucleotide exchange factor (GEF) for Rac and leads to Rac activation. Activation of Rac by this means can lead to activation of the p38 and JNK stress-signaling MAPK pathways, which generally are not activated by nonhematopoietic growth factors acting directly on RTKs. Thus, mitogenic signaling in hematopoietic cells uses a variety of cytoplasmic tyrosine kinases that activate the same Ras, Rac, Rho, PI3K, and PLCγ pathways as RTKs but with different emphasis on particular pathways to direct cellular responses.

Growth Factors That Bind G-Protein Coupled Receptors

A number of ligands that bind to G-protein coupled receptors (GPCRs), including lysophosphatidic acid (LPA) neuropeptides (e.g., bombesin, bradykinin, endothelin, and vasopressin) and other peptides (cholecystokinin, thrombin, and gastrin), are known primarily for reasons other than their ability to stimulate cell proliferation. Activation of GPCRs leads to the activation of one or more trimeric G-proteins by charging the α subunit with GTP and liberating the βγ subunits.

Some mitogenic ligands (e.g., bombesin) activate G_q proteins, leading to PLCβ activation and subsequent activation of a MAPK cascade and activation of PI3K by PKC *(78,79)*. Ligands (e.g., LPA or thrombin) that couple to G_i receptors, by contrast, can activate ERK by Ras activation and involve tyrosine phosphorylation *(80)*. One possible scenario is that activated βγ recruits PI3Kγ (an isoform that does not associate with p85) to the membrane, resulting in activation *(81)*. In some manner PI3Kγ kinase activity stimulates the activity of a Src-family tyrosine kinase, perhaps through its protein kinase activity *(82)*. Src activation promotes the phosphorylation of RTKs (e.g., EGFR) and of Shc, which then act as adapter proteins to recruit Grb2 and Sos to the membrane and activate Ras *(83,84)*. Several GPCR ligands also couple to G_{12} and G_{13}, which can activate a guanine nucleotide exchange factor for Rho and stimulate cytoskeletal changes and the JNK MAPK cascade *(85–87)*.

Extracellular Matrix

Growth and survival of normal cells in tissue culture generally is dependent on adhesion to a surface that accumulates, or is coated by, an extracellular matrix (ECM) that includes proteins such as fibronectin, laminin, and collagen *(88)*. In other cases, terminal differentiation depends on interactions with the ECM *(89)*. These diverse contributions of the ECM are reminiscent of growth factors. In vivo, the ECM can contribute to growth factor-signaling pathways in several ways. These include binding and retention of growth factors, obligatory association of heparin sulfate proteoglycans with FGFs to form an active FGFR ligand, and direct stimulation of signal transduction by ECM protein receptors (e.g., integrin).

An important aspect of integrin–ECM interactions is their concentration at a limited number of focal adhesion sites *(79,90)*. This concentration is dependent on the activity of Rho family GTPases governing the cytoskeleton and on the cell–ECM interactions themselves for tension *(91)*. Various proteins become associated with integrins at focal adhesions, including a tyrosine kinase called focal adhesion kinase (FAK), Src, and the adapter proteins, p130CAS and Paxillin. The assembly of this complex is initiated by FAK autophosphorylation and probably results from clustering of integrins in response to the binding of a ligand (e.g., fibronectin). This stimulates further tyrosine phosphorylations and recruitment of SH2-domain proteins, including Shc and Grb2/Sos, leading to Ras activation. The stimulation of many different integrins can activate FAK.

A subset of integrins can stimulate Ras through another pathway that is independent of FAK *(92)*. These integrins are linked to the Src-family tyrosine kinase Fyn by the transmembrane protein, caveolin. Integrin ligation stimulates Fyn activity and leads to phosphorylation of Fyn-associated Shc and recruitment of Grb2–Sos and Ras activation *(93)*. In addition to directly activating Ras, integrins may potentiate other growth factor signaling pathways, in some cases by contributing to receptor activation (perhaps by clustering) and in others by potentiating downstream events, perhaps by promoting association of Raf with membranes, or by providing a scaffold for the Ras–ERK pathway.

Activation of some integrins stimulates an associated serine/threonine kinase, integrin-linked kinase (ILK), leading to nuclear accumulation of β-catenin–Lef-1, an effector of the Wnt signaling pathway *(94)*. Clearly, ECM interactions contribute through growth factor-signaling pathways to maintaining cells in an appropriate proliferating or differentiated state. ECM-derived signals may be important for ensuring that a cell's behavior is appropriate to its environment. Thus, complete loss of ECM contact generally leads to apoptosis, whereas migration to a different ECM environment may, for example, induce a proliferating cell to differentiate. These effects would no doubt be amplified by the localized distribution of growth factors.

Information Content of Tyrosine Kinase Signaling Pathways

Many ligands that can influence proliferation can connect to a restricted group of signaling pathways that involve tyrosine kinase phosphorylation at an early step and focus on Ras. These ligands also use Ras-independent branches to activate other key signaling molecules (e.g., PLC, PI3K, Ca^{2+}, and Rac/Rho-family GTPases). The widespread use of Ras-centered pathways to regulate growth (among other events) means that most cell types contain the signal transduction machinery that could translate mutational activation of these signaling pathways into a proliferative response. The common use of Ras-centered pathways is consistent with the association of activated Ras with many tumor types. However, activation of these pathways can lead to outcomes other than growth. It is therefore important to ask whether the extent of activation of a given pathway or the relative balance of different pathways is instrumental in determining the cellular response.

Some tissue culture models suggest that quantitative aspects of the Ras–ERK pathway determine whether Ras–ERK activation is interpreted as a proliferation signal. The pheocytochroma cell line, PC12, can be induced to proliferate by activation of EGFRs or to differentiate by stimulation of NGFRs. Each RTK activates various signaling pathways, but activated MEK (the intermediate between Ras and ERK) is sufficient to phenocopy each of these responses, inducing differentiation of PC12 cells and proliferation of fibroblasts *(2)*. EGFR is more rapidly internalized and down-regulated than NGFR in PC12 cells and leads to a more short-lived stimulation of activated Ras. If EGFR is overexpressed, EGF can elicit PC12 cell differentiation. Conversely, variant PC12 cells selected to proliferate in response to NGF have reduced numbers of NGFRs. These results have been interpreted as defining the duration of Ras–ERK signaling critical for determining the choice between proliferation and differentiation, drawing attention to the observation that only sustained activation leads to discernible nuclear accumulation of ERKs *(2)*. However, separating the contribution of the duration of signaling from that of signal magnitude is difficult, and in all cases of Ras–ERK signaling, at least some ERK probably reaches the nucleus to act on transcription factors and elicit a response.

Studies using conditionally expressed activated versions of the Raf family in NIH3T3 cells corroborated the general observation that excessive Ras–ERK signaling in established cell lines can promote quiescence in preference to proliferation. Overexpressed activated A-Raf induced smaller changes in ERK activity than other family members, Raf1 or B-Raf, but it was unique in stimulating proliferation. Moreover, a hyperactivated form of A-Raf was a more potent activator of ERK than the parent protein, but it failed to induce proliferation. Excessive Raf activity made the NIH3T3 cells refractory to PDGF growth stimulation. These artificial situations show that the magnitude of Ras–ERK signaling can be used to choose between a proliferative response and a growth arrest response consistent with cell differentiation.

In several established cell lines, the ERK pathway alone cannot stimulate proliferation (at any degree of activation tested), but it can be complemented by other pathways, including activation of PI3K or Rho family GTPases *(47,66)*. Similarly, activation of the ERK pathway can stimulate apoptosis, limiting induced proliferation, unless complemented by the antiapoptotic activities of the PI3K/PKB pathway *(3)*. In these situations, the ability of Ras (and mitogens) to stimulate the ERK and PKB pathways in a balanced manner is crucial to producing a strong proliferative response.

In primary cell lines even Ras activation (leading to ERK and PI3K activation) is not sufficient to stimulate growth. Instead it induces a senescent state in which cells remain alive but quiescent and refractory to the actions of mitogens *(1)*. Clearly it is necessary to understand the regulation of the cell cycle and how cells differentiate, senesce, and die to understand how and why the contribution of different branches of growth factor-signaling pathways to cell proliferation is cell type specific (Figure 4).

TGF β Family Signaling

Members of the TGFβ family can stimulate proliferation of some cells in culture but more often exert an inhibitory role that can prevent growth, even of some tumor-derived cells *(95)*. The BMP subfamily in particular has many roles in vertebrate and invertebrate development that have a number of interesting characteristics, including dose-dependent responses, which allow them to act as morphogens, instructing cell fate according to spatial concentration gradients *(8,96)*.

All TGFβ family proteins are active as dimers, but a variety of heterodimeric partnerships are permissible, including association with ligands that form an inactive complex. The expression of BMPs is highly regulated, but in many cases production of inhibitory ligands is also a key spatially restricted developmental event. Thus, the

Spemann organizer (the most dorsal and earliest invaginating mesoderm of *Xenopus*) produces molecules, such as Chordin and Noggin, that bind to BMP4 and inhibit induction of epidermal cells, thereby leading to adoption of the default neural fate *(97–99)*. Furthermore, extracellular Chordin and related molecules can be cleaved by specific proteases whether alone or in complex with BMPs, modifying the spatial distribution of Chordin and providing a means to transport inactive complexed BMPs before activation at a distant site.

In many developmental contexts, TGFβ proteins regulate cell fate choices, but clear examples also exist of their role in promoting apoptosis, for example, to eliminate webbing between limb digits *(100),* and in maintaining the proliferation of several cell types, including stem cells *(101).*

Two types of receptor serine threonine kinases (types I and II) are required to respond to TGFβ *(102)*. Initial binding of ligand to the type II receptor (sometimes enhanced by an ancillary receptor) recruits type I receptor, which also binds to the ligand. The type II receptor is constitutively active and phosphorylates the type I receptor within a ligand–receptor complex that leads to its activation. Mutationally activated type I receptor is sufficient to propagate the signal; its key targets are proteins of the Smad family. The receptor-regulated subfamily of Smads have a conserved N-terminal MH1 domain and a conserved C-terminal MH2 domain, which interact and are inert before phosphorylation of the C-terminus by the activated type I receptor *(8)*. This activation step promotes heterodimerization with a second type of Smad protein, Smad4, which does not interact directly with receptors; it also promotes entry of the Smad complex into the nucleus. Both events are essential to elicit a transcriptional response *(103)*. In some cases, the Smad complex associates with another DNA-binding protein (e.g., FAST-1 for a specific functional site on the activin-responsive *Mix-1* gene promoter) *(104);* in other cases, the DNA-binding activity of the MH1 domain suffices to target the complex to important promoter regulatory elements *(8,105)*. In each case, the MH2 domains of the Smads provide an essential transcription activation function. Inhibitory Smads often are transcriptionally induced by TGFβ family signaling. These Smads can act by competing with receptor-regulated Smads for association with type-I receptor or by inhibiting heterodimerization of activated Smads with Smad4 *(8)*.

Different TGFβ family members can have very different effects on the same cell, largely as a result of activation of different type-I receptors and the consequent activation of specific Smads *(106)*. For example, BMP2–4 complexes activate BMPRI and BMPRIB, and hence activate Smad5 and 8, whereas TGFβ ligands activate Smad 2 and 3 by TβRI. A single ligand (i.e., BMP4) can elicit many different responses as development proceeds. These responses probably result from association of activated Smads with different DNA-binding proteins and a changing array of other transcription factors that act on BMP target genes. Smads can be phosphorylated by MAPKs, leading to inactivation *(107),* but also can be activated by MAPKs *(108),* providing the potential for interaction with tyrosine kinase signaling pathways *(109)*.

Several types of mutations affecting TGFβ signaling have been implicated in carcinogenesis. The most frequent mutation associated with human tumors is loss of Smad4 function. This would be expected to stimulate proliferation in many cell types because of the essential role of Smad4 as a partner for all receptor-activated Smads and the generally growth inhibitory role of TGF-β signaling. Loss of heterozygosity (LOH) for the genomic region, including Smad4, is seen very frequently in human pancreatic carcinomas and in colorectal tumors *(110,111).* In the intestinal crypts, TGFβI and TGFβII receptor are expressed in cells near the lumen, implying a possible role in slowing proliferation and inducing differentiation as cells move and mature from the base of the crypts toward the lumen. Mutations affecting TGFβ type II receptors have been found in tumors, especially when genomic instability was induced by the absence of DNA repair enzymes in hereditary nonpolyposis colorectal cancer (HNPCC) *(112,113).* Also, mice lacking Smad3, an effector for TGFβ1, develop lethal colorectal adenocarcinomas before 6 months, implying that failure of TGFβ signaling can suffice to promote tumor formation *(114).* Mice that are heterozygous for Smad4 (homozygotes die early) do not develop tumors at an enhanced rate but can exacerbate the effects of heterozygosity for the tumor suppressor, adenomatous polyposis coli (APC) (see Wnt signaling, next section) *(115).* Thus, loss of TGFβ signaling can contribute to tumor initiation and progression, although the range of cell types affected is not as great as for tyrosine kinase signaling *(115,116).*

Wnt Signaling

The Wnt name stems from the realization that *Drosophila wingless,* which affects many developmental decisions, and *int-1,* which can induce tumors if overexpressed in response to insertion of a retrovirus, were similar in sequence and action *(7).* The mechanisms of Wnt signaling have been studied largely in a developmental context in *Drosophila, Caenorhabditis elegans,* and *Xenopus.* As for TGFβ family members, Wnt proteins can act as morphogens, indicating dose-dependent signal transduction. Their activity can be regulated not only by controlling their expression and diffusion but also through the production of secreted homologues of Wnt receptors that can bind Wnts and inhibit their actions *(117).*

The receptors for Wnts are transmembrane proteins of the Frizzled (Fz) family. Although these receptors have seven transmembrane domains, characteristic of G-protein-coupled receptors, it has not been shown directly that they can activate G-proteins. Two types of signal-transduction pathways may be elicited by Wnts. The best-studied pathway involves Disheveled, glycogen synthase kinase 3 (GSK3), β-catenin, and T-cell factor–lymphoid enhancer factor (Tcf–Lef) family transcription factors (discussed later). Some Wnts can signal without using β-catenin and LEF, but instead stimulate release of intracellular calcium ions by a pathway that requires G-protein function and involves phosphatidylinositol signaling *(118,119).*

The central regulatory step in the major Wnt-signaling pathway is the regulation of ubiquitin-mediated proteolysis of β-catenin *(7).* β-Catenin associates with the homophilic, calcium-binding transmembrane adhesion molecule, cadherin, and with α-catenin, which can bind actin. This adhesion complex can link the actin cytoskeletons of apposed cells. When β-catenin is present in excess of cadherins, it is rapidly degraded by the ubiquitin proteolysis pathway *(120).* Degradation most likely is triggered by phosphorylation of the N-terminal region of β-catenin by GSK3 and can be inhibited by mutational alteration of the key phosphorylation sites or by inhibiting GSK3 activity. Wnt signaling reduces degradation of β-catenin, although the mechanism is unclear. Transduction of the Wnt signal from Fz requires the activity of a protein, Disheveled, that has no known biochemical activity but that may bind to Fz, and can lead to reduced GSK3 activity and stabilization of β-catenin. The stabilized cytoplasmic β catenin can move to the nucleus and associate with Tcf–Lef transcription factors. Tcf–Lef proteins cannot activate transcription alone, but β-catenin includes a strong transcription activation domain at its C-terminus. Hence, the β-catenin–Tcf complex can bind specific sites on DNA and stimulate transcription *(121)*. Accordingly, some Wnt-responsive genes include crucial Tcf-binding sites.

This simple model for converting a Wnt signal into a specific transcriptional response has, in reality, some additional complexity *(122)*. First, interaction of β-catenin with Tcf proteins does not always lead to gene activation. Wnt-like signaling in early *Xenopus* embryos defines future dorsal regions and prevents repression of the *siamois* gene in dorsal regions *(123)*. Wnt signaling in the four-cell *C. elegans* embryo opposes the normal activity of the Tcf family protein, Pop-1 *(124)*. Thus, β-catenin might, in some cases, act to sequester Tcf proteins rather than actively stimulate transcription. Second, the regulation of β-catenin phosphorylation involves several additional players. Axin can bind both GSK3 and β-catenin and promotes phosphorylation of β-catenin *(125)*. Accordingly, axin promotes β-catenin degradation and opposes Wnt signaling *(126)*. Another GSK3 binding protein (GBP) inhibits GSK-3 activity; accordingly, in *Xenopus* embryos, GBP can stabilize β-catenin ectopically, and GBP is essential for normal dorsoventral polarity *(127)*. In this context, GBP responds to a signal generated by fertilization-dependent cortical rotation rather than to an extracellular Wnt signal.

The APC protein is the most interesting additional Wnt-signaling pathway component with respect to cancer. APC mutations are found in familial adenomatous polyposis (FAP) and many sporadic colonic tumors *(4)*. Loss of APC function may be one of the earliest steps in tumor formation in these cases. APC can bind to β-catenin through well-defined repetitive motifs in each protein, and most APC mutations in cancer cells truncate the protein to remove some or all of these binding sites. APC-mutant colon cancer cell lines have high amounts of β-catenin in complex with Tcf proteins, and β-catenin levels can be reduced by transfection of wild-type APC. Thus, in the colon, APC is important for maintaining low levels of β-catenin *(128);* however, this may not be true universally. In both *Xenopus* embryos and in four-cell *C. elegans* embryos, APC promotes Wnt like signaling (implying stabilization of β-catenin) *(122)*. APC is a very good substrate for GSK3, and several of the interactions among GSK3, β-catenin, and APC are phosphorylation dependent. Thus, APC may help to target β-catenin for phosphorylation and degradation in the absence of a Wnt signal, but the association between APC and β-catenin also may stabilize β-catenin in the absence of GSK3 activity or titrate low amounts of GSK3 activity during Wnt signaling. As a result, APC might affect β-catenin degradation in either direction, depending on circumstance.

APC is a large molecule and might have other significant interactions. APC can associate with microtubules and may regulate or respond to changes in cell shape or contacts that affect the coordination of migrations in the colonic villi with proliferation and differentiation *(129)*. In colon carcinomas and in melanomas, β-catenin is stabilized not only by APC mutations but also by mutations affecting the N-terminus of β-catenin, suggesting that stabilization of β-catenin is key to the tumor-promoting activity of APC mutations *(128)*.

Hedgehog Signaling Pathways

The Hh family of proteins was first discovered in *Drosophila,* where its principal role is to control cell fate by inducing changes in gene transcription *(6)*. Hh signaling also can lead to proliferation, in some cases directly. Vertebrate Hh proteins control many aspects of development, including patterning of the neural tube, somites, and limbs. Excessive or inappropriate Hh signaling can produce tumors and, in humans, is associated principally with basal cell carcinoma *(130)*.

Hh signal transduction involves the relief of multiple inhibitory constraints on the activity of transcriptional activators of the GLI family of zinc finger DNA-binding proteins (originally identified as being amplified in gliomas). The signaling pathway is best understood in *Drosophila,* where the GLI homolog is called Ci *(6)*. Binding of Hh to its receptor, Patched (Ptc), releases an inhibitory constraint on the seven-pass transmembrane protein, Smoothened (Smo). Smo is similar in structure to Fz proteins and, as for Fz, it is unclear whether it activates G-proteins. Somehow Smo activation leads to multiple regulatory events that affect Ci activity.

In the absence of Hh, the primary Ci translation product (Ci-155) forms complexes with various proteins, binds to microtubules, and undergoes partial proteolysis that produces a relatively stable product, Ci-75. Ci-75 may be a transcriptional repressor, and activity of the Ci-155 precursor probably is constrained by microtubule association and the effects of complexing proteins. Hh signaling inhibits proteolysis of Ci-155 to Ci-75, frees Ci-155 from microtubules, and facilitates the conversion of Ci-155 into a transcriptional activator, in opposition to the action of one of the complexing proteins (Suppressor of fused). How Smo activation accomplishes these feats is unknown, but the process undoubtedly involves several regulated phosphorylations. The proteolysis of Ci-155 can be regulated by phosphorylation of Ci at protein kinase (PKA) sites, a kinesin-like molecule (Costal-2) that complexes with Ci is hyperphosphorylated in response to Hh, and a protein kinase (Fused) that associates with Ci is required to counter the effects of Suppressor of fused. Several of these signaling interactions are conserved in vertebrates. However, selective transcriptional induction and repression of different GLI genes is also an important mechanism for enhancing the initial Hh response in vertebrates.

Loss of function mutations in *ptc,* activating mutations in *Smo,* and overexpression of GLI proteins have each been associated with human cancers *(131–133)*. Overexpression of Hh from a keratin promoter in mice leads to very rapid and widespread development of basal cell carcinomas, indicating the sufficiency of this pathway to promote overproliferation *(134)*. Such tumors, however, rarely progress further and do not show evidence of genomic instability.

How Do Growth Factor-Signaling Pathways Impinge on Cell Growth?

Cell proliferation requires cell division and growth without extensive cell death. Although some relationships between cell division and cell growth for mammalian cells exist, the linkage between the two processes does not appear strict *(135)*. Thus, the rate of cell-cycle progression can be altered without affecting growth to produce populations of cells of abnormal size. Similarly, cell cycle decisions are not tightly linked, at least temporarily, to cell death decisions. The contribution of growth factors to cell division, growth, and death are therefore discussed separately before examining interactions among regulators of these processes.

Cell-Cycle Regulation

G_1 Restriction Point Control by Rb and Cyclin D-dependent Kinases

Numerous studies in cell culture, where environmental conditions can be manipulated, have led to the view that there is a single point in late G_1 phase (before DNA replication in S-phase), known as the restriction point, at which cells commit to undergoing a complete cell cycle on the basis of environmental cues *(136)*. In other words, environmental signals (e.g., growth factors, adhesion to the ECM, and cell contact) cannot influence the decision to cycle at a stage after the restriction point. The molecular basis of this restriction point in normal cells is the phosphorylation of Rb beyond a critical threshold by CDKs *(137)*. Under normal circumstances (in tissue culture cells) this event triggers an inexorable series of events, including dissociation of the transcription factor, E2F-1 from Rb, activation and derepression of E2F-dependent genes, and successive accumulation and activation of cyclin-E-dependent kinases, followed by cyclin A-dependent protein kinases *(138)*. The latter two kinase activities are essential for entry into S-phase, generally 1–2 h after the restriction point is passed.

The G_1 CDK inhibitors of two families counteract the activation and the activities of these kinases *(139)*. The INK4a family (p15, p16, p18, and p19) bind only to the partners of D-cyclins (viz, cdk4 and cdk6), inhibiting both assembly and activity of cycD–cdk4/6 complexes. The Kip family (p21, p27, and p57) inhibits cyclin A, D, and E kinase activities when present in stoichiometric excess in the complex. Cyclin D normally is required for cell-cycle progression and increasing cyclin D concentrations can shorten G_1 *(140)*. These effects of cyclin D are observed only if functional Rb protein is present, suggesting that the key contribution of cyclin D to cell-cycle progression is mediated by Rb phosphorylation *(138)*.

In a cyclin D-regulated cell cycle in the presence of functional Rb, phosphorylation of Rb and activation of E2F-1 leads to transcriptional activation of cyclin E, cyclin A, and E2F-1, reinforcing the initial activation of E2F. The transcriptionally induced cyclin E-cdk2 can phosphorylate Rb further, ensuring continued release of E2F-1. Also, the increased cyclin D kinase levels that triggered Rb phosphorylation can now titrate Kip family inhibitors away from other CDKs, further promoting the increase of cyclin E–cdk2 activity. Cells do not normally arrest in G_1 with hyperphosphorylated Rb, implying that the changes consequent to increasing cyclin D kinase activity beyond a critical threshold are sufficient to activate cyclin E and cyclin A kinase activities beyond the inhibitory capacity of Kips and ensure entry into S-phase. The patterns of activity of CDKs during the cell cycle are consistent with this model. Cyclin D kinase activity gradually increases during G_1 phase and is largely maintained through S-phase, whereas cyclin E and A kinases exhibit sharp peaks of activity in late G_1 and at the G_1–S-phase border, respectively. Thus, the regulation of cyclin D kinase activity is clearly a key focus for the action of mitogens *(141)*.

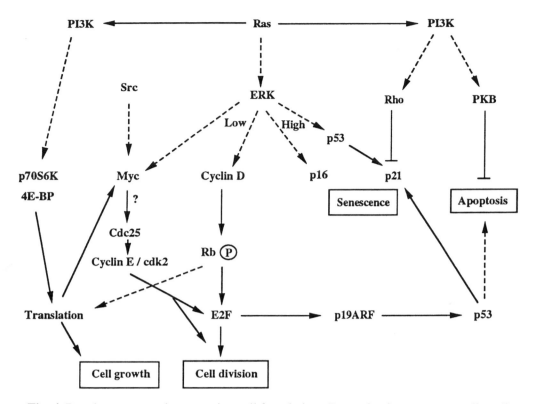

Fig. 4. Regulatory networks governing cell fate choices. Ras activation promotes cell cycling by inducing cyclin D via the MAPK, ERK. Strong Myc induction depends on additional pathways, including translational consequences of PI3K activation. Myc also promotes cell cycling, in part through activation of cyclin E-dependent kinase, perhaps mediated by Cdc25 induction. High ERK activity induces the cyclin-dependent kinase inhibitors, p16 and p21, which can induce senescence. The senescent response can be alleviated in some cases by activation of Rho, which prevents p21 induction, or by mutations inactivating p16, p53, or p21. Phosphorylation of Rb leads to release of E2F, which promotes entry into S-phase and which also induces p19ARF, and hence stabilizes p53. The p53 may prevent passage into S-phase through p21 induction but otherwise will promote apoptosis. Apoptosis may be inhibited by PI3K-dependent activation of PKB. PI3K also activates p70S6K and inactivates 4E-BP, promoting general translation and stimulating cell growth. Indirect effects are indicated by *dashed lines.*

Additional G₁ Controls: Cyclin E and A Kinases and Their Inhibitors

The requirement for multiple kinase activities to enter S-phase provides additional potential points of regulation. Artificially overexpressed cyclin E can enhance the effect of excess cyclin D on shortening G_1 *(138)*. Furthermore, one can imagine various circumstances in which the cyclin D kinase restriction point is passed but cyclin E kinase activity now becomes rate-limiting and in some cases insufficient for passage into S-phase. One such circumstance, common in cancers, is when Rb or p16Ink4a is inactivated by mutation. In *Rb* mutant cells in tissue culture cell-cycle progression shows a residual dependence on growth factor stimulation. Also, protein levels of p27Kip decrease considerably during G_1 after mitogen stimulation, implying that p27 levels can be regulated by mitogens. Mice lacking p27 function are viable but all their tissues show increased proliferation, manifested as excessive numbers of undersized cells (142). Thus, in most tissues, p27 regulates the rate of entry into S-phase.

Only late-onset pituitary tumors are seen in p27-mutant mice. However, the absence of p27 enhances the rate of appearance of tumors in Rb-heterozygous mice, suggesting an important default role for maintaining regulated quiescence in the absence of Rb control of the restriction point. Therefore growth factor-signaling pathways are expected to act on cycE/cdk2 or Kip-family inhibitors and that such pathways can contribute to carcinogenesis.

G_1 Checkpoint Controls

Even if environmental cues provide the appropriate inputs for entry into S-phase, various checkpoint controls that monitor DNA damage, chromosome and centrosome number, or other cellular stresses can prevent this transition. A key pathway for sensing prereplicative problems is the activation of p53, followed by transcriptional induction of the cdk inhibitor, p21 (139). Very rapid passage through G_1 promoted by mutation of growth factor-signaling pathways, Rb, or the cdk inhibitors, p16 and p27, possibly might not allow sufficient time for S-phase preparations, such as DNA repair, placing a greater burden on the p53–p21 checkpoint control as a key cell-cycle control point.

Terminal Differentiation

Terminally differentiated cells often remain quiescent even in environments that would stimulate proliferation of their precursors. In myoblasts, MyoD is essential for induction of terminally differentiated muscle-specific genes and also induces p21 in a p53-independent manner (143). Conversely, overexpression of p21 induces muscle cell differentiation. If the myoblast cell cycle is artificially maintained by cyclin D1 overexpression, terminal differentiation and MyoD-responsive gene expression are inhibited (144). Thus, there are mutually inhibitory interactions between two types of regulators; those that promote differentiation and those that promote cell cycling. Histologic examination of expression patterns suggest that increased amounts of p21 or other cdk inhibitors may be a general mechanism of maintaining quiescence of terminally differentiated cells. Thus, the expression of key transcriptional regulators of cell differentiation (e.g., MyoD) may limit cell-cycle progression despite mitogenic inputs that would otherwise bypass the restriction point.

Senescence

Senescence was originally described as a stable G_1 growth-arrested state seen in primary cells that had undergone a characteristic (high) number of replicative cycles (145). Senescence has several defining features, including a characteristic gene expression profile (e.g., high acidic β-galactosidase and low c-fos) and resistance to both apoptosis and growth stimulation by mitogens. Replication-dependent senescence may be triggered in nondifferentiated cells by shortening of telomeres beyond a critical threshold (146) and is accompanied by elevated expression of cdk inhibitors, principally p21 and p16 (145,147). Rodent cells can escape senescence through mutations in the p16 INK4a locus or p53 (which normally induces p21), whereas only oncogenes (e.g., adenovirus E1a and SV40 large-T) that affect both p53 and the key p16 target, Rb, can immortalize human cells *(148)*. How shortening of telomeres provokes increases in cdk inhibitors is unknown; however, many or all of the features of senescence, including increased p16 and p21 expression, can be triggered prematurely by Ras activation in primary rodent or human cells *(1)*. Thus, senescence, like differentiation and proliferation, represents a distinct program that can be initiated by growth factor signaling pathways. Induction of senescence hinges on the regulation of cdk inhibitors: forced expression of cdk inhibitors can suffice to induce senescence *(149)*, and INK4a or p53 mutations can abrogate Ras-induced senescence *(1)*.

Cell Growth

The rates of ribosomal RNA and protein synthesis, ribosome assembly, and general translation are key determinants of cell growth. Stimulation of general translation through p70^{S6K} activation and 4E-BP inactivation accompanies most tyrosine kinase signals and is undoubtedly an important feature for stimulating sufficient growth to allow continued cell cycling. Many additional interactions probably link cell-cycle progression to the cell's biosynthetic rate. Indeed, the Rb protein not only regulates cell-cycle entry by E2F activity but also represses transcription by RNA polymerase I and III *(150,151)*, consistent with an observation that most cell growth takes place after passing the G_1 restriction point *(152)*.

Signaling Pathways That Activate the Cell Cycle

Tyrosine Kinase Pathways

Transcriptional control of cyclin D1 can link growth factors to cell cycling. Activation of RTKs, Ras, Raf, or ERK, can activate cyclin D1 transcription, such that mRNA levels increase up to 20-fold, generally peaking about 6 h after mitogen stimulation *(138,141)*. Furthermore, Ras inhibition prevents increased cyclin D1 transcription in response to mitogen and inhibits progression to S-phase in an Rb-dependent manner *(153)*. Induction of cyclin D1 by the Ras–ERK pathway is therefore an important contribution to passage through the G_1 restriction point. The delay between mitogen stimulation and cyclin D induction implies a delayed immediate-early effect (i.e., one mediated principally by the immediate-early response genes, such as *jun, fos,* and *myc*). Indeed, mitogen induction requires an AP-1 site in the cyclin D1 promoter *(154)*. Also, c-*myc* overexpression can stimulate cyclin D1 overexpression (and entry into S-phase) in collaboration with a defective RTK that retains the ability to induce *jun* and *fos* *(155,156)*; however, additional observations imply that regulation of the cyclin D1 promoter probably is quite complex. For example, mitogenic induction can act through a promoter region that contains an Ets site and no AP-1 sites, and cyclin D mRNA can be induced by serum in the absence of protein synthesis, both indications of an immediate-early effect *(154,157)*.

Overexpression of cyclin D is often found in human tumors, in some cases as a result of amplification of the gene or of translocations that elevate transcription *(138)*. Artificially induced overexpression of cyclin D1 in mouse mammary epithelia initially induces overproliferation and eventually tumors, showing that altered regulation of cyclin D levels can promote growth and contribute to tumor formation.

Cyclin D induction by mitogens may not be sufficient for passing the cell cycle restriction point, however. In quiescent cells, synthetic overexpression of cyclin D and cdk4 does not produce active cyclin D kinase complexes or Rb phosphorylation until cells are further stimulated to proliferate, implying regulated assembly of active CDKs *(158,159)*. Cyclin D kinase inhibitors (e.g., p27) may prevent assembly and activation of cyclin D dependent kinase and therefore may sometimes account for the insufficiency of cyclin D accumulation in promoting growth.

The levels of p27Kip generally are regulated posttranslationally through the cell cycle and in response to mitogens *(160)*. In macrophages, CSF-1 elicits a reduction in p27 *(161)*. Increasing p27 by altering cAMP levels blocks the mitogenic response to CSF-1. In quiescent T cells, Ag-receptor stimulation induces CDK complexes that remain inactive. Further stimulation by IL-2 reduces p27 amounts and elicits proliferation *(162)*. The IL-2-mediated decrease in p27 is blocked by rapamycin, suggesting the involvement of mTOR-dependent translational mechanisms. Thus, in some cases, transcriptional induction of cyclin D through the Ras–ERK pathway may be complemented by translational reductions in p27 mediated by the PI3K–mTOR–p70^{S6K}–4E-BP branch of tyrosine kinase signaling.

Activation of cyclin E–cdk2 and cyclinA–cdk2 complexes requires phosphorylation by a CDK-activating kinase (CAK) and dephosphorylation of inhibitory residues on cdk2 by the cdc25 phosphatase *(163,164)*. c-*myc* can induce transcription of cdc25A and B and stimulate cyclin E-cdk2 activity without altering its abundance *(37,164)*. c-*myc* is not always effectively induced by Ras–ERK pathways, so this effect of *myc* may contribute to the observed requirement of *myc* overexpression to complement proliferation induced by Ras–ERK activity under some circumstances *(38,165)*.

Other Pathways

Specific links between cell-cycle control and signaling pathways used by Wnts and Hh proteins have not been defined clearly; however, transcriptional induction of key target genes probably provide at least some of the links. A relevant target of the Wnt pathway in colon cancer may be the c-*myc* gene. Expression of *myc* is high in APC mutant cells (that constitutively produce β-catenin–Tcf-4) but can be reduced by introduction of wild-type APC *(166)*. This effect on the *myc* promoter requires Tcf-4 sites and can be mediated by oligomerized synthetic Tcf-4 binding sites, suggesting direct activation by β-catenin–Tcf4.

Signaling Pathways Leading to Inhibition of the Cell Cycle TGFβ Pathways

TGFβ Pathways

Inhibition of cell proliferation by TGFβ may be accompanied by decreased amounts of cdk4 *(167–169)*, increased Ink-family inhibitor p15 *(170)*, or increased Kip-family inhibitors p27 *(171–172)* or p21 *(173)*. These observations suggest that there are diverse pathways for reducing the activity of CDK. In fact, the primary responses to TGFβ may be more limited and subsequent interactions among CDKs and their inhibitors may ramify this response *(173)*. In cycling mink lung epithelial cells, the first effect of TGFβ is to increase p15 mRNA levels. The induced p15 binds to cyclin D kinases, displacing p27, which inhibits cyclin E kinases and leads to rapid cessation of cell cycling. In this quiescent state, cdk4/6 levels subsequently decline. In keratinocytes, a similar induction of p15 occurs, but p21 mRNA levels also increase, leading to direct inhibition of cyclin D- and E-dependent kinases. Thus, the primary effects of TGFβ may be to induce transcription of cdk inhibitors.

Ras Pathways

Activated Ras, Raf, or ERK can induce elevated levels of CDK inhibitors in primary cells and also in some immortalized, established tissue culture cell lines *(1,174–176)*. Ras-induced cell-cycle arrest in primary cells is accompanied by other manifestations of the senescence program. In some cell types, p16 (Ink 4a) is induced *(176)*. In other cells, p21 (Kip family) also is induced by p53 activation. Cell-cycle inhibition is not observed in the absence of either p21 or p53 function *(1,174)*. In some cases, induction of these cdk inhibitors requires higher or more prolonged activation of the Ras–ERK pathways than, for example, induction of cyclin D1 *(175,176)*. Furthermore, activation of Rho, which frequently accompanies Ras activation during mitogen stimulation, blocks induction of p21 by Ras *(177)*.

A normal mitogenic signal might activate Ras sufficiently to stimulate cyclin D expression but not enough to induce cdk inhibitors, particularly in the context of other (PI3K, Rho GTPase) pathways that are activated. A strong Ras–ERK signal may be used to promote differentiation, but this signal generally will be in the context of specific transcription factors, such as MyoD that contribute to the induction of cdk inhibitors. A persistent, strong Ras–ERK signal in cells that are not transcriptionally primed to differentiate may not arise in normal development or physiology and may be used as an alarm signal that elicits senescence to protect the organism from inappropriate cell proliferation in response to mutations. The requirement for p53 in inducing senescence is in keeping with the idea that senescence is a protective checkpoint mechanism.

Apoptosis

During normal development many cells die, especially in the nervous and immune systems, in a characteristic, self-contained manner termed apoptosis *(178)* (*see* Chapter 9). In some cases, such as the elimination of self-reactive lymphocytes, activation of a specific receptor for a member of the tumor necrosis factor (TNF) family, CD95 (Fas), triggers apoptosis. In other cases, particularly in the nervous system, apoptosis may be a default action in the absence of specific trophic cues from target cells, and therefore mandates functional connections for survival. A general requirement for antiapoptotic signals can be inferred from the findings that many cells removed from their natural environment undergo apoptosis but can be rescued from this state by supplying adhesive or soluble signals.

Antiapoptotic Growth Factor-Signaling Pathways

Stimulation of RTKs, especially by IGF-1, PDGF, or NGF, can elicit antiapoptotic signals in various cells *(179,180)*. These antiapoptotic effects may be blocked by inhibitors of PI3K activity or dominant negative forms of PKB. Activated forms of PI3K and PKB can protect cells from apoptosis induced by a variety of stimuli, including loss of anchorage and deprivation of growth factors *(43,181)*. Ras activation also can protect against apoptosis. In PC12 cells, ERK activation can protect from apoptosis *(182),* but in most fibroblasts and epithelial cells examined, activation of PI3K accounts for the survival activity of Ras *(183–184)*. In fibroblasts, activation of the ERK pathway actually promotes apoptosis *(3)*.

One crucial target of PKB may be the Bcl-2 family protein, BAD *(185,186)*. Bcl-2 and Bcl-XL are survival proteins that promote continued function of mitochondria and prevent the aggregation-induced activation of procaspases. Procaspase proteolysis produces an active caspase and results in catalytic amplification of a cascade of activation of different caspases, initiating the varied manifestations of apoptosis. BAD is one member of a Bcl-2-related subfamily that can inactivate the Bcl-2 survival proteins by direct binding. However, PKB phosphorylation of BAD promotes interaction with a 14–3–3 protein and prevents BAD from binding Bcl-2 or Bcl-XL. BAD-induced cell death cannot be prevented by PKB in the absence of its target phosphorylation site, suggesting that BAD phosphorylation is a key antiapoptotic action of the PI3K pathway.

Proapoptotic Growth Factor-Signaling Pathways

The activation of some aspects of growth factor-signaling pathways also can promote apoptosis. Activation has been observed for the Ras–ERK pathway in fibroblasts and in a number of contexts if c-*myc* is overexpressed in the absence of additional strong growth factor inputs (that might promote survival through the PI3K–PKB pathway) *(3,187)*. Since cell-cycle activation involves activation of E2F-1, which itself can induce apoptosis, the proapoptotic properties of c-*myc* may be attributable, at least in part, to E2F-1. For both c-*myc* and E2F-1, apoptosis generally depends on p53 function *(187,188)*, but several exceptions have been found, including situations in which CD95 activation is critical *(189,190)*. This leads to a postulate whereby c-*myc*, and perhaps E2F-1, sensitize a cell to other apoptotic signals, such as DNA damage (mediated by p53) or autocrine production of CD95 ligand.

Both Myc and E2F-1 affect p53 activity by increasing levels of the p19ARF protein *(191,192)*. The p19ARF protein derives from the same locus, INK4A, as the CDK inhibitor, p16, but it shares no amino acid sequences despite sharing a coding exon (which is translated in an alternative reading frame [ARF]) *(193)*. The level and activity of p53 are normally decreased by binding to MDM2 (a p53-inducible gene product). The p19ARF protein can bind MDM2 and prevent it from inhibiting p53 *(194)*. Hence c-*myc* and E2F-1 can activate p53 via p19ARF. Furthermore, primary mouse embryo fibroblasts that lack either p53 or p19ARF are resistant to c-*myc*-induced apoptosis. In the absence of p19ARF, other stimuli, such as DNA damage, can still induce p53 activity and elicit checkpoint responses of growth arrest or apoptosis. Thus, c-*myc* and E2F-1 probably trigger p53-mediated apoptosis by inducing p19ARF, and p19ARF can be regarded as a checkpoint input for p53 that monitors growth factor-signaling pathways. Consistent with this idea, p19ARF null fibroblasts, like p53 nulls, do not show replicative senescence and are stimulated to proliferate rather than undergo senescence in response to activated Ras.

Synthesis

Normal Cells

A cell is normally subject to numerous environmental inputs that regulate its behavior, including ligands that activate tyrosine kinase and TGFβ pathways, and ECM and lateral cell interactions (at least in epithelia). In a quiescent cell, the summation of these inputs is insufficient to trigger passage through the G_1 cell-cycle restriction point, but does effectively counter the cell's inherent apoptotic tendency if the cell maintains its position. Proliferation most commonly will be stimulated by novel presentation or increased concentration of a ligand that induces an increase in cyclin D kinase components. A common way to achieve proliferation is through modest stimulation of the Ras–ERK pathway; however, this proliferation will be sufficient to trigger the cell cycle only if the levels of CDK inhibitors are exceeded. TGFβ family proteins, transcriptional regulators of terminal differentiation (e.g., MyoD), and ERK activation itself induce CDK inhibitors, in part by p19ARF–p53-dependent mechanisms. Other features of tyrosine kinase signaling (e.g., Rho activation and ERK-independent induction of *myc*) may be important to counter these actions and allow a net increase in CDK activity sufficient for cell cycling. Both Myc and Rho can oppose cell-cycle arrest that is imposed by high levels of Kip family inhibitors and may act primarily on cyclin E kinase to promote passage through the G_1 restriction point *(164,177,195)*. Myc induction by ERK activity may be supplemented through translational effects of the PI3K pathway *(56)*, but other important mechanisms probably exist for inducing Myc *(38,141)*.

Once the G_1 restriction point is traversed, Myc and E2F will both be active and may activate p53 by p19ARF, which would promote apoptosis. Several antiapoptotic pathways probably can counter this effect. The PI3K–PKB–BAD-mediated pathway is stimulated by Ras, tyrosine kinase activation, and continued interactions with the ECM. Hence, more than one branch of tyrosine kinase signaling pathways and ECM interactions often may be essential to stimulate cell proliferation in the appropriate environment. In some environments, in which cells lack ECM inputs, or TGFβ signaling is high, or cells are poised to undergo terminal differentiation, stimulation of tyrosine kinase signaling pathways may not induce proliferation but instead may lead to apoptosis, terminal differentiation, or continued quiescence.

Cancer Cells

Key Mutagenic Changes

Tumor formation involves the accumulation of mutations that allow a cell to proliferate autonomously. Initially the cell may take advantage of existing ECM and growth factor inputs that promote survival and cell cycling, but it must overcome inhibitory constraints imposed by its environment. Eventually the tumor cell will be deprived of normal environmental inputs and will have to compensate for this loss. To gain this autonomy, cancer cells generally must undergo several relevant mutations *(4,110)*. To some extent, the need for several mutations can be made according to the known interactions among regulators of cell cycle and apoptotic and senescence programs.

The cyclin D kinase–Rb restriction point can be bypassed by mutations in Rb or cyclin D-kinase inhibitors, such as p16Ink4a, or by amplification of cyclin D genes. One of these changes (but generally not more than one) can be found in most cancers *(138)*. Mechanistically, Ras activation can achieve the same ends by activating cyclin D expression. However, Ras mutations and Rb–p16–cyclin D mutations often are found in the same cancer cell, and Ras mutations generally are not an early occurrence in the progression toward cancer. Thus, Ras probably has additional essential carcinogenic functions, and Rb–cyclin D–p16 alterations may be more effective than Ras at bypassing the Rb restriction point, perhaps because excessive Ras–ERK signaling induces cdk inhibitors and senescence.

Complete bypass of the restriction point also may require stimulation of cyclin E kinase activity in the face of increased levels of Kip-family cdk inhibitors. In some cases stimulation of cyclin kinase may require increased Myc activity induced by gene amplification or by mutagenic activation of signaling pathways (Ras, Wnt, Abl). In other situations, mutagenic inactivation of TGFβ signaling pathways may be required to limit cdk inhibitor levels.

The above mutagenic changes will lead (at least through E2F and Myc) to induction of p53 by p19ARF *(191,192,194)*. Increased p53 activity will induce p21Kip and may lead to cell-cycle arrest and senescence *(138)*. If p21 induction is not sufficient to arrest the cell cycle (e.g., because of the effects of Myc or titration by cyclin D kinases *[1,165,174,176]*) the activation of p53, E2F, and Myc instead may promote apoptosis. The most common means to counter these effects is through mutation of p53 or genes that regulate its activity, including Mdm2 and p19ARF. The p53 and Ink4a mutations (that mostly affect p16 and p19ARF) are extremely common in cancers *(196)*.

Myc and E2F also can trigger p53-independent apoptosis, so even in the absence of p53, tumor cells must have some additional protection from apoptosis. Protection could be provided by the PI3K–PKB pathway, which can be activated by Ras alone in most cells *(43)*. Thus, activating Ras mutations may be important as much for their antiapoptotic role as for their effects on the cell cycle. The induction of autocrine growth factors (e.g., TGFα) or excessive or ectopic receptors (e.g., ErbB2) in response to Ras activation may further enhance the effects of Ras on the cell cycle and cell survival.

The control of the cell cycle by CDKs and their inhibitors, the induction of senescent and apoptotic responses through p53, and the regulatory relationships among CDK effectors, p53, and growth factor-signaling pathways provide a number of obstacles to continued proliferation. Whether this circuitry is in place deliberately to counter carcinogenesis is unclear, but its existence necessitates the accumulation of multiple mutations to produce a cancer.

Development of a Cancer Cell

Although we can observe that cancer cells do accumulate multiple mutations, and we can rationalize the need for these mutations to allow autonomous growth, it is remarkable that this process can occur, especially as replicative senescence normally limits a human cell to about 100 doublings *(145)*. To accumulate three, or often as many as seven, specific mutations in a single cell *(4)* without incurring a significant number of additional mutations that might lead to cell lethality requires a large number of target cells, some mutagenic activity, and a strong selection system. DNA replication is inherently mutagenic. Continued cell division coupled to survival can generate huge numbers of progeny from a single founder cell, and both cell division and escape from cell death can be used as efficient selection strategies. A situation in which one or two mutations permit mild overproliferation and survival of a cell is possible. For this cell and its progeny, proliferation may be limited by occasionally triggering senescence or apoptosis. Thus, if a new mutation reduces or eliminates senescent or apoptotic responses, that cell will now proliferate at the expense of its sisters and produce an even larger population that can incur further mutations and grow more aggressively and more independently of its environment. This process can be repeated, in each case selecting for a new property, including metastasis and angiogenesis. However, this scenario leaves several points unexplained. How does a cell first acquire enough mutations to start behaving differently? How does a cell accumulate so many mutations if only normal errors in DNA replication and environmental mutagens are responsible? Finally, how does a cancer cell extend its life beyond the limit that is normally set by telomere shortening?

To find the answers to these questions, the progressive formation of cancers must be studied. Unfortunately there are very few situations in which progressive genetic changes and changes in behavior can be correlated during the development of the cancer. In spontaneous (noninherited) colorectal cancer, a progression from hyperproliferation, through adenomas of increasing size, carcinoma, and metastasis correlates in many cases with a defined series of genetic changes in the aberrant tissue *(4)*. This progression provides a framework from which to derive speculative ideas.

Loss or mutation of both copies of APC is an extremely prevalent early change in colorectal cancer and is associated with hyperproliferation and early adenomas. In many cases in which APC is unaffected, mutations are found that stabilize β-catenin, its binding partner *(197)*. Tcf is invariably expressed in the APC or β-catenin mutant tissue, implying that activation of β-catenin–Tcf is an important consequence of these mutations. Myc induction may, in turn, be an important response to β-catenin–Tcf, perhaps inducing some additional inappropriate cell cycles *(166)*. However, APC mutations must do more than induce Myc, otherwise *myc* amplification would be expected as an early step in colorectal cancer. Heterozygous APC mutations do predispose individuals to other cancers, but the connection between APC and coloerctal cancer is particularly robust, implying that APC normally has a key role in regulating the behavior of colonic epithelial cells *(4)*. Different cancers may be initiated by mutation of different key genes that have been termed gatekeepers.

Why APC is key in the colon is unclear. Introduction of wild-type APC into mutant cells induces apoptosis, and APC has been implicated in directing migrations from the crypt to the tip of a villus *(129)*. Perhaps the most pressing need for a future cancer cell in the colonic epithelium is to avoid the normal migration toward inevitable cell death at the tips of villi. Mutation of APC may prevent this migration while simultaneously inducing changes that contribute to cell division or survival *(198)*. Continued proliferation of APC mutant cells may rely as much on environmental signals in the crypt, where cell proliferation is abundant, as on the consequences of APC mutation.

In other cancers, the situation may be very different. In hematopoietic cells, a primary mutagenic change may involve stimulation of proliferation from a quiescent state (e.g., by activation of a cytoplasmic tyrosine kinase) *(74)*. p27Kip-mutant mice selectively develop pituitary tumors, implying that changes in cell-cycle control can be key initiators for cells of the intermediate lobe of the pituitary, which normally are found in a quiescent, fully differentiated state in adults *(142)*.

As APC mutant adenomas grow, they probably lose essential growth stimulatory and antiapoptotic signals derived from the base of the crypt. Activating Ras mutations commonly are found in larger adenomas and might provide essential compensation for these missing environmental signals (by induced cyclin D and PI3K–PKB-mediated protection from apoptosis) that otherwise would limit the size of the adenoma.

The next mutation commonly suffered is loss of Smad4. This loss may prevent induction of cdk inhibitors by TGFβ1, which is released from luminal regions of the villi. At this stage we would expect the Ras pathway and induced Myc to drive the cell cycle despite environmental signals that normally would specify quiescence. However, the p19ARF/p53 checkpoint response might be activated, inciting apoptosis. p53 mutations are the next known change suffered in these cells, leading to the generation of carcinomas.

The earliest steps in the carcinoma pathway (loss of two wild-type APC alleles) occur with a frequency and in a time scale commensurate with normal mutation rates *(4)*; however, the subsequent accumulation of mutations (two in *smad4,* two in *p53,* and one in *ras*) is more rapid, suggesting that genomic stability is undergoing changes, most likely induced by a specific mutational event. Colonic tumors almost invariably do display genomic instability, predominantly aneuploidy, which could underlie LOH for the tumor suppressors, p53 and Smad4.

Even if mutations occur at increasingly rapid rates, the accumulation of six key mutations subsequent to an initial APC mutation (perhaps in a stem cell) normally takes many years and would exceed the normal lifespan of a human cell. At some stage, however, many tumor cells acquire telomerase activity *(146)*. Only a few stem cells normally express telomerase. Thus, human cellular life-span is normally limited by replicative shortening of telomeres. This limits growth because it induces senescence and because vital telomeric functions (and subsequently essential genes) are lost. A tumor cell escapes both problems by inactivating instigators of the senescence program (e.g., through p53 mutations) and by activating telomerase. It is interesting to speculate whether these are linked phenomena. For immortal cells (e.g., germline stem cells [GSCs]) telomere shortening conceivably induces telomerase and that response is specifically blocked in other mortal cells by the actions of p53 in favor of inducing p21 and other agents that promote senescence. Perhaps in p53 mutant cells the short telomere signal, or even activated Ras, which can mimic this signal, now activates telomerase.

Many aspects of normal cell proliferation regulation act as double-edged swords in carcinogenesis. Apoptosis and senescence programs demand multiple mutagenic changes to achieve autonomous replication, but they also automatically provide selective pressure for the amplification of populations that have suffered mutations in key regulatory genes (e.g., CDK inhibitors, p53, p19ARF). In some cases mutations in these key reporting genes might further accelerate carcinogenesis, because such mutations (p53 especially) encourage genomic instability or (more speculatively) loss of replicative senescence. The precise way in which cancers exploit these selection systems and their original growth environment to mature slowly toward the disease state is not well understood, but the way is clearly cell type specific. It is important to understand these different strategies to exploit the specific weaknesses of incipient tumors before they develop further mutations that make them less sensitive to interventions.

References

1. Serrano M, Lin AW, McCurrach ME, Beach D, Lowe SW. Oncogenic *ras* provokes premature cell senescence associated with accumulation of *p53* and *p16INK4a*. *Cell.* 1997; 88:593–602.

2. Marshall CJ. Specificity of receptor tyrosine kinase signaling: transient versus sustained extracellular signal-regulated kinase activation. *Cell.* 1995; 80:179–85.

3. Kauffmann-Zeh A, Rodriguez-Viciana P, Ulrich E, et al. Suppression of c-Myc-induced apoptosis by Ras signalling throgh PI(3)K and PKB. *Nature.* 1997; 385:544–8.

4. Kinzler KW, Vogelstein B. Lessons from hereditary colorectal cancer. *Cell.* 1996; 87:159–70.

5. Schweitzer R, Shilo BZ. A thousand and one roles for the *Drosophila* EGF receptor. *Trends Genet.* 1997; 13:191–6.

6. Ingham PW. Transducing Hedgehog: the story so far. *EMBO J.* 1998; 17:3505–11.

7. Cadigan KM, Nusse R. Wnt signalling: a common theme in animal development. *Genes Dev.* 1997; 11:3286–305.

8. Whitman M. Smads and early developmental signaling by the TGFβ superfamily. *Genes Dev.* 1998; 12:2445–62.

9. Clandinin TR, DeModena JA, Sternberg PW. Inositol trisphosphate mediates a Ras-independent response to Let-23 receptor tyrosine kinase activation in *C. elegans. Cell.* 1998; 92:523–33.

10. Blair SS. Compartments and appendage development in *Drosophila. Bioessays.* 1995; 17:299–309.

11. Dominguez M, Brunner M, Hafen E, Basler K. Sending and receiving the Hedgehog signal-control by the *Drosophila* Gli protein Cubitus interruptus. *Science.* 1996; 272:1621–25.

12. Brook WJ, Cohen SM. Antagonistic interactions between Wingless and Decapentaplegic responsible for dorsal–ventral pattern in the *Drosophila* leg. *Science.* 1996; 273:1373–76.

13. Meier P, Evan G. Dying like flies. *Cell.* 1998; 95:295–8.

14. Kumar JP, Tio M, Hsiung F, et al. Dissecting the roles of the EGF receptor in eye development and MAP kinase activation. *Development.* 1998; 125:3875–85.

15. Freeman M. Cell determination strategies in the *Drosophila* eye. *Development.* 1997; 124:261–70.

16. Kumar J, Moses K. Transcription factors in eye development; a gorgeous mosaic. *Genes Dev.* 1997; 11:2023–28.

17. Weiss A, Schlessinger J. Switching signals on or off by receptor dimerization. *Cell.* 1998; 94:277–80.

18. Kavanaugh WM, Williams LT. An alternative to SH2 domains for binding tyrosine-phosphorylated proteins. *Science.* 1994; 266:1862–65.

19. Pawson T. Protein molecules and signalling networks. *Nature.* 1995; 373:573–80.

20. Songyang Z, Shoelson SE, Chaudhuri M, et al. SH2 domains recognize specific phospho-peptide sequences. *Cell.* 1993; 72:767–8.

21. Heldin CH. Simultaneous induction of stimulatory and inhibitory signals by PDGF. *FEBS Lett.* 1997; 410:17–21.

22. Kazlauskas A. Receptor tyrosine kinases and their targets. *Curr Opin Genet Dev.* 1994; 4:5–14.

23. Egan SE, Giddings BW, Brooks MW, Buday L, Sizeland AM, Weinberg RA. Association of Sos Ras exchange protein with Grb2 is implicated in tyrosine kinase signal transduction and transformation. *Nature.* 1993; 363:5–51.

24. Rozakis-Adcock M, McGlade J, Mbamalu G, et al. Association of the Shc and Grb2/Sem5 SH2-containing proteins is implicated in activation of the Ras pathway by tyrosine kinases. *Nature.* 1992; 360:689–92.

25. Baltensperger K, Kozma LM, Cherniack AD, et al. Binding of the Ras activator Son of Sevenless to insulin receptor substrate-1 signaling complexes. *Science.* 1993; 260:1950–52.

26. Kouhara H, Hadari YR, Spivak-Kroizman T, et al. A lipid-anchored Grb2-binding protein

that links FGF-receptor activation to the Ras/MAPK signaling pathway. *Cell.* 1997; 89:693–702.

27. Tzivion G, Luo Z, Avruch J. A dimeric 14-3-3 protein is an essential cofactor for Raf kinase activity. *Nature.* 1998; 394:88–92.

28. Morrison D, Cutler RE. The complexity of Raf-1 regulation. *Curr Opin Cell Biol.* 1997; 9:174–9.

29. Sternberg PW, Alberola-Ila J. Conspiracy theory: Ras and Raf do not act alone. *Cell.* 1998; 95:447–50.

30. Tzivion X, Luo Z, Avruch J. A dimeric 14-3-3 protein is an essential cofactor for Raf kinase activity. *Nature.* 1998; 394:88–92.

31. Lewis TS, Shapiro PS, Ahn NG. Signal transduction through MAP kinase cascades. *Adv Cancer Res.* 1998; 74:49–139.

32. Robinson MJ, Cobb MH. Mitogen-activated protein kinase pathways. *Curr Opin Cell Biol.* 1997; 9:180–6.

33. Elion EA. Routing MAP kinase cascades. *Science.* 1998; 281:1625–6.

34. Wasylyk B, Hagman J, Gutierrez-Hartmann A. Ets transcription factors: nuclear effectors of the Ras–MAP-kinase signaling pathway. *Trends Biochem Sci.* 1998; 23:213–6.

35. Xing J, Ginty DD, Greenberg ME. Coupling of the Ras–MAPK pathway to gene activation by RSK2, a growth factor-regulated CREB kinase. *Science.* 1996; 273:959–63.

36. Roussel MF, Davis JN, Cleveland JL, Ghysdael J, Hiebart SW. Dual control of *myc* expression through a single DNA binding site targeted by ets family proteins and E2F. *Oncogene.* 1994; 9:405–15.

37. Bouchard C, Staller P, Eilers M. Control of cell proliferation by Myc. *Trends Cell Biol.* 1998; 8:202–6.

38. Barone MV, Courtneidge SA. Myc but not Fos rescue of PDGF signalling block caused by kinase-inactive Src. *Nature.* 1995; 378:509–2.

39. Ip YT, Davis RJ. Signal transduction by the c-*jun* N-terminal kinase (JNK)—from inflammation to development. *Curr Opin Cell Biol.* 1998; 10:205–19.

40. Sonenberg N, Gingras AC. The mRNA 5′ cap-binding protein eIF4E and control of cell growth. *Curr Opin Cell Biol.* 1998; 10:268–75.

41. Carpenter CL, Cantley LC. Phosphoinositide kinases. *Curr Opin Cell Biol.* 1996; 8:153–8.

42. Pullen N, Dennis PB, Andjelkovic M, et al. Phosphorylation and activation of p70S6K by PDK1. *Science.* 1998; 279:707–10.

43. Downward J. Mechanisms and consequences of activation of protein kinase B/Akt. *Curr Opin Cell Biol.* 1998; 10:262–7.

44. Alessi DR, Kozlowski MT, Weng QP, Morrice N, Avruch J. 3-Phosphoinositide-dependent protein kinase 1 (PDK1) phosphorylates and activates the p70 S6 kinase in vivo and in vitro. *Curr Biol.* 1997; 8:69–81.

45. Downward J. Lipid-regulated kinases: some common themes at last. *Science.* 1998; 279:673–4.

46. Le Good JA, Ziegler WH, Parekh DB, Alessi DR, Cohen P, Parker PJ. Protein kinase C isotypes controlled by phosphoinositide 3-kinase through the protein kinase PKD1. *Science.* 1998; 281:2042–45.

47. Rodriguez-Viciana P, Warne PH, Khwaja A, et al. Role of phosphoinositide 3-OH kinase in cell transformation and control of the actin cytoskeleton by Ras. *Cell.* 1997; 89:457–67.

48. Nimnual AS, Yatsula BA, Bar-Sagi D. Coupling of Ras and Rac guanosine triphosphatases through the Ras exchanger Sos. *Science.* 1998; 279:560–62.

49. Han J, Luby-Phelps K, Das B, et al. Role of substrates and products of PI 3-kinase in

regulating activation of Rac-related guanosine triphosphatases by Vav. *Science.* 1998; 279:558–60.

50. Hawkins PT, Eguinoa A, Qiu RG, et al. PDGF stimulates an increase in GTP–Rac via activation of phosphoinositide 3-kinase. *Curr Biol.* 1995; 5:393–405.

51. Van Aelst L, D'Souza-Schorey C. Rho GTPases and signaling networks. *Genes Dev.* 1997; 11:2295–322.

52. Reif K, Nobes CD, Thomas G, Hall A, Cantrell DA. Phosphatidylinositol 3-kinase signals activate a selective subset of Rac/Rho-dependent effector pathways. *Curr Biol.* 1996; 6:1445–55.

53. Chou MM, Blenis J. The 70 kDa S6 kinase complexes with and is activated by the Rho family G proteins Cdc42 and Rac1. *Cell.* 1996; 85:573–83.

54. Mendes R, Kollmorgen G, White MF, Rhoads RE. Requirement of protein kinase Cζ for stimulation of protein synthesis by insulin. *Mol Cell Biol.* 1997; 17:5184–92.

55. Proud CG. p70 S6 kinase: an enigma with variations. *Trends Biochem Sci.* 1996; 21:181–5.

56. West MJ, Stonely M, Willis AE. Translational induction of the c-*myc* oncogene via activation of the FRAP/TOR signalling pathway. *Oncogene.* 1998; 17:769–80.

57. Burnett PE, Barrow RK, Cohen NA, Snyder SH, Sabatini DM. RAFT1 phosphorylation of the translational regulators p70 S6 kinase and 4E–BP1. *Proc Natl Acad Sci USA.* 1998; 95:1432–37.

58. Hara K, Yonezawa K, Weng QP, Kazlowski MT, Belham C, Avruch J. Amino acid sufficiency and mTOR regulate p70 S6 kinase and eIF–4E BP1 through a common effector mechanism. *J Biol Chem.* 1998; 273:14484–94.

59. Marais R, Light Y, Mason C, Paterson H, Olson MF, Marshall CJ. Requirement of Ras–GTP–Raf complexes for activation of Raf-1 by protein kinase C. *Science.* 1998; 280:109–12.

60. Darnell JE. STATs and gene regulation. *Science.* 1997; 277:1630–35.

61. Scharenberg AM, Kinet JP. PtdIns-3,4,5-P3: a regulatory nexus between tyrosine kinases and sustained calcium signals. *Cell.* 1998; 94:5–8.

62. Rodriguez-Viciana P, Warne PH, Dhand R, et al. Phosphatidylinositol-3-OH kinase as a direct target of Ras. *Nature.* 1994; 370:527–32.

63. Klinghofer RA, Duckworth B, Valius M, Cantley L, Kazlauskas A. PDGF-dependent activation of PI3-kinase is regulated by receptor binding of SH2-domain-containing proteins which influence Ras activity. *Mol Cell Biol.* 1996; 16:5905–14.

64. Hu Q, Klippel A, Muslin AJ, Fantl WJ, Williams LT. Ras-dependent induction of cellular responses by constitutively active phosphatidylinositol-3 kinase. *Science.* 1995; 268:100–2.

65. King AJ, Sun H, Diaz B, et al. The protein kinase Pak3 positively regulates Raf-1 activity through phosphorylation of serine 338. *Nature.* 1998; 396:180–3.

66. White MA, Nicolette C, Minden A, et al. Multiple Ras functions can contribute to mammalian cell transformation. *Cell.* 1995; 80:533–41.

67. Todaro GJ, DeLarco JE, Cohen S. Transformation by murine and feline sarcoma viruses specifically blocks binding of epidermal growth factors to cells. *Nature.* 1976; 264:26–31.

68. Tzahar E, Yarden Y. The ErbB-2/HER2 oncogenic receptor of adenocarcinomas: from orphanhood to multiple stromal ligands. *Biochem Biophys Acta.* 1998; 1377:M25–M37.

69. McCarthy SA, Samuels ML, Pritchard CA, Abraham JA, McMahon M. Rapid induction of heparin-binding epidermal growth factor/diphtheria toxin receptor expression by *Raf* and *Ras* oncogenes. *Genes Dev.* 1995; 9:1953–64.

70. Lenferink AE, Pinkas-Kramarski R, van de Pol, ML, et al. Differential endocytic routing of homo- and hetero-dimeric ErbB tyrosine kinases confers signaling superiority to receptor heterodimers. *EMBO J.* 1997; 17:3385–97.

71. Tzahar E, Pinkas-Kramarski R, Moyer JD, et al. Bivalence of EGF-like ligands drives the ErbB signaling network. *EMBO J.* 1997; 16:4934–50.

72. Watowich SS, Wu H, Socolovsky M, Klingmuller U, Constantinescu SN, Lodish HF. Cytokine receptor signal transduction and the control of hematopoietic cell development. *Annu Rev Cell Dev Biol.* 1996; 12:91–128.

73. Ihle JN. Cytokine receptor signalling. *Nature.* 1995; 377:591–4.

74. Bolen JB, Brugge JS. Leukocyte protein tyrosine kinases: potential for drug discovery. *Annu Rev Immunol.* 1997; 15:371–404.

75. Tybulewicz VL. Analysis of antigen receptor signalling using mouse gene targeting. *Curr Opin Cell Biol.* 1998; 10:195–204.

76. Weiss A, Littman DR. Signal transduction by lymphocyte antigen receptors. *Cell.* 1994; 76:263–74.

77. Cantrell D. The real LAT steps forward. *Trends Cell Biol.* 1998; 8:180–2.

78. Hawes BE, van Biesen T, Koch WJ, Lutrell LM, Lefkowitz RJ. Distinct pathways of Gi- and Gq-mediated mitogen-activated protein kinase activation. *J Biol Chem.* 1995; 270:17148–53.

79. Rozengurt E, Rodriguez-Fernandez JL. Tyrosine phosphorylation in the action of neuropeptides and growth factors. *Essays Biochem.* 1997; 32:73–86.

80. Kranenburg O, Verlaan I, Hordijk PL, Moolenaar WH. Gi-mediated activation of the Ras/MAP kinase pathway involves a 100 kDa tyrosine-phosphorylated Grb2 SH3 binding protein, but not Src or Shc. *EMBO J* 1997; 16:3097–105.

81. Lopez-Ilasaca M, Crespo P, Pellici PG, Gutkind JS, Wetzker R. Linkage of G protein-coupled receptors to the MAPk signaling pathway through PI 3-kinase γ. *Science.* 1997; 275:394–7.

82. Bondeva T, Pirola L, Bulgarelli-Leva G, Rubio I, Wetzker R, Wymann MP. Bifurcation of lipid and protein kinase signals of PI3Kγ to the protein kinases PKB and MAPK. *Science.* 1998; 282:293–6.

83. Dikic I, Tokiwa G, Lev S, Courtneidge SA, Schlessinger J. A role for Pyk2 and Src in linking G-protein-coupled receptors with MAP kinase activation. *Nature.* 1996; 383:547–50.

84. Luttrell LM, Della Rocca GJ, van Biesen T, Luttrell DK, Lefkowitz RJ, Gβγ subunits mediate Src-dependent phosphorylation of the epidermal growth factor receptor. *J Biol Chem.* 1997; 272:4637–44.

85. Hall A. G proteins and small GTPases: distant relatives keep in touch. *Science.* 1998; 280:2074–5.

86. Hart MJ, Jiang X, Kozasa T, et al. Direct stimulation of the guanine nucleotide exchange activity of p115 RhoGEF by Ga13. *Science.* 1998; 280:2112–4.

87. Kozasa T, Jiang X, Hart MJ, et al. P115 RhoGEF, a GTPase activating protein for Ga12 and Ga13. *Science.* 1998; 280:2109–11.

88. Varner JA, Cheresh DA. Integrins and cancer. *Curr Opin Cell Biol.* 1996; 8:724–30.

89. Lin CQ, Bissell MJ. Multi-faceted regulation of cell differentiation via extracellular matrix. *FASEB J.* 1993; 7:737–43.

90. Clark EA, Brugge JS. Integrins and signal transduction pathways: the road taken. *Science.* 1995; 268:233–9.

91. Howe A, Aplin AE, Alahari SJ, Juliano RL. Integrin signaling and cell growth control. *Curr Opin Cell Biol.* 1998; 10:220–31.

92. Wary KK, Mainiero F, Isakoff SJ, Marcantonio EE, Giancotti FG. The adapter protein Shc couples a class of integrins to the control of cell cycle progression. *Cell.* 1996; 87: 733–43.

93. Wary KK, Mariotti A, Zurzolo C, Giancotti FG. A requirement for caveolin-1 and associated kinase Fyn in integrin signaling and anchorage-dependent cell growth. *Cell.* 1998; 94:625–34.

94. Novak A, Hsu SC, Leung-Hagenstein C, et al. Cell adhesion and the integrin-linked kinase regulate the LEF-1 and β-catenin signaling pathways. *Proc Natl Acad Sci USA.* 1998; 95:4374–9.

95. Roberts AB, Sporn MB. Physiological actions and clinical applications of transforming growth factor-β. *Growth Factors.* 1993; 8:1–9.

96. Sasai Y, De Robertis EM. Ectodermal patterning in vertebrate embryos. *Dev Biol.* 1997; 182:5–20.

97. Zimmerman LB, De Jesus-Escobar LJ, Harland RM. The Spemann organizer signal noggin binds and inactivates bone morphogenetic protein 4. *Cell.* 1996; 86:599–606.

98. Wilson PA, Lagna G, Suzuki A, Hemmati-Brivanlou A. Concentration-dependent patterning of the *Xenopus* ectoderm by BMP4 and its signal transducer Smad1. *Development.* 1997; 124:3177–84.

99. Piccolo S, Sasai Y, Lu B, DeRobertis E. Dorsoventral patterning in *Xenopus* inhibition of ventral signals by binding of chordin to BMP-4. *Cell.* 1996; 86:589–98.

100. Zou H, Niswander L. Requirement for BMP signaling in interdigital apoptosis and scale formation. *Science.* 1996; 272:738–41.

101. Xie T, Spradling AC. Decapentaplegic is essential for the maintenance and division of germline stem cells in the *Drosophila* ovary. *Cell.* 1998; 94:251–60.

102. Wrana JL, Attisano L, Wieser R, Ventura F, Massague J. Mechanism of activation of the TGFβ receptor. *Nature.* 1994; 370:341–7.

103. Liu F, Pouponnot C, Massague J. Dual role of the Smad4/DPC4 tumor suppressor in TGFβ inducible transcriptional complexes. *Genes Dev.* 1997; 11:3157–67.

104. Chen X, Weisber E, Vridmacher V, Watanabe M, Naco G, Whitman M. Smad4 and FAST-1 in the assembly of activin-response factor. *Nature.* 1997; 389:85–9.

105. Kim J, Johnson K, Chen H, Carroll S, Laughon A. *Drosophila* Mad binds to DNA and directly mediates activation of vestigial by Decapentaplegic. *Nature.* 1998; 388:304–8.

106. Feng XH, Derynck R. A kinase subdomain of transforming growth factor-β (TGFβ) type I receptor determines the TGFβ intracellular signaling specificity. *EMBO J.* 1997; 16:3912–23.

107. Kretzschmar M, Doody J, Massague J. Opposing BMP and EGF signalling pathways converge on the TGFβ family mediator Smad1. *Nature.* 1997; 389:618–22.

108. de Caestecker C, Parks W, Frank C, et al. Smad2 transduces common signals from receptor serine-threonine and tyrosine kinases. *Genes Dev.* 1998; 12:1587–92.

109. Neubuser A, Peters H, Balling R, Martin G. Antagonistic interactions between FGF and BMP signaling pathways: a mechanism for positioning the sites of tooth formation. *Cell.* 1997; 90:247–55.

110. Vogelstein B, Fearon ER, Hamiltaon SR, et al. Genetic alterations during colorectal-tumor development. *N Engl J Med.* 1988; 319:525–32.

111. Hahn SA, Schutte M, Hoque AT, et al. DPC4, a candidate tumor suppressor gene at human chromosome 18q21.1. *Science.* 1996; 271:350–53.

112. Lu S, Kawabata M, Imamura T, et al. HNPCC associated with germline mutation in the TGFβ type II receptor gene. *Nat Genet.* 1998; 19:17–8.

113. Markowitz S, Wang J, Myeroff L, et al. Inactivation of the type II TGFβ receptor in colon cancer cells with microsatellite instability. *Science.* 1995; 268:1336–8.

114. Zhu Y, Richardson JA, Parada LF, Graff JM. Smad3 mutant mice develop metastatic colorectal cancer. *Cell.* 1998; 94:703–14.

115. Takaku K, Oshima M, Miyoshi H, Matsui M, Seldin JF, Taketo MM. Intestinal tumorigenesis in compound mutant mice of both *Dpc4* (*Smad4*) and *Apc* genes. *Cell.* 1998; 92:645–56.

116. Cui W, Fowlis DJ, Bryson S, et al. TGFβ 1 inhibits the formation of benign skin tumors, but enhances progression to invasive spindle carcinomas in transgenic mice. *Cell.* 1996; 86:531–42.

117. Brown JD, Moon RT. Wnt signaling: why is everything so negative? *Curr Opin Cell. Biol.* 1998; 10:182–7.

118. Kengaku M, Capdevila J, Rodriguez-Esteban C, et al. Distinct WNT pathways regulating AER formation and dorsoventral polarity in the chick limb bud. *Science.* 1998; 280:1274–7.

119. Slusarski DC, Corces VG, Moon RT. Interaction of Wnt and a Frizzled homologue triggers G-protein-linked phosphatidylinositol signalling. *Nature.* 1997; 390:410–3.

120. Aberle H, Bauer A, Stappert J, Kispert A, Kemler R. β-Catenin is a target for the ubiquitin-proteasome pathway. *EMBO J.* 1997; 16:3797–804.

121. Cavallo R, Rubenstein D, Peifer M. Armadillo and dTCF: a marriage made in the nucleus. *Curr Opin Gen Dev.* 1997; 7:459–66.

122. Cox RT, Peifer M. Wingless signaling: the inconvenient complexities of life. *Curr Biol.* 1998; 8:R140–4.

123. Brannon M, Gomperts M, Sumoy L, Moon RT, Kimelman D. A β-catenin/XTcf-3 complex binds to the siamois promoter to regulate dorsal axis specification in *Xenopus. Genes Dev.* 1997; 11:2359–70.

124. Han M. Gut reaction to Wnt signaling in worms. *Cell.* 1997; 90:581–4.

125. Ikeda S, Kishida S, Yamamoto H, Murai H, Koyama S, Kikuchi A. Axin, a negative regulator of the Wnt signaling pathway, forms a complex with GSK-3β and β-catenin and promotes GSK-3β-dependent phosphorylation of β-catenin. *EMBO J.* 1998; 17:1371–84.

126. Zeng L, Fagotto F, Zhang T, et al. The mouse Fused locus encodes Axin, an inhibitor of the Wnt signaling pathway that regulates embryonic axis formation. *Cell.* 1997; 90:181–92.

127. Yost C, Farr GH, Pierce SB, Ferkey DM, Chen MM, Kimelman D. GBP, an inhibitor of GSK-3, is implicated in *Xenopus* development and oncogenesis. *Cell.* 1998; 93:1031–41.

128. Gumbiner BM. Carcinogenesis: a balance between β-catenin and APC. *Curr Biol.* 1997; 7:R443–6.

129. Barth AI, Pollack AL, Altschuler Y, Mostov KE, Nelson WJ. Amino-terminal deletion of β-catenin results in stable co-localization of mutant β-catenin with APC protein and altered MDCK cell adhesion. *J Cell Biol.* 1997; 136:693–706.

130. Ingham PW. The patched gene in development and cancer. *Curr Opin Genet Dev.* 1998; 8:88–94.

131. Dahmane N, Lee J, Robins P, Heller P, Ruiz i Altaba A. Activation of the transcription factor Gli 1 and the Sonic hedgehog signalling pathway in skin tumours. *Nature.* 1997; 389:876–81.

132. Johnson RL, Rothman AL, Xie JW, et al. Human homolog of patched, a candidate gene for the basal cell nevus syndrome. *Science.* 1996; 272:1668–71.

133. Xie J. Murone M, Luoh SM, et al. Activating smoothened mutations in sporadic basal-cell carcinoma. *Nature.* 1998; 391:90–2.

134. Oro AE, Higgins KM, Hu Z, Bonifas JM, Epstein EH, Scott MP. Basal cell carcinoma in mice overexpressing Sonic hedgehog. *Science.* 1997; 276:817–9.

135. Larsson O, Dafgard E, Engstrom W, Zetterberg A. Immediate effects of serum depletion on dissociation between growth in size and cell division in 3T3 cells. *J Cell Physiol.* 1986; 127:267–73.

136. Sherr CJ. G1 phase progression: cycling on cue. *Cell.* 1994; 79:551–5.

137. Weinberg RA. The retinoblastoma protein and cell cycle control. *Cell.* 1995; 81:323–30.

138. Sherr CJ. Cancer cell cycles. *Science.* 1996; 274:1672–7.

139. Sherr CJ, Roberts JM. Inhibitors of mammalian G1 cyclin-dependent kinases. *Genes Dev.* 1995; 9:1149–63.

140. Quelle DE, Ashmun RA, Shurtleff SA, et al. Overexpression of mouse D-type cyclins accelerates G1 phase in rodent fibroblasts. *Genes Dev.* 1993; 7:1559–71.

141. Roussel MF. Key effectors of signal transduction and G1 progression. *Adv Cancer Res.* 1998; 65:1–25.

142. Kiyokawa H, Kineman RD, Manova-Todorova KO, et al. Enhanced growth of mice lacking the cyclin-dependent kinase inhibitor function of p27Kip1. *Cell.* 1996; 85:721–32.

143. Halevy O, Novitch BG, Spicer DB, et al. Correlation of terminal cell cycle arrest of skeletal muscle with induction of p21 by MyoD. *Science.* 1995; 267:1018–21.

144. Skapek SX, Rhee J, Spicer DB, Lasser AB. Inhibition of myogenic differentiation in proliferating myoblasts by cyclin D-dependent kinase. *Science.* 1995; 267:1022–44.

145. Campisi J. Replicative senescence: an old lives' tale? *Cell.* 1996; 84:497–500.

146. de Lange T. Telomeres and senescence: ending the debate. *Science.* 1998; 279:334–5.

147. Serrano M, Lee HW, Chin L, Gordon-Cardo C, Beach D, De Pinho RA. Role of the INK4a locus in tumor suppression and immortality. *Cell.* 1996; 85:27–37.

148. Weinberg RA. The cat and mouse games that genes, viruses, and cells play. *Cell.* 1997; 88:573–5.

149. McConnell BB, Starborg M, Brookes S, Peters G. Inhibitors of cyclin-dependent kinases induces features of replicative senescence in early passage human diploid fibroblasts. *Curr Biol.* 1998; 8:351–4.

150. White RJ, Trouche D, Martin K, Jackson SP, Kouzarides T. Repression of RNA polymerase III transcription by the retinoblastoma protein. *Nature.* 1996; 382:8–90.

151. Cavanaugh AH, Hempel WM, Taylor LJ, Rogalsky V, Todorov G, Rothblum LI. Activity of RNA polymerase I transcription factor UBF blocked by RB gene product. *Nature.* 1995; 374:177–80.

152. Zetterberg A, Engstrom W, Dafgard E. The relative effects of different types of growth factor on DNA replication, mitosis and cellular enlargement. *Cytometry.* 1984; 5:368–75.

153. Peeper DS, Upton TM, Ladha MH, et al. RAS signalling linked to the cell cycle machinery by the retinoblastoma protein. *Nature.* 1997; 386:177–81.

154. Albanese C, Johnson J, Watanabe G, et al. Transforming p21ras mutants and c-Ets-2 activate the cyclin D promoter through distinguishable regions. *J Biol Chem.* 1995; 270:23589–97.

155. Afar DE, McLaughlin L, Sherr CJ, Witte ON, Roussel MF. Signaling by *abl* oncogenes through cyclin D1. *Proc Natl Acad Sci USA.* 1995; 92:9540–4.

156. Roussel MF, Theodoras AM, Pagano M, Sherr CJ. Rescue of defective mitogenic signaling by D-type cyclins. *Proc Natl Acad Sci USA.* 1995; 92:6837–41.

157. Winston JT, Pledger WJ. Growth regulation of cyclin D1 mRNA expression through protein synthesis-dependent and -independent mechanisms. *Mol Biol Chem.* 1993; 4:1133–44.

158. Winston JT, Coats SR, Wang YZ, Pledger WJ. Regulation of the cell cycle machinery by oncogenic ris. *Oncogene.* 1996; 12:127–34.

159. Matsushime H, Quelle DE, Shurtleff SA, Shibuya M, Sherr CJ, Kato J. D-type cyclin dependent kinase activity in mammalian cells. *Mol Cell Biol.* 1994; 14:2066–76.

160. Hengst L, Reed SI. Translational control of p27Kip1 accumulation during the cell cycle. *Science.* 1996; 271:1851–64.

161. Kato J, Matsuoka M, Polyak K, Massague J, Sherr CJ. Cyclic AMP induced G1 arrest mediated by an inhibitor (p27Kip1) of cyclin dependent kinase 4 activation. *Cell.* 1994; 79:487–96.

162. Nourse J, Firpo E, Flanagan WM, et al. Interleukin-2 mediated elimination of p27Kip1 cyclin-dependent kinase inhibitor prevented by rapamycin. *Nature.* 1994; 372:570–3.

163. Fisher RP, Morgan DO. A novel cyclin associates with MO15/cdk7 to form the cdk-activating kinase. *Cell.* 1994; 78:713–24.

164. Galaktinov K, Chen X, Beach D. Cdc25 cell-cycle phosphatase as a target of c-*myc*. *Nature.* 1996; 382:511–7.

165. Ruley HE. Transforming collaborations between *ras* and nuclear oncogenes. *Cancer Cells.* 1990; 2:258–68.

166. He TC, Sparks AB, Rago C, et al. Identification of c-*MYC* as a target of the APC pathway. *Science.* 1998; 281:1509–12.

167. Ewen ME, Oliver CJ, Sluss HK, Miller SJ, Peeper DS. p53-dependent repression of CDK4 translation in TGFβ1 induced cell cycle arrest. *Genes Dev.* 1995; 9:204–17.

168. Ewen ME, Sluss HK, Whitehouse LL, Livingston DM. TGFβ inhibition of cdk4 synthesis is linked to cell cycle arrest. *Cell.* 1993; 74:1009–20.

169. Geng Y, Weinberg RA. Transforming growth factor β effects on expression of G1 cyclins and cyclin-dependent protein kinases. *Proc Natl Acad Sci USA.* 1993; 89:5547–51.

170. Hannon GJ, Beach D. p15INK4b is a potential effector of TGFβ induced cell cycle arrest. *Nature.* 1994; 371:257–61.

171. Slingerland JM, Hengst L, Pan C, Alexander D, Stampfer M, Reed SI. A novel inhibitor of cyclin-cdk activity detected in transforming growth factor-β arrested epithelial cells. *Mol Cell Biol.* 1994; 14:3683–94.

172. Polyak K, Kato JY, Solomon MJ, et al. p27Kip1, a cyclin dependent kinase inhibitor, links transforming growth factor β and contact inhibition to cell cycle arrest. *Genes Dev.* 1994; 8:9–22.

173. Reynisdottir I, Polyak K, Ivarone A, Massague J. Kip/Cip and Ink4 cdk inhibitors cooperate to induce cell cycle arrest in response to TGFβ. *Genes Dev.* 1995; 9:1831–45.

174. Lin A, Barradas M, Stone JC, van Aelst L, Serrano M, Lowe SW. Premature senescence involving p53 and p16 is activated in response to constitutive MEK/MAPK mitogenic signaling. *Genes Dev.* 1998; 12:3008–19.

175. Woods D, Parry D, Cherwinski H, Bosch E, Lees E, McMahon M. Raf-induced proliferation or cell cycle arrest is determined by the level of Raf activity with arrest mediated by p21 Cip1. *Mol Cell Biol.* 1997; 17:5598–611.

176. Zhu J, Woods D, McMahon M, Bishop JM. Senescence of human fibroblasts induced by oncogenic Raf. *Genes Dev.* 1998; 12:2997–3007.

177. Olson MF, Paterson HF, Marshall CJ. Signals from Ras and Rho GTPases interact to regulate expression of p21Waf1/Cip1. *Nature.* 1998; 394:295–9.

178. Jacobson MD, Weil M, Raff MC. Programmed cell death in animal development. *Cell.* 1997; 88:347–54.

179. Stewart CE, Rotwein P. Growth, differentiation and survival; multiple physiological functions for insulin-like growth factors. *Physiol Rev.* 1996; 76:1005–26.

180. Segal RA, Greenberg ME. Intracellular signaling pathways activated by neurotrophic factors. *Annu Rev Neurosci.* 1996; 19:463–89.

181. Khwaja A, Rodriguez-Viciana P, Weenstrom S, Warne PH, Downward J. Matrix adhesion and Ras transformation both activate a phosphoinositide 3-OH and protein kinase B/Akt cellular survival pathway. *EMBO J.* 1997; 16:2783–93.

182. Xia Z, Dickens M, Raingeaud J, Davis RJ, Greenberg ME. Opposing effects of ERK and JNK-p38 MAP kinases on apoptosis. *Science.* 1995; 270:1326–31.

183. Dudek H, Datta SR, Franke TF, et al. Regulation of neuronal survival by the serine–threonine protein kinase Akt. *Science.* 1997; 275:661–5.

184. Marte BM, Downward J. PKB/Akt: connecting phosphoinositide 3-kinase to cell survival and beyond. *Trends Biochem Sci.* 1997; 22:355–8.

185. Datta SR, Dudek H, Tao X, et al. Akt phosphorylation of BAd couples survival signals to the cell-intrinsic death machinery. *Cell.* 1997; 91:231–41.

186. del Peso L, Gonzalez-Garcia M, Page C, Herrera R, Nunez G. Interleukin-3-induced phosphorylation of BAD through the protein kinase Akt. *Science.* 1997; 278:687–9.

187. Thompson EB. The many roles of c-*myc* in apoptosis. *Annu Rev Physiol.* 1998; 60:575–600.

188. Wu X, Levine AJ. p53 and E2F-1 cooperate to mediate apoptosis. *Proc Natl Acad Sci USA.* 1994; 91:3602–6.

189. Hueber AO, Zornig M, Lyon D, Suda T, Shigekazu N, Evan GI. Requirement for the CD95 receptor-ligand pathway in c-*Myc*-induced apoptosis. *Science.* 1997; 278:1305–9.

190. Evan G, Littlewood T. A matter of life and cell death. *Science.* 1998; 281:1317–22.

191. Zindy F, Eischen CM, Randle D, et al. *Myc* signaling via the ARF tumor suppressor regulates p53-dependent apoptosis and immortalization. *Genes Dev.* 1998; 12:2424–34.

192. de Stanchina E, McCurrach ME, Zindy F, et al. E1A signaling to p53 involves the p19ARF tumor suppressor. *Genes Dev.* 1998; 12:2435–43.

193. Chin L, Pomerantz J, DePinho RA. The INK4a/ARF tumor suppressor: one gene—two products—two pathways. *Trends Biochem Sci.* 1998; 23:291–6.

194. Pomerantz J, Schreiber-Agus N, Liegeois NJ, et al. The Ink4a tumor suppressor gene product p19ARF interacts with MDM2 and neutralizes MDM2's inhibition of p53. *Cell.* 1998; 9:713–23.

195. Vlach J, Hennecke S, Alevizopoulos K, Conti D, Amati B. Growth arrest by the cyclin dependent kinase inhibitor p27Kip1 is abrogated by c-*myc*. *EMBO J.* 1996; 15:6595–604.

196. Sherr CJ. Tumor surveillance via the ARF–p53 pathway. *Genes Dev.* 1998; 12:2984–91.

197. Sparks AB, Morin PJ, Vogelstein B, Kinzler KW. Mutational analysis of the APC/β-catenin/Tsf pathway in colorectal cancer. *Cancer Res.* 1998; 58:1130–34.

198. Peifer M. β-Catenin as oncogene: the smoking gun. *Science.* 1997; 275:1752–3.

7

Estrogen Action and Breast Cancer

Hong Liu and V. Craig Jordan

Introduction

Worldwide, breast cancer is the most common cancer affecting women, accounting for 19% of all malignancies in women *(1)*. The growth of breast tumors can be regulated by multiple factors (Fig. 1) including steroid hormones such as estrogens *(2,3)*, progesterones *(4,5)*, and androgens *(6)*; growth factors such as epidermal growth factor (EGF) *(7)*; insulin; and insulin-like growth factor-I (IGF-I) *(8)*. Epidemiological studies and animal models of carcinogenesis demonstrated that ovarian hormones play a critical role in the etiology of breast cancer *(9–14)*.

In 1896 George Beatson demonstrated that removal of the ovaries in a premenopausal patient with breast cancer could lead to a dramatic improvement in the course of the disease. However, by 1900 Stanley Boyd had demonstrated, in perhaps the first clinical trial, that only one in three premenopausal women could anticipate disease control after oophorectomy. Unfortunately, the reason for the selective hormonal sensitivity of breast cancer would remain obscure for the next 60 yr until Jensen and Jacobson *(15)* described the target-site specificity of estradiol in the immature rat. Their classic experiment showed that after an injection of [³H]estradiol, the radioactive steroid was bound to, and retained by, known estrogen target tissues including the uterus, vagina, and pituitary gland. In contrast, estradiol was not retained by nontarget tissues such as skeletal muscle. Jensen suggested that an estrogen receptor (ER) must be present in estrogen target tissues to sequester the steroid specifically and to initiate the cascade of biochemical events associated with estrogen action in that tissue. Because ER is not only a critical predictor of hormone sensitivity in breast cancer but also a key target for drug action, this signal-transduction pathway is described in great detail.

Biology of Estrogen Receptors

Estrogens play a pivotal role in controlling breast tumor growth. The mechanism of estrogen action was unknown until an estrogen-binding protein called ER, now renamed as ER-α, was identified in the 1960s and was postulated to be a ligand-activated transcription modulator *(16,17)*. Since the cloning of the *ER*-α gene *(18,19)*, significant progress has been made in identifying the structure of ER-α and elucidating the mechanism of ER-α-mediated gene transcription.

From: *Principles of Molecular Oncology*
Edited by: M. H. Bronchud, M. A. Foote, W. P. Peters, and M. O. Robinson © Humana Press Inc., Totowa, NJ

EPITHELIAL CELLS   **STROMAL CELLS**

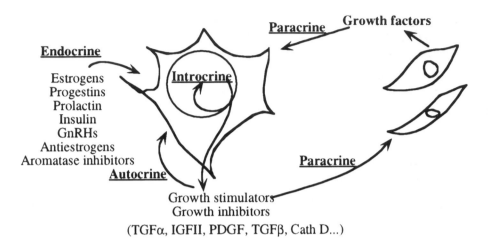

Fig. 1. Growth regulation of breast tumors: the growth of breast tumors can be regulated through endocrine, autocrine, paracrine, and introcrine pathways.

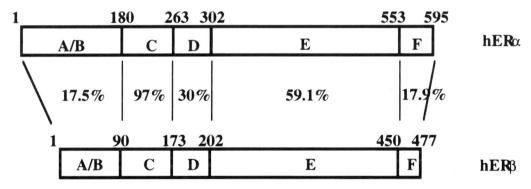

Fig. 2. Schematic diagram of human ER-α and ER-β coding amino acid sequences *(27–29)*. The DNA-binding domains of ER-α and ER-β are highly conserved.

Structure of ER-α

ER-α is a member of the nuclear hormone-receptor superfamily that includes steroid hormone receptors, thyroid and retinoid hormone receptors, vitamin D receptor, and a large number of orphan receptors for which no ligands have been identified to date *(13,20–22)*. These receptors function as ligand-activated transcription factors. The human *ER-α* gene encompasses nearly 140 kb on chromosome 6q24–27 and has eight exons. It encodes a protein of 595 amino acids with a molecular mass of approximately 67 kDa *(23–25)* localized in cell nuclei *(26)*. Like all members of the nuclear hormone-receptor superfamily, ER-α has A–F domains from the N-terminus to the C-terminus (Fig. 2).

The N-terminal A–B domain is composed of 180 amino acids and is not highly conserved among the nuclear hormone-receptor superfamily. This region has autonomous activation function (AF1) in a cell- and promoter-specific manner *(30–32)*. For example, the transactivation activity of AF1 is approx 5% and 58% of the full ER-α activity in transfected into HeLa cervical carcinoma cells and chicken embryo fibroblasts, respectively. Although AF1 can act independent of AF2 (localized to the E domain) *(33)*, AF1 synergizes with AF2 and is required for the full activity of ER-α under most circumstances such as in MDA–MB-231 human breast cancer cells and in HEC-1 human endometrial cancer cells *(32,34,35)*. Although it is unclear how AF1 potentiates AF2 activity, it is reported that AF1 interacts with AF2 directly or indirectly in the presence of 17β-estradiol (estradiol) or the antiestrogen tamoxifen. Steroid receptor coactivator-1 (SRC-1) enhances this interaction *(36)*. AF1 also contributes to the partial agonist activity of tamoxifen. Results from a deletion mutagenesis study *(35)* have shown that the first 40 amino acids do not affect the transcriptional activity of ER-α. Amino acids 41 to 64 are absolutely required for the tamoxifen-induced transactivation activity of ER-α but not for the estradiol-induced effect. The A–B domain has been reported to interact directly with c-Jun in vitro and crosstalk with the activating protein 1 (AP-1) signal transduction pathway *(37)*, which might be one of the mechanisms for tamoxifen resistance/tamoxifen-stimulated growth. In addition, EGF can stimulate the hormone-independent activation of ER-α through the mitogen-activated protein kinase (MAPK)-mediated phosphorylation of serine 118 in the A–B domain *(38,39)*. However, it is still unclear how AF1 interacts with the transcriptional initiation complex and initiates transcription.

The C domain (amino acids 180–262) is the DNA-binding domain (DBD), which is highly conserved throughout the entire nuclear hormone-receptor superfamily. It contains the 66-amino-acid core sequence (cysteine 185 to methionine 250) which forms the two zinc fingers known to be important for the high DNA-binding affinity and the site-specific DNA recognition of ER-α. However, deletion mutagenesis studies *(40)* have shown that the zinc finger core does not bind to DNA and an intact C domain is the minimal requirement for ER-α binding to the perfect palindromic estrogen response element (ERE) with a consensus sequence of (5′GGTCANNNTGACC-3′). In addition, amino acids up to serine 282 in the D domain can stabilize the DBD–ERE complex and are required for ER-α binding to imperfect palindromic ERE such as the pS2 and *Xenopus* vitellogenin B1–2. In the resolved crystal structure of the DBD bound to an ERE *(41)*, two molecules of DBD sit in the adjacent major grooves from one side of the DNA double helix. The side chains of glutamic acid 203, lysine 206, lysine 210, and arginine 33 interact with the central four base pairs of AGGTCA by hydrogen bonds (Fig. 3). Tyrosine 195, histidine 196, tyrosine 197, arginine 211, arginine 234, lysine 235, glutamine 238, and arginine 241 contact the phosphate backbone of the ERE. The crystal structure data further support the results from biochemical and mutational studies. There is also weak dimerization activity within the minimal region for DNA binding *(42)*, which is also observed in the DBD crystal structure (Fig. 3).

The border of the C–D domain is referred to as the hinge region and interacts with heat shock protein 90 (hsp90). The association of hsp90 with ER-α may be responsible for the inactive status and stability of unoccupied ER-α and be important for the high hormone-binding affinity of the receptor. Recently, the hinge region has been shown

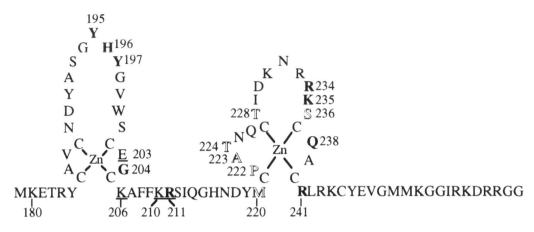

Fig. 3. DNA-binding domain of ER-α: <u>underlined,</u> interact with base pairs; **bolded,** interact with phosphate backbone; outlined, dimer interface *(41)*.

to associate with a coactivator L7/SPA in the presence of the antiestrogen tamoxifen *(43),* which might explain the partial agonist activity of tamoxifen.

Domain E (amino acids 302–553) is the largest region in ER-α and most conserved in the nuclear hormone-receptor superfamily. This domain contains motifs that are responsible for hormone-binding activity, receptor dimerization *(44),* and hormone-dependent association of ER-α with coactivators such as estrogen receptor-associated protein (ERAP) 160/140 *(45),* SRC-1 *(46),* cointegrator-associated protein (p/CIP) *(47)*–amplified in breast cancer-1(AIB1) *(48),* /RAC3 *(49),* /ACTR *(50),* receptor-interacting protein (RIP)140 *(51),* p300/CBP *(52–55),* transcriptional mediators or intermediary factors (TIF)1 *(56),* TIF2 *(57)*–glucocorticoid receptor interacting protein (GRIP)1 *(58–60),* and thyroid hormone receptor-interacting protein 1 (TRIP1) *(61)* and has hormone-dependent transactivation activity (AF2). The crystal structure of the estradiol-occupied and raloxifene (an antiestrogen)-occupied hormone-binding domain (HBD) of ER-α has been solved *(62),* giving us a clear view of how ER-α agonists and ER-α antagonists induce different conformational changes of the HBD. The HBD of ER-α has 12 α-helices (H1–H12) that form a three-layered α-helical sandwich and two-stranded antiparallel β-sheets (S1 and S2). The hydrophobic hormone-binding pocket is in contact with parts of H3, H6, H8, the loop between H7 and H8, H11, H12, and the loop between S1 and S2. When estradiol binds to ER-α, the 3-hydroxy group of estradiol forms hydrogen bonds with glutamic acid 353 in H3 and arginine 394 in H6 (Fig. 4A). The 17β-hydroxy group contacts histidine 524 in H11 by a hydrogen bond. H12 then forms a lid covering the hydrophobic pocket and facilitates the interaction with coactivators such as SRC-1. Raloxifene can also bind to ER-α, but induces a very different conformation of the HBD. In the raloxifene–ER-α complex, a hydroxy group interacts with glutamic acid 353 and arginine 394 just like the 3-hydroxy group of estradiol (Fig. 4B). The 11-hydroxy group of raloxifene also forms a hydrogen bond with histidine 524. However, the association with raloxifene results in a rotation of the imidazole ring of histidine 524. In addition, the long side chain of raloxifene interacts with H3, H5/H6, H11, and the loop between H11 and H12 and forms a

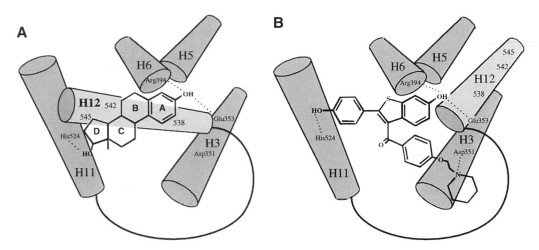

Fig. 4. Schematic representation of estradiol **(A)** and raloxifene **(B)** occupied ER-α. **(A)** When estradiol binds to ER-α, H12 forms a lid covering the hormone-binding pocket. **(B)** When raloxifene occupies the receptor, H12 is pushed away from the hydrophobic hormone-binding pocket.

hydrogen bond between N26 of raloxifene and aspartate 351 in H3, pushing H12 away from the binding pocket. As a result, H12 positions itself between H5 and H3, and masks lysine 362 which is critical for the association of ER-α with SRC-1 *(63)*. The conformational change induced by raloxifene binding destroys the interacting surface for coactivators such as SRC-1, thus providing the structural basis for the mechanism of antiestrogenic activity of raloxifene. As the alkylaminoethoxy side chain is the common structural feature for ER antagonists *(64)*, the raloxifene-induced conformational change might be the model for understanding the molecular mechanism for the action of the other antiestrogens. Indeed, 4-hydroxytamoxifen, the active metabolite of tamoxifen, also binds to ER-α and induces a conformational change analogous to the raloxifene–ER-α complex (GL Greene, *personal communication*).

The C-terminal F domain is not conserved in the nuclear-receptor superfamily. Although the F domain might be involved in differentially regulating transcription responsive to estrogens and antiestrogens in a cell-type dependent manner *(65)*, the function of this domain needs to be clarified.

A third activation domain (AF2a) located between amino acids 282 and 351 has been identified within the boundary of the D and E domains of ER-α *(66,67)*. An in vitro study showed that the human TATA-binding protein associated factor (TAFII30) directly interacted with ER-α at the AF2a region in a hormone-independent manner and enhanced ER-α-mediated transcription *(68)*, thus providing a possible mechanism for the autonomous transactivation activity of AF2a in yeast and mammalian cell systems *(66,67)*.

Hormone-Dependent Activation of ER-α

ER-α can activate gene expression by both the classic ERE and the non-ERE pathways. The classic ERE pathway has been studied in the greatest detail to elucidate

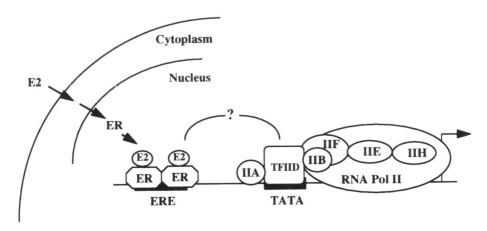

Fig. 5. The classic schematic diagram of the mechanism of ER-mediated transcription through the ERE-dependent pathway.

hormone-dependent gene transactivation by ER-α. In the classic ERE pathway, estrogens such as estradiol and its synthetic analog, diethylstrilbestrol (DES), diffuse into cell nuclei and bind to ER-α. Estrogen-occupied ER allosterically changes its conformation that leads to the dissociation from hsp90. The association with coactivators subsequently forms a homodimer on ERE and activates transcription (Fig. 5).

The questions arise, How does estrogen-occupied ER-α regulate gene expression? What is the bridge between the estradiol–ER-α complex and the basal transcriptional machinery or general transcription factors (GTF) that recognizes the core promoter and successfully initiates transcription? These questions have been addressed after the discovery of ERAP in 1994 *(45)*. Pull-down assays that used glutathione *S*-transferase (GST)–HBD(ER-α) as the bait showed that several proteins with appropriate molecular masses of 300 kDa, 150–170 kDa (at least three protein bands on sodium dodecyl sulfate-polyacrylamide gel electrophoresis [SDS-PAGE] gel), 140 kDa, 90–110 kDa, 80 kDa, and 36 kDa *(45,51,53)* were associated with the ER-α HBD in a hormone-dependent manner. Since then, a growing number of nuclear hormone-receptor-associated proteins have been characterized or cloned. These proteins have some common characteristics: they interact with ER-α HBD in the presence of estrogens; antiestrogens such as tamoxifen, ICI164,384 and ICI182,780 inhibit the interaction of ERAP; and ER-α interaction with ERAP is dependent upon the integrity of the AF2 domain (H12) in the HBD. Some transcriptionally inactive mutants do not interact with ERAP. The receptor interaction domains (RIDs) of most of these proteins such as CBP/p300, RIP140, and SRC-1/ACTR/AIB1/p/CIP have LXXLL motifs which are both necessary and sufficient for the ER-α–ERAP interaction *(47,69)*. The hormone-dependent association of ER-α with ERAP correlates with hormone-dependent ER-α-mediated transcription, suggesting that ERAP might function as the coactivators of ER-α. These proteins can be divided into groups according to their amino acid sequences (Table 1).

So far, the SRC family contains three subgroups: SRC-1, TIF2–GRIP1, and p/CIP/AIB1/RAC3/ACTR. p/CIP and GRIP1 are the mouse homologues of RAC3 and TIF2,

Table 1
ER-α Coactivators

Coactivators		Molecular mass	Reference
	SRC-1	120 kDa[a]/170 kDa	46,55
SRC	p/CIP/AIB1/RAC3/ACTR	152/155/154/154 kDa	47–50
	TIF2/GRIP1	160/158.5 kDa	57–59
TIF1		112 kDa	56,70,71
RIP140		140 kDa	72
ERAP140		140 kDa	45
TRAP1/SUG1		45.6 kDa	70
CBP/p300		300 kDa	52–55
SWI/SNF			73–76

[a]N-terminal truncated form.

respectively. RAC3, ACTR, and AIB1 are highly homologous to each other (97% to >99%) and might be the variant forms of the same protein. SRC-1 and TIF2 have the most profound enhancement on ER-α-mediated transcription. The SRC share a structure of a highly conserved N-terminal basic helix–loop–helix (bHLH) domain and PAS domains (Fig. 6A). bHLH and PAS domains have been shown to be involved in DNA binding and protein–protein interaction *(77–79)*. However, the functions of these domains in the coactivators are not clear because they are not required for SRC to interact with receptors nor do they enhance the transactivational activity of receptors *(46,55)*. SRC interact with ER-α through RIDs in a hormone-dependent fashion. In addition, SRC-1 and p/CIP/ACTR also bind to CBP/p300 *(46,47,50,55)*.

CBP and p300 are two large proteins that have similar sequence and functions. They function as global transcriptional coactivators for many signaling pathways by directly

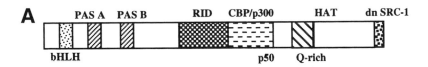

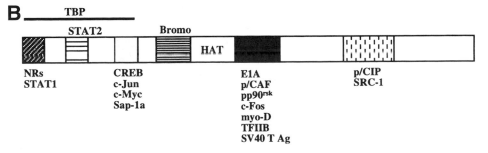

Fig. 6. Schematic structures of SRC-1 (A) and CBP/p300 (B).

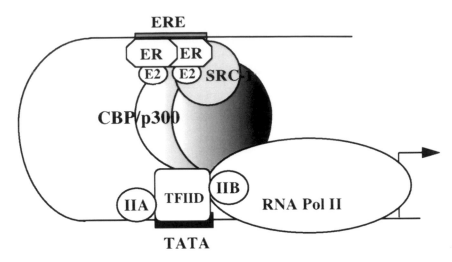

Fig. 7. A new dimension of the molecular mechanism of ER-mediated transcription: coactivators form the bridge between ER and general transcriptional factors.

interacting with many sequence-specific activators (Fig. 6B), including nuclear receptors *(53–55)*, STAT *(80,81)*, CREB *(75)*, AP1 *(54)*, c-Myb *(82–84)*, E1A *(52,85)*, P/CAF *(85–87)*, pp90^{rsk} *(88)*, MyoD *(89,90)*, TFIIB *(75)*, TBP *(81,91–93)*, p/CIP *(47)*, SRC-1 *(53–55)*, and p53 *(94,95)*. CBP/p300 interacts with ER-α in a hormone-dependent fashion and enhances estrogen-induced ER-α-mediated transcription. Because CBP/p300 interacts with ER-α, SRC, and GTF, it may function as the bridge between an estrogen-occupied ER-α complex and the basal transcriptional machinery, thus providing a new dimension to the molecular mechanism of ER-α-mediated transcription (Fig. 7). Because CBP–p300 is involved in so many signaling pathways, it may be a key factor in ER-α crosstalk with other signal transduction pathways. Nevertheless, what may be more significant is the finding that SRC-1 *(96)*, ACTR *(50)*, and CBP/p300 have intrinsic histone acetyltransferase (HAT) activities *(87,97)*. CBP/p300 also interacts with another HAT: p/CAF *(55,87,97)*.

Cellular DNA is tightly bound to histones and other nuclear proteins, which are packed into very compact chromatin. This structural stability restricts the accessibility of GFT to DNA and adds a layer of complexity to the regulation of gene function. The basic structural component of chromatin is the nucleosome, which is composed of 180–200 base pair (bp) DNA, 146 bps of which are wrapped around a histone octamer composed of two molecules of histone 2A, histone 2B, histone 3, and histone 4 *(98)*. Highly positively charged histone tails protrude from the octamer and interact with the negatively charged DNA, thus restricting the accessibility of DNA to transcription factors *(99,100)*. Nucleosomes strongly inhibit transcription *(101–103)*. More than 30 yr ago, it was found that histone acetylation can affect gene expression *(104)*. The histones of transcriptionally inactive genes are hypoacetylated *(105–107)*, but upon acetylation, the histone tails are neutralized and released from the negatively charged DNA. As a result, the nucleosomal structure is relaxed and made accessible to transcrip-

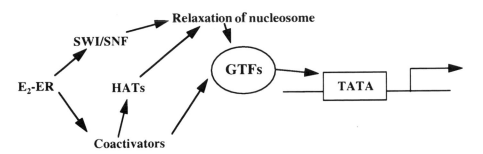

Fig. 8. A two-step model *(112):* First, estrogen-occupied ER recruits HAT that loosen the chromatin; second, transcriptional factors bind on the exposed promoter sites followed by gene transcription.

tion factors *(108)*. ER-α coactivators such as SRC-1 and CBP/p300 have intrinsic HAT activities. ER-α is reported to interact with chromatin components such as histone 2B and histone 4 *(109)*, and SWI/SNF *(73,76)*, which is a component of the RNA polymerase II holoenzyme complex. Histone 2B, histone 4, and other modified histones might facilitate ER-α binding to nucleosomal DNA *(109)*, and SWI/SNF, which has DNA-dependent ATPase activity, is involved in chromatin disassembly, and may facilitate transcription factor to bind to DNA *(74,110)*. After binding to DNA, ER-α may recruit coactivators into the ER–DNA complex. The coactivators with HAT activities would acetylate histone tails and relax the chromatin structure. GTF would then gain access to DNA and form a preinitiation complex (PIC) at the start site. As discussed earlier, ER-α interacts with GTF through coactivators and stabilizes PIC to initiate gene transcription *(111)*. The discovery that coactivators possess HAT activity now divides ER-mediated transcription into two steps as first suggested for the progesterone-receptor (PR) model *(112)* (Fig. 8). Initial HAT activity will loosen the chromatin followed by assembly of transcriptional factors on the exposed promoter sites.

ER-α can also activate the expression of genes by directly interacting with other sequence-specific transcriptional activators when the promoter regions do not contain palindromic ERE sites (Fig. 9). For instance, transforming growth factor (TGF)-β3 is up-regulated by estradiol and raloxifene through ER-α *(113,114)*, and the DBD of ER-α is unnecessary, as ER-α does not directly bind to the enhancer sequence (called raloxifene-responsive element or RRE) or related element in the TGF-β3 promoter, which is important for estradiol–raloxifene-induced ER-α-mediated transcription. However, ER-α was found in the RRE complex when the other cellular proteins were present, suggesting that ER-α binds to some factor(s) in the cell that directly binds to the RRE (Fig. 9A). Unfortunately, the RRE and related element-binding factor(s) have not been identified. ER-α can also activate the expression of ovalbumin in a similar way (protein–protein interaction), although a putative ERE site in the promoter of ovalbumin has recently been found *(115)*. The promoter region of ovalbumin contains AP-1 sites, and ER-α has been found in AP-1–DNA complexes (Fig. 9B). Studies in vitro indicate that the N-terminal domain of ER-α can interact directly with c-Jun in the AP-1 complex *(37)*. The transcription factor Sp1 can also interact with ER-α in

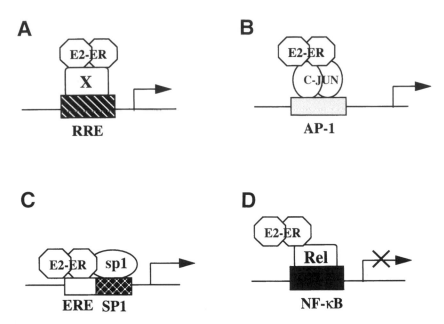

Fig. 9. ER regulates gene expression through ERE-independent pathways. **(A)** ER regulates TGF-β3 gene expression through RRE site; **(B)** ER interacts with AP-1 complex on AP-1 site; **(C)** ER forms ER–Sp1 complex on ERE–SP1 site; and **(D)** ER directly interacts with NF–κB subunit and blocks NF-κB-dependent gene expression such as IL-6.

vitro. ER-α enhances the expression of cathepsin D *(116–118)*, hsp27 *(119,120)*, and RAR *(121–123)* through Sp1 interaction (Fig. 9C). ER-α also interacts with NF-κB and inhibits NF-κB-mediated interleukin (IL)-6 gene expression *(124–126)* (Fig. 9D).

Hormone-Independent Activation of ER-α

In addition to hormone-dependent activation, ER-α can be activated by a broad spectrum of factors including dopamine *(127)*, heregulin *(128,129)*, TGF-α *(130,131)*, insulin and IGF-I *(38,132–135)*, and cAMP *(127,132,136–139)*. The concept of cross-talk between different signal-transduction pathways was initiated when EGF was found to mimic estrogen-stimulated growth in the mouse uterus *(140)*. It was shown that EGF can phosphorylate serine 118 in the A–B region of ER-α through a MAPK pathway, thereby activating ER-α-mediated gene transcription in the absence of estradiol *(38,39,140)*. ER-α can also be phosphorylated in vitro between amino acids 82–121 by the cyclin A–CDK2 complex, and cyclin A is known to increase hormone-dependent and hormone-independent transactivation of ER-α *(141)*. In addition, cyclin D1 plays an important role in the development of the normal mammary gland and the proliferation of mammary epithelium during pregnancy *(142,143)*. Cyclin D1 is overexpressed in some breast tumors *(144–146)*, and MMTV–cyclin D1 transgenic mice are known to be predisposed to mammary carcinoma *(147)*. Cyclin D1 can bind to the HBD of ER-α directly and has been found to activate ER-α independent of estradiol and potentiate the transcriptional activity of the E$_2$–ER complex *(148,149)*.

ER-β

ER-β is a novel ER that was first cloned from rat prostate *(154),* and the human *(27)* and mouse *(150)* ER-β receptors were subsequently cloned. Although human ER-α and ER-β are coded by two different genes, mapped to chromosome 6q24–27 *(23,25)* and 14q22–24 *(28),* respectively, they are highly conserved in the DBD (97%) and HBD (59%) *(27,28)* (Fig. 2). ER-β is a 54-kDa protein *(29)* that binds to estradiol with an affinity (0.5 n*M*) similar to ER-α (0.2 n*M*) *(151).* ER-β binds to DNA *(29,150,152,153),* associates with SRC-1 *(150,152),* and activates ERE-dependent reporter gene expression in transient transfection experiments in a hormone-dependent fashion *(27,150,152–154)* in a manner similar to ER-α. In addition, ER-β can form heterodimers with ER-α on DNA that enhance ERE-containing promoter activity *(152).* However, differential activation of ER-α- and ER-β-mediated gene expression has also been reported at AP-1 sites *(155).* ER-α induces AP-1 promoter activity in the presence of estradiol and DES *(37,155).* In contrast, estrogens either have no effect or inhibit AP-1-mediated transcription, whereas antiestrogens stimulate AP-1-mediated gene expression through ER-β *(155).* The different effect of ER-α and ER-β might be due to the differences in the N-terminal A–B domains. ER-α interacts with c-Jun through the N-terminus of the receptor *(37)* and forms a complex with AP-1 on DNA *(156).* No data currently exist to suggest that ER-β can interact with c-Jun in a similar manner. Although the physiological significance of the existence of two or more ERs is not clear, the differences in activity and tissue/cell distribution might explain the wide range of activity of estrogen and the tissue-specific effects of antiestrogen drugs such as tamoxifen and raloxifene *(28,157).*

Antiestrogens

It is well established that estradiol plays a key role in the development and growth of breast cancer through the ER-α signal-transduction pathway. Clinically, two-thirds of breast cancers are ER-α positive, thus making ER-α a good target for anti-breast cancer drugs and the strategic use of antiestrogens as preventives. An impressive list of antiestrogens is being evaluated clinically, primarily because of the enormous success of tamoxifen as a breast cancer treatment (Fig. 10). These compounds all bind to ER-α and inhibit estrogen-induced effects under certain circumstances.

Tamoxifen as an Antitumor Agent

Tamoxifen, a nonsteroidal antiestrogen, competes with estradiol to bind to ER-α with a binding affinity (K_o) of 20 n*M* *(158).* Tamoxifen-occupied ER-α still binds to the ERE, but the binding triggers a different conformational change than that of the estradiol–ER-α complex *(42,159,160).* The alkylaminoethoxy side chain of tamoxifen prevents the correct folding of the ER-α HBD *(160–162)* and blocks estradiol-induced association of the ER-α HBD with coactivators that are essential for estradiol-induced ER-α transactivational activity *(45,46,51).*

Tamoxifen was developed for the treatment of breast cancer because of its known antiestrogenicity in the laboratory. Tamoxifen has proven to be the endocrine treatment of choice for all stages of breast cancer in pre- and postmenopausal patients *(163).*

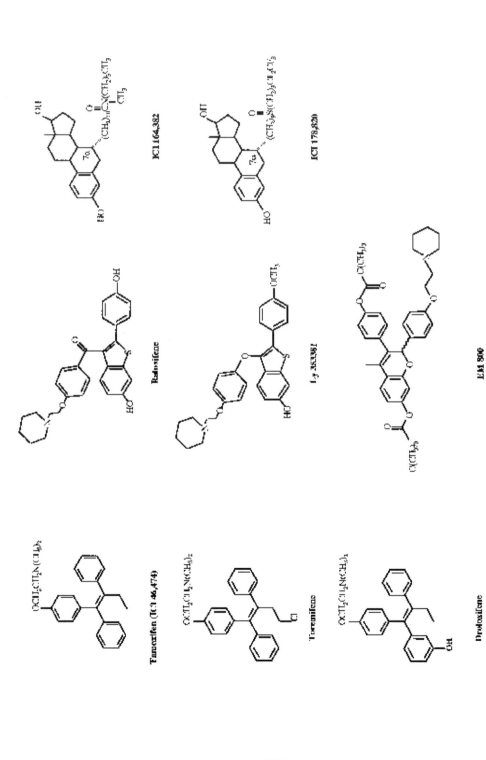

Fig. 10. Structures of some antiestrogens: tamoxifen-like antiestrogens such as tamoxifen, toremifene, and droloxifene; raloxifene-like antiestrogens such as raloxifene, Ly 353381, and EM 800; and pure antiestrogens such as ICI 164,384 and ICI 178820.

About two-thirds of ER-α-positive breast cancer patients initially respond to tamoxifen treatment. Overall, tamoxifen treatment reduces the incidence of contralateral breast cancer and produces a survival advantage in both node-positive and node-negative breast cancer patients *(164)*. However, tamoxifen cannot be viewed as a cure for breast cancer because some tumors predicted to respond do not, and responding tumors eventually become resistant.

Tamoxifen Resistance and Tamoxifen-Stimulated Breast Tumors

Understanding the mechanisms of tamoxifen resistance will contribute to the design of new and more effective therapies. Multiple mechanisms have been proposed for tamoxifen resistance, including estrogen availability and local metabolism of tamoxifen; loss and mutation of the ER; activation of alternative signal-transduction pathways; and agonist/antagonist balance of tamoxifen.

Estrogen Availability and Local Metabolism of Tamoxifen

Tamoxifen is reported to cause an increase in circulating estradiol levels in premenopausal patients *(165–168)*. Because tamoxifen and estradiol compete with each other for ER, a high concentration of estradiol could potentially block the inhibitory effect of tamoxifen. This hypothesis is supported by the clinical observation that patients with stage IV disease who initially respond to tamoxifen and subsequently develop tamoxifen resistance can respond to oophorectomy *(169)*.

The pharmacokinetics and metabolism of tamoxifen have been extensively studied in patients *(170–172)*. There is no evidence for reduced absorption or distribution or high levels of estrogenic metabolites in sera produced during long-term tamoxifen treatment *(172)*. However, local metabolism of tamoxifen in tumor cells or stromal components might contribute to tamoxifen resistance and tamoxifen-stimulated tumor growth. It was reported that the intratumoral tamoxifen concentration was reduced in tamoxifen-resistant patients compared with short-term tamoxifen-treated patients *(173)*. A similar phenomenon was observed earlier in MCF-7 breast tumors in animal models *(174)*, suggesting that local metabolism does play a role in tamoxifen resistance. The main metabolite of tamoxifen *N*-desmethyl tamoxifen (*N*-dMT) *(175,176)* is a weak antiestrogen having a potency, efficacy, and affinity for the ER similar to that of tamoxifen. Tamoxifen is also metabolized to 4-hydroxytamoxifen (Z isomer) which is a potent antiestrogen with an affinity for ER-α comparable to estradiol *(177)*. However, the Z isomer is unstable *(178,179)* and can be converted to the weakly antiestrogenic E isomer of 4-hydroxytamoxifen *(180–182)*, which will result in decreased antiestrogenicity of tamoxifen. A low level of metabolite E (tamoxifen without the dimethylaminoethane side chain) is detected in human tumors during tamoxifen therapy *(183)*. The Z isomer of metabolite E is very weakly estrogenic *(170,182)*. However, this is unstable and can be converted to the E isomer, a potent estrogen *(182)*. It was suggested that the E isomer of 4-hydroxytamoxifen with weak antiestrogenicity causes tamoxifen resistance and the E isomer of metabolite E with potent estrogenicity stimulates tumor growth. This hypothesis was addressed by using a fixed-ring version of tamoxifen that is incapable of the isomerization of the Z isomer to the E isomer. It has been demonstrated that both the fixed-ring version of tamoxifen and tamoxifen support the growth of tamoxifen-dependent tumors *(184)*, suggesting that mechanisms other than local metabolism should be considered for tamoxifen resistance and tamoxifen-stimulated tumor growth.

Loss or Mutation of the ER-α

ER-α plays a pivotal role in the estrogen responsiveness of tissues and tumors. About two-thirds of all human breast tumors expressing both ER-α and PR respond favorably to tamoxifen treatment and <10% of ER-α-negative breast tumors respond *(185,186)*. The inhibitory effects of tamoxifen are manifested predominantly through the ER-α signal transduction pathway. Because most ER-α-negative breast tumors do not respond to tamoxifen therapy and some advanced tumors become ER-α negative *(187)*, it is reasonable to hypothesize that the loss of ER-α is one of the mechanisms of tamoxifen resistance. Because breast tumors are heterogeneous, and there may be ER-negative cells before tamoxifen treatment, these resistant cells may selectively grow and become the dominant cell population in the tumors, resulting in tamoxifen-resistant growth *(188)*. Unfortunately, the drift from ER-positive to ER-negative tumors does not seem to be the major mechanism to explain the development of drug resistance to tamoxifen *(189)*. Apparently it is difficult to lose ER by hormone deprivation under laboratory conditions *(190)*. In addition, clinical studies have shown that breast tumors that eventually fail tamoxifen therapy remain ER positive *(191)* and laboratory models of tamoxifen drug resistance remain ER positive *(192,193)*.

However, there has been much interest in the possibility that alterations in ER-α structure and function can affect cellular responsiveness to tamoxifen. To determine the role of ER-α mutations in tamoxifen resistance, Karnik and co-workers *(194)* examined 20 tamoxifen-sensitive and 20 tamoxifen-resistant breast tumors using single-strand conformation polymorphism (SSCP) analysis. Ten percent of the tamoxifen-resistant tumors were found mutated in exon 6, which encodes part of the ER-α HBD. Although the rate is quite low, mutation of ER-α is a possible mechanism for tamoxifen resistance. By screening ER-α cDNA from four tamoxifen-stimulated MCF-7 tumors, we found a single-point mutation in ER from one of the tumors *(195)*. The mutation occurred in the codon for amino acid 351, resulting in the replacement of an aspartic acid with a tyrosine in the HBD of ER-α *(196)*. This mutation increased the estrogenic activity of a tamoxifen analog and converted the antiestrogenic pharmacology of raloxifene to a partial estrogenic activity *(197,198)*. The crystal structure of the raloxifene-occupied ER-α demonstrated that raloxifene directly contacted with ER at aspartic acid 351 through a hydrogen bond with the long side chain of raloxifene. Raloxifene binding resulted in a conformation change of the ER-α HBD that prevented coactivators such as SRC-1 from binding to ER-α and blocked estrogen-induced ER-α transactivation *(62)*. When aspartate 351 is mutated to tyrosine, the interactions between the ER-α HBD and raloxifene will be different and the resulting conformational change of the hormone-binding pocket of the raloxifene-occupied mutated ER-α may be similar to that of estradiol-induced, and may facilitate the association of ER-α with coactivators. This hypothesis is under investigation in our laboratory.

Loss and mutation of ER-α may account for some forms of tamoxifen resistance, but 50% of tamoxifen-resistant tumors have normal amounts of wild-type ER-α. Other mechanisms of tamoxifen resistance remain to be characterized *(189)*.

Alternative Signal-Transduction Pathways

AP-1 is a transcription factor composed of a Fos–Jun heterodimer or Jun–Jun homodimer. AP-1 binds to its cognate AP-1 binding site and activates gene expression. It has been shown that long-term tamoxifen treatment increases AP-1 activity in MCF-7 cells *(199)*. Growth of MCF-7 tumors in athymic mice under estradiol-deficient conditions results in a tumor phenotype that is still responsive to estradiol but is also stimulated by tamoxifen; AP-1 activity is increased *(200)*. AP-1 activity can be induced through a variety of signal transduction pathways, such as the MAPK and protein kinase C (PKC) pathways. However, these studies did not address how AP-1 activity was enhanced and whether AP-1 protein synthesis was required for the increased AP-1 activity. It has been proposed that ER-α directly interacts with c-Jun and activates AP-1 *(37)*. However, there is no direct evidence that the interaction between ER-α and AP-1 is hormone dependent. Therefore, the mechanism of how tamoxifen activates AP-1 is still unknown.

Agonist/Antagonist Balance of Tamoxifen

Tamoxifen and raloxifene have estrogenic activity in certain cells such as MDA–MB-231 ER-negative human breast cancer cells transfected with ER-α *(35,197,201)*, Hep G2 human hepatoma cells *(202)*, and in certain tissues such as uterus and bone *(163)*. The cell- and tissue-specific agonist/antagonist activity of tamoxifen suggests that the factors that are required for these activities may be differentially expressed in various cells and tissues.

Increases in protein kinase A (PKA) activity have been shown to augment the agonist activity of tamoxifen *(203)*. Therefore it is important to study how PKA activity correlates to the agonist activity of tamoxifen in different cells or tissues and whether tamoxifen up-regulates PKA activity in the cells or tissues where it acts as an agonist.

Deletion mutagenesis studies have shown that amino acids 41–64 of the ER-α are required for the agonist activity of tamoxifen in MDA–MB-231 cells and HEC-1 human endometrial cancer cells transfected with ER-α *(35)*. This suggests that tamoxifen induces the binding of some transcription factor(s) to this region of ER-α. These transcription factor(s) may be expressed only in cells or tissues where tamoxifen manifests its estrogenic activity. The regulation of transcription factor(s) by tamoxifen may be another possible mechanism for tamoxifen resistance or tamoxifen-stimulated tumor growth.

Other coactivators have been reported to enhance the agonist activity of tamoxifen. Using a yeast two-hybrid screening system, L7/SPA, a 27-kDa protein *(204)*, was found to bind to the hinge-HBD region of PR in the presence of the PR partial agonist RU486 *(43)*. Although the hinge region is not conserved among members of the nuclear-receptor superfamily, L7/SPA was also shown to bind to the hinge-HBD of ER-α and enhance ER-α-mediated transcription in the presence of tamoxifen. A study of the tissue distribution of L7/SPA may help to elucidate the cell- and tissue-specific agonist activity of tamoxifen. In addition, the known ER coactivator, SRC-1, also augments the agonist activity of tamoxifen *(205)*. However, tamoxifen does not induce but blocks estradiol-induced SRC-1 binding to ER-α HBD in vitro *(45)*. The region where SRC-1 binds to the tamoxifen-occupied ER and how SRC-1 enhances the agonist activity of tamoxifen is still unclear, although it has been shown that SRC-1 binds to the

N-terminus of ER in vitro *(206)*. Two nuclear hormone-receptor corepressors have been cloned that bind to unliganded thyroid receptor (TR), SMRT (silencing mediator for RAR and TR) *(207,208)*, and retinoic acid receptor (RAR), N-CoR (nuclear receptor-corepressor). The binding of SMRT and N-CoR is required for the repressive effects of the unliganded receptors. Ligand binding induces conformational changes of the receptors that release the bound corepressors and recruit coactivators to induce gene expression. Interestingly, SMRT was reported to bind to full-length ER in vitro in a hormone-independent manner *(205)*. SMRT and N-CoR significantly inhibited tamoxifen-induced ER-α-mediated transcription. Moreover, L7/SPA and SRC-1 can partially restore the agonist activity of tamoxifen that is inhibited by the corepressors *(43,205)*. These observations raise an important issue, that is, the balance between coactivators and corepressors may control the agonist and antagonist activities of tamoxifen in a system. A study of the differential expression and the regulation of these and other coactivators/corepressors will contribute to our understanding of the diverse pharmacological effects of tamoxifen.

Future Perspectives: Molecular Biology

Extensive studies have already been conducted on tumor resistance to tamoxifen and tamoxifen-stimulated growth. As a result, many hypotheses have been proposed to explain the multiple actions of antiestrogens. However, very few studies have focused on cell- or tissue-specific transcription factors that may be essential to understand the agonist activity of tamoxifen. We believe it will be extremely important to determine whether there are any specific proteins associated with ER-α in the presence of tamoxifen in a cell-/tissue-specific manner.

The AF1 domain of ER-α shows transactivational activity in a cell- and promoter-specific manner which correlates with tamoxifen's agonist activity, suggesting that the AF1 domain might play a role in tamoxifen-stimulated growth. It has been demonstrated that tamoxifen induces AP-1 activity in certain cell lines through the AF1 domain *(37)*, but it is still unknown as to how tamoxifen enhances ER transactivation activity on ERE containing promoter.

The coactivators SRC-1 and L7/SPA are known to increase and the corepressors SMRT and N-CoR are known to inhibit tamoxifen's agonist activity in some cell lines *(43,205)*. However, there are no data showing that ER-α directly interacts with these factors in the presence of tamoxifen. Further studies are needed to establish the roles of coactivators and corepressors in tamoxifen-induced ER-α transcriptional activity. Coactivators such as SRC-1 and CBP/p300 seem to be ubiquitous, but the question can be asked as to whether the expression of these genes is regulated and whether tamoxifen plays a role in that regulation. Taking the question one step further, can tamoxifen regulate other coactivators such as L7/SPA and corepressors such as N-CoR and SMRT?

Finally, there may be a role for ER-β in the target site-specific effect of tamoxifen. ER-β is highly homologous to ER-α in both DBD and HBD. However, it is very different at the AF1 domain (only 17% homology between the two receptors). Because it is believed that ER ligands regulate AF1 activity and the ER-α and ER-β receptor complexes can regulate AP-1 activation differently *(155)*, one can ask the question of whether ER-β plays a role in tamoxifen resistance and tamoxifen-stimulated growth.

Although the issue of the molecular mechanism of selective ER modulation is complex, at present there is an enormous incentive to elucidate the transduction pathway because of the value of antiestrogens as established therapeutic agents.

Future Strategies: Clinical Applications

During the past 25 yr, enormous changes have occurred in the strategic application of antiestrogens. Originally their action as antifertility agents in animals held the promise of an application as a "morning after" pill. However, studies in the 1960s demonstrated that the drugs induced ovulation so the goal changed to a therapy for infertility. The discovery of ER, and the knowledge that estrogen controlled breast tumor growth, focused attention on antiestrogens to treat breast cancer. Tamoxifen is now the gold standard for the treatment of all stages of breast cancer. Millions of women are taking tamoxifen because of the unequivocal observation that the drug confers numerous advantages with few side effects.

The finding in 1987 that "antiestrogens" maintain bone density completely changed the prospects for the prevention of breast cancer in postmenopausal women. Tamoxifen and raloxifene both maintain bone density, prevent mammary carcinogenesis, and have antiuterotropic activity although raloxifene is less estrogenic at the latter target site *(209,210)*. Clearly an application to prevent osteoporosis could have the advantage of preventing breast and endometrial cancer as an added beneficial side effect *(211)*. All of the pieces are in place to realize this goal clinically. Raloxifene is available for the prevention of osteoporosis *(212),* and the pharmacologies of raloxifene and tamoxifen are very similar. The knowledge that raloxifene can prevent breast cancer will come from the implementation of two strategies: the evaluation of epidemiological data on the incidence of breast cancer in users and nonusers of raloxifene to prevent osteoporosis and, most importantly, the clinical evaluation of the worth of tamoxifen vs raloxifene in the prevention of breast cancer in high-risk women. Confirmation of the hypothesis that targeted antiestrogenic drugs can prevent breast cancer will not only establish the topic as a textbook example of successful translational research but also will lead to a revolution in women's health. For the future, a whole range of new agents will be available to target different risk factors for osteoporosis, coronary diseases, and uterine and breast cancer.

References

1. Parkin DM, Pisani P, Ferlay J. Estimates of the worldwide incidence of eighteen major cancers in 1985. *Int J Cancer.* 1993; 54:594–606.
2. Lippman ME, Bolan G. Oestrogen-responsive human breast cancer in long term culture. *Nature.* 1975; 256:592–3.
3. Lippman ME, Huff KK, Jakesz T, et al. Estrogens regulate production of specific growth factors in hormone-dependent human breast cancer, In: *Estrogen/Antiestrogen Action and Breast Cancer Therapy* (Jordan VC, ed.), The University of Wisconsin Press, Madison, 1986, pp. 237–247.
4. Catherino WH, Wolf D, Jordan VC. A naturally occurring estrogen receptor mutation results in increased estrogenicity of a tamoxifen analog. *Mol Endocrinol.* 1995; 9:1053–63.
5. Groshong SD, Owen GI, Grimison B, et al. Biphasic regulation of breast cancer cell

growth by progesterone: role of the cyclin-dependent kinase inhibitors, p21 and p27. *Mol Endocrinol.* 1997; 11:1593–607.

6. Birrell SN, Bentel JM, Hickey TE, et al. Androgens induce divergent proliferative responses in human breast cancer cell lines. *J Steroid Biochem Mol Biol.* 1995; 52:459–67.

7. Osborne CK, Hamilton B, Titus G, Livingston RB. Epidermal growth factor stimulation of human breast cancer cells in culture. *Cancer Res.* 1980; 40:2361–6.

8. Nolan MK, Jankowska L, Prisco M, Xu S, Guvakova MA, Surmacz E. Differential roles of IRS-1 and SHC signaling pathways in breast cancer cells. *Int J Cancer.* 1997; 72:828–34.

9. Feinleib M. Breast cancer and artificial menopause: a cohort study. *J Natl Cancer Inst.* 1968; 41:315–29.

10. Trichopoulos D, MacMahon B, Cole P. The menopause and breast cancer risk. *J Natl Cancer Inst.* 1972; 48:605–13.

11. Dao TL. The role of ovarian steroid hormones in mammary carcinogenesis. In: *Hormones and Breast Cancer* (Pike MC, Siiteri PK, and Welsch CW, eds.), Cold Spring Harbor Laboratory Press, Cold Spring Harbor, New York, 1981, 281 pp.

12. Henderson BE, Ross RK, Castagrande JT. Breast cancer and the estrogen window hypothesis. *Lancet.* 1981; 2:363.

13. Beato M. Gene regulation by steroid hormones. *Cell.* 1989; 56, 325–44.

14. Pike M, Spicer DV, Dahmoush L, Press MF. Estrogens, progestogens, normal breast cell proliferation, and breast cancer risk. *Epidemiol Rev.* 1993; 15:17–35.

15. Jensen EV, Jacobson HI. Basic guides to the mechanism of estrogen action. *Recent Prog Horm Reg.* 1962; 18:387–414.

16. Toft DO, Gorski J. A receptor molecule for estrogens: isolation from the rat uterus and preliminary characterization. *Proc Natl Acad Sci USA.* 1966; 57:1574–81.

17. Jensen EV, Sujuki T, Kawashima T, Stumpt WE, Jungblut PW, Desombre ER. A two-step mechanism for the interaction of estrodial with rat uterus. *Proc Natl Acad Sci USA.* 1968; 59:632–8.

18. Green S, Walter P, Greene G, et al. Cloning of the human estrogen receptor cDNA. *J Steroid Biochem.* 1986; 24:77–83.

19. Greene G, Gilna P, Waterfield M, Baker A, Hort Y, Shine J. Sequence and expression of human estrogen receptor complementary DNA. *Science.* 1986; 231:1150–4.

20. Evans RM. The steroid and thyroid hormone superfamily. *Science.* 1988; 240:889–95.

21. Green S, Chambon P. Nuclear receptors enhance our understanding of transcription regulation. *Trends Gene.* 1988; 4:309–14.

22. Tsai MJ, O'Malley BW. Molecular mechanisms of action of steroid/thyroid receptor superfamily members. *Annu Rev Biochem.* 1994; 63:451–86.

23. Gosden JR, Middleton PG, Rout D. Localization of the human oestrogen receptor gene to chromosome 6q24–q27 by in situ hybridization. *Cytogenet Cell Genet.* 1986; 43:218–20.

24. Ponglikitmongkol M, Green S, Chambon P. Genomic organization of the human oestrogen receptor gene. *EMBO J.* 1988; 7:3385–8.

25. Menasce LP, White GR, Harrison CJ, Boyle JM. Localization of the estrogen receptor locus (ESR) to chromosome 6Q25.1 by FISH and a simple post-FISH banding technique. *Genomics.* 1993; 17:263–5.

26. Ylikomi T, Bocquel MT, Berry M, Gronemeyer H, Chambon P. Cooperation of proto-signals for nuclear accumulation of oestrogen and progesterone receptors. *EMBO J.* 1992; 11:3681–94.

27. Mosselman S, Polman J, Dijkema R. ER-β: identification and characterization of a novel human estrogen receptor. *FEBS Lett.* 1996; 392:49–53.

28. Enmark E, Pelto-Huikko M, Grandien K, et al. Human estrogen receptor β—gene structure,

chromosomal localization and expression pattern. *J Clin Endocrinol Metab.* 1997; 82:4258–65.

29. Pace P, Taylor J, Suntharalingam S, Coombes RC, Ali S. Human estrogen receptor β binds DNA in a manner similar to and dimerizes with estrogen receptor α. *J Biol Chem.* 1997; 272:25832–8.

30. Kumar V, Green S, Stack G, Berry M, Jin JR, Chambon P. Functional domains of the human estrogen receptor. *Cell.* 1987; 51:941–51.

31. Parker MG, Lehman JA, Martin DE. Identification of constitutive and steroid-dependent transactivation domains in the mouse oestrogen receptor. *J Steroid Biochem.* 1989; 34:33–39.

32. Tora L, White J, Brou C. The human estrogen receptor has two independent nonacidic transcriptional activation functions. *Cell.* 1989; 59:477–87.

33. Brou C, Wu J, Ali S, et al. Different TBP-associated factors are required for mediating the stimulation of transcription in vitro by the acidic transactivator GAL VP16 and the two nonacidic activation functions of the estrogen receptor. *Nucleic Acids Res.* 1993; 21:5–12.

34. McDonnell DP, Vegeto E, O'Malley BW. Identification of a negative regulatory function for steroid receptors. *Proc Natl Acad Sci USA.* 1992; 89:10563–7.

35. McInerney EM, Katzenellenbogen BS. Different regions in activation function-1 of the human estrogen receptor required for antiestrogen- and estradiol-dependent transcription activation. *J Biol Chem.* 1996; 271:24172–8.

36. McInerney EM, Tsai MJ, O'Malley BW, Katzenellenbogen BS. Analysis of estrogen receptor transcriptional enhancement by a nuclear hormone receptor coactivator. *Proc Natl Acad Sci USA.* 1996; 93:10069–73.

37. Webb P, Lopez GN, Uht RM, Kushner PJ. Tamoxifen activation of the estrogen receptor/ AP-1 pathway: potential origin for the cell-specific estrogen-like effects of antiestrogens. *Mol Endocrinol.* 1995; 9:443–56.

38. Kato S, Endoh H, Masuhiro Y. Activation of the estrogen receptor through phosphorylation by mitogen-activated protein kinase. *Science.* 1995; 270:1491–4.

39. Bunone G, Briand PA, Miksicek RJ, Picard D. Activation of the unliganded oestrogen receptor by EGF involves the MAP kinase pathway and direct phosphorylation. *EMBO J.* 1996; 15:2174–83.

40. Mader S, Chambon P, White JH. Defining a minimal estrogen receptor DNA binding domain. *Nucleic Acids Res.* 1993; 21:1125–32.

41. Schwabe JW, Chapman L, Finch JT, Rhodes D. The crystal structure of the estrogen receptor DNA-binding domain bound to DNA: how receptors discriminate between their response element. *Cell.* 1993; 75:567–78.

42. Kumar V, Chambon P. The estrogen receptor binds tightly to its responsive element as a ligand-induced homodimer. *Cell.* 1988; 55:145–56.

43. Jackson TA, Richer JK, Bain DL, Takimoto GS, Tung L, Horwitz KB. The partial agonist activity of antagonist-occupied steroid receptors is controlled by a novel hinge domain-binding coactivator L7/SPA and the corepressors N-CoR or SMART. *Mol Endocrinol.* 1997; 11:693–705.

44. Fawell SE, Lees JA, White R, Parker MG. Characterization and colocalization of steroid binding and dimerization activities in the mouse estrogen receptor. *Cell.* 1990; 60:953–62.

45. Halachmi S, Marden E, Martin G, MacKay H, Abbondanza C, Brown M. Estrogen receptor-associated proteins: possible mediators of hormone-induced transcription. *Science.* 1994; 264:1455–8.

46. Onate SA, Tsai SY, Tsai MJ, O'Malley BW. Sequence and characterization of a coactivator for the steroid hormone receptor superfamily. *Science.* 1995; 270:1354–7.

47. Torchia J, Rose DW, Inostroza J., et al. The transcriptional co-activator p/CIP binds CBP and mediates nuclear-receptor function. *Nature.* 1997; 387:677–84.

48. Anzick SL, Kononen J, Walker RL, et al. AIB1, a steroid receptor coactivator amplified in breast and ovarian cancer. *Science.* 1997; 277:965–8.

49. Li H, Gomes PJ, Chen JD. RAC3, a steroid/nuclear receptor-associated coactivator that is related to SRC-1 and TIF2. *Proc Natl Acad Sci USA.* 1997; 94:8479–84.

50. Chen H, Lin RJ, Schiltz RL, et al. Nuclear receptor coactivator ACTR is a novel histone acetyltransferase and forms a multimeric activation complex with P/CAF and CBP/p300. *Cell.* 1997; 90:569–80.

51. Cavailles V, Dauvois S, Danielian PS, Parker MG. Interaction of proteins with transcriptionally active estrogen receptors. *Proc Natl Acad Sci USA.* 1994; 91:10009–13.

52. Chakravarti D, LaMorte VJ, Nelson MC, et al. Role of CBP/P300 in nuclear receptor signalling. *Nature.* 1996; 383:99–103.

53. Hanstein B, Eckner R, DiRenzo J, et al. p300 is a component of an estrogen receptor coactivator complex. *Proc Natl Acad Sci USA.* 1996; 93:11540–5.

54. Kamei Y, Xu L, Heinzel T, et al. A CBP integrator complex mediates transcriptional activation and AP-1 inhibition by nuclear receptors. *Cell.* 1996; 85:403–14.

55. Yao TP, Ku G, Zhou N, Scully R, Livingston DM. The nuclear hormone receptor coactivator SRC-1 is a specific target of p300. *Proc Natl Acad Sci USA.* 1996; 93:10626–31.

56. Le Douarin B, Zechel C, Garnier J, et al. The N-terminal part of TIF1, a putative mediator of the ligand-dependent activation function (AF-2) of nuclear receptors, is fused to B-raf in the oncogenic protein T18. *EMBO J.* 1995; 14:2020–33.

57. Voegel JJ, Heine MJ, Zechel C, Chambon P, Gronemeyer H. TIF2, a 160 kDa transcriptional mediator for the ligand-dependent activation function AF-2 of nuclear receptors. *EMBO J.* 1996; 15:3667–75.

58. Hong H, Kohli K, Garabedian MJ, Stallcup MR. GRIP1, a transcriptional coactivator for the AF-2 transactivation domain of steroid, thyroid, retinoid and vitamin D receptors. *Mol Cell Biol.* 1997; 17:2735–44.

59. Hong H, Kohli K, Trived A, Johnson DL, Stallcup MR. GRIP1, a novel mouse protein that serves as a transcriptional coactivator in yeast for the hormone binding domains of steroid receptors. *Proc Natl Acad Sci USA.* 1996; 93:4948–52.

60. Walfish PG, Yoganathan T, Yang Y, Hong H, Butt TR, Stallcup MR. Yeast hormone response element assays detect and characterize GRIP1 coactivator-dependent activation of transcription by thyroid and retinoid nuclear receptors. *Proc Natl Acad Sci USA.* 1997; 94:3697–702.

61. Lee JW, Ryan F, Swaffield JC, Johnston SA, Moore DD. Interaction of thyroid-hormone receptor with a conserved transcriptional mediator. *Science.* 1995; 374:91–4.

62. Brzozowski AM, Pike AC, Dauter Z, et al. Molecular basis of agonism and antagonism in the oestrogen receptor. *Nature.* 1997; 389:735–8.

63. Pirkko MAH, Kalkhoven E, Parker MG. AF-2 activity and recruitment of steroid receptor coactivator 1 to the estrogen receptor depend on a lysine residue conserved in nuclear receptors. *Mol Cell Biol.* 1997; 17:1832–9.

64. Jordan VC. Biochemical pharmacology of antiestrogen action. *Pharmacol Rev.* 1984; 36:245–76.

65. Montano MM, Muller V, Trobaugh A, Katzenellenbogen BS. The carboxy-terminal F domain of the human estrogen receptor: role in the transcriptional activity of the receptor and the effectiveneses of antiestrogens as estrogen antagonists. *Mol Endocrinol.* 1995; 9:814–25.

66. Pierrat B, Heery DM, Chambon P, Losson R. A highly conserved region in the hormone-

binding domain of the human estrogen receptor functions as an efficient transactivation domain in yeast. *Gene.* 1994; 143:193–200.

67. Norris JD, Fan D, Kerner SA, McDonnell DP. Identification of a third autonomous activation domain within the human estrogen receptor. *Mol Endocrinol.* 1997; 11:747–54.

68. Jacq X, Brou C, Lutz Y, Davidson I, Chambon P, Tora L. Human TAFII30 is present in a distinct TFIID complex and is required for transcriptional activation by the estrogen receptor. *Cell.* 1994; 79:107–17.

69. Heery DM, Kalkhoven E, Hoare S, Parker MG. A signature motif in transcriptional coactivators mediates binding to nuclear receptors. *Nature.* 1997; 387:733–6.

70. vom Baur E, Zechel C, Heery D, et al. Differential ligand-dependent interactions between the AF-2 activating domain of nuclear receptors and the putative transcriptional intermediary factors mSUG1 and TIF1. *EMBO J.* 1996; 15:110–24.

71. Thénot S, Heriquet C, Rochefort H, Cavaillès V. Differential interaction of nuclear receptors with the putative human transcriptional coactivator hTIF1. *J Biol Chem.* 1997; 272:12062–8.

72. Joyeux A, Cavaillès V, Balaguer P, Nicolas JC. RIP140 enhances nuclear receptor-dependent transcription in vivo in yeast. *Mol Endocrinol.* 1997; 11:193–202.

73. Chiba H, Muramatsu M, Nomoto A, Kato H. Two human homologues of *Saccharomyces cerevisiae* SWI2/SNF2 and *Drosophila brahma* are transcriptional coactivators cooperating with the estrogen receptor and the retinoic acid receptor. *Nucleic Acids Res.* 1994; 22:1815–20.

74. Imbalzano AN, Kwon H, Green MR, Kingston RE. Facilitated binding of TATA-binding protein to nucleosomal DNA. *Nature.* 1994; 370:481–5.

75. Kwok RP, Lundblad JR, Chrivia JC, et al. Nuclear protein CBP is a coactivator for the transcription factor CREB. *Nature.* 1994; 370:223–6.

76. Ichinose H, Garnier JM, Chambon P, Losson R. Ligand-dependent interaction between the estrogen receptor and the human homologues of *SWI2/SNF2*. *Gene.* 1997; 188:95–100.

77. Burbach KM, Poland A, Bradfield CA. Cloning of the Ah-receptor cDNA reveals a distinctive ligand-activated transcription factor. *Proc Natl Acad Sci USA.* 1992; 89:8185–9.

78. Reyes H, Reisz-Porszasz S, Hankinson O. Identification of the Ah receptor nuclear translocator protein (Arnt) as a component of the DNA binding form of the Ah receptor. *Science.* 1992; 256:1193–5.

79. Lindebro MC, Poellinger L, Whitelaw ML. Protein–protein interaction via PAS domains: role of the PAS domain in positive and negative regulation of the bHLH/PAS dioxin receptor-Arnt transcription factor complex. *EMBO J.* 1995; 14:3528–39.

80. Horvai AE, Xu L, Korzus E, et al. Nuclear integration of JAK/STAT and Ras/AP-1 signaling by CBP and p300. *Proc Natl Acad Sci USA.* 1997; 94:1074–9.

81. Korzus E, Torchia J, Rose DW, et al. Transcription factor-specific requirements for coactivators and their acetyltransferase functions. *Science.* 1998; 279:703–7.

82. Swope DL, Mueller CL, Chrivia JC. CREB-binding protein activates transcription through multiple domains. *J Biol Chem.* 1996; 271:28138–45.

83. Goldman PS, Tran VK, Goodman RH. The multifunctional role of the co-activator CBP in transcriptional regulation. *Recent Prog Horm Res.* 1997; 52:103–20.

84. Yang C, Shapiro LH, Rivera M, Kumar A, Brindle PK. A role for CREB binding protein and p300 transcriptional coactivators in Ets-1 transactivation functions. *Mol Cell Biol.* 1998; 18:2218–29.

85. Yang XJ, Ogryzko VV, Nishikawa J, Howard BH, Nakatani Y. A p300/CBP-associated factor that competes with the adenoviral oncoprotein E1A. *Nature.* 1996; 382:319–24.

86. Baniahmad C, Nawaz Z, Baniahmad A, Gleeson MAG, Tsai MJ, O'Malley BW. Enhance-

ment of human estrogen receptor activity by SPT6: a potential coactivator. *Mol Endocrinol.* 1995; 9:34–43.

87. Ogryzko VO, Schiltz RL, Russanova V, Howard BH, Nakatani Y. The transcriptional coactivators p300 and CBP are histone acetyltransferases. *Cell.* 1996; 87:953–9.

88. Nakajima T, Fukamizu A, Takahashi J, et al. The signal-dependent coactivator CBP is a nuclear target for pp90RSK. *Cell.* 1996; 86:465–74.

89. Puri PL, Avantaggiati ML, Balsano C, et al. p300 is required for MyoD-dependent cell cycle arrest and muscle-specific gene transcription. *EMBO J.* 1997; 16:369–83.

90. Sartorelli V, Huang J, Hamamori Y, Kedes L. Molecular mechanisms of myogenic coactivation by p300: direct interaction with the activation domain of MyoD and with the MADS box of MEF2C. *Mol Cell Biol.* 1997; 17:1010–26.

91. Dallas PB, Yaciuk P, Moran E. Characterization of monoclonal antibodies raised against p300: both p300 and CBP are present in intracellular TBP complexes. *J Virol.* 1997; 71:1726–31.

92. Dallas PB, Cheney IW, Liao DW, et al. p300/CREB binding protein-related protein p270 is a component of mammalian SWI/SNF complexes. *Mol Cell Biol.* 1998; 18:3596–603.

93. Sang N, Avantaggiati ML, Giordano A. Roles of p300, pocket proteins, and hTBP in E1A-mediated transcriptional regulation and inhibition of p53 transactivation activity. *J Cell Biochem.* 1997; 66:277–85.

94. Avantaggiati ML, Ogryzko V, Gardner K, Giordano A, Levine AS, Kelly K. Recruitment of p300/CBP in p53-dependent signal pathways. *Cell.* 1997; 89:1175–84.

95. Gu W, Shi XL, Roeder RG. Synergistic activation of transcription by CBP and p53. *Nature.* 1997; 387:819–27.

96. Spencer TE, Jenster G, Burcin MM, et al. Steroid receptor coactivator-1 is a histone acetyltransferase. *Nature.* 1997; 389:194–8.

97. Bannister AJ, Kouzarides T. The CBP coactivator is a histone acetyltransferase. *Nature.* 1996; 384:641–3.

98. Arents G, Moudrianakis EN. Topography of the histone octamer surface: repeating structural motifs utilized in the docking of nucleosomal DNA. *Proc Natl Acad Sci USA.* 1993; 90:10489–93.

99. King RW, Jackson PK, Kirschner MW. Mitosis in transition. *Cell.* 1994; 79:563–71.

100. Nurse P. Ordering S phase and M phase in the cell cycle. *Cell.* 1994; 79:547–50.

101. Jeong S, Stein A. Micrococcal nuclease digestion of nuclei reveals extended nucleosome ladders having anomalous DNA lengths for chromatin assembled on non-replicating plasmids in transfected cells. *Nucleic Acids Res.* 1994; 22:370–5.

102. Felsenfeld G, Boyes J, Chung J, Clark D, Studitsky V. Chromatin structure and gene expression. *Proc Natl Acad Sci USA.* 1996; 93:9384–8.

103. Roth SY, Allis CD. Histone acetylation and chromatin assembly: a single escort, multiple dances? *Cell.* 1996; 87:5–8.

104. Allfrey VG, Faulkner R, Mirsky AE. Acetylation and methylation of histones and their possible role in the regulation of RNA synthesis. *Proc Natl Acad Sci USA.* 1964; 51:786–94.

105. Wolffe AP. Nucleosome positioning and modification: chromatin structures that potentiate transcription. *Trends Biochem Sci.* 1994; 19:240–4.

106. Brownell JE, Allis CD. Special HATs for special occasions: linking histone acetylation to chromatin assembly and gene activation. *Curr Opin Genet Dev.* 1996; 6:176–84.

107. Wolffe AP, Pruss D. Targeting chromatin disruption: transcription regulators that acetylate histones. *Cell.* 1996; 84:817–9.

108. Wolffe AP. Histone deacetylase: a regulator of transcription. *Science.* 1996; 272:371–2.

109. Ruh MF, Cox LK, Ruh TS. Estrogen receptor interaction with specific histones. Binding to genomic DNA and an estrogen response element. *Biochem Pharmacol.* 1996; 52:869–78.

110. Kwon H, Imbalzano AN, Khavari PA, Kingston RE, Green MR. Nucleosome disruption and enhancement of activator binding by a human SWI/SNF complex. *Nature.* 1994; 370:477–81.

111. Ing NH, Beekman JM, Tsai SY, Tsai MJ, O'Malley BW. Members of the steroid hormone receptor superfamily interact with TFIIB (S300-II). *J Biol Chem.* 1992; 267:17617–23.

112. Jenster G, Spencer TE, Burcin MM, Tsai SY, Tsai MJ, O'Malley BW. Steroid receptor induction of gene transcription: a two-step model. *Proc Natl Acad Sci USA.* 1997; 94:7879–84.

113. Yang NN, Bryant HU, Hardikar S, et al. Estrogen and raloxifene stimulate transforming growth factor-β 3 gene expression in rat bone: a potential mechanism for estrogen- or raloxifene-mediated bone maintenance. *Endocrinology.* 1996; 137:2075–84.

114. Yang NN, Venugopalan M, Hardikar S, Glasebrook A. Correction: raloxifene response needs more than an element. *Science.* 1997; 275:1249.

115. Klinge CM, Silver BF, Driscoll MD, Sathya G, Bambara RA, Hilf R. Chicken ovalbumin upstream promoter-transcription factor interacts with estrogen receptor, binds to estrogen response elements and half-sites, and inhibits estrogen-induced gene expression. *J Biol Chem.* 1997; 272:31465–74.

116. Krishnan V, Wang X, Safe S. Estrogen receptor–Sp1 complexes mediate estrogen-induced *cathepsin D* gene expression in MCF-7 human breast cancer cells. *J Biol Chem.* 1994; 269:15912–7.

117. Wang F, Porter W, Xing W, Archer TK, Safe S. Identification of a functional imperfect estrogen-responsive element in the 5′-promoter region of the human *cathepsin D* gene. *Biochemistry.* 1997; 36:7793–801.

118. Wang F, Hoivik D, Pollenz R, Safe S. Functional and physical interactions between the estrogen receptor Sp1 and nuclear aryl hydrocarbon receptor complexes. *Nucleic Acids Res.* 1998; 26:3044–52.

119. Porter W, Saville B, Hoivik D, Safe S. Functional synergy between the transcription factor Sp1 and the estrogen receptor. *Mol Endocrinol.* 1997; 11:1569–80.

120. Porter W, Wang F, Wang W, Duan R, Safe S. Role of estrogen receptor/Sp1 complexes in estrogen-induced heat shock protein 27 gene expression. *Mol Endocrinol.* 1996; 10:1371–8.

121. Augereau P, Miralles F, Cavailles V, Gaudelet C, Parker M, Rochefort H. Characterization of the proximal estrogen-responsive element of human *cathepsin D* gene. *Mol Endocrinol.* 1994; 8:693–703.

122. Rishi AK, Shao ZM, Baumann RG, et al. Estradiol regulation of the human retinoic acid receptor alpha gene in human breast carcinoma cells is mediated via an imperfect half-palindromic estrogen response element and Sp1 motifs. *Cancer Res.* 1995; 55:4999–5006.

123. Sun G, Porter W, Safe S. Estrogen-induced retinoic acid receptor alpha 1 gene expression: role of estrogen receptor–Sp1 complex. *Mol Endocrinol.* 1998; 12:882–90.

124. Ray A, Prefontaine KE, Ray P. Down-modulation of interleukin-6 gene expression by 17 β-estradiol in the absence of high affinity DNA binding by the estrogen receptor. *J Biol Chem.* 1994; 269:12940–6.

125. Ray P, Ghosh SK, Zhang DH, Ray A. Repression of *interleukin-6* gene expression by 17 β-estradiol: inhibition of the DNA-binding activity of the transcription factors NF-IL6 and NF-kappa β by the estrogen receptor. *FEBS Lett.* 1997; 409:79–85.

126. Stein B, Yang MX. Repression of the interleukin-6 promoter by estrogen receptor is mediated by NF-kappa β and C/EBP β. *Mol Cell Biol.* 1995; 15:4971–9.

127. Smith CL, Conneely OM, O'Malley BW. Modulation of the ligand-independent activation

of the human estrogen receptor by hormone and antihormone. *Proc Natl Acad Sci USA.* 1993; 90:6120–4.

128. Pietras RJ, Arboleda J, Reese DM, et al. HER-2 tyrosine kinase pathway targets estrogen receptor and promotes hormone-independent growth in human breast cancer cells. *Oncogene.* 1995; 10:2435–46.

129. Tang CK, Perez C, Grunt T, Waibel C, Cho C, Lupu R. Involvement of heregulin-β 2 in the acquisition of the hormone-independent phenotype of breast cancer cells. *Cancer Res.* 1996; 56:3350–8.

130. Ignar-Trowbridge DM, Pimentel M, Parker MG, McLachlan JA, Korach KS. Peptide growth factor cross-talk with the estrogen receptor requires the A/B domain and occurs independently of protein kinase C or estradiol. *Endocrinology.* 1996; 137:1735–44.

131. Ignar-Trowbridge DM, Pimentel M, Teng CT, Korach KS, McLachlan JA. Cross talk between peptide growth factor and estrogen receptor signaling systems. *Environ Health Perspect.* 1995; 103:35–8.

132. Aronica SM, Katzenellenbogen BS. Stimulation of estrogen receptor-mediated transcription and alteration in the phosphorylation state of the rat uterine estrogen receptor by estrogen, cyclic adenosine monophosphate, and insulin-like growth factor-I. *Mol Endocrinol.* 1993; 7:743–52.

133. Ma ZQ, Santagati S, Patrone C, Pollio G, Vegeto E, Maggi A. Insulin-like growth factors activate estrogen receptor to control the growth and differentiation of the human neuroblastoma cell line SK-ER3. *Mol Endocrinol.* 1994; 8:910–8.

134. Hafner F, Holler E, von Angerer E. Effect of growth factors on estrogen receptor mediated gene expression. *J Steroid Biochem Mol Biol.* 1996; 58:385–93.

135. Lee AV, Weng CN, Jackson JG, Yee D. Activation of estrogen receptor-mediated gene transcription by IGF-I in human breast cancer cells. *J Endocrinol.* 1997; 152:39–47.

136. Cho H, Katzenellenbogen BS. Synergistic activation of estrogen receptor-mediated transcription by estradiol and protein kinase activators. *Mol Endocrinol.* 1993; 7:441–52.

137. Ince BA, Montano MM, Katzenellenbogen BS. Activation of transcriptionally inactive human estrogen receptors by cyclic adenosine 3′,5′-monophosphate and ligands including antiestrogens. *Mol Endocrinol.* 1994; 8:1397–406.

138. Ince BA, Schodin DJ, Shapiro DJ, Katzenellenbogen BS. Repression of endogenous estrogen receptor activity in MCF-7 human breast cancer cells by dominant negative estrogen receptors. *Endocrinology.* 1995; 136:3194–9.

139. El-Tanani MK, Green CD. Two separate mechanisms for ligand-independent activation of the estrogen receptor. *Mol Endocrinol.* 1997; 11:928–37.

140. Ignar-Trowbridge D, Nelson KG, Bidwell MC, et al. Coupling of dual signaling pathways: epidermal growth factor action involves the estrogen receptor. *Proc Natl Acad Sci USA.* 1992; 89:4658–62.

141. Trowbridge JM, Rogatsky I, Garabedian MJ. Regulation of estrogen receptor transcriptional enhancement by the cyclin A/Cdk2 complex. *Proc Natl Acad Sci USA.* 1997; 94:10132–37.

142. Fantl V, Stamp G, Andrews A, Rosewell I, Dickson C. Mice lacking cyclin D1 are small and show defects in eye and mammary gland development. *Genes Dev.* 1995; 9:2364–72.

143. Sicinski P, Donaher JL, Parker SB, et al. Cyclin D1 provides a link between development and oncogenesis in the retina and breast. *Cell.* 1995; 82:621–30.

144. Lammie GA, Fantl V, Smith R, et al. *D11S287,* a putative oncogene on chromosome 11q13, is amplified and expressed in squamous cell and mammary carcinomas and linked to BCL-1. *Oncogene.* 1991; 6:439–44.

145. Schuuring E, Verhoeven E, Mooi WJ, Michalides RJ. Identification and cloning of two overexpressed genes, *U21B31/PRAD1* and *EMS1,* within the amplified chromosome 11q13 region in human carcinomas. *Oncogene.* 1992; 7:355–61.

146. Bartkova J, Lukas J, Muller H, Strauss M, Gusterson B, Bartek J. Cyclin D1 protein expression and function in human breast cancer. *Int J Cancer.* 1995; 57:353–61.

147. Wang TC, Cardiff RD, Zukerberg L, Lees E, Arnold A, Schmidt EV. Mammary hyperplasia and carcinoma in MMTV–cyclin D1 transgenic mice. *Nature.* 1994; 369:669–71.

148. Neuman E, Ladha MH, Lin N, et al. Cyclin D1 stimulation of estrogen receptor transcriptional activity independent of cdk4. *Mol Cell Biol.* 1997; 17:5338–47.

149. Zwijsen RM, Wientjens E, Klompmaker R, van der Sman J, Bernards R, Michalides RJ. CDK-independent activation of estrogen receptor by cyclin D1. *Cell.* 1997; 88:405–15.

150. Tremblay GB, Tremblay A, Copeland NG, et al. Cloning, chromosomal localization, and functional analysis of the murine estrogen receptor β. *Mol Endocrinol.* 1997; 11:353–65.

151. Kuiper GG, Gustafsson JA. The novel estrogen receptor-β subtype: potential role in the cell- and promoter-specific actions of estrogens and anti-estrogens. *FEBS Lett.* 1997; 410:87–90.

152. Cowley SM, Hoare S, Mosselman S, Parker MG. Estrogen receptors α and β form heterodimers on DNA. *J Biol Chem.* 1997; 272:19858–62.

153. Pettersson K, Grandien K, Kuiper GG, Gustafsson JÅ. Mouse estrogen receptor β forms estrogen response element-binding heterodimers with estrogen receptor α. *Mol Endocrinol.* 1997; 11:1486–96.

154. Kuiper GG, Enmark E, Pelto-Hulkko M, Nilsson S, Gustafsson J. Cloning of a novel estrogen receptor expressed in rat prostate and ovary. *Proc Natl Acad Sci USA.* 1996; 93:5925–30.

155. Paech K, Webb P, Kuiper GG, et al. Differential ligand activation of estrogen receptors ER-α and ER-β at AP1 sites. *Science.* 1997; 277:1508–10.

156. Gaub MP, Bellard M, Scheuer I, Chambon P, Sassone-Corsi P. Activation of the ovalbumin gene by the estrogen receptor involves the *fos–jun* complex. *Cell.* 1990; 63:1267–76.

157. Kuiper GG, Carlsson B, Grandien K, et al. Comparison of the ligand binding specificity and transcript tissue distribution of estrogen receptors α and β. *Endocrinology.* 1997; 138:863–70.

158. Lippman M, Bolan G, Huff K. Interactions of antiestrogens with human breast cancer in long-term tissue culture. *Cancer Treat Rep.* 1976; 60:1421–9.

159. Brown M, Sharp PA. Human estrogen receptor forms multiple protein–DNA complexes. *J Biol Chem.* 1990; 265:11238–43.

160. Beekman JM, Allan GF, Tsai SY, Tsai MJ, O'Malley BW. Transcriptional activation by the estrogen receptor requires a conformational change in the ligand binding domain. *Mol Endocrinol.* 1993; 7:1266–74.

161. Giambiagi N, Pasqualini JR. Immunological differences between the estradiol-, tamoxifen- and 4-hydroxytamoxifen-estrogen receptor complexes detected by two monoclonal antibodies. *J Steroid Biochem.* 1988; 30:213–7.

162. McDonnell DP, Clemm DL, Hermann T, Goldman ME, Pike JW. Analysis of estrogen receptor function in vitro reveals three distinct classes of antiestrogens. *Mol Endocrinol.* 1995; 9:659–69.

163. Jordan VC. "Studies on the estrogen receptor in breast cancer"—20 years as a target for the treatment and prevention of cancer. *Breast Cancer Res Treat.* 1995; 36:267–85.

164. Early Breast Cancer Trialists' Collaborative Group. Tamoxifen for early breast cancer: an overview of the randomized trials. *Lancet.* 1998; 351:1451–67.

165. Groom GV, Griffiths K. Effect of the anti-estrogen tamoxifen on plasma levels of luteinizing hormone, follicle stimulating hormone, prolactin, estradiol and progesterone in normal premenopausal women. *J Endocrinol.* 1976; 70:421–8.

166. Manni A, Pearson OH. Antiestrogen-induced remissions in premenopausal women with stage IV breast cancer: effects on ovarian function. *Cancer Treat Rep.* 1980; 64:779–85.

167. Ravdin PM, Fritz NF, Tormey DC, Jordan VC. Endocrine status of premenopausal node positive breast cancer patients after adjuvant chemotherapy and long-term tamoxifen. *Cancer Res.* 1988; 48:1026–9.

168. Jordan VC, Fritz NF, Langan-Fahey S, Thompson M, Tormey DC. Alteration of endocrine parameters in premenopausal women with breast cancer during long-term adjuvant tamoxifen therapy. *J Natl Cancer Inst.* 1991; 83:1488–91.

169. Sawka CA, Pritchard KI, Paterson DJ, et al. Role and mechanism of action of tamoxifen in premenopausal women with metastatic breast cancer. *Cancer Res.* 1996; 46:3152–6.

170. Jordan VC, Bian RR, Brown RR, Gosden B, Santos MA. Determination and pharmacology of a new hydroxylated metabolite of tamoxifen observed in patient sera during therapy for advanced breast cancer. *Cancer Res.* 1983; 43:1446–50.

171. Lien EA, Solheim E, Kvinnsland S, Veland PM. Identification of 4-hydroxy-*N*-desmethylta-moxifen as a metabolite of tamoxifen in human bile. *Cancer Res.* 1988; 48:2304–8.

172. Langan-Fahey SM, Tormey DC, Jordan VC. Tamoxifen metabolites in patients on long-term adjuvant therapy for breast cancer. *Eur J Cancer.* 1990; 26:883–8.

173. Johnston SR, Haynes BP, Smith IE, et al. Acquired tamoxifen resistance in human breast cancer and reduced intra-tumoral drug concentration. *Lancet.* 1993; 342:1521–2.

174. Osborne CK, Coronado E, Allred DC, Wiebe V, DeGregorio M. Acquired tamoxifen resistance: correlation with reduced breast tumor levels of tamoxifen and isomerisation of trans-4-hydroxytamoxifen. *J Natl Cancer Inst.* 1991; 83:1477–82.

175. Jordan VC. Metabolites of tamoxifen in animals and men: identification, pharmacology and significance. *Breast Cancer Res Treat.* 1982; 2:123–8.

176. Jordan VC. Estrogen receptor antagonists. In: *Reproductive Endocrinology, Surgery and Technology.* (Adashi EY, Rock JA, and Rosenwaks Z, eds.), Lippincott-Raven, Philadelphia, 1996, pp. 528–45.

177. Jordan VC, Collins MM, Rowsby L, Prestwich G. A monohydroxylated metabolite of tamoxifen with potent antiestrogenic activity. *J Endocrinol.* 1977; 75:305–6.

178. Katzenellenbogen BS, Norman MJ, Eckert RL, Peltz SW, Mangel WF. Bioactivities, estrogen receptor interactions and plasminogen activator-inducing activities of tamoxifen and hydroxytamoxifen isomers in MCF-7 human breast cancer cells. *Cancer Res.* 1984; 44:112–9.

179. Katzenellenbogen JA, Carlson KE, Katzenellenbogen BS. Facile geometric isomerization of phenolic nonsteroidal estrogens and antiestrogens: limitations to the interpretation of experiments characterizing the activity of individual isomers. *J Steroid Biochem.* 1985; 22:589–96.

180. Jordan VC, Haldeman B, Allen KE. Geometric isomers of substituted triphenylethylenes and antiestrogen action. *Endocrinology.* 1981; 108:1353–61.

181. Lieberman ME, Gorski J, Jordan VC. An estrogen receptor model to describe the regulation of prolactin synthesis by antiestrogens in vitro. *J Biol Chem.* 1983; 258:4741–5.

182. Murphy CS, Langan-Fahey SM, McCague R, Jordan VC. Structure–function relationships of hydroxylated metabolites of tamoxifen that control the proliferation of estrogen-responsive T47D breast cancer cells. *Mol Pharmacol.* 1990; 38:737–43.

183. Wiebe VJ, Osborne CK, McGuire WL, DeGregorio M. Identification of estrogenic tamoxi-

fen metabolite(s) in tamoxifen-resistant human breast tumors. *J Clin Oncol.* 1992; 10:990–4.

184. Wolf DM, Langan-Fahey SM, Parker CP, McCague R, Jordan VC. Investigation of the mechanism of tamoxifen stimulated breast tumor growth with non-isomerizable analogues of tamoxifen and its metabolites. *J Natl Cancer Inst.* 1993; 85:806–12.

185. King RJ, Stewart JF, Millis RR, Rubens RD, Hayward JL. Quantiative comparison of estrogen and progesterone receptor contents of primary and metastatic human breast tumors in relation to response to endocrine treatment. *Breast Cancer Res Treat.* 1982; 2:339–46.

186. Clark GM, McGuire WL. Steroid receptors and other prognostic factors in primary breast cancer. *Semin Oncol.* 1988; 15:20–5.

187. Nomura Y, Tashiro H, Shinozuka K. Changes of steroid hormone receptor content by chemotherapy and/or endocrine therapy in advanced breast cancer. *Cancer.* 1985; 55:546–51.

188. Clarke R, Lippman ME. Acquisition of antiestrogen resistance in breast cancer. In: *Drug Resistance in Oncology,* (Teicher BA, ed.), Marcel Dekker, New York, 1993, pp. 501–36.

189. Tonnetti DA, Jordan VC. The role of estrogen receptor mutations in tamoxifen-stimulated breast cancer. *J Steroid Biochem Mol Biol.* 1997; 62:119–128.

190. Pink JJ, Jordan VC. Models of estrogen receptor regulation by estrogens and antiestrogens in breast cancer cell lines. *Cancer Res.* 1996; 56:2321–30.

191. Robertson JF. Oestrogen receptor: a stable phenotype in breast cancer. *Br J Cancer.* 1996; 73:5–12.

192. Osborne CK, Coronado EB, Robinson JP. Human breast cancer in the athymic nude mouse: cytostatic effects of long-term antiestrogen therapy. *Eur J Cancer Clin Oncol.* 1987; 23:1189–96.

193. Gottardis MM, Jordan VC. Development of tamoxifen-stimulated growth of MCF-7 tumors in athymic mice after long-term antiestrogen administration. *Cancer Res.* 1988; 48:5183–7.

194. Karnik PS, Kulkarni S, Liu XP, Budd T, Bukowski RM. Estrogen receptor mutations in tamoxifen-resistant breaset cancer. *Cancer Res.* 1994; 54:349–53.

195. Wolf CM, Jordan VC. Characterization of tamoxifen stimulated MCF-7 tumor variants grown in athymic mice. *Breast Cancer Res Treat.* 1994; 31:117–28.

196. Wolf CM, Jordan VC. The estrogen receptor from a tamoxifen stimulated MCF-7 tumor variant contains a point mutation in the ligand binding domain. *Breast Cancer Res Treat.* 1994; 31:129–38.

197. Levenson AS, Catherino WH, Jordan VC. Estrogenic activity is increased for an antiestrogen by a natural mutation of the estrogen receptor. *J Steroid Biochem Mol Biol.* 1997; 60:261–8.

198. Levenson AS, Jordan VC. The key to the antiestrogenic mechanism of raloxifene is amino acid 351 (aspartate) in the estrogen receptor. *Cancer Res.* 1998; 58:1872–5.

199. Astruc ME, Chabret C, Bali P, Gagne D, Pons M. Prolonged treatment of breast cancer cells with antiestrogens increases the activating protein-1-mediated response: involvement of the estrogen receptor. *Endocrinology.* 1995; 136:824–32.

200. Dumont JA, Bitonti AJ, Wallace CD, Baumann RJ, Cashman EA, Cross-Doersen DE. Progression of MCF-7 breast cancer cells to antiestrogen-resistant phenotype is accompanied by elevated levels of AP-1 DNA binding activity. *Cell Growth Different.* 1996; 7:51–9.

201. Levenson AS, Tonetti DA, Jordan VC. The oestrogen-like effect of 4-hydroxytamoxifen on induction of transforming growth factor-α mRNA in MDA-MB-231 breast cancer cells stably expressing the oestrogen receptor. *Br J Cancer.* 1998; 18:12–19.

202. Tzukerman MT, Esty A, Santiso-Mere D, et al. Human estrogen receptor transactivational

capacity is determined by both cellular and promoter context and mediated by two functionally distinct intramolecular regions. *Mol Endocrinol.* 1994; 94:21–30.

203. Fujimoto N, Katzenellenbogen BS. Alteration in the agonist/antagonist balance of antiestrogens by activation of protein kinase A signaling pathways in breast cancer cells: antiestrogen selectivity and promoter dependence. *Mol Endocrinol.* 1994; 8:296–304.

204. Lin A, Chan YL, McNally J, Peleg D, Meyuhas O, Wool IG. The primary structure of rat ribosomal protein L7. *J Biol Chem.* 1987; 262:12665–71.

205. Smith CL, Nawaz Z, O'Malley BW. Coactivator and corepressor regulation of the agonist/antagonist activity of the mixed antiestrogen, 4-hydroxytamoxifen. *Mol Endocrinol.* 1997; 11:657–66.

206. Onate SA, Boonyaratanakornkit V, Spencer TE, et al. The steroid receptor coactivator-1 contains multiple receptor interacting and activation domains that cooperatively enhance the activation function 1 (AF1) and AF2 domains of steroid receptors. *J Biol Chem.* 1998; 273:12101–8.

207. Chen JD, Evans RM. A transcriptional co-repressor that interacts with nuclear hormone receptors. *Nature.* 1995; 377:454–7.

208. Chen JD, Umesono K, Evans RM. SMRT isoforms mediate repression and anti-repression of nuclear receptor heterodimers. *Proc Natl Acad Sci USA.* 1996; 93:7567–71.

209. Gottardis MM, Jordan VC. The antitumor action of keoxifene and tamoxifen in the *N*-nitrosomethylurea-induced rat mammary carcinoma model. *Cancer Res.* 1987; 47:4020–4.

210. Jordan VC, Phelps E, Lindgren JU. Effects of antiestrogens on bone in castrated and intact female rats. *Breast Cancer Res Treat.* 1987; 10:31–5.

211. Lerner LJ, Jordan VC. Development of antiestrogens and their use in breast cancer: Eighth Cain Memorial Lecture. *Cancer Res.* 1990; 50:4177–89.

212. Delmas PD, Bjarnason NH, Mitlak BH, et al. Effects of raloxifene on bone mineral density, serum cholesterol concentrations, and uterine endometrium in postmenopausal women. *N Engl J Med.* 1997; 337:1641–7.

8

Cyclin-Dependent Kinases and Their Regulators as Potential Targets for Anticancer Therapeutics

Leonardo Brizuela, Jeno Gyuris, and Muzammil Mansuri

Introduction

A number of complex changes take place between the time a cell is generated and the time the cell divides into two new daughter cells. This process is known as the cell division cycle or cell cycle. The morphological changes associated with particular stages of the cell cycle are well known; however, a detailed understanding of the regulatory mechanisms controlling cell-cycle progression has only recently been elucidated. Understanding the biochemical and genetic mechanisms that control these cellular changes is fundamental to cell biology because it impinges on processes such as cell transformation, cell differentiation, and cell growth. Clearly a greater knowledge of the molecular mechanisms underlying the transformation of mammalian cells offers the opportunity of designing inhibitors of the specific biochemical processes responsible for abnormal cell proliferation or cancer.

The core of the cell-cycle machinery has been preserved through evolution. As organisms evolved, cells adapted to respond to a larger and more complex number of stimuli that dictate their proliferative activity. This evolution has usually been achieved by the addition of more layers of control over the same basic cell-cycle circuitry. The use of yeast models and cell biology of invertebrate systems has provided invaluable information and powerful experimental tools to aid our understanding of cell-cycle regulation *(1,2)*. This chapter deals with the group of proteins most directly involved in the regulation of the mammalian cell division cycle. These regulatory proteins belong to a unique family of kinases named cyclin-dependent kinases (CDKs). The identification of the CDK has also led to a number of other related and important discoveries of the molecular mechanisms involved in the regulation of cell-cycle progression. A number of proto-oncogenes (cyclin D1, CDC25, CDK4) and tumor suppressors (pRb, p53, p16) have been identified in the context of cell-cycle regulation. Together, these discoveries have enhanced our overall understanding of cell transformation and tumor biology.

Chapter 6 introduced many of the concepts discussed in this chapter, including cell-cycle regulation by CDK. This chapter assesses the current knowledge concerning CDKs, and their role in cell transformation and cancer. The potential applications of CDKs in rational drug design for the development of new antiproliferative agents for

From: *Principles of Molecular Oncology*
Edited by: M. H. Bronchud, M. A. Foote, W. P. Peters, and M. O. Robinson © Humana Press Inc., Totowa, NJ

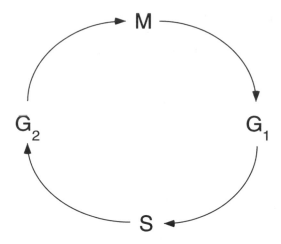

Fig. 1. Cell cycle phases. See text for description of G_1, S, G_2, and M.

oncology and other proliferative disorders is discussed. Inhibition of CDK represents one of the first mechanistic approaches to the development of therapies for cancer.

CDKs and Their Role in Cell-Cycle Progression

Each cell division cycle consists of two major periods of morphophysiological activity (Fig. 1). The first period of activity, or S-phase, involves DNA replication in which the cell duplicates its genetic material. The second period, or M-phase, occurs when the sister chromatids separate and nuclear division takes place, generating two nuclei with identical and complete sets of genetic material. In mammalian cells, the M phase is also kinetically linked to the process of cytoplasmic division or cytokinesis. The S and M phases are separated by two Gap phases (G_1 and G_2). The complete cell cycle proceeds through G_1 to S to G_2 and finally to M-phase. The transition through these phases of the cell cycle is regulated by the CDKs. Other important events, including checkpoint controls (checkpoint controls ensure fidelity in the completion of the critical processes in the preceding phases), occur during the G_1 and G_2 phases. The G_1 and G_2 processes ensure proper cell growth and accumulation of critical cellular components required for the advancement of the cell to the next phase. The restriction point or "R" point, located in late G_1, is critical to cell-cycle progression. "R" defines the point beyond which cell-cycle progression becomes independent from external growth factors and thereby committed to that round of cell division *(3)*.

Protein phosphorylation is a reversible modification that has been widely implicated in cellular regulation of protein structure and activity; this occurs by phosphorylation of specific residues through ATP hydrolysis and phosphoester bond formation. The CDKs are heteromultimeric kinases *(4,5)* that phosphorylate specific serine/threonine residues adjacent to prolines in their protein substrates. There is also a strong preference for other basic residues to surround these two positions (S/T-P). The primary sequence is not the only determinant for CDK substrate utilization *(6,7)*. For example, CDK4/

cyclin D1 and CDK 2 cyclin E both phosphorylate pRb but show preference for different positions on the substrate *(8)*. The activities of the CDK complexes can themselves also be modulated by phosphorylation (*see* Posttranslational Modifications of CDF).

In their simplest form, CDKs are dimeric complexes composed of a catalytic (CDK) subunit, which contains the ATP-binding pocket, and a regulatory (cyclin) subunit. The composition and stoichiometry of the specific complexes vary depending on the individual components (CDK and cyclins), the stage of the cell cycle, the cell type, and the transformation state of the cell *(9)*. To be catalytically competent, the catalytic subunit (CDK1–9) and a regulatory subunit (cyclin A–H and cyclin T) must combine and also be in the correct phosphorylation state. Figure 2A shows the combinations of the catalytic and regulatory subunits which furnish functionally discrete CDK complexes. Alternative spliced forms (i.e., cyclin E) and additional subtypes (i.e., cyclins D1–3 or cyclins A1–2) enlarge the number of cyclins and hence the complexity of the functional CDK/cyclin combinations. The activity of most of the CDK complexes can be associated with specific points during cell-cycle progression *(5)* (Fig. 3); however, some family members are associated with processes that do not involve proliferation. CDK 5, for example, is involved with neuronal processes and not proliferation *(10)* and other CDK complexes are clearly involved in transcriptional control *(11)*.

Whereas the levels of the catalytic CDK subunits remain relatively constant throughout the cell cycle, the amounts of the regulatory cyclin subunits oscillate. These oscillations mean that specific cyclins will be present only at certain times during the cell division cycle. Consequently, the cyclins regulate CDK complex formation and activity and also confer substrate specificity and cellular compartmentalization (*see* Other Mechanisms of Regulation). The cyclins contain an amino acids motif (approx 100 amino acids) known as the cyclin box; this cyclin box is also found in pRb and TFIIB. This motif is a critical element at the CDK–cyclin interface and defines a 5α helix bundle is repeated twice in the cyclin subunit *(12,13)*. The cyclins show high structural similarity but their overall level of identity is very low (Fig. 2B). Although the smallest kinases known, the CDK catalytic subunits contain all the usual kinase subdomains plus a characteristic signature sequence (variations of the "PSTAIRE" sequence) that define a key element for interaction with the cyclins. Experiments indicate that some of the CDK/cyclin complexes may show some level of redundancy. For example, despite the decreased size and defects in mammary epithelial and retina cells displayed by the cyclin D1 knockout mice, cyclin D1 deletion does not result in embryonic lethality or any major postembryonic collapse *(14)*. Figure 3 shows the distribution and activities of a number of the CDK complexes involved in cell-cycle regulation. The CDK integrate signals from the cell and its environment to either initiate or inhibit cell cycle progression. Granulocyte-macrophage colony-stimulating factor (GM-CSF), for example, induces increased cyclin D1 synthesis in a fashion that parallels the stimulatory activity of this growth factor *(15)*. Other signals such as the mitogen antagonists cAMP and transforming growth factor-β (TGF-β) have a negative effect on CDK and cell-cycle progression *(16,17)*. DNA-damaging agents and differentiation factors also induce cell cycle arrest through CDK modulation *(18,19)*.

A number of other proteins are known to interact with these subunits: the proliferating cell nuclear antigen (Ag) (PCNA), CDK inhibitor proteins (CIP–KIP and INK4 family

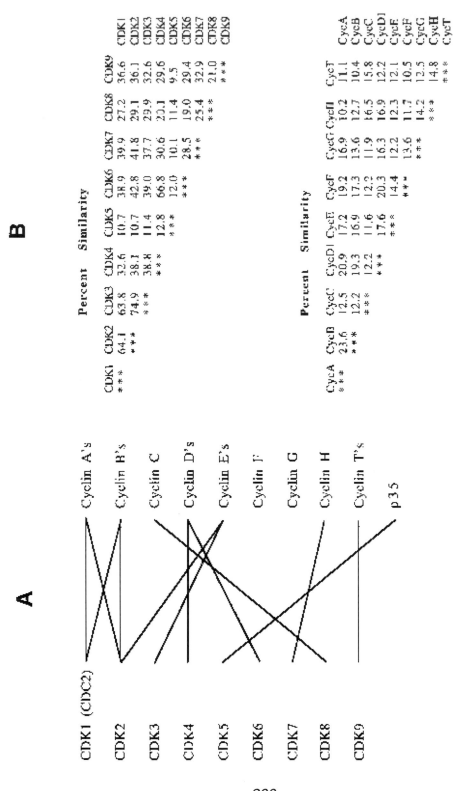

Fig. 2. CDKs and cyclins. (**A**) CDK and cyclin combinations found in vivo. (**B**) Similarity between CDK family members.

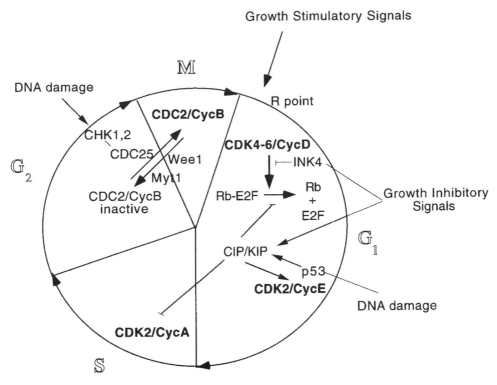

Fig. 3. CDK control of cell cycle regulation.

members), the members of the retinoblastoma (Rb) family (p107/p130/p300), CKS family members, transcription factors, and various transforming viral proteins *(5,9)*. The significance of every one of these interactions is not completely understood at present.

Checkpoint controls monitor the state of completion and fidelity of the critical molecular and macromolecular processes preceding critical commitment points in the cell-division cycle. CDKs play a critical role in the execution of the cell-cycle checkpoints. To date, two cell-cycle checkpoints have been characterized. The first precedes DNA synthesis (S-phase) and ensures replication of undamaged DNA *(18,19)*. The second immediately precedes mitosis (G_2/M-phase) and is also affected by DNA damage, incomplete DNA replication, or spindle microtubule polymerization *(20)*. CDK1 (CDC2) has been identified as the final mediator of the G_2/M checkpoint *(21)*. Finally, deregulation of checkpoint elements has been reported to be associated with virally induced oncogenesis *(22)*.

There is also a strong association between the execution of the restriction point and the activation of CDKs (CDK4 and CDK6). CDK4/CDK6 activity is absolutely required for entry into G_1 and subsequent cell-cycle progression *(23)* (Fig. 3). CDK 4–cyclin D phosphorylates the Rb tumor suppressor gene that leads to its dissociation from the E2F transcription group of proteins. This dissociation allows the E2F–DP complexes to initiate the transcription of a large number of genes required for DNA synthesis. Whereas pRb contains 16 potential CDK phosphorylation sites, CDK 4/cyclin D preferentially phosphorylates S-795 *(8)*. Whereas the elimination of the CDK 4/cyclin D

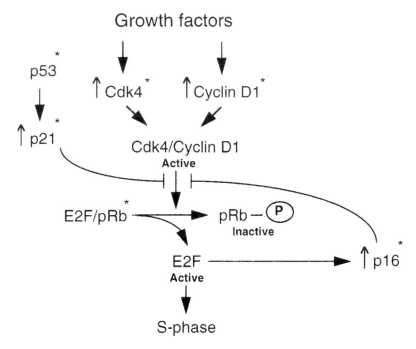

Fig. 4. The *CDK 4/Cyclin D/pRp/p16* pathway. *Asterisk* indicates that alterations in the respective genes have been associated with cellular transformation and tumorigenesis.

complex arrests cell cycle progression in Rb wild-type cells, it has no effect on cells lacking functional pRb *(23)*. These results support the hypothesis that pRb is the only physiologically relevant substrate of CDK4. Other elements involved in the pRb pathway are the CDK inhibitors p16 (and related members) and p21 (and related members), as well as tyrosine kinase(s) involved in negative regulation of CDK4 *(24)*. Multiple oncogenic alterations have been associated with the Rb pathway, including activation of several oncogenes and inactivation of diverse tumor suppressors (Fig. 4), highlighting its central role in the regulation of cell proliferation and transformation.

CDK2/cyclin E is also required for G_1 progression; pRb is again a key substrate. As in the case of cyclin D, ectopic expression of cyclin E shortens G_1. It appears that pRb must be phosphorylated by CDK4/cyclin D before pRb phosphorylation by CDK2/cyclin E *(25)*. Moreover, elimination of the pRb function does not eliminate the need of CDK2/cyclin E for cell-cycle progression *(26,27)*. This suggests that substrate(s), other than pRb, may mediate the cell-cycle regulatory role of CDK2/cyclin E. In mammalian cells, CDK2/cyclin A has been associated with control of DNA synthesis. Cyclin A localization to the nucleus is associated with the start of S-phase. Microinjection of antibodies (Abs) against cyclin A, as well as expression of antisense constructs, inhibit DNA synthesis *(28)*. CDK1/cyclin B activity is responsible for induction of mitosis in all eukaryotic cells. This activity is also known as maturation promoting factor (MPF) and also constitutes the cellular histone H1 kinase *(29–31)*. MPF is a dominant activity able to induce mitotic events in cells regardless of their position in the cell cycle *(32)*. Not only is CDK1/cyclin B activation absolutely required for entry into mitosis but its elimination or degradation is necessary also for cells to exit mitosis. Cyclin B mutants devoid of the destruction box sequence necessary for degradation cannot eliminate cyclin B and hence induce a mitotic block *(33)*. Cyclin B degradation occurs through ubiquitin-mediated degradation by the anaphase-promoting complex (APC) *(34)*. Substrates other than histone H1 for CDK1/cyclin B have been identified and consist of a wide range of structural proteins and enzymes that are involved in the morphological changes that take place during mitosis, including lamins, vimentin, caldesmon, microtubule-associated proteins, CDC25 (as part of a feedback loop control), cABL, and CKII, among others *(35)*.

Regulation of CDK Activity

The molecular and biochemical basis of CDK regulation is best understood through familiarity of the three-dimensional structures of these molecules and their regulators. Atomic models, obtained by crystallographic and nuclear magnetic resonance (NMR) analysis of CDK2, CDK6, cyclin A, cyclin H, and some of their inhibitors (p27, p19, p18, and p16) in various monomeric and bound forms, have provided valuable information regarding the structural implications of their primary sequences, as well as the role of critical posttranslational modifications and atomic and structural effects of their interactions.

The catalytic CDK subunits form a bilobular structure typical of known protein kinases (Fig. 5) *(13,36–38)*. The smaller lobe of the catalytic subunit contains approximately the first 100 residues of the protein and comprises of a five-stranded β sheet and a unique α helix. The α helix contains the signature CDK PSTAIRE motif and is responsible for the interaction with the regulatory cyclin subunit (red domain in Fig. 5) *(13)*. The larger lobe, defined by approx 200 residues of the C-terminal mainly comprises α helices and is predicted to contain the peptide-binding site. The ATP-binding site lies in the cleft between the two lobes of the catalytic subunit *(36,39)*. The small lobe contains (1) the highly conserved glycine loop that provides the backbone amides that hydrogen bond to the β- and γ-phosphate of ATP and (2) the highly conserved lysine residue (E51 in CDK2) involved in ion pairing with the α and β phosphates of ATP. Key threonine and tyrosine residues (T-14 and Y-15, respectively, in CDK2) involved in the negative regulation of CDK activity lie in the glycine-rich region. The large lobe encodes the critical aspartic acid (D146 in CDK2) that establishes salt bridges with E51 and defines the correct configuration of the ATP-binding pocket. Another important motif of the CDKs is the T loop, which contains the CDK-activating kinase (CAK) phosphorylation site (T-160 in CDK2) (orange motif of Figs. 5 and 6) required for kinase activation.

The monomeric catalytic CDK subunit is catalytically incompetent. Binding the regulatory subunit induces a number of changes that allow proper ATP binding and catalysis to occur *(13,36)*. The signature PSTAIRE loop rearranges to bring the E51 into proximity to the ATP-binding site. This stabilizes the position of the active site lysine to allow proper orientation of the ATP. In a second conformational change, the T loop moves away from the catalytic cleft (compare the position of the T loop in Figs. 5 and 6). CAK phosphorylation of the T-160 residue also further stabilizes the T loop by eliminating the steric hindrance that the T loop places on the catalytic site and allowing access to the substrate *(40)*.

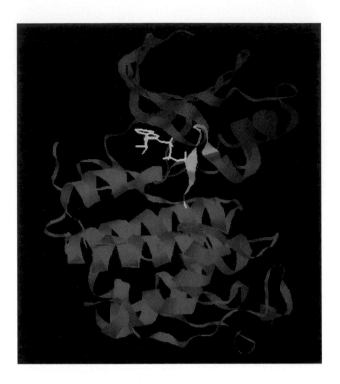

Fig. 5. Crystal structure of monomeric CDK 2. *Purple,* small lobe; magenta, large lobe; red, PSTAIRE helix; orange, T loop; green, ATP.

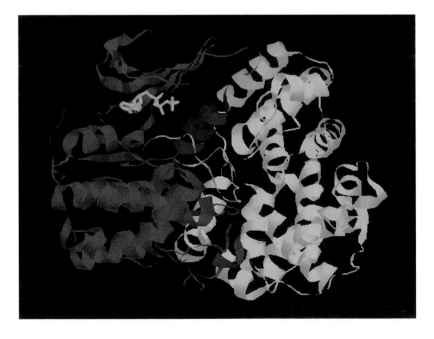

Fig. 6. Crystal structure of CDK 2 bound to cyclin A. Magenta, CDK 2; *blue,* cyclin A; Red, PSTAIRE helix; orange, T loop; Green, ATP.

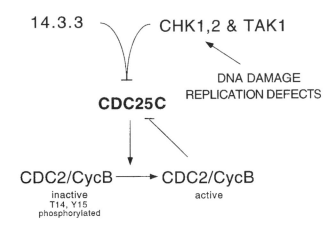

Fig. 7. Regulation of CDC25 C.

Posttranslation Modifications of CDK

As with other protein kinases, the activity of CDK is regulated by phosphorylation/ dephosphorylation events. To be catalytically competent, the newly formed CDK–cyclin complex must be correctly phosphorylated at position T-160 in the T loop. The kinase responsible for T-160 phosphorylation is CAK *(41)*. CAK (CDK7/cyclin H), while a member of the CDK family *(see* Fig. 2A), does not show cell cycle-dependent activity. CAK has been associated with the transcriptional machinery as part of the TFIIH complex involved in the phosphorylation of the C-terminal repeat of the RNA polymerase II *(42)*. In budding yeast, the dimeric CAK homologue (CDK7/cyclin H) has been associated only with transcriptional control, while a novel monomeric kinase CAK1 (unrelated to CAK) has been associated with positive regulation of its substrate, CDC28 *(43)*.

Phosphorylation can also play a negative role in the regulation of the CDKs. Phosphorylation of residues T-14 and Y-15 of CDK 2 (and equivalent residue on other CDKs, when applicable) has a negative effect on CDK activity *(44)*. The T-14 and Y-15 residues are located in the glycine-rich loop of the kinase that forms the roof of the ATP-binding site and is involved in critical interactions with the ATP. At the G_2–M transition, the dephosphorylation of T-14 and Y-15 residues of CDK1/cyclin B complex is the limiting step for activation of this kinase and for induction of mitosis *(45)*. The phosphorylation of the T-14 and Y-15 positions is performed by Myt-1 (a dual specific kinase) or Wee-1 (a tyrosine kinase) *(46,47)*. The inhibitory effect of T-14 and Y-15 phosphorylation can be reversed by the CDC25 family of dual specific phosphatases *(45)*. There are three members of the CDC25 family: CDC25A, B, and C. The oncogenic potential of CDC25A and B has recently been described *(48)*, but CDC25C is the best understood of these three phosphatases. CDC25C has been associated with dephosphorylation and activation of CDK1/cyclin B at mitosis. The activity of the CDC25C phosphatase is itself regulated by two different mechanisms (Fig. 7). As part of a positive feedback loop, CDC25C becomes phosphorylated by its substrate, the CDK1/ cyclin B kinase *(49,50)*. Also, CDC25C is regulated by its interaction with the 14–3–3 proteins *(51,52)*. Interaction of the phosphatase with the 14–3–3 proteins requires

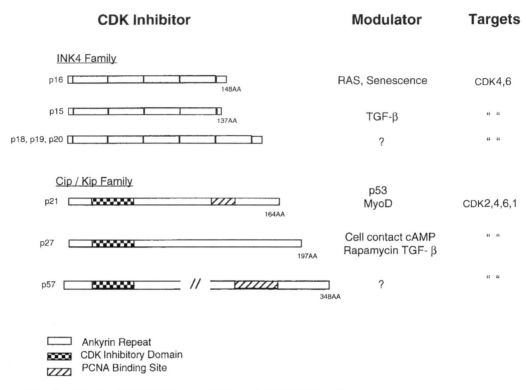

Fig. 8. Cellular CDK inhibitors: INK4 and CIP/KIP families.

phosphorylation of the former at position 416 by Chk 1, Chk 2, and the c-TAK1 *(53–55)*. This results in down-regulation of the CDC25 activity and/or in its altered cellular localization *(51,52)*.

Cellular Inhibitors

A large number of proteins have been identified that bind to and inhibit the CDK–cyclin complexes. These proteins are generically referred to as cyclin-dependent kinase inhibitors (CKIs) *(56)*. CKIs can be divided into two separate groups: the INK4 and CIP–KIP families of inhibitors (Fig. 8). The INK4 (inhibitors of CDK 4 or 6 kinases) family members, p15, p16, p18, and p19, are structurally highly conserved. They bind and inhibit CDK4- and CDK6-associated kinases specifically *(57)*. Although the INK4 members behave identically in vitro, their cellular expression patterns differ and they respond to different signals. Up-regulation of p16 levels has been observed in cells by activated Ras and during senescence *(58)*. p15 levels change the response of cells to TGF-β or other antimitogenic agents *(59)*. The expression of p18 and p19 is regulated in a cell cycle-dependent manner with maximum expression at S-phase *(60)*. The analysis of the recently solved CDK 6–p19 structure *(37,38)* (Fig. 9) suggests that p19 exerts its inhibitory activity by changing the structure of the CDK-6 molecule. The INK4a locus encodes two proteins, p16 and p19[ARF], which regulate two important tumor-suppressor pathways involved in human cancers. p16 regulates the pRb pathway (through the modulation of cyclin D-dependent kinases) *(57)*. p19[ARF], which is generated

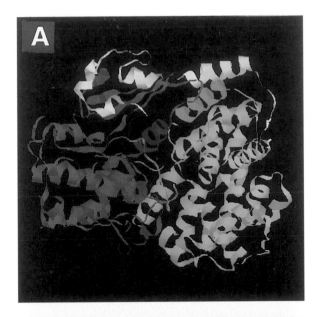

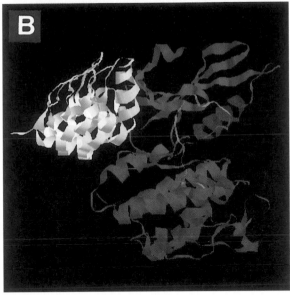

Fig. 9. (A) Crystal structure of CDK 2–cyclin A bound to p27. Magenta, CDK 2; blue, cyclin A; white, p27 N-terminal domain. **(B)** Crystal structure of CDK 6 bound to p19. Magenta, CDK6; white, p19.

by an alternative reading frame (ARF) within this locus, induces p53 stabilization *(61)*. Mice originally engineered to eliminate the p16 expression, but that also eliminate p19[ARF], develop sporadic tumors at an early stage and show hypersensitivity to chemical carcinogenesis *(62)*. Mice lacking the function of only p19[ARF] also develop sporadic tumors, validating it as a bona fide tumor suppressor *(63)*.

Members of the CIP–KIP family inhibit all the CDK complexes and show little structural similarity. CIP–KIP members (Fig. 8) play an important role in the control of cell proliferation in response to antimitogenic agents. For example, p21 and/or p27 can regulate cell-cycle arrest induced by differentiation factors (in a p53-independent fashion) *(64)*, DNA-damaging agents (in a p53-dependent fashion) *(18,19)*, and antimitogenic conditions such as cell-to-cell contact and loss of cell anchorage *(64)*. Modulation of p27 levels regulate cell proliferation *(65)*. Correlation of low levels of p27 expression in tumor samples with poor patient survival indicates that p27 regulation has an impact in normal development and in aberrant cell growth, as described below. Several reports indicate that the cellular levels of p27 are regulated at the transcriptional, translational, and posttranslational levels *(56)*. The phosphorylation and ubiquitin-mediated degradation *(66)* have also been reported to be involved in regulating p27 stability.

The structure of CDK2/cyclin A in the presence of the inhibitory domain of p27 has been reported *(67)*. This structure shows that the N-terminal region of p27 interacts with the small lobe of CDK2, thereby altering the conformation of this region and the ATP-binding site. One of the key interactions outside the ATP-binding pocket involves the N-terminal coil of p27 and a highly conserved shallow groove on the cyclin molecule. This interaction is defined by the RRLFG motif of p27 which is also present in other proteins known to interact with CDK/cyclin complexes *(68)*. Structural information derived from a CDK2/cyclin A/p27 complex corroborates genetic and biochemical data indicating that motifs of p21 and p27 interact with both the CDK and cyclin subunits *(69)*. A role for CIP members in modulation of complex formation of cyclin D-dependent kinases has been proposed based on this observation. Finally, reshuttling of p27, from cyclin D complexes to cyclin E complexes, as cells are subjected to mitotic stimuli has also been reported *(70)*.

Other Mechanisms of Regulation

CDK activity is also regulated by mechanisms other than posttranslational modifications and interaction with cellular inhibitors. As discussed earlier, synthesis and degradation of the regulatory cyclin subunit is another important factor. Ubiquitin-mediated protein degradation has a central role in regulating cyclin levels. This was originally shown for cyclin B and later observed with cyclins E and D *(71–73)*. Likewise ubiquitination has been linked to p27 degradation. Phosphorylation at specific positions is believed to be the trigger for this degradative pathway. Another level of regulation takes place on the transcriptional level. Up-regulation of cyclin D transcription in response to growth factors and induction of p21 and p15 in response to antimitogenic signaling are examples. Cellular localization of the enzymes with respect to the relevant substrate(s) is another level of regulation. For example, cyclin B1 is found in the cytoplasm until the initiation of mitosis when it moves to the nucleus. A specific sequence, the cytoplasmic retention signal (CRS), is responsible for sequestering cyclin B1 in the cytoplasm *(74)*.

Another level of regulation is represented by modulation of the CDK/cyclin complex assembly. CDK4/cyclin D complex formation requires mitogenic signals. The necessary serum stimulation can be mimicked by ectopic expression of MEK1 and is likely to involve modulation of interaction of CDK 4 with molecular chaperons such as CDC37 *(75,76)*. Also, a phosphatase candidate for the T-loop dephosphorylation has been cloned *(77)* and has been suggested to preferentially use uncomplexed, T-loop phosphorylated CDKs as substrates *(78)*. However, no clear indication of its regulatory nature with respect to cell-cycle control have been described.

Finally, it is important to mention that regulation of the interaction between CDK complexes and a subset of cellular and viral proteins (including CDK substrates) is based on the use of a common motif present in a number of CDK-interacting proteins, including p21 family members, E2F, CDC25, and p107 *(78)*. This is the "RRLFG" motif, in the context of the p27 and CDK2/cyclin A interaction. As discussed, differential CDK inhibition has been shown with peptides containing this sequence *(69)*. Cellular effects of such peptides are described later.

Oncogenic Alterations of the Cell-Cycle Regulators

In the previous section, the molecular mechanisms that tightly control the transition through the G_1/S and G_2/M checkpoints were discussed. Normal cells transition from G_1 to S in response to extracellular signals such as growth factors, hormones, or cytokines, or after contacts with other cells and the extracellular matrix (ECM). In the absence of these extracellular signals, the cells withdraw to quiescence (G_0) from which they may either reenter into the cell division cycle or differentiate. Again, both of these decisions are made in response to specific extracellular signals. This mechanism ensures the correct balance of growth of the various tissues. It has been long recognized that the breakdown in these growth control processes is a hallmark of cancer *(79)*.

In contrast to G_1–S, the G_2–M transition is regulated mainly by intracellular signals (such as the completion of DNA synthesis). The role of the G_2–M checkpoint is to prevent mitosis when the DNA is damaged and not yet repaired. Alterations that abrogate the G_2–M checkpoint control allow cells with damaged genomes to undergo mitosis and result in the transmission of mutated genomes. From these altered genomes, new mutations may arise that contribute to the selection of cancer cells. This genomic instability is another hallmark of cancer *(79)*.

Since the discovery of the various mammalian cell-cycle regulators, many reports have examined the expression of various cell-cycle regulators in human tumors. The inherent problem of this approach is that it can only suggest a correlation. It is difficult to differentiate whether cells proliferate uncontrollably because they contain abnormal amounts of the specific cell-cycle regulatory protein or if protein is present in abnormal quantities only because the cells have divided uncontrollably. This section focuses on those molecular alterations of the cell-cycle regulators in which the genetic alteration in the gene itself is detected or in which the abnormal RNA or protein levels may have diagnostic/prognostic value for the treatment of the tumor.

Alterations of Cyclin D1 *in Human Tumors*

Molecular analysis of tumors in the past decade have revealed a number of different mechanisms that lead to the deregulated expression of *cyclin D1* gene. Indeed, the extreme number of tumors that show alteration in the cyclin D pathway (either in the cyclins themselves or their upstream regulators or downstream targets, Fig. 4) consistently implicate *cyclin D1* in the development of a variety of human tumors. These data suggest that the deregulation of this pathway is extremely important for the development of human cancers and holds great promise for therapeutic intervention.

Chromosomal Translocations Affecting Cyclin D1

The *cyclin D1* gene (*CCND1*) maps to 11q13, a region that is altered in a variety of proliferative disorders *(80)*. In a number of hematologic malignancies, reciprocal chromosomal translocation is a common feature. These translocations result in either the deregulated expression of a gene lying close to the breakpoint or the fusion of the coding information from the two chromosomal partners *(81)*. One of the characteristic translocations in a group of B-cell neoplasms (now collectively called mantle-cell lymphoma, MCL) is the t(11;14) translocation in which the *BCL-1* locus on chromosome 14 becomes juxtaposed with the *CCND1* gene on chromosome 11. As a result, most tumors with the t(11;14) translocations show increased expression of the cyclin D1 RNA, protein, or both, arguing that the primary target gene activated by the translocation is *CCND1 (82)*. It is now clear that most MCLs, which account for approx 5% of all non-Hodgkin's lymphomas (NHLs), show cytogenetic or molecular evidence for the t(11;14) translocation *(83,84)*. However, significant number of MCLs without the apparent translocations expresses increased amounts of *cyclin D1 (85,86)*. The mechanism(s) responsible for the overexpression in the latter situation remain unknown. Interestingly, none of the translocations that have been examined so far affected the coding region of *cyclin D1,* suggesting that the normal gene product contributes to tumorigenesis.

Other Chromosomal Rearrangements Affecting Cyclin D1

Another type of chromosomal rearrangement that also activates *cyclin D1* expression is an inversion of part of chromosome 11 (inv[11][p15;q13]) that places the *CCND1* locus at the band q13 adjacent to the parathyroid hormone gene (PTH) at band p15 *(87)*. This rearrangement has been reported in only three cases of benign parathyroid adenomas, but the impact of these rearrangement had been enormous, as it led to the discovery of *cyclin D1* as the candidate *PRAD1* oncogene *(88)*. In each case, the rearrangement resulted in a dramatic increase in the expression of cyclin D1 RNA, thereby contributing to the formation of the adenoma.

Gene Amplifications Affecting Cyclin D1

The most frequent chromosomal abnormality that affects *cyclin D1* is the amplification of the 11q13 region that had been observed in a significant portion of breast and squamous cell carcinomas. The amplification of this region suggest that a potential oncogene(s) lies in the area providing a selection pressure for the maintenance of the amplicon. Several lines of evidence suggest that this candidate oncogene is *CCND1*. First, as the consequence of the amplification, *CCND1* is expressed at higher levels *(89–91)*. Second, in most 11q13 amplifications, *CCND1* lies at the center of the amplification unit and is amplified *(92,93)*. The average amplification frequency of *CCND1* in primary breast tumors is 13–24% and the cyclin D1 protein is overexpressed in approx 50% of the tumors *(94–98)*.

High-frequency *CCND1* amplifications and *cyclin D1* overexpression are also observed with squamous cell carcinomas of the head, neck, oral cavity, larynx, and esophagus *(99–102)*. Cyclin D1 overexpression has been observed in ~50% of these cases and *CCND1* amplification has been detected in 23–40% of the cases. The *CCND1* locus is amplified in 32% of non-small-cell lung carcinomas (NSCLCs) and 44% of the tumors overexpress *cyclin D1 (103)*. In pancreatic carcinomas, the data are more controversial. One study finds *CCND1* amplification in 25% of the samples and detects *cyclin D1* overexpression in 68% of the samples. This study also finds correlation between the nuclear overexpression of *cyclin D1* and the poor prognosis of the tumor *(104)*. In a similar study, no *CCND1* amplification is detected *(105)*.

CDK4 *Amplification in Human Sarcomas and Gliomas*

The *CDK4* gene encoding the catalytic partner of cyclin D1 is located on chromosome 12q13 *(106)* and lies in a region that is frequently amplified in human sarcomas and gliomas *(107,108)*. Several genes, such as *WNT1, MDM2, GADD153, GLI, OS4, GAS16, GAS27, GAS41, GAS56, GAS64, GAS89,* and *SAS*, are implicated in the development of subsets of cancers and lie in this region *(109)*. However, several studies argue that *CDK4* amplification is the key event *(110–112)*. It has been demonstrated that *CDK4* is overexpressed as the result of amplification *(112,113)*. *CDK4* amplification and overexpression shows reciprocal correlation with the deletion of its inhibitor p16 and its regulatory subunit cyclin D1 *(114–118)*. The reported amplification frequency of *CDK4* in sarcomas is 8–36% *(113,119)* while in gliomas and astrocytomas this frequency is approx 10% *(112,120)*.

Mutations in the p16 *Binding-Domain* of CDK4 *in Familial Melanomas*

The analysis of familial melanoma patients have revealed an interesting mutation in the coding region of *CDK4* that also illustrates the intimate relationship between *CDK4* and *p16* and the spectacular diversity of molecular alterations that affect the cyclin D1/CDK4/p16/Rb pathway in human tumors. In approx 5% of the familial melanomas, the *R24* in CDK4 is mutated to *C24 (121–123);* the X-ray structure shows that the *R24* is buried in the protein–protein interface. This mutation, that functionally maps to the p16-binding domain of CDK4, disrupts the interaction between CDK4 and the p16 family of inhibitors, leading to the deregulation of the D1/CDK4/p16/Rb pathway.

Deletion and Point Mutations that Inactivate p16[Ink4a/MTS1/CDKN2A] *Gene in Human Tumors*

Two independent lines of research led to the discovery of p16 as an inhibitor of the CDK4/cyclin D kinase *(57)* and also implicated it as a candidate tumor suppressor located at the chromosomal position 9p21 *(124,125)*. This chromosomal region is frequently deleted in many human tumors and it is linked to the hereditary susceptibility to melanoma *(126,127)*. It is now evident that *p16[Ink4a/MTS1/CDKN2A]* alone, but not its close relative *p15[Ink4b/MTS2/CDKN2B]*, can sustain tumor-specific mutations in a large number of tumors. The *p16[Ink4a/MTS1/CDKN2A]* locus encodes two overlapping genes, each regulated by its own promoter. The transcript generated from the distal promoter encompasses exons 1α–2–3 encoding p16. The transcript generated by the proximal promoter is formed by exons 1β–2–3 in a different reading frame and encodes a completely different protein, p19[ARF]. The N-terminal 64 amino acids of p19[ARF] is encoded by the unique exon 1β while the C-terminal 105 amino acids are encoded by an ARF in exon 2 *(128)*. As discussed in the previous section, 19[ARF] overexpression induces p53-dependent growth arrest, plays a role in the regulation of p53, and is a bona fide tumor suppressor in mice *(61,129,130)*.

There are three major mechanisms of inactivation of the *INK4a* locus in human cancers: (1) deletion of both alleles, deletion of one allele, and either (2) intragenic mutation of the remaining allele or (3) methylation of the remaining allele *(131–135)*. Deletions remove both p16 and p19^{ARF} (and occasionally p15) while intragenic point mutations that are frequent in the unique exon 1a of *p16$^{Ink4a/MTS1/CDKN2A}$* or in the common exon 2 appear to inactivate p16 function only *(136)*. Therefore, deletions and intragenic mutations must be functionally distinct. Point mutations lead to the inactivation of the pRb pathway while deletions inactivate both the pRb and p53 pathways. One of the most striking differences between human tumors is the relative frequency of deletions and mutations in this locus.

Homozygous deletions appear to predominate in gliomas (57%), mesotheliomas (56%), leukemias (40%), nasopharyngeal carcinomas (42%), sarcomas (8%), ovarian carcinomas (16%), and bladder carcinomas (18%). In contrast, esophageal (30%) and biliary tract cancers (58%) sustain only intragenic point mutations. Both deletions and mutations have been detected in head and neck (8% mutations, 6% deletions) and NSCLCs (16%) mutations, 14% deletions) *(131–133,137)*. Ninety-eight percent of the pancreatic cancers have inactivated p16: 48% homozygous deletion, 34% hemizygous deletion and intragenic mutation, and 16% hemizygous deletion and methylation mediated silencing *(131–137)*. Neither deletion nor mutation is detected in breast cancers, neuroblastomas, colorectal tumors, and non-acute lymphocytic leukemia (ALL) leukemias.

Mutually Exclusive Alterations of Cyclin D1, p16 *and* pRb

The only known physiological substrate of the CDK4/cyclin D1 kinase is pRb. Progression through G_1 requires the phosphorylation and inactivation of pRb by the CDK4/cyclin D1 kinase and the liberation of the pRb-associated transcription factors (Fig. 4). The implication of this functional link is that perturbation in any of the genes involved in this pathway will likely have similar negative consequences. There is a great deal of evidence suggesting that the CDK4/cyclin D1/p16/pRb pathway behaves as a single mutagenic target during tumorigenesis. The amplification or overexpression of *cyclin D1* and/or *CDK 4* or *CDK 4* mutation will promote pRb phosphorylation and inactivation, leading to unrestrained cell proliferation. The inactivation of p16 will have the same effect. In tumors with a mutated or deleted Rb gene, there is no need for additional selection for the alteration of the upstream genes. Consequently, in *pRb*-negative cells there is reduced level of cyclin D1 and high levels of wild-type p16. *Rb*-positive cells frequently have *CDK4–cyclin D1* amplification/overexpression and/or mutation of *p16$^{Ink4a/MTS1/CDKN2A}$*. Mutually exclusive inactivation of p16 or pRb has been observed in gliomas *(113,118,120)*. Small-cell lung carcinomas (SCLCs) generally express wild-type p16 and have mutated pRb, while NSCLCs show frequent loss of p16 and have wild-type pRB *(138)*. This inverse correlation also applies to *CDK4* amplifications vs *p16$^{Ink4a/ME1/CDKN2A}$* inactivation in sarcomas and gliomas *(113,118,120)*. In familial melanoma, ~50% of the families carry inactive alleles of *p16$^{Ink4a/ME1/CDKN2A}$* while ~5% carry the CDK4 *R24C* mutation that disrupts the interaction of CDK4 with p16 *(123)*. As more data become available, it is becoming increasingly evident that the deregulation of the CDK4/cyclinD1/p16/pRb pathway is deregulated in most human tumors and the deregulation of this pathway is a common theme in tumor development.

This exquisite balance of these genes supports the idea that the pathway can be considered as a single mutagenic target.

Reduced Levels of p27 Protein in Human Tumors

The *p27^{Kip1}* gene is not mutated in human cancers although the gene itself is localized to the chromosome band 12p13, a locus known to be altered in leukemias and mesotheliomas. Further analysis of tumor samples did not reveal tumor-specific mutations in the coding region of the *p27^{kip1}* gene *(139,140)*. However, p27 protein levels appear to be reduced in human tumors. More significantly, this reduction of p27 protein levels strongly correlates with tumor progression and poor survival in patients with breast, colon, or gastric carcinomas *(141–144)*. In breast cancer samples, p27 consistently decreased with increasing tumor grade and is a strong predictor of reduced disease-free survival and appears to be an independent prognostic indicator *(142,145)*. The value of p27 as a prognostic marker is even higher when it is used in combination with cyclin E. Combinatorial analysis of p27 and cyclin E expression levels showed that patients with low cyclin E and high p27 levels have considerably longer survival rate than patients with high cyclin E and low p27^{Kip1} levels *(143)*. In colorectal and gastric carcinomas, low p27 levels correlate significantly with poor survival *(141,144)*. The subset of patients whose tumor lacked any detectable p27 exhibited a uniformly poor prognosis. In addition, in prostate adenocarcinomas, low p27 expression predicts poor disease-free survival and is an independent predictor of treatment failure after radical retropubic prostatectomy *(146,147)*. Similarly, in Barrett's-associated adenocarcinomas of the esophagus, the loss of p27 is associated with parameters of aggressive behavior such as higher histological grade, depth of invasion, presence of lymph node metastasis, and survival *(148)*.

In normal cells, p27 regulates the progression from G_1 into S-phase by binding to and inhibiting the activity of the CDK 2–cyclin E complex (Fig. 9). In p27-negative tumors, there is an increase in cyclin A- and cyclin E-associated kinase activity but no significant correlation between p27 expression levels and proliferative status *(141,142)*. These data may suggest an additional role for p27. For example, p27 has been shown to play a role in adhesion-dependent cell growth, and the loss of p27 may confer the ability to grow in an environment with altered ECM properties, thus facilitating metastasis *(149,150)*. p27^{Kip1} may also regulate the exit from the cell cycle and the initiation of cell differentiation. In this regard, it is noteworthy that in colon carcinomas the well or moderately differentiated carcinomas had high p27 levels while the poorly differentiated carcinomas had lower expression of p27 *(151)*. The various studies demonstrated no correlation between *p27^{Kip1}* mRNA and protein levels, suggesting that a posttranscriptional mechanism(s) is responsible for the reduction of p27 in tumor cells *(141,142,148,151)*. p27 protein levels are regulated by the ubiquitin-mediated degradation of p27 by the proteosome *(66)*. It has been suggested that the increased activity of a *p27^{Kip1}*-specific degradative pathway may be responsible for the reduction of p27 in tumor cells *(141)*.

Alterations in Other Cell-Cycle Regulators

There have been reports of *cyclin E* overexpression in high proportion of breast cancers, but the *cyclin E* gene itself is amplified in a small number of cases *(90,152–154)*. Together with p27, cyclin E overexpression has prognostic value for the outcome of the disease. Although historically very important, there is only one example of a human liver carcinoma in which the *cyclin A* gene was overexpressed as a result of hepatitis B virus (HBV) integration *(155,156)*. However, it is important to point out that both cyclin E- and cyclin A-associated kinase activity may become deregulated as the direct consequence of increased p27 degradation in human tumors.

Another mechanism that may lead to deregulated cyclin D-, cyclin E-, and cyclin A-associated kinase activity is the overexpression of the putative activating phosphatases CDC25A and CDC25B. It has been observed that CDC25B mRNA is overexpressed in 32% of human breast cancers and its overexpression was most frequent in high histological grade cancers with poor prognosis although the prognostic value of these findings is currently unclear *(48,157,158)*.

Inhibitors of Cyclin-Dependent Kinases as Therapeutic Agents

One of the reasons that the cell cycle is such a compelling drug discovery target is that it represents one of the most downstream signals that must be deranged before cell-cycle disruption. The central role of the p16/CDK4/cyclin D/pRb pathway supports this hypothesis (Fig. 4). Many different technologies have been used as potential therapeutic options. Reports exist of gene therapy, protein therapy, antisense, and small molecule approaches to correct cell cycle alterations. This section is not a comprehensive review of the known inhibitors; rather it is designed to give some indication of the types of approaches and current status of inhibitor development. Because this area of research is relatively new, most data are in preclinical stages. No compound specifically designed to inhibit the cell cycle has yet been through the clinic.

Small-Molecule Approaches

As outlined previously, CDKs play a central role in the initiation and orchestration of cell-cycle events. There are several examples where alterations in these key CDKs lead to tumor development. Specifically, up-regulation of the CDKs has been linked to transformation. Considerable effort has been devoted, therefore, to developing inhibitors of these CDKs. The CDKs require that several biochemical steps must be coordinated and occur in a linear sequence for these enzymes to function correctly. Each of these steps represents, in theory, a viable drug discovery target *(159)*. Despite the wide range of possibilities, the vast majority of the effort has been devoted to finding inhibitors of the catalytic activity of the CDK enzymes. This focus on the catalytic activity is driven by the recent success the pharmaceutical industry has enjoyed in finding specific inhibitors of various kinase enzymes. Parke–Davis (PD 153035, Fig. 10) have reported on an epidermal growth factor receptor (EGFR) antagonist that has 5pM activity with apparent exquisite selectivity *(160)*. These inhibitors of kinase catalytic activity tend, in the main, to be ATP-competitive inhibitors.

ATP-competitive inhibitors pose two problems, both of which are related to specificity. The first relates to "chemical specificity." Because there are a very large number

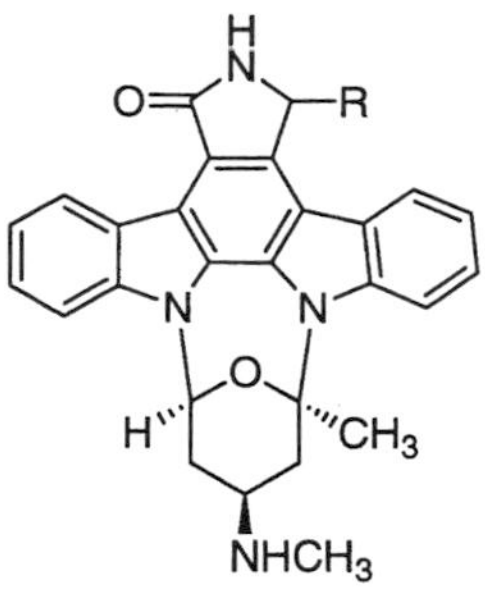

R = H Staurosporine
R = OH UCN-01

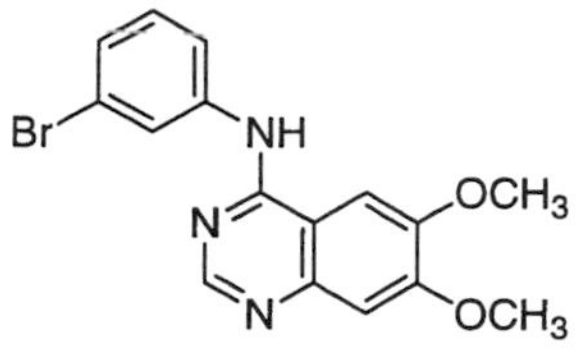

PD 153035

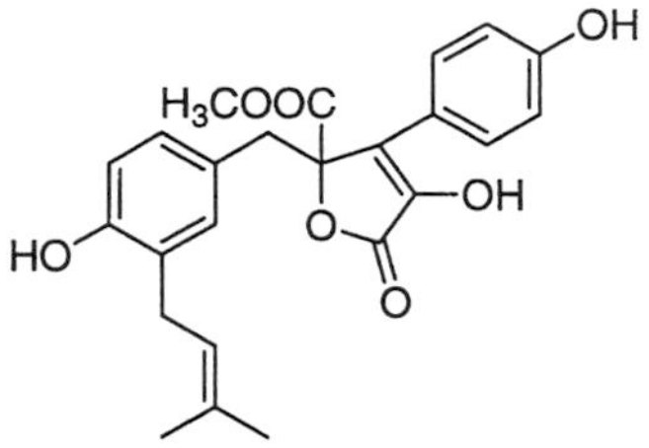

Butryolactone

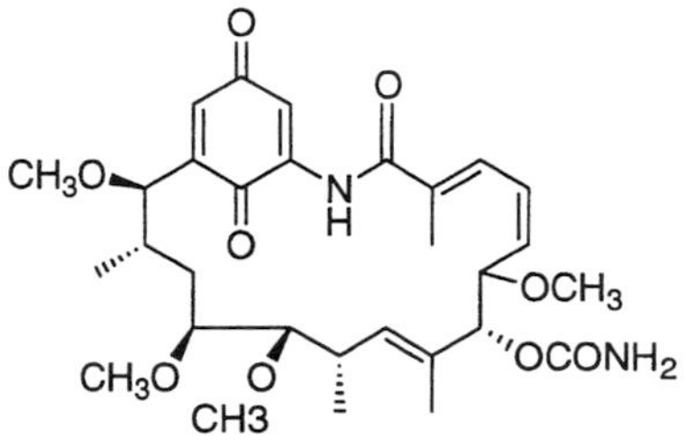

Herbamycin

Fig. 10. Kinase inhibitors identified from screening.

of kinases present in a cell, research groups screen against representatives of different kinase families. Because these assays are not comprehensive this makes it very difficult to know whether the cellular effect or phenotype observed with a specific inhibitor is due to inhibition of the kinase of interest of some other totally unrelated kinase. An example of this relates to staurosporine and UCN-01; both are bis-indole compounds and have very closely related structures (Fig. 10). Both of these analogues are broad-spectrum kinase inhibitors and show cell-growth inhibitory effects. In addition, both alter the ratio of phosphorylated and unphosphorylated pRb, but this ratio is different for the two compounds. The cellular effects observed for these two compounds may be due to inhibition of other unrelated kinases and not inhibition of CDKs themselves or a combination of CDK inhibition along with inhibition of a second kinase *(161)*.

This lack of biological specificity can be very important, especially in tracking side effects of various compounds. Cellular markers that follow the mechanism of action of the specific kinases of interest do provide data that give some insight into the phenotype. The specific phosphorylation sites on the Rb protein modified by individual CDKs are known *(8)*. The CDK4/cyclin D enzyme is preferentially phosphorylates pRb on S-795, while CDK 2–cyclin E and A phosphorylates on S-821 *(8)*. The phosphorylation at these positions can be taken as a qualitative indication that some part of the biological effect is due to inhibition of CDKs. Given their role in driving cell-cycle progression, compounds that inhibit all CDKs would be expected to induce both G_1 and G_2 arrests.

General Classes of CDK Inhibitors

The potential inhibitors of CDKs can come from natural product screening, compound libraries, and combinatorial chemistry. Any kinase inhibitor from an unrelated kinase program can also be used as a starting point for a potential CDK inhibitor. Several classes of kinase inhibitors such as staurosporine, naphthalene sulfonamides, isoquinoline derivatives, and sphingosine have been reported *(162,163)*. A number of these have been tested against the CDKs and shown to be active *(164,165)*. In general, these compounds display broad specificity *(162,163)*. Figures 10 and 11 show some of the initial lead structures from various screening approaches that have been identified as CDK inhibitors.

The natural product butryolactone was discovered by screening against murine CDK 1–cyclin B and is an ATP-competitive inhibitor (Fig. 10) *(166–168)*. It shows some selectivity among the CDKs, being more potent against CDK1 and CDK2 and showing little effect against CDK4/cyclin D (Table 1). It was also shown to inhibit Rb phosphorylation in vitro and in vivo. Butryolactone shows activity in WI38 cells and causes a G_1–S arrest. The compound also inhibited histone–H1 phosphorylation and caused concomitant G_2–M arrest. This pattern of G_1–S and G_2–M arrest will be seen many times with inhibitors that are active against several of the different CDK enzymes. Herbamycin (Fig. 10) has been shown to decrease levels of CDK 6 but has no effect on the closely related CDK4 complex or CDK2 levels *(169)*. This is very unusual selectivity. Because the CDKs are so well regulated, this compound could well be involved in some pathway that controls CDK 6 levels without exerting a direct effect on CDK 6 itself.

By contrast, other well-known inhibitors of kinases such as staurosporine (Fig. 10) tend to inhibit all kinases equally well. For CDK selectivity this "pan-kinase" activity requires that the chemists design away off-target kinase activity while keeping the CDK activity. This can be achieved; the purine analogues isopentenyladenine and 6-dimethylaminopurine (6-DMAP) (Fig. 11) are nonselective kinase inhibitors; however, olomoucine and roscovitine, which are derived from these leads do offer selectivity (Table 2). These purines are discussed later in greater depth.

The final class of inhibitors covered are flavones. This class of compounds are known to inhibit receptor protein kinases *(162)*. In routine testing of compounds in the National Cancer Institute (NCI) panel of human tumor cell lines (leukemia, NSCLC, colon, renal, prostate, and breast cancer cell lines) *(170)*, L 86-8275 was shown to be active in cells (Fig. 12). When the mechanism of action of this flavone was examined, it transpired that this compound inhibited the CDKs *(171)*. L 86-8275 has been taken into development by Aventis and is currently in phase 2 clinical trials. Again, the flavones are discussed in greater depth later in the chapter.

Purines as CDK Inhibitors

Isopentenyladeneine and 6-DMAP are nonselective CDK inhibitors (Fig. 11). Examination of the structures of these two compounds clearly shows the relation to the structure of adenine. Several purine analogues including isopentenyladenine and 6-DMAP have been shown to be ATP-competitive kinase inhibitors *(172)*. Screening has led to the discovery of olomoucine as a selective CDK inhibitor (Table 2). Olomoucine is a selective inhibitor for CDK2 and CDK1 and shows little activity against CDK4

R1 = R2 = H   Olomoucine

R1 = C2H5 R2 = CH3
Roscovitine

R = NH-CH2-CH=C(CH3)2
Isopentenyladenine

R = N(CH3)2   6-DMAP

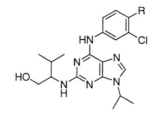

CVT 313

R = H   Purvalanol A
R = COOH Purvalanol B

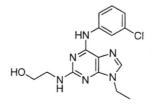

Roscovitine

Structure 1

Fig. 11. Purine CDK inhibitors.

or other protein kinases such as protein kinase A (PKA) and protein kinase C (PKC) (Table 2). An understanding of the reasons for this selectivity may allow the preparation of CDK-specific inhibitors. As described earlier, a number of the CDK and cyclin subunits have been crystallized individually or as complexes. Various groups have crystallized a number of the small molecular weight inhibitors in the active site of the CDK subunit. Among the bound complexes is one with olomoucine, isopentenyladenine, Flavopirdol, and purvalanol B in the active site of CDK2. It is important to note

Table 1
CDK Specificity of Known Kinase Inhibitors

Target	Staurosporine	UCN-01	Butyrolactone	Flavopiridol	Olomoucine	Roscovitine
CDK1	0.003–0.009	0.031	0.60	0.40	7	0.65
CDK2	0.007	0.030	1.5	0.40	7	0.70
CDK4	<10.0	0.032	>1000	0.40	>1000	>100
PKA	0.008	—	200	145	>2000	>1000
PKC	0.005	0.007	160	—	>1000	>100

Table 2
Purine CDK Inhibitors

Enzyme/Cpd	CVT-313	Purvalanol A	Purvalanol B	Roscovitine	Structure 1
CDK 2/E	0.5	35	9	0.70	—
CDK 1/B	4.2	4	6	0.25	0.08
CDK 4/D$_1$	215	850	>10,000	>100	—
PKA	1250	9000	3800	>1000	180
PKC	1250	>10,000	>100,000	>100	31.5
Mech'n	ATP	ATP	ATP	ATP	

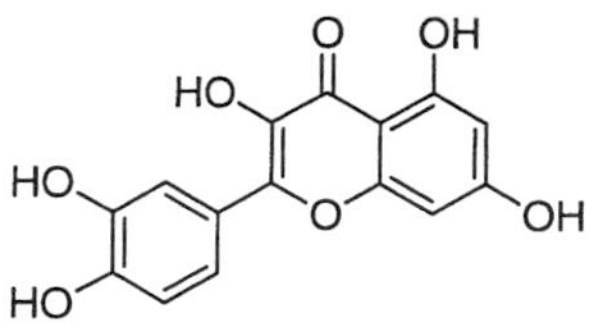

Quercitin

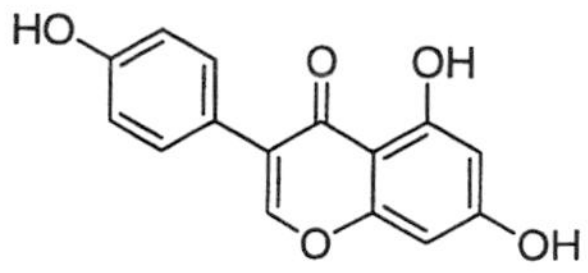

Genestein

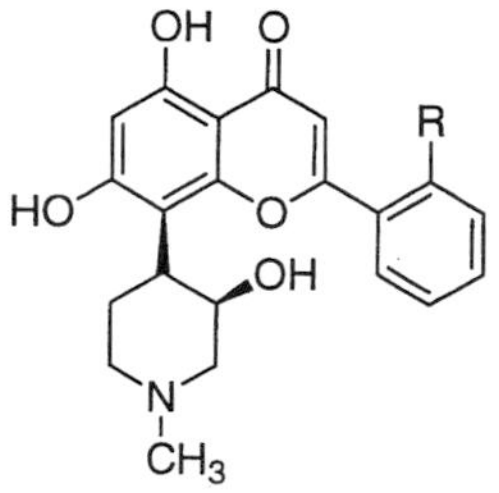

R = H   L 86-8275

R = Cl   L 86-8275 Flavopiridol

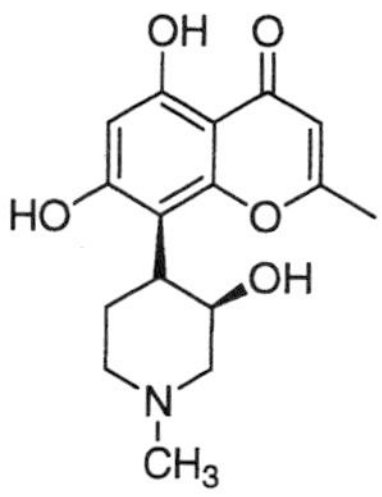

Rohitukine

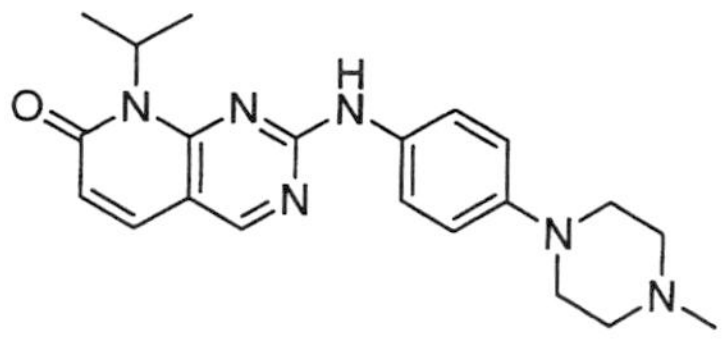

PD-172803

Fig. 12. Flavone CDK inhibitors.

that all the co-crystals, to date, have been with the monomeric (and thus inactive) CDK subunit.

Examination of the co-crystals of the CDK subunit with ATP, olomoucine, and isopentenyladenine offers insights into the observed selectivity *(173)*. The three purine rings in these three different analogues bind in the same portion of the ATP-binding cleft, but their three orientations are very different. In ATP the N-6 amino group is pointed toward the deepest part of the ATP-binding pocket. The larger N-6 substituents in olomoucine and isopentenyladenine (Fig. 11) make it sterically impossible to sit in exactly the same manner as ATP. In these two analogues, the N-6 groups occupy the space occupied by the ATP ribose and phosphate groups. With isopentenyladenine, the bulky N-6-isopentenyl group takes the position of the ribose ring of ATP and with olomoucine this space is occupied by the N-2-hydroxyethyl group. The selectivity observed with olomoucine is explained by the position of the N-6 benzyl group. In olomoucine this group binds toward the outside of the ATP-binding pocket in a region not occupied in the ATP–CDK2 complex or the isopentenyladenine–CDK2 complex.

One of the advantages that these purine derivatives offer is their synthetic accessibility. There is a vast knowledge base of nucleic acid chemistry, and the purine scaffold is amenable to combinatorial chemistry approaches. The purine nucleus has three positions amenable to combinatorial chemistry approaches; all three positions have been studied in both combinatorial and traditional approaches *(174–179)* (Fig. 11). The structure–activity relationships from all these and related approaches suggest that the substituent on N-9 should be a small alkyl group; the substituent at the 6-position is optimal if it is an aryl, aralkyl, or substituted aryl. The C_2-position is best as a substituted ethanolamine group.

One of these combinatorial studies has led to the synthesis of purvalanol B, one of the more selective CDK2 antagonists to date (Fig. 11) *(180)*. This compound is very closely related to olomoucine and shows similar selectivity (Table 2). An X-ray structure of purvalanol B with CDK2 shows that the selectivity of this compound again arises from the unique interactions of the N-6-group substituent. CVT-313 also shows selectivity for CDK2 compared with other kinases as do roscovitine and structure 1 (Fig. 11; Table 2). The cellular effects of CVT-313 *(181)*, olomoucine *(182)*, and purvalanol A have also been examined. CVT-313 and olomoucine both show a G_1–S arrest at lower concentrations and both a G_1–S and G_2–M arrest at higher concentrations. No cell cycle arrest data are available for purvalanol A. In terms of cellular potency, CVT-313 shows an average IC_{50} (50% inhibitory concentration) for growth inhibition ranging from 1.5 to 2.0 µM in nine cell lines *(181)*. Purvalanol A and olomoucine have been tested against the NCI panel of human tumor cell lines (leukemia, NSCLC, colon, renal, prostate, and breast cancer cell lines) *(170)* and show an average IC_{50} of 2 µM and 60 µM, respectively. CVT-313 has also been tested in a rat carotid artery model of restenosis and results show that at 1.25 mg/kg for 15 min under pressure, the compound can reduce neointima formation by 80%.

Flavones as CDK Inhibitors

A natural product screen for antiinflammatory compounds at Hoechst in the 1980s led to the discovery of rohitukine (Fig. 12). Further testing of rohitukine and its analogues for inhibition of the EGFR and for cytotoxicity on selected tumor cell lines showed flavopiridol to be the derivative with the strongest inhibitory and cytotoxic activity in vitro (Fig. 13). Flavopiridol also exhibited in vivo growth inhibition of human tumors xenografted onto *nu/nu* mice *(183)*. The average potency of Flavopiridol in the NCI tumor cell-line panel was 66 nM *(171)*. These cell experiments showed that the effects of flavopiridol are far greater on tumor cell than normal bone marrow cells.

The antitumor activity of flavopiridol in vitro and in cells was much higher than would be predicted from its activity against known kinases. The cell-cycle effects of flavopiridol show that the compound can give both G_1 and G_2 arrest in asynchronous cells *(184)*. Testing against the individual kinases showed that inhibition of CDK1/ cyclin B can account for the G_2 arrest phenomena observed *(185)*. The progression

Peptide 1 : K A C R R L F G P V D S E Q L S R D C D

Peptide 2 : K R R Q T S M T D F Y H S K R R L I F S

Peptide 3 : K R R L I F S K

Peptide 4 :   A C R R L F G P V D S E

Peptide 5 : P V K R R L D L

Peptide 6 : D A A R E G F L D T L V V L H R A G A R

Peptide 7 :   F L D T L V V L H R

Fig. 13. Non-ATP-competitive peptide CDK inhibitors. Letters are symbols for amino acids.

through G_1–S phase is controlled by both CDK4 and CDK2. Flavopiridol inhibits both these enzymes (Table 3), and this can account for the observed G_1 arrest *(186)*. The structural activity relationships around Flavopiridol has been reported elsewhere *(171)*.

The X-ray structure of a Flavopiridol analogue L 86-8275 (Fig. 12) bound in CDK 2 has also been reported. As with the earlier analogues discussed, Flavopiridol occupies the ATP-binding pocket with the benzopyran ring occupying approximately the same space as the purine ring of ATP. This benzopyran ring is again rotated to accommodate the molecule. As earlier, the aromatic ring is pointed to an area of the ATP-binding pocket not normally used by ATP. The appended nitrogen containing the piperidine ring occupies the phosphate-binding region of the binding pocket *(187,188)*. Flavopiridol has also been tested in various preclinical and pharmacokinetic models. The dose limiting toxicities are shown in Table 3. It is entering phase 2 trials using a 72-h continuous-infusion dosing schedule at 50 mg/m^2/day. The dose-limiting toxicity that has been identified is secretory diarrhea that can be managed by administering Imodium® (loperamide HCl). A second phase 1 trial is planned, and synergy studies are reported to be underway (Senderowicz, personal communication; 189).

All the compounds mentioned have been CDK2-selective inhibitors. To date, very few CDK4-selective compounds have been disclosed. Parke–Davis have reported that PD-172803 is 10-fold selective for CDK4 (Fig. 12).

Non-ATP-Based Approaches

Finding compounds that inhibit the activity of the CDKs by a non-ATP-competitive mechanism have the advantage of obviating the chemical and biological specificity issues discussed earlier. Several different groups have examined proteins that interact with the CDKs to ascertain whether these interactions can be copied with small molecules.

A systematic study of the p21 protein was undertaken by several groups. These studies identified two separate domains responsible for binding to the CDK and the cyclin subunit. In studies using overlapping peptides spanning the whole of p21, two 20-amino-acids peptides (peptides 1 and 2; Fig. 13) were reported to bind and inhibit the catalytic activity of both CDK4/cyclin D and CDK2/cyclin A or E (Fig. 13) *(190)*.

Table 3
Subacute Toxicities of Flavopiridol

Species	Application	Dose schedule	Results		Conclusions
Rats (Fischer 344)[a] (10/sex/dose)	9 × iv (every 8 h for 72 h)	0.5;1;2 mg/kg/injection (1.5;3;6 mg/kg/d)	≥1.5 mg/kg/d ≥3.0 mg/kg/d	Soft or loose stools reversible atrophy of thymus splenic lymphoid follicle and bone marrow; decrease of RBC, Hb, leukocytes, platelets	Maximal tolerated dose: 1 mg/kg/injection (3 mg/kg/d– 18 mg/m²/d)
			≥6.0 mg/kg/d	Lethal (1/10)	
Rats (Fischer 344)[a] (5 male/dose)	9 × iv (every 8 h for 72 h)	2;4;6;10 mg/kg/injection (6;12;18;30 mg/kg/d)	≥6.0 mg/kg/d	Soft or loose stools reversible atrophy of thymus, splenic lymphoid follicle and bone marrow; decrease of RBC, Hb, leukocytes, platelets	
			≥12.0 mg/kg/d	Lethal (5/5)	
Dogs (Beagle)[a] (2/sex/dose)	1 × 72 h continuous infusion	0.8;1.3 mg/kg/d	0.8 mg/kg/d 1.3 mg/kg/d	No sign of toxicity; increased soft stool; decrease in food consumption; increase in ck and ap; multifocal congestion of mucosal vasculature of the gut	Tolerated dose: 0.8 mg/kg/d (16 mg/m²/d)
Dogs (Beagle)[b] (1 male/dose)	72-h infusion	1.9;2.8 mg/kg/d	≥2.8 mg/kg/d	Lethal	Toxic dose low: 1.3 mg/kg/d (26 mg/m²/d)

[a]Ameson D et al. *Proc Am Assoc Cancer Res* 1995; 36: Abst 366
[b]Southern Research Institute (Birmingham AI) sponsored by the NCI-DTP.
iv = intravenous; RBC = red blood cells; Hb = hemoglobin

One of 20-mer was truncated to an 8-mer (peptide 3; Fig. 13) that still showed activity in the relevant assays. The same two interacting domains (peptides 3–5) were identified by a separate group using a different starting point *(69,191)*.

The similar approach has been described for p16 *(192,193)*. Again, a 20-amino-acid peptide (peptide 6; Figure 13) has been identified as being inhibitory to CDK4/cyclin D. Note from Fig. 13 that this peptide spans the 84–103 stretch of p16. An independent analysis also identified this region as necessary for p16 function. An alanine scan was conducted and a truncated peptide of 10 amino acids (peptide 7; Fig. 13) shown to be active against CDK4/cyclin D. The peptides from p16 do not contain the cyclin-binding motif identified in all the other approaches.

In an interesting proof of principle series of experiments the 16-amino-acid sequence from *Antennapedia* responsible for the internalization across the membrane (called Penetrin) was linked to peptides 2, 3, 6, and 7 *(190,192,193)*. The internalization sequence should enable these peptides to cross the cell membrane and exert a cellular effect that can be observed. The chimeric peptide produced from peptides 2 (M92A) and 3 with Penetrin was tested on HaCaT cells. In both cases G_1 arrest and a reduction in pRb levels occurred, suggesting that the cellular effect is by the expected mechanism. The chimera with peptide 2 is effective at 25 μ*M* while the peptide 3 chimera shows comparable effects at 50 μ*M*. The p16-derived chimeric peptides were tested in a similar manner. Peptide 6 (D92A mutation) linked to Penetrin showed good activity at 12 μ*M;* it efficiently blocks serum-deprived HaCaT cells from entering S-phase and gives near complete G_1 arrest. This effect lasts 36–48 h. This chimeric peptide was also tested in six different cell lines at 20 μ*M*. It again blocked S-phase entry in four of these cell lines.

Interestingly, this chimeric peptide had no effect on an pRb-negative cell line, suggesting that the phenotype being observed is mechanism related. Peptide 7 linked to Penetrin also blocks cell-cycle progression.

A yeast two-hybrid approach has been developed to identify random peptides, called aptamers, that are dominant inhibitors of protein function *(194)*. The aptamers are *Escherichia coli* thioredoxin molecules that display 20-amino-acid long random peptides in their active site loops. Aptamer libraries are used in the two-hybrid system to identify peptides that bind to a target protein. Aptamers that bind specifically to the target are tested for their ability to interfere with the function of the target protein. For example, aptamers have been identified that are capable of binding to CDK2 tightly (dissociation constant as low as 38 n*M*) and selectively (most of them bind to CDK2 only and not to other CDK family members). Several inhibit CDK2 activity in vitro. One of them (pep8) binds to CDK2 near its active site and selectively inhibits the phosphorylation of histone H1 (IC$_{50}$: 5 n*M*) but not pRb by CDK2/cyclin E. This distinct substrate specificity is not observed with natural inhibitors. The mode of inhibition is competitive, suggesting that pep8 interferes with the interaction of CDK2 with histone H1 but not pRb. Expression of pep8 in cells blocks the cell cycle at the G_1–S transition, possibly because pep8 interferes with the phosphorylation of substrates required to pass through G_1 *(195)*. These aptamers may help to dissect the functions of different CDK2 substrates and aid the development of highly specific, nonpeptidic inhibitors of CDK2.

Gene Therapy Applications

The natural CKIs are highly potent and specific inhibitors of CDKs. The overproduction of CKIs in both normal and tumor cells leads to cell-cycle arrest and inhibition of cell proliferation. These observations suggest a use for CKIs as cytostatic agents for the treatment of proliferative diseases. In this approach, the gene encoding a CKI protein is linked to a vector DNA that facilitates the uptake and high level expression of the transgene. The most popular vector system used for the delivery of CKIs is based on human adenoviruses (Ads). These replication deficient Ad vectors infect a variety of cell types both in vitro and in vivo and can program high levels of transgene expression for several weeks after infection.

Ad vectors that direct the expression of p16, p21, and p27 (Ad-p16, Ad-p21, and Ad-p27) have been constructed and tested both in tissue culture and animal models. As expected, the overexpression of CKIs inhibits CDK activity, G_1 arrest, and cell proliferation both in normal and tumor cells *(191,196,197)*. Ad–p16 inhibits only the proliferation of cells that express wild-type pRb (*Rb*⁺) while it has little or no effect on the proliferation of cells with mutant pRb (*Rb*⁻) *(198)*. Ad-p21 and Ad-p27 constructs inhibit both *Rb*⁺ and *Rb*⁻ cells equally well. In addition to their cytostatic effect, a varying degree of cytotoxicity is associated with Ad–CKI infections. It has been demonstrated that p27 overexpression in normal and cancer cells induces apoptosis *(199–201)*, although the apoptotic effect may be due to the collaboration of p27 and the *E4* gene product of the adenovirus vector (S. Patel and J. McArthur, *personal communication*).

Intratumoral injections of Ad–CKI vectors into tumor xenografts result in inhibition of tumor growth. However, in accordance with its cytotoxic effect, Ad–p27 injections into breast xenografts cause tumor regression *(202)*. The co-delivery of p16 and p53, but not p16 or p53 alone, into tumor cells reportedly induces apoptosis and tumor regression in xenografts *(203)*. These results suggest that optimal antitumor effect may be achieved only with Ad–CKIs in intratumoral injections when the cytostatic effect of the inhibitors is combined with cytotoxicity and apoptosis through the cooperation of the CKIs with another gene product(s), or possibly with chemotherapeutic agent(s). However, it is feasible to deliver the vector constructs directly to endothelial cells in the tumor vasculature resulting in inhibition of endothelial cell proliferation and migration, causing the inhibition of tumor-specific angiogenesis (Chapter 11 further discusses angiogenesis). In this scenario, the disruption of the tumor vasculature by Ad–CKI infection would lead to tumor cell apoptosis due to hypoxia, starvation, and increased concentration of toxic metabolites in the tumor.

Protein Therapy Applications

The inhibitory effects of CKIs depend on their relative abundance to their respective CDK/cyclin targets. The concentration of CKIs must exceed that of the target CDKs to inhibit their activity completely. As discussed earlier, this can be achieved in vivo by the ectopic overexpression of CKIs using gene therapy. Theoretically, the cellular concentration of CKIs can also be elevated by direct delivery of the inhibitor proteins. The inherent problem with this approach is that CKIs are intracellular proteins and exogenous CKIs are unable to cross the cell membrane and localize to the nucleus. Fortunately, a number of proteins have been described with the demonstrated ability to penetrate cell membranes and carry covalently linked cargo proteins inside the cell. These proteins include the products of two viral genes, the HIV-1 tat *(204)* and HSV-1 VP22 *(205)* proteins, as well as peptides derived from the *Drosophila melanogaster antennapedia (206)* and the human fibroblast growth factor (FGF) proteins *(207)*. These polypeptides can function as "delivery tags" facilitating the cellular uptake of cargo proteins from the extracellular space. To use these delivery tag-inhibitor fusions for the treatment of cancer and other proliferative diseases, the proteins must be delivered locally to the site of the diseased tissue in sustained-release formulations.

It has been demonstrated that Penetrin (a 16-amino-acid long peptide of *D. melanogaster antennapedia* protein) can mediate the delivery of p16- and p21-derived peptides into cells resulting in inhibition of cell proliferation, although at relatively high concentrations (IC_{50}: 10–50 mM) (*see above*). Different size peptides of the HIV-1 tat protein have been used to deliver p16 and p27 into normal and tumor cells. These experiments have identified two short peptides of tat (amino acids 48–60 and 47–58) that, when fused to p16 or p27, efficiently mediate their cellular uptake and nuclear localization. These exogenously added tat–p16 and tat–p27 proteins are potent inhibitors of cell proliferation. For example, the IC_{50} of the various tat–p27 fusion proteins is in the 0.8–5 mM range when added to human primary coronary artery smooth muscle cells (*208;* Lamphere L, Wick S, Gyuris J, *manuscript in preparation*).

Antisense Approaches

Because CDKs and cyclins are essential for cell proliferation they are popular targets for approaches using antisense oligonucleotides. Antisense oligonucleotides are short (15–25 nucleotides) nucleic acids segments that are complementary to the target mRNA. Inside the cell, antisense oligonucleotides hybridize to the complementary mRNA according to the Watson–Crick pairing rules. It is thought that this heteroduplex is degraded by RNase H leading to the inhibition of gene function *(209)*.

As expected, the ablation of CDK or cyclin functions inhibits the proliferation of all cell types (with the exception of cyclin D1 inhibition in *Rb⁻* cells). The inhibition of p27 with an antisense oligonucleotide in a three-dimensional culture of tumor cells sensitizes slowly proliferating tumors to chemotherapeutic agents and to radiation by increasing cell proliferation and reducing intercellular adhesion. This observation suggests that p27 antagonists potentially may be useful chemosensitizers in conjunction with traditional chemotherapeutic agents *(149)*.

The use of antisense oligonucleotides as therapies against disease-causing genes is a very attractive idea, as theoretically a 15-nucleotide oligonucleotides has the basepairing specificity to interact with only one target within the entire human genome. Unfortunately, a number of issues hinder the development of antisense-based therapies including the nonspecific and non-antisense mechanism of action, intracellular stability, the affinity to the target sequence, cell permeation, and delivery of the oligonucleotides. Significant advances must be made in these areas before this approach lives up to its potential.

Conclusion

CDKs play a fundamental role in the regulation of normal cell-cycle progression by controlling critical transition points. They are also integral parts of checkpoint control mechanisms that to ensure proper segregation of the genetic information with high fidelity. Deregulation of the CDKs has been implicated in cellular transformation and in the development of many different tumor types. Understanding the enzymology and structural biology of the CDKs, as well as that of their regulators, allows the exploitation of these important molecules as targets for drug discovery. Although this chapter has focussed on the discussion of the CDKs themselves, any one of the effectors are potential drug targets also. A number of the other regulatory targets (Chk-1, Plk, CDC25, etc.) are currently being investigated in several laboratories.

Already a large effort has been made in the identification of small molecular weight inhibitors for CDKs. A number of compounds are nearing clinical trials. As the case with efforts on other kinases, specificity of ATP-competitive agents remains an issue. Because there are so many regulators of the CDKs, in addition to the small-molecule approaches, different treatment modalities (gene therapy, protein therapy, etc.) remain viable and exciting possibilities.

Acknowledgment

We would like to thank Ms. Jill Fregoe for administrative support and patience and Dr. Xu Xu for help with the program used for the generation of the crystal structure pictures.

References

1. Hartwell LH, Culotti J, Reid B. Genetic control of the cell-division cycle in yeast. I. Detection of mutants. *Proc Natl Acad Sci USA.* 1970; 66:352–9.
2. Masui Y, Markert CL. Cytoplasmic control of nuclear behavior during meiotic maturation of frog oocytes. *J Exp Zool.* 1971; 177:129–45.
3. Pardee AB. G1 events and regulation of cell proliferation. *Science.* 1989; 246:603–8.
4. Morgan DO. Principles of CDK regulation. *Nature.* 1995; 374:131–5.
5. Hunter T, Pines J. Cyclins and cancer. II. Cyclin D and CDK inhibitors come of age. *Cell.* 1994; 79:573–82.
6. Marin O, Meggio F, Draetta G, Pinna LA. The consensus sequences for cdc2 kinase and for casein kinase-2 are mutually incompatible. A study with peptides derived from the β-subunit of casein kinase-w. *FEBS Lett.* 1992; 301:111–4.
7. Songyang Z, Blechner S, Hoagland N, Hoekstra MF, Piwnica-Worms H, Cantley LC. Use of an oriented peptide library to determine the optimal substrates of protein kinases. *Curr Biol.* 1994; 4:973–82.
8. Connell-Crowley L, Harper JW, Goodrich DW. Cyclin D1/Cdk4 regulates retinoblastoma protein-mediated cell cycle arrest by site-specific phosphorylation. *Mol Biol Cell.* 1997; 8:287–301.
9. Xiong Y, Zhang H, Beach D. Subunit rearrangement of the cyclin-dependent kinases is associated with cellular transformation. *Genes Dev.* 1993; 7:1572–83.
10. Tsai LH, Delalle I, Caviness VS Jr, Chae T, Harlow E. p35 is a neural-specific regulatory subunit of cyclin-dependent kinase 5. *Nature.* 1994; 371:419–23.
11. Jones KA. Taking a new TAK on tat transactivation. *Genes Dev.* 1997; 11:2593–9.
12. Lees EM, Harlow E. Sequences within the conserved cyclin box of human cyclin A are sufficient for binding to and activation of cdc2 kinase. *Mol Cell Biol.* 1993; 13:1194–201.
13. Jeffrey PD, Russo AA, Polyak K, et al. Mechanism of CDK activation revealed by the structure of a cyclinA-CDK2 complex. *Nature.* 1995; 376:313–20.
14. Sicinski P, Donaher JL, Parker SB, et al. Cyclin D1 provides a link between development and oncogenesis in the retina and breast. *Cell.* 1995; 82:621–30.
15. Matsushime H, Roussel MF, Ashmun RA, Sherr CJ. Colony-stimulating factor 1 regulates novel cyclins during the G1 phase of the cell cycle. *Cell.* 1991; 65:701–13.

16. Kato JY, Matsuoka M, Polyak K, Massague J, Sherr CJ. Cyclic AMP-induced G1 phase arrest mediated by an inhibitor (P27Kip1) of cyclin-dependent kinase 4 activation. *Cell.* 1994; 79:487–96.

17. Massague J, Polyak K. Mammalian antiproliferative signals and their targets. *Curr Opin Genet Dev.* 1995; 5:91–6.

18. Dulic V, Kaufmann WK, Wilson SJ, et al. p53-dependent inhibition of cyclin-dependent kinase activities in human fibroblasts during radiation-induced G1 arrest. *Cell.* 1994; 76:1013–23.

19. El-Deiry WS, Tokino T, Waldman T, et al. Topological control of p21WAF1/CIP1 expression in normal and neoplastic tissues. *Cancer Res.* 1995; 55:2910–9.

20. Rudner AD, Murray AW. The spindle assembly checkpoint. *Curr Opin Cell Biol.* 1996; 8:773–80.

21. O'Connor PM. In *Checkpoint Controls and Cancer* (Kastan MB, ed.), Imperial Cancer Research Fund, Cold Spring Harbor Press, Plainview, NY, 1997, pp. 151–182.

22. Jin DY, Spencer F, Jeang KT. Human T cell leukemia virus type 1 oncoprotein tax targets the human mitotic checkpoint protein MAD1. *Cell.* 1998; 93:81–91.

23. Draetta GF. Mammalian G-1 cyclins. *Curr Opin Cell Biol.* 1994; 6:842–6.

24. Terada Y, Tatsuka M, Jinno S, Okayama H. Requirement for tyrosine phosphorylation of Cdk4 in G1 arrest induced by ultraviolet irradiation. *Nature.* 1995; 376:358–62.

25. Ohtsubo M, Roberts JM. Cyclin-dependent regulation of G1 in mammalian fibroblasts. *Science.* 1993; 259:1908–12.

26. Lukas J, Herzinger T, Hansen K, et al. Cyclin E-induced S phase without activation of the pRb/E2F pathway. *Genes Dev.* 1997; 11:1479–92.

27. Alevizopoulos K, Vlach J, Hennecke S, Amati B. Cyclin E and c-Myc promote cell proliferation in the presence of p16INK4a and of hypophosphorylated retinoblastoma family proteins. *EMBO J.* 1997; 16:5322–33.

28. Papano M, Pepperkok R, Verde F, Ansorge W, Draetta GF. Cyclin A is required at two points in the human cell cycle. *EMBO J.* 1992; 11:961–71.

29. Dunphy WG, Brizuela L, Beach D, Newport J. The *Xenopus* cdc2 protein is a component of MPF, a cytoplasmic regulator of mitosis. *Cell.* 1988; 54:423–31.

30. Gautier J, Norbury C, Lohka M, Nurse P, Maller J. Purified maturation-promoting factor contains the product of a *Xenopus* homolog of the fission yeast cell cycle control gene *cdc2+. Cell.* 1988; 54:433–9.

31. Arion D, Meijer L, Brizuela L, Beach D. cdc2 is a component of the M phase-specific histone H1 kinase: evidence for identity with MPF. *Cell.* 1988; 55:371–8.

32. Rao PN, Johnson RT. Mammalian cell fusion: studies on the regulation of DNA synthesis and mitosis. *Nature.* 1970; 225:159–64.

33. Murray AW, Solomon MJ, Kirschner MW. The role of cyclin synthesis and degradation in the control of maturation promoting factor activity. *Nature.* 1989; 339:280–86.

34. Peters JM, King RW, Hoeoeg C, Kirschner MW. Identification of BIME as a subunit of the anaphase-promoting complex. *Science.* 1996; 274:1199–201.

35. Basi G, Draetta G. The cdk2 kinase: structure, activation, and its role at mitosis in vertebrate cells. In *Cell Cycle Control* (Hutchinson C and Glover DM, eds.), ILR Press, Oxford, UK, 1995, pp. 107–143.

36. De Bondt HL, Rosenblatt J, Jancarik J, Jones HD, Morgan DO, Kim SH. Crystal structure of cyclin-dependent kinase 2. *Nature.* 1993; 363:595–602.

37. Brotherton DH, Dhanaraj V, Wick S, et al. Crystal structure of the complex of the cyclin D-dependent kinase Cdk6 bound to the cell-cycle inhibitor p19INK4d. *Nature.* 1998; 395:244–50.

38. Russo AA, Tong L, Lee JO, Jeffrey PD, Pavletich NP. Structural basis for inhibition of the cyclin-dependent kinase Cdk6 by the tumour suppressor p16INK4a. *Nature*. 1998; 395:237–43.

39. Pines J. Cell cycle. Confirmation change. *Nature*. 1995; 376:294–5.

40. Russo AA, Jeffrey PD, Pavletich NP. Structural basis of cyclin-dependent kinase activation by phosphorylation. *Nat Struct Biol*. 1996; 3:696–700.

41. Fisher RP, Morgan DO. A novel cyclin association with MO15/CDK7 to form the CDK-activating kinase. *Cell*. 1994; 78:713–24.

42. Serizawa H, Maekelae TP, Conaway JW, Conaway RC, Weinberg RA, Young RA. Association of Cdk-activating kinase subunits with transcription factor TFIIH. *Nature*. 1995; 374:280–2.

43. Espinoza FH, Farrell A, Erdjument-Bromage H, Tempst P, Morgan DO. A cyclin-dependent kinase-activating kinase (CAK) in budding yeast unrelated to vertebrate CAK. *Science*. 1996; 273:1714–7.

44. Lew DJ, Kornbluth S. Regulatory roles of cyclin dependent kinase phosphorylation in cell cycle control. *Curr Opin Cell Biol*. 1996; 8:795–804.

45. Coleman TR, Dunphy WG. Cdc2 regulatory factors. *Curr Opin Cell Biol*. 1994; 6:877–82.

46. Mueller PR, Coleman TR, Kumagai A, Dunphy WG. Myt1: a membrane-associated inhibitory kinase that phosphorylates Cdc2 on both threonine-14 and tyrosine-15. *Science*. 1995; 270:86–90.

47. Parker LL, Piwnica-Worms H. Inactivation of the p34cdc2–cyclin B complex by the human WEE1 tyrosine kinase. *Science*. 1992; 257:1955–7.

48. Galaktionov K, Lee AK, Eckstein J, et al. CDC25 phosphatases as potential human oncogenes. *Science*. 1995; 269:1575–7.

49. Hoffmann I, Clarke PR, Marcote MJ, Karsenti E, Draetta GF. Phosphorylation and activation of human cdc25-C by cdc2–cyclin B and its involvement in the self-amplification of MPF at mitosis. *EMBO J*. 1993; 12:53–63.

50. Kumagai A, Dunphy WG. Regulation of the cdc25 protein during the cell cycle in *Xenopus* extracts. *Cell*. 1992; 70:139–51.

51. Kumagai A, Yakowec PS, Dunphy WG. 14–3–3 Proteins act as negative regulators of the mitotic inducer Cdc25 in *Xenopus* egg extracts. *Mol Biol Cell*. 1998; 9:345–54.

52. Lopez-Girona A, Furnari B, Mondesert O, Russel P. Nuclear localization of Cdc25 is regulated by DNA damage and a 14–3–3 protein. *Nature*. 1999; 397:172–5.

53. Matsuoka S, Huang M, Elledge SJ. Linkage of ATM to cell cycle regulation by the Chk2 protein kinase. *Science*. 1998; 282:1893–7.

54. Sanchez Y, Wong C, Thoma RS, et al. Conservation of the Chk1 checkpoint pathway in mammals: linkage of DNA damage of Cdk regulation through Cdc25. *Science*. 1997; 277:1497–501.

55. Peng CY, Graves PR, Ogg S, et al. C-TAK1 protein kinase phosphorylates human Cdc25C on serine 216 and promotes 14-3-3 protein binding. *Cell Growth Different*. 1998; 9:197–208.

56. Harper JW. In *Checkpoint Controls and Cancer*. (Kastan MB, ed.), ICRF, Cold Spring Harbor Press, Plainview, NY, 1997, pp. 91–107.

57. Serrano M, Hannon GJ, Beach D. A new regulatory motif in cell-cycle control causing specific inhibition of cyclin D/CDK4. *Nature*. 1993; 366:704–7.

58. Serrano M, Lin AW, McCurrach ME, Beach D, Lowe SW. Oncogenic *ras* provokes premature cell senescence associated with accumulation of p53 and p16INK4a. *Cell*. 1997; 88:593–602.

59. Hannon GJ, Beach D. p15INK4B is a potential effector of TGF-β-induced cell cycle arrest. *Nature.* 1994; 371:257–61.

60. Hirai H, Roussel MF, Kato JY, Ashmun RA, Sherr CJ. Novel INK4 proteins, p19 and p18, are specific inhibitors of the cyclin D-dependent kinases CDK4 and CDK6. *Mol Cell Biol.* 1995; 15:2672–81.

61. Kamijo T, Weber JD, Zambetti G, Zindy F, Roussel MF, Sherr CJ. Functional and physical interactions of the ARF tumor suppressor with p53 and Mdm2. *Proc Natl Acad Sci USA.* 1998; 95:8292–7.

62. Serrano M, Lee H, Chin L, Cordon-Cardo C, Beach D, DePinho RA. Role of the INK4a locus in tumor suppression and cell mortality. *Cell.* 1996; 85:27–37.

63. Kamijo T, Zindy F, Roussel MF, et al. Tumor suppression at the mouse INK4a locus mediated by the alternative reading frame product p19ARF. *Cell.* 1997; 91:649–59.

64. Halevy O, Novitch BG, Spicer DB, et al. Correlation of terminal cell cycle arrest of skeletal muscle with induction of p21 by MyoD. *Science.* 1995; 267:1018–21.

65. Polyak K, Kato J, Solomon C, et al. p27Kip1, a cyclin-Cdk inhibitor, links transforming growth factor-β and contact inhibition to cell cycle arrest. *Genes Dev.* 1994; 8:9–22.

66. Pagano M, Tam SW, Theodoras AM, et al. Role of the ubiquitin-proteasome pathway in regulating abundance of the cyclin-dependent kinase inhibitor p27. *Science.* 1995; 269:682–5.

67. Vlach J, Hennecke S, Amati B. Phosphorylation-dependent degradation of the cyclin-dependent kinase inhibitor p27. *EMBO J.* 1997; 16:5334–44.

68. Russo AA, Jeffrey PD, Patten AK, Massague J, Pavletich NP. Crystal structure of the p27Kip1 cyclin-dependent-kinase inhibitor bound to the cyclin A–Cdk2 couples. *Nature.* 1996; 382:325–31.

69. Adams PD, Sellers WR, Sharma SK, Wu AD, Nalin CM, Kaelin WG. Identification of a cyclin–cdk2 recognition motif present in substrates and p21-like cyclin-dependent kinase inhibitors. *Mol Cell Biol.* 1996; 16:6623–33.

70. Chen J, Saha P, Kornbluth S, Dynlacht BD, Dutta A. Cyclin-binding motifs are essential for the function of p21CIP1. *Mol Cell Biol.* 1996; 16:4673–82.

71. Reynisdottir I, Massague J. The subcellular locations of p15(Ink4b) and p27(Kip1) coordinate their inhibitory interactions with cdk4 and cdk2. *Genes Dev.* 1997; 11:492–503.

72. Glotzer M, Murray AW, Kirschner MW. Cyclin is degraded by the ubiquitin pathway. *Nature.* 1991; 349:132–8.

73. Clurman BE, Sheaff RJ, Thress K, Groudine M, Roberts JM. Turnover of cyclin E by the ubiquitin-proteasome pathway is regulated by cdk2 binding and cyclin phosphorylation. *Genes Dev.* 1996; 10:1979–90.

74. Diehl JA, Zindy F, Sherr CJ. Inhibition of cyclin D1 phosphorylation on threonine-286 prevents its rapid degradation via the ubiquitin–proteasome pathway. *Genes Dev.* 1997; 11:957–72.

75. Pines J, Hunter T. The differential localization of human cyclins A and B is due to a cytoplasmic retention signal in cyclin B. *EMBO J.* 1994; 13:3772–81.

76. Cheng M, Sexl V, Sherr CJ, Roussel MF. Assembly of cyclin D-dependent kinase and titration of p27Kip1 regulated by mitogen-activated protein kinase kinase (MEK1). *Proc Natl Acad Sci USA.* 1998; 95:1091–6.

77. Lamphere L, Fiore F, Xu X, et al. Interaction between Cdc37 and Cdk4 in human cells. *Oncogene.* 1997; 14:1999–2004.

78. Gyuris J, Golemis E, Chertkov H, Brent R. Cdi1, a human G1 and S phase protein phosphatase that associates with Cdk2. *Cell.* 1993; 75:791–803.

79. Hartwell LH, Kastan MB. Cell cycle control and cancer. *Science.* 1994; 266:1821–8.

80. Lammie GA, Peters G. Chromosome 11q13 abnormalities in human cancer. *Cancer Cells.* 1991; 3:413–20.

81. Rabbitts TH. Chromosomal translocations in human cancer. *Nature.* 1994; 372:143–9.

82. Shivdasani RA, Hess JL, Skarin AT, Pinkus GS. Intermediate lymphocytic lymphoma: clinical and pathologic features of a recently characterized subtype of non-Hodgkin's lymphoma. *J Clin Oncol.* 1993; 11:802–11.

83. Withers DA, Harvey RC, Faust JB, Melnyk O, Carey K, Meeker TC. Characterization of a candidate *bcl-1* gene. *Mol Cell Biol.* 1991; 11:4846–53.

84. Rosenberg CL, Wong E, Petty EM, et al. *PRAD1,* a candidate *BCL1* oncogene: mapping and expression in centrocytic lymphoma. *Proc Natl Acad Sci USA.* 1991; 88: 9638–42.

85. Bosch F, Jares P, Campo E, et al. *PRAD-1/cyclin D1* gene overexpression in chronic lymphoproliferative disorder: a highly specific marker of mantle cell lymphoma. *Blood.* 1994; 84:2726–32.

86. de Boer CJ, van Krieken JH, Kluin-Nelemans HC, Kluin PM, Schuuring E. Cyclin D1 messenger RNA overexpression as a marker for mantle cell lymphoma. *Oncogene.* 1995; 10:1833–40.

87. Arnold A, Kim HG, Gaz RD, et al. Molecular cloning and chromosomal mapping of DNA rearranged with the parathyroid hormone gene in a parathyroid adenoma. *J Clin Invest.* 1989; 83:2034–40.

88. Motokura T, Bloom T, Kim HG, et al. A novel cyclin encoded by a *bcl1*-linked candidate oncogene. *Nature.* 1991; 350:512–5.

89. Lammie GA, Fantl V, Smith R, et al. *D11S287,* a putative oncogene on chromosome 11q13, is amplified and expressed in squamous cell and mammary carcinomas and linked to *BCL-1. Oncogene.* 1991; 6:439–44.

90. Buckley MF, Sweeney KJ, Hamilton JA, et al. Expression and amplification of cyclin genes in human breast cancer. *Oncogene.* 1993; 8:2127–33.

91. Fantl V, Smith R, Brookes S, Dickson C, Peters G. Chromosomes 11q13 abnormalities in human breast cancer. *Cancer Surveys.* 1993; 18:77–94.

92. Gaffey MJ, Frierson HF Jr, Williams ME. Chromosome 11q13, c-*erB-2,* and c-*myc* amplification in invasive breast carcinoma: clinicopathologic correlations. *Mod Pathol.* 1993; 6:654–9.

93. Parise O Jr, Janot F, Guerry R, et al. Chromosome 11q13 gene amplifications in head and neck squamous cell carcinomas: relation with lymph node invasion. *Int J Oncol.* 1994; 5:309–13.

94. Pacilio C, Germano D, Addeo R, et al. Constitutive overexpression of *cyclin D1* does not prevent inhibition of hormone-responsive human breast cancer cell growth by antiestrogens. *Cancer Res.* 1998; 58:871–6.

95. Barbareschi M, Pelosio P, Caffo O, et al. *Cyclin-D1*-gene amplification and expression in breast carcinoma: relation with clinicopathologic characteristics and with retinoblastoma gene product, p53 and p21WAF1 immunohistochemical expression. *Int J Cancer.* 1997; 74:171–4.

96. Frierson HF Jr, Gaffey MJ, Zukerberg LR, Arnold A, Williams ME. Immunohistochemical detection and gene amplification of *cyclin D1* in mammary infiltrating ductal carcinoma. *Mod Pathol.* 1996; 9:725–30.

97. Champerne MH, Bieche I, Lizard S, Lidereau R. 11q13 amplification in local recurrence of human primary breast cancer. *Genes Chromos Cancer.* 1995; 12:128–33.

98. Zhang SY, Caamano J, Cooper F, Guo X, Klein-Szanto AJ. Immunohistochemistry of cyclin D1 in human breast cancer. *Am J Clin Pathol.* 1994; 102:695–8.

99. Rubin JS, Qiu L, Etkind P. Amplification of the *Int-2* gene in head and neck squamous cell carcinoma. *J Laryngol Otol.* 1995; 109:72–6.

100. Xu L, Davidson BJ, Murty VV, et al. *TP53* gene mutations and *CCND1* gene amplification in head and neck squamous cell carcinoma cell line. *Int J Cancer.* 1994; 59:383–7.

101. Adelaide J, Monges G, Derderian C, Seitz JF, Birnbaum D. Oesophageal cancer and amplification of the human *cyclin D* gene *CCND1/PRAD1. Br J Cancer.* 1995; 71:64–8.

102. Yoshida K, Kawami H, Kuniyasu H, et al. Coamplification of *cyclin D, hst-1* and *int-2* genes is a good biological marker of high malignancy for human esophageal carcinomas. *Oncol Rep.* 1994; 1:493–6.

103. Marchetti A, Doglioni C, Barbareschi M, et al. *Cyclin D1* and retinoblastoma susceptibility gene alterations in non-small cell lung cancer. *Int J Cancer.* 1998; 75:187–92.

104. Gansauge S, Gansauge F, Ramadani M, et al. Overexpression of *cyclin D1* in human pancreatic carcinoma is associated with poor prognosis. *Cancer Res.* 1997; 57:1634–7.

105. Huang L, Lang D, Geradts J, et al. Molecular and immunochemical analyses of RB1 and cyclin D1 in human duct pancreatic carcinomas and cell lines. *Mol Carcinogen.* 1996; 15:85–95.

106. Demetrick DJ, Zhang H, Beach DH. Chromosomal mapping of human CDK2, CDK4, and CDK5 cell cycle kinase genes. *Cytogenet Cell Genet.* 1994; 66:72–4.

107. Mandahl N, Heim S, Johansson B, et al. Lipomas have characteristic structural chromosomal rearrangements of 12q13-q14. *Int J Cancer.* 1987; 39:685–8.

108. Turc-Carel C, Limon J, Dal Cin P, Rao U, Karakousis C, Sandberg AA. Cytogenetic studies of adipose tissue tumors. II. Recurrent reciprocal translocation t(12;16)(q13;p11) in myxoid liposarcomas. *Cancer Genet Cytogenet.* 1986; 23:291–9.

109. Fischer U, Meltzer P, Meese E. Twelve amplified and expressed genes localized in a single domain in glioma. *Hum Genet.* 1996; 98:625–8.

110. Berner JM, Forus A, Elkahloun A, Meltzer PS, Fodstad O, Myklebost O. Separate amplified regions encompassing CDK4 and MDM2 in human sarcomas. *Genes Chromos Cancer.* 1996; 17:254–9.

111. Ladanyi M, Lewis R, Jhanwar SC, Gerald W, Huvos AG, Healey JH. *MDM2* and *CDK4* gene amplification in Ewing's sarcoma. *J Pathol.* 1995; 175:211–7.

112. Reifenberger G, Reifenberger J, Ichimura K, Meltzer PS, Colllins VP. Amplification of multiple genes from chromosomal region 12q13-14 in human malignant gliomas: preliminary mapping of the amplicons shows preferential involvement of CDK4, SAS, and MDM2. *Cancer Res.* 1994; 54:4299–303.

113. Maelandsmo GM, Berner JM, Florenes VA, et al. Homozygous deletion frequency and expression levels of the *CDKN2* gene in human sarcomas—relationship to amplification and mRNA levels of CDK4 and CCND1. *Br J Cancer.* 1995; 72:393–8.

114. Kovar H, Jug G, Aryee DN, et al. Among genes involved in the RB dependent cell cycle regulatory cascade, the *p16* tumor suppressor gene is frequently lost in the Ewing family of tumors. *Oncogene.* 1997; 15:2225–32.

115. Sonoda Y, Yoshimoto T, Sekiya T. Homozygous deletion of the *MTS1/p16* and *MTS2/p15* genes and amplification of the *CDK4* gene in glioma. *Oncogene.* 1995; 11:2145–9.

116. He J, Olson JJ, James CD. Lack of p16INK4 or retinoblastoma protein (pRb), or amplification-associated overexpression of cdk4 is observed in distinct subsets of malignant glial tumors and cell lines. *Cancer Res.* 1995; 55:4833–6.

117. Petronio J, He J, Fults D, Pedone C, James CD, Allen JR. Common alternative gene alterations in adult malignant astrocytomas, but not in childhood primitive neuroectodermal tumors: *P16ink4* homozygous deletions and *CDK4* gene amplifications. *J Neurosurg.* 1996; 84:1020–3.

118. Schmidt EE, Ichimura K, Reifenberger G, Collins VP. *CDKN2 (p16/MTS1)* gene deletion or CDK4 amplification occurs in the majority of glioblastomas. *Cancer Res.* 1994; 54:6321–4.

119. Cordon-Cardo C, Latres E, Drobnjak M, et al. Molecular abnormalities of *mdm2* and *p53* genes in adult soft tissue sarcomas. *Cancer Res.* 1994; 54:794–9.

120. He J, Allen JR, Collins PV, et al. *CDK4* amplification is an alternative mechanism to *p16* gene homozygous deletion in glioma cell lines. *Cancer Res.* 1994; 54:5804–7.

121. Hussussian CJ, Struewing JP, Goldstein AM, et al. Germline *p16* mutations in familial melanoma. *Nat Genet.* 1994; 8:15–21.

122. Woelfel T, Hauer M, Schneider J, et al. A p16INK4a-insensitive *CDK4* mutant targeted by cytolytic T lymphocytes in a human melanoma. *Science.* 1995; 269:1281–4.

123. Zuo L, Weger J, Wang Q, et al. Germline mutations in the p16INK4a binding domain of CDK4 in familial melanoma. *Nat Genet.* 1996; 12:97–9.

124. Kamb A, Gruis NA, Weaver-Feldhaus J, et al. A cell cycle regulator potentially involved in genesis of many tumor types. *Science.* 1994; 264:436–40.

125. Nobori T, Miura K, Wu DJ, Lois A, Takabayashi K, Carson DA. Deletions of the cyclin-dependent kinase-4-inhibitor gene in multiple human cancers. *Nature.* 1994; 368:753–6.

126. Einhorn S, Heyman M. Chromosome 9 short arm deletions in malignant diseases. *Leuk Lymphoma.* 1993; 11:191–6.

127. Cannon-Albright LA, Goldgar DE, Meyer LJ, et al. Assignment of a locus for familial melanoma, MLM, to chromosome 9p13–p22. *Science.* 1992; 258:1148–52.

128. Quelle DE, Zindy F, Ashmun RA, Sherr CJ. Alternative reading frames of the INK4A tumor suppressor gene encode two unrelated proteins capable of inducing cell cycle arrest. *Cell.* 1995; 83:993–1000.

129. Pomerantz J, Schreiber-Agus N, Liegeois NJ, et al. The *Ink4a* tumor suppressor gene product, p19Arf, interacts with MDM2 and neutralizes MDM2's inhibition of p53. *Cell.* 1998; 92:713–23.

130. Zhang Y, Xiong Y, Yarbrough WG. ARF promotes MDM2 degradation and stabilizes p53: ARF-INK4a locus deletion impairs both the Rb and p53 tumor suppression pathways. *Cell.* 1998; 92:725–34.

131. Hirama T, Koeffler HP. Role of the cyclin-dependent kinase inhibitors in the development of cancer. *Blood.* 1995; 86:841–54.

132. Palmero I, Peters G. Perturbation of cell cycle regulators in human cancer. *Cancer Surv.* 1996; 27:351–67.

133. Foulkes WD, Flanders TY, Pollock PM, Hayward NK. The *CDKN2A (p16)* gene and human cancer. *Mol Med.* 1997; 3:5–20.

134. Merlo A, Herman JG, Mao L, et al. 5′ CpG island methylation is associated with transcriptional silencing of the tumour suppressor *p16/CDKN2/MTS1* in human cancers. *Nat Med.* 1995; 1:686–92.

135. Herman JG, Merlo A, Mao L, et al. Inactivation of the *CDKN2/p16/MTS1* gene is frequently associated with aberrant DNA methylation in all common human cancers. *Cancer Res.* 1995; 55:4525–30.

136. Quelle DE, Cheng M, Ashmun RA, Sherr CJ. Cancer-associated mutations at the *INK4a* locus cancel cell cycle arrest by p16INK4a but not by the alternative reading frame protein p19ARF. *Proc Natl Acad Sci USA.* 1997; 94:669–73.

137. Hall M, Peters G. Genetic alterations of cyclins, cyclin-dependent kinases, and Cdk inhibitors in human cancer. *Adv Cancer Res.* 1996; 68:67–108.

138. Shapiro GI, Edwards CD, Kobzik L, et al. Reciprocal Rb inactivation and p16INK4 expression in primary lung cancers and cell lines. *Cancer Res.* 1995; 55:505–9.

139. Pietenpol JA, Bohlander SK, Sato Y, et al. Assignment of the human *p27Kip1* gene to 12p13 and its analysis in leukemias. *Cancer Res.* 1995; 55:1206–10.

140. Ponce-Castaneda MV, Lee MH, Latres E, et al. *p27Kip1*: chromosomal mapping to 12p12–12p13.1 and absence of mutations in human tumors. *Cancer Res.* 1995; 55:1211–14.

141. Loda M, Cukor B, Tam SW, et al. Increased proteasome-dependent degradation of the cyclin-dependent kinase inhibitor p27 in aggressive colorectal carcinomas. *Nat Med.* 1997; 3:231–4.

142. Catzavelos C, Bhattacharya N, Ung YC, et al. Decreased levels of the cell-cycle inhibitor p27Kip1 protein: prognostic implications in primary breast cancer. *Nat Med.* 1997; 3:227–31.

143. Porter PL, Malone KE, Heagerty PJ, et al. Expression of cell-cycle regulators p27Kip1 and cyclin E, alone and in combination, correlate with survival in young breast cancer patients. *Nat Med.* 1997; 3:222–5.

144. Mori M, Mimori K, Shiraishi T, et al. *p27* expression and gastric carcinoma (letter). *Nat Med.* 1997; 3:593.

145. Tan P, Cady B, Wanner M, et al. The cell cycle inhibitor *p27* is an independent prognostic marker in small (T1a,b) invasive breast carcinomas. *Cancer Res.* 1997; 57:1259–63.

146. Yang RM, Naitoh J, Murphy M, et al. Low *p27* expression predicts poor disease-free survival in patients with prostate cancer. *J Urol.* 1998; 159:941–5.

147. Tsihlias J, Kapusta LR, DeBoer G, et al. Loss of cyclin-dependent kinase inhibitor *p27Kip1* is a novel prognostic factor in localized human prostate adenocarcinoma. *Cancer Res.* 1998; 58:542–8.

148. Singh SP, Lipman J, Goldman H, et al. Loss or altered subcellular localization of *p27* in Barrett's associated adenocarcinoma. *Cancer Res.* 1998; 58:1730–5.

149. St. Croix B, Florenes VA, Rak JW, et al. Impact of the cyclin-dependent kinase inhibitor *p27Kip 1* on resistance of tumour cells to anticancer agents. *Nat Med.* 1996; 2:1204–10.

150. Zhu X, Ohtsubo M, Boehmer RM, Roberts JM, Assoian RK. Adhesion-dependent cell cycle progression linked to the expression of *cyclin D1,* activation of cyclin E-cdk2, and phosphorylation of the retinoblastoma protein. *J Cell Biol.* 1996; 133:391–403.

151. Ciaparrone M, Yamamoto H, Yao Y, et al. Localization and expression of p27KIP1 in multistage colorectal carcinogenesis. *Cancer Res.* 1998; 58:114–22.

152. Keyomarsi K, O'Leary N, Molnar G, Lees E, Fingert HJ, Pardee AB. Cyclin E, a potential prognostic marker for breast cancer. *Cancer Res.* 1994; 54:380–5.

153. Keyomarsi K, Pardee AB. Redundant cyclin overexpression and gene amplification in breast cancer cells. *Proc Natl Acad Sci USA.* 1993; 90:1112–6.

154. Leach FS, Elledge SJ, Sherr CJ, et al. Amplification of cyclin genes in colorectal carcinomas. *Cancer Res.* 1993; 53:1986–9.

155. Wang J, Chenivesse X, Henglein B, Brechot C. Hepatitis B virus integration in a *cyclin A* gene in a hepatocellular carcinoma. *Nature.* 1990; 343:555–7.

156. Wang J, Zindy F, Chenivesse X, Lamas E, Henglein B, Brechot C. Modification of *cyclin A* expression by hepatitis B virus DNA integration in a hepatocellular carcinoma. *Oncogene.* 1992; 7:1653–6.

157. Gasparotto D, Maestro R, Piccinin S, et al. Overexpression of *CDC25A* and *CDC25B* in head and neck cancers. *Cancer Res.* 1997; 57:2366–8.

158. Wu W, Fan YH, Kemp BL, Walsh G, Mao L. Overexpression of *cdc25A* and *cdc25B* is

frequent in primary non-small cell lung cancer but is not associated with overexpression of c-*myc*. *Cancer Res.* 1998; 58:4082–5.

159. Meijer L. Chemical inhibitors of cyclin-dependent kinases. *Trends Cell Biol.* 1996; 6:393–7.

160. Fry DW, Kraker AJ, McMichael A, et al. A specific inhibitor of the epidermal growth factor receptor tyrosine kinase. *Science.* 1994; 265:1093–5.

161. Shimizu E, Zhao MR, Nakanishi H, et al. Differing effects of staurosporine and UCN-01 on RB protein phosphorylation and expression of lung cancer cell lines. *Oncology.* 1996; 53:494–504.

162. Chang CJ, Gaehlen R. Protein-tyrosine kinase inhibition: mechanism-based discovery of antitumor agents. *J Nat Prod.* 1992; 55:1529–60.

163. Hidaka H, Kobayashi R. Pharmacology of protein kinase inhibitors. *Annu Rev Pharmacol Tociol.* 1992; 32:377–97.

164. Cui CB, Kakeya H, Osada H. Spirotryprostatin B, a novel mammalian cell cycle inhibitor produced by *Aspergillus fumigatus*. *J Antibiot (Tokyo).* 1996; 49:832–5.

165. Kleinberger-Doron N, Shelah N, Capone R, Gazit A, Levitzki A. Inhibition of Cdk2 activation by selected tyrophositins causes cell arrest at late G1 and S phase. *Exp Cell Res.* 1998; 241:340–51.

166. Kitagawa M, Okabe T, Ogino H, et al. Butyrolactone 1A selective inhibitor of CDK2 and CDC2 kinase. *Oncogene.* 1993; 8:2425–32.

167. Kitagawa M, Higahashi H, Takahashi IS, et al. A cyclin-dependent kinase inhibitor, butyrolactone I, inhibits phosphorylation of RB protein and cell cycle progression. *Oncogene.* 1994; 9:2549–57.

168. Someya A, Tanaka N, Okuyama A. Inhibition of cell cycle oscillation of DNA replication by a selective inhibitor of the cdc2 kinase family, butyrolactone I, in *Xenopus* egg extracts. *Biochem Biophys Res Commun.* 1994; 198:536–45.

169. Akagi T, Ono H, Shimotohno K. Tyrosine kinase inhibitor herbimycin A reduces the stability of cyclin-dependent kinase Cdk6 protein in T-cells. *Oncogene.* 1996; 13:399–405.

170. Paull K, Shoemaker RH, Hodes L, et al. Display and analysis of patterns of differential activity of drugs against human tumor cell lines: development of mean graph and COMPARE algorithm. *J Natl Cancer Inst.* 1989; 81:1088–92.

171. Sedlacek HH, Czech J, Naik R, et al. Flavopiridol (L86 8275; NSC 649890), a new kinase inhibitor for tumor therapy. *Int J Oncol.* 1996; 9:1143–68.

172. Rebhun LI, White D, Sander G, Ivy N. Cleavage inhibition in marine eggs by puromycin and 6-dimethylaminopurine. *Exp Cell Res.* 1973; 77:312–8.

173. Schulze-Gahmen U, Brandsen J, Jones HD, et al. Multiple modes of ligand recognition: crystal structures of cyclin-dependent protein kinase 2 in complex with ATP and two inhibitors, olomoucine and isopentenyladenine. *Proteins.* 1995; 22:378–91.

174. Norman TC, Gray NS, Koh JT, Schultz PG. A structure-based library approach to kinase inhibitors. *J Am Chem Soc.* 1996; 118:7430–1.

175. Gray NS, Kwon S, Schultz PG. Combinatorial synthesis of 2,9-substituted purines. *Tetrahedr Lett.* 1997; 38:1161–4.

176. Nugiel DA, Cornelius LAM, Corbett JW. Facile preparation of 2,6-disubstituted purines using solid-phase chemistry. *J Org Chem.* 1997; 62:201–3.

177. Imbach P, Capraro HG, Furet P, Mett H, Meyer T, Zimmermann J. 2,6,9-Trisubstituted purines: optimization towards highly potent and selective CDK1 inhibitors. *Bioorg Med Chem Lett.* 1999; 9:91–6.

178. Havlicek L, Hanus J, Vesely J, et al. Cytokinin-derived cyclin-dependent kinase inhibitors:

synthesis and cdc2 inhibitory activity of olomoucine and related compounds. *J Med Chem.* 1997; 40:408–11.

179. Schow SR, Mackman RL, Blum C, et al. Synthesis and activity of 2,6,9-trisubstituted purines. *Bioorg Med Chem Lett.* 1997; 7:2697–702.

180. Gray NS, Wodicka L, Thunnissen AM, et al. Exploiting chemical libraries, structure, and genomics in the search for kinase inhibitors. *Science.* 1998; 281:533–8.

181. Brooks EE, Gray NS, Joly A, et al. CVT-313, a specific and potent inhibitor of CDK2 that prevents neointimal proliferation. *J Biol Chem.* 1997; 272:29207–11.

182. Vesely J, Havlicek L, Strnad M, et al. Inhibition of cyclin-dependent kinases by purine analogues. *Eur J Biochem.* 1994; 224:771–86.

183. Sedlacek HH, Hoffmann D, Czech J, Kolar C, Seemann G, Gussow D, Bosslet K. *Chimia.* 1991; 45:311–6.

184. Kaur G, Stetler-Stevenson M, Sebers S, et al. Growth inhibition with reversible cell cycle arrest of carcinoma cells by flavone L86-8275. *J Natl Cancer Inst.* 1992; 84: 1736–40.

185. Losiewicz MD, Carlson BA, Kaur G, Sausville EA, Worland PJ. Potent inhibition of CDC2 kinase activity by the flavonoid L86-8275. *Biochem Biophys Res Commun.* 1994; 201:589–95.

186. Carlson BA, Dubay MM, Sausville EA, Brizuela L, Worland PJ. Flavopiridol induces G1 arrest with inhibition of cyclin-dependent kinase (CDK) 2 and CDK4 in human breast carcinoma cells. *Cancer Res.* 1996; 56:2973–8.

187. De Azevedo WF Jr, Mueller-Dieckmann HJ, Schulze-Gahmen U, Worland PJ, Sausville EA, Kim SH. Structural basis for specificity and potency of a flavonoid inhibitor of human CDK2, a cell cycle kinase. *Proc Natl Acad Sci USA,* 1996; 93:2735–40.

188. Kim SH, Schulze-Gahmen U, Brandsen J, de Azevedo WF Jr. Structural basis for chemical inhibition of CDK2. *Prog Cell Cycle Res.* 1996; 2:137–45.

189. Bible KC, Kaufmann SH. Cytotoxic synergy between flavopiridol (NSC 649890, L86-8275) and various antineoplastic agents: the importance of sequence of administration. *Cancer Res.* 1997; 57:3375–80.

190. Ball KL, Lain S, Fahraeus R, Smythe C, Lane DP. Cell-cycle arrest and inhibition of Cdk4 activity by small peptides based on the carboxy-terminal domain of p212WAF1. *Curr Biol.* 1997; 7:71–80.

191. Chen J, Willingham T, Shuford M, Nisen PD. Tumor suppression and inhibition of aneuploid cell accumulation in human brain tumor cells by ectopic overexpression of the cyclin-dependent kinase inhibitor p27-KIP1. *J Clin Invest.* 1996; 97:1983–8.

192. Fahraeus R, Paramio JM, Ball KL, Lain S, Lane DP. Inhibition of pRb phosphorylation and cell-cycle progression by a 20-residue peptide derived from p16CDKN2/INK4A. *Curr Biol.* 1996; 6:84–91.

193. Fahraeus R, Lain S, Ball KL, Lane DP. Characterization of the cyclin-dependent kinase inhibitory domain of the INK4 family as a model for a synthetic tumour suppressor molecule. *Oncogene.* 1998; 16:587–96.

194. Colas P, Cohen B, Jessen T, Grishina I, McCoy J, Brent R. Genetic selection of peptide aptamers that recognize and inhibit cyclin-dependent kinase 2. *Nature.* 1996; 380:548–50.

195. Cohen BA, Colas P, Brent R. An artificial cell-cycle inhibitor isolated from a combinatorial library. *Proc Natl Acad Sci USA.* 1998; 95:14272–7.

196. Jin X, Nguyen D, Zhang WW, Kyritsis AP, Roth JA. Cell cycle arrest and inhibition of tumor cell proliferation by the *p16INK4* gene mediated by an adenovirus vector. *Cancer Res.* 1995; 55:3250–3.

197. Yang ZY, Perkins ND, Ohno T, Nabel EG, Nabel GJ. The p21 cyclin-dependent kinase inhibitor suppresses tumorigenicity in vivo. *Nat Med.* 1995; 1:1052–6.

198. Craig C, Kim M, Ohri E, et al. Effects of adenovirus-mediated *p16INK4A* expression on cell cycle arrest are determined by endogenous *p16* and *Rb* status in human cancer cells. *Oncogene.* 1998; 16:265–72.

199. Gotoh A, Kao C, Ko SC, Hamada K, Liu TJ, Chung LW. Cytotoxic effects of recombinant adenovirus p53 and cell cycle regulator genes (*p21 WAF1/CIP1* and *p16CDKNH4*) in human prostate cancer. *J Urol.* 1997; 158:636–41.

200. Katayose Y, Kim M, Rakkar AN, Li Z, Cowan KH, Seth P. Promoting apoptosis: a novel activity associated with the cyclin-dependent kinase inhibitor p27. *Cancer Res.* 1997; 57:5441–5.

201. Wang X, Gorospe M, Huang Y, Holbrook NJ. *P27Kip1* overexpression causes apoptitic death of mammalian cells. *Oncogene.* 1997; 15:2991–7.

202. Rakkar ANS, Li ZW, Katayose Y, Kim M, Cowan KH, Seth P. Adenoviral expression of the cyclin-dependent kinase inhibitor *p27* (*Kip1*): a strategy for breast cancer gene therapy. *J Natl Cancer Inst.* 1998; 90:1836–8.

203. Sandig V, Brand K, Herwig S, Lukas J, Bartek J, Strauss M. Adenovirally transferred *p16-INK4/CDKN2* and *p53* genes cooperate to induce apoptotic tumour cell death. *Nat Med.* 1997; 3:313–9.

204. Frankel AD, Pabo CO. Cellular uptake of the tat protein from human immunodeficiency virus. *Cell.* 1988; 55:1189–94.

205. Elliott G, O'Hare P. Intercellular trafficking and protein delivery by a herpesvirus structural protein. *Cell.* 1997; 88:223–33.

206. Derossi D, Joliot AH, Chassaing G, Prochiantz A. The third helix of the *Antennapaedia* homeodomain translocates through biological membranes. *J Biol Chem.* 1994; 269: 10444–50.

207. Peters KG, Marie J, Wilson E, et al. Point mutation of an FGF receptor abolishes phosphatidylinositol turnover and Ca^{2+} flux but not mitogenesis. *Nature.* 1992; 358:678–81.

208. Nagahara H, Vocero-Akbani AM, Snyder EL, et al. Transduction of full-length TAT fusion proteins into mammalian cells: TAT-p27(Kip1) induces cell migration. *Nat Med.* 1998; 4:1449–52.

209. Wagner RW. Gene inhibition using antisense oligodeoxynucleotides. *Nature* 1994; 372: 333–5.

9

Apoptosis Pathways
Clinical Relevance

Caroline Archer, Peter Trott, and Mitchell Dowsett

Introduction

Apoptosis is a closely regulated, energy-dependent form of cell death. Apoptosis was noted by pathologists for many years, but >25 yr ago Kerr, Wyllie, and Currie derived the term "apoptosis" to describe the characteristic morphological features of a process separate from necrosis *(1)*. Apoptosis is Greek for "dropping off," and was used by Homer to refer to the falling of leaves from a tree in autumn, thus aptly describing the cellular loss.

Apoptotic cell death has been shown to be important in the steady-state kinetics of normal tissues *(2)* and accounts for the focal deletion of cells during normal embryonic development *(3)*. Apoptotic cell death has a potential pathogenic role in many conditions as well as cancer, such as acquired immunodeficiency syndrome (AIDS) *(4)* and neurodegenerative disorders *(5)*, and can be induced in cells by a wide variety of stimuli in vitro. Importantly for cancer medicine, apoptosis is seen after chemotherapy and ionizing radiation radiotherapy.

Histologically, the presence of mitoses has been important in the diagnosis of malignant conditions. For example, a high mitotic index can distinguish a benign uterine fibroid from a leiomyosarcoma. A high mitotic index in tumors may correlate with a poor outcome, important in the diagnosis and prognosis of cancer. In a study of 288 breast carcinomas, a high apoptotic index was correlated with high mitotic rate and high tumor grade *(6)*.

Thus, tumor growth is not just a problem of uncontrolled proliferation, but also of reduced apoptosis; the balance between apoptosis and proliferation is crucial in determining overall growth or regression. Therefore, knowledge of the biochemical and molecular events that control apoptosis and their regulation is essential in understanding tumor-growth dynamics and also to discover ways of manipulating and enhancing apoptosis to clinical advantage. Chapter 6 of this volume also discusses some basic principles of apoptosis in relation to growth-factor signaling.

From: *Principles of Molecular Oncology*
Edited by: M. H. Bronchud, M. A. Foote, W. P. Peters, and M. O. Robinson © Humana Press Inc., Totowa, NJ

Cell Morphology

The process of apoptosis involves a cell dying in the midst of surviving cells, in contrast to necrosis, which involves clusters of cells dying in an area associated with an inflammatory infiltrate. The morphological changes can be seen on light microscopy, and have been characterized further by electron microscopy.

The earliest morphological change is that of nuclear condensation, with the chromatin forming clumps that gather adjacent to the nuclear membrane. The cytoplasm condenses, causing contraction of the cell, loss of volume, and loss of adhesion to surrounding cells. In vitro, the cell surface has been shown to become irregular with numerous surface protrusions that eventually round up and break off as membrane-bound apoptotic bodies. These bodies usually contain condensed nuclear chromatin and, once released into the extracellular space, are rapidly ingested by phagocytic cells or neighboring cells *(7)*.

Condensation and fragmentation of nuclear chromatin occurs in the early stages of necrosis, but the chromatin is not packaged into specific membrane-bound fragments. Other morphological differences between the two processes are that the cytoplasm in necrosis swells rather than contracts as the cell bursts, spilling cytoplasmic contents that excite a neutrophil response and an inflammatory exudate. The entire cell becomes eosinophilic histologically with chromatin structures. The process of apoptosis is further distinguished from necrosis by being energy dependent.

Methods of Detection

Visualization of apoptosis by electron microscopy is the "gold standard" technique, but it is not applicable to the study of large numbers of cells and is not widely available. Light microscopy is useful but apoptotic cells and bodies can sometimes be difficult to recognize.

DNA fragmentation is a characteristic biochemical marker of apoptosis. Internucleosomal cleavage of DNA creates fragments that are multiples of 180–200 basepairs (bps), creating the classic "DNA ladder" on agarose gel electrophoresis *(8)*. However, these short lengths are not a universal feature and fragments of 50–300 bps in length have also been identified after induction of apoptosis *(9)*.

The knowledge of DNA fragmentation has enabled the development of histochemical techniques that incorporate biotinylated nucleotides onto the exposed ends of the DNA fragments. *In situ* end labeling (ISEL) uses DNA polymerase 1 which preferentially labels 3′-hydroxyl ends *(10)*, and terminal deoxynucleotidyltransferase-mediated bio-dUTP nick-end labeling (TUNEL) uses terminal transferase *(11)*. These techniques have allowed the study of apoptosis to be readily applied to formalin-fixed paraffin-embedded tissue, and have shown equivalent results on comparison in breast cancer sections *(12)*.

The breakup of DNA in necrosis means necrotic areas also stain positively, but these can generally be distinguished from apoptosis that occurs as a single cell death surrounded by healthy cells. It must be recognized that assessment of apoptosis by this method (and most others) provides only a "snapshot" of a very dynamic process. The number of apoptotic cells and bodies seen in a tissue sections depends on the rate of phagocytosis by surrounding cells. Histochemistry-based methods allow semiquantitation only; different studies report differing methods of quantitation. This difference needs to be taken into consideration when interpreting studies using an apoptotic index.

Similar end-labeling techniques are applicable to single-cell suspensions using flow cytometry *(13)*, and this has also been demonstrated using fine-needle aspirates from clinical specimens *(14)*. Cell membrane changes can be exploited using annexin V-fluorescein isothiocyanate conjugate (FITC), a calcium-dependent phospholipid-binding protein with high affinity for phosphatidylserine. Phosphatidylserine is exposed on the cell membrane in the early stages of the apoptotic process. On flow cytometry, the annexin V-stained cells appear as a sub-G_1 peak in the DNA histogram *(15)*. The presence of DNA laddering on agarose gel electrophoresis is often used to indicate apoptosis in in vitro systems.

Components of the Apoptotic Pathway

Over the years, many of the components of the apoptotic pathway have been characterized, revealing apoptosis to be a highly complex process. However, a pattern is emerging of a series of early events depending on the stimulus to the cell followed by a common pathway involving a series of cysteine proteases, the caspases. This common pathway ultimately results in DNA fragmentation and morphological changes associated with apoptosis. Mitochondria have emerged as having a central role in the process and its regulation, with the BCL-2 family of proteins playing a particularly important part.

It is thought that all mammalian cells have the capacity to undergo apoptosis, but much of our current understanding of the mechanism has been derived from studies on an invertebrate system, the nematode *Caenorhabditis elegans*. Three genes in *C. elegans* seem to be most important: *ced-3, ced-4,* and *ced-9. ced-3* and *ced-4* appear to be essential for apoptosis and *ced-9* appears to antagonize their action *(16)*. These genes have mammalian homologues: *ced-3*, a family of serine proteases named "caspases" *(17)*; *ced-9*, the *BCL-2* family *(18)*; and *ced-4*, the apoptotic protease-activating factor-1 (Apaf-1) *(19)*.

Caspases

The *ced-3* gene encodes a product similar to the mammalian enzyme interleukin (IL)-1β-converting enzyme, ICE *(20)*, artificial activation of which causes cell death in cultured mammalian cells *(21)*. ICE itself does not appear to be involved in apoptosis in mammalian tissues but a series of ICE-like proteases, at present numbering around 10, have been identified that feature strongly in the apoptotic pathway. These are termed caspases (cyteine-containing aspartate-specific proteases), so named as they all contain the amino acid cysteine in their active site and cleave their substrate after an aspartate residue. They exist as inactive cytosolic zymogens and are cleaved into one or more active subunits, which activate other caspases and themselves, resulting in a proteolytic cascade (reviewed in ref. *22*). The family of caspases has been subdivided into initiator caspases, which are activated in response to a cell death signal, and executioner caspases, which progress the signal activating the cascade that results in DNA fragmentation and cell death.

Cytochrome c

It has recently been found that the key step in activating executioner caspases in cytochrome *c*, a component of the mitochondria known to be involved the respiratory chain. Cytochrome c was found to be a necessary factor of a cell-free extract that could activate one of the central executioner caspases, caspase-3 (CPP32/apopain/Yama) and cause nuclear fragmentation in HeLa cells *(23)*. The treatment of HeLa cells with staurosporine, a potent proapoptotic agent, causes the release of cytochrome c from the mitochondria into the cytosol and this could be blocked by the antiapoptotic protein BCL-2 *(24)*. Others have shown that apoptosis can be induced in different cell types after the microinjection of cytochrome c compared with a control microinjection *(25)*.

Cytochrome c needs another cytosolic factor to initiate apoptosis; this factor was initially designated Apaf-1. This actually appears to be two factors; one a 130-kDa protein that has close sequence homology to *ced-4*, now itself termed Apaf-1, and a 35-kDa protein, termed Apaf-3 (Apaf-2 is synonymous with cytochrome c). Apaf-1 interacts with cytochrome c to cause caspase-3 activation in vitro *(19)* and Apaf-3 has now been identified in vitro systems as caspase-9 *(26)*.

The current model is then that cytochrome c is released from the mitochondria in response to various apoptotic signals, and interacts with Apaf-1 in conjunction with ATP to activate procaspase-9 to caspase-9, which then activates caspase-3, the key protease involved. The result of caspase activation is DNA fragmentation and degradation of components of the cytoskeleton, actins, and lamins (Fig. 1).

A caspase-activated deoxyribonuclease (CAD) was identified in mouse cells that appears to exist with an inhibitor, I-CAD (also termed DNA fragmentation factor, DFF). Caspase activation results in separation of the inhibitor from the active enzyme so the latter can pass into the nucleus and cause the internucleosomal DNA degradation seen in apoptotic cell death *(27,28)*.

Although it appears that release of cytochrome c initiates the caspase cascade and represents an irreversible step in the pathway to cell death, it may not be a universal requirement and may vary according to stimulus to the cell. Cytochrome c release can be seen in cells after staurosporine treatment, which induces apoptosis, but not with BMD188, another apoptosis inducer in the same cells *(29)*. One mechanism known to be able to induce apoptosis without cytochrome c release is that induced by FAS ligand activation of the FAS receptor.

FAS-Mediated Apoptosis

FAS receptor

FAS (also known as CD95 or Apo1) is a cell-surface receptor, part of the tumor necrosis factor (TNF) family. It mediates cell death after binding by its ligand, FasL. FasL is a cell-surface protein produced mainly by activated T cells, but both FAS and FasL can be expressed on a variety of cell types. The FAS/FasL system is involved in immune regulation, mainly in eliminating unwanted activated T cells *(30)*, thereby down-regulating immune reactions, and is one of the pathways of cytotoxic-mediated killing *(31)*.

FAS Signaling

Once activated, FAS binds an adaptor protein called FADD or Mort1 through a death domain (DD) positioned in the cytoplasmic portion of the receptor *(32)*. This binding produces a so-called death-inducing signaling complex (DISC) that then medi-

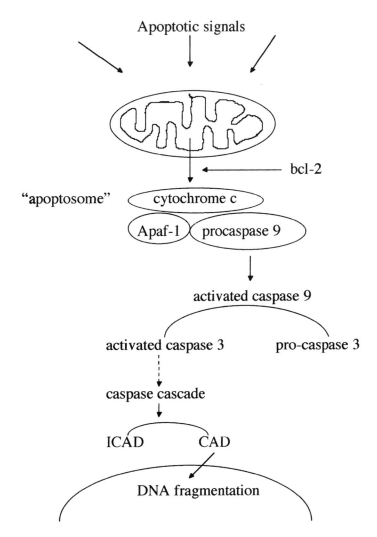

Fig. 1. Role of cytochrome *c*. Cytochrome *c* is released from mitochondria in response to various apoptotic signals. Cytochrome *c* interacts with Apaf-1 in conjunction with ATP to activate procaspase-9 to caspase-9. This, in turn, activates caspase-3. Caspase activation causes DNA fragmentation and degradation of the components of the cytoskeleton. ICAD, DNA fragmentation factor; CAD, caspase-activated deoxyribonuclease.

ates apoptosis by binding and directly activating caspase-8 (also termed FLICE, MACH, or Mch5), leading to further downstream caspase activation *(33,34)* (Fig. 2). Other receptors of the TNF family can also interact with FADD *(35,36)* and TNF itself has its own adapter protein, TRADD *(37)*.

Although direct activation of caspase-8, and consequent caspase-cascade activation, appears to allow signaling by FAS to bypass mitochondrial influence, the mitochondria may still have a part to play in FAS-mediated apoptosis. In some cells BCL-xl, an antiapoptotic member of the BCL-2 family, can inhibit FAS-mediated apoptosis *(38)*. BCL-xl, however, is localized to the outer mitochondrial membrane, endoplasmic

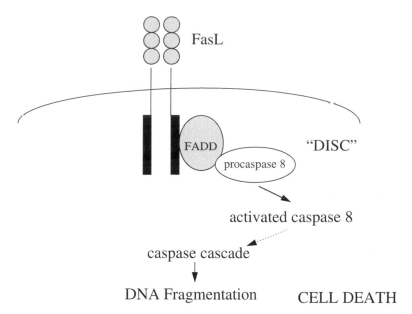

Fig. 2. Role of FAS signaling. FasL (FAS bound to its ligand) binds to an adapter protein, FADD, that mediates apoptosis through binding and activating caspase-8. Activated caspase-8 causes further caspase activation and finally apoptosis. DISC, death-inducing signaling complex.

reticulum (ER), and outer nuclear membrane *(39)* rather than the plasma membrane where caspase-8 is bound and activated. In FAS- or TNF-expressing MCF-7 cells, apoptosis triggered by respective ligand binding has been seen to be associated with a shift of cytochrome *c* from the mitochondria to the cytosol as measured by immunohistochemistry *(40)*. Cells expressing BCL-xl showed no cytochrome *c* changes and apoptosis was inhibited, although caspase-8 was apparently activated. This result suggests that BCL-xl can act downstream of caspase-8 to inhibit FAS-induced apoptosis. This inhibition is cell specific, indicating that as well as the recruitment of different apoptotic pathways depending on the stimulus, different pathways in different cell types may be activated after exposure to the same stimulus. It may be that in some cells cytochrome *c* release and caspase activation may be needed in addition to direct activation of caspase-8 to mediate apoptosis through FAS.

Clinical Role of FAS, Immune Regulation, and Cell Death

The study of hematopoietic tumors has revealed much of the role of the FAS- and TNF-receptor systems, but there are other tumors where the immune system is known to be important, such as melanoma, in which FAS could play a role. In solid tumors, the role of this pathway is less clear, although FAS does seem to be expressed on certain solid tumors, for example, lung carcinoma *(41)*. The presence of FAS could be a therapeutic target to encourage the cell to undergo apoptosis, but this may be an oversimplistic extrapolation. In vitro resistance to FAS-stimulated apoptosis is seen in cell lines despite cell-surface expression of FAS *(42)*. Up-regulation of FAS has been seen after chemotherapeutic agents in cell lines *(43)*. The FAS pathway therefore may be important in tumors as a mechanism for drug-induced apoptosis.

The role of the FAS pathway in immune regulation could also contribute to tumor death through cytotoxic T-cell killing, but tumor production of FasL may oppose any T-cell-mediated response by destroying circulating T cells. This phenomenon can be seen in melanoma cell lines which have been shown to express FasL. In vitro, these cells cause apoptosis of FAS-sensitive target cells. When injected into FAS-deficient mice, whose immune cells cannot be killed by FasL binding, the FAS-expressing melanoma cells cause greater tumor growth than in mice with immune cells vulnerable to FAS activation *(44)*. Cytotoxic T-cell killing of tumor cells occurs mainly through FAS activation, but there are other mechanisms that may be important *(45)*, and there exist resistance mechanisms. An inhibitor, FLIP (Flice-inhibitory protein, also called Casper, CASH, and MRIT), has been characterized that may interfere with FAS-mediated apoptosis. FLIP is seen in large amounts in melanoma cell lines and malignant melanoma tumors *(46)*.

Another slightly different role has been suggested for the FAS system: it may be involved in the development of cancer from premalignant states, malignant transformation in T-cell malignancies, and possibly chemoresistance *(47)*.

Clearly, there is more to learn. As our knowledge of immunotherapy and the apoptotic pathways and resistance mechanisms increase, these "death receptors" may be used to greater effect.

BCL-2 Family—Regulators of Apoptosis

Background

The mitochondria, as previously described, act in most situations as a focal point in the apoptotic pathway and provide a convenient position for regulatory molecules to intervene. The BCL-2 family of proteins appear to be involved here, acting to both enhance and oppose the apoptotic process. In cell-free systems, nuclear condensation and DNA fragmentation were found to be dependent on the presence of mitochondria and be inhibitable by BCL-2 *(48)*.

BCL-2 is an acronym for the B-cell lymphoma/leukemia-2 gene which was identified at the site of the t(14;18) chromosomal translocation, occurring in 85% of diffuse B-cell lymphomas *(49)*. The involvement of *BCL-2* in apoptosis was first seen indirectly when it was noted to prolong cell survival. Immature pre-B cells dependent on IL-3 for survival in culture were noted to persist despite IL-3 withdrawal when the cells were transfected with BCL-2, an effect that seemed to occur without cell proliferation *(50)*. This persistence was later formally shown to be due to the ability of BCL-2 to block apoptosis *(51)*.

Structure of the BCL-2 Family

The 24-kDa protein encoded by the *BCL-2* gene contains a stretch of hydrophobic amino acids required for insertion into membranes *(52)*. Immunolocalization has shown *BCL-2* to be present on the outer mitochondrial membrane, nuclear membrane, and the ER.

At present about 15 members of the *BCL-2* family of genes have been identified and there will probably be more. Some of the proteins are antiapoptotic, for example, BCL-2 and BCL-xl; and others proapoptotic, for example, bax *(53)*. BCL-x has two splice variants, BCL-xl and BCL-xs. The larger, BCL-xl, has very close sequence homology to BCL-2 and has been shown, like BCL-2, to prevent cell death in IL-3-dependent cells after growth factor withdrawal; BCL-xs appears to act in a proapoptotic manner *(54)*. All members possess at least one of four conserved motifs known as BCL-2 homology domains (BH1, BH2, BH3, and BH4). Most proapoptotic members have at least BH1 and BH2. Small proteins incorporating only the BH3 sequence, such as BAK, appear to be able to bind to antiapoptotic proteins, such as BCL-2, and suppress the antiapoptotic effect *(55)*. A similar small protein, bik, when overexpressed commits the cell to apoptosis by interacting with BCL-2, BCL-xl, and its smaller splice variant BCL-xs *(56)*. These small proteins may mediate their effects through interaction with BCL-2 only and thus act in a dominant negative manner.

Dimerization and Pore Formation

The ability of the family members to bind with each other seems to be an important part of their function. Bax, a proapoptotic protein, can form homodimers and heterodimers with BCL-2, and the ratio of BCL-2/bax within the cell could be a determinant of cell survival or death *(57)*. The BH domains that individual proteins have in common appear to be key in the ability of these proteins to bind with each other, as seen when mutations in either the BH1 or BH2 domains prevent BCL-2 from blocking apoptosis and binding bax *(58)*. What is not known is how dimer formation is regulated, but phosphorylation may be involved; BCL-2 is known to be inactivated by phosphorylation *(59)*.

Hypotheses on the mechanism of action of the BCL-2 family have been influenced by the observation that the three-dimensional structure of BCL-xl contained a region structurally similar to the pore-forming domains of bacterial toxins, such as diphtheria toxin *(60)*. These pore-forming domains can create ion channels in biological membranes; BCL-xl has been shown to display this ability. The channel formed by BCL-xl is pH sensitive and cation sensitive at physiological pH *(61)*. BCL-2 and bax have been shown to form ion channels when added to synthetic membranes *(62,63)*. As well as interacting with each other to form pores, the BCL-2 members also antagonize the process; BCL-2 can inhibit the pore-forming capacity of bax *(64)*. These channels may cause movement of ions sufficient to influence mitochondrial membrane potential, which is an early apoptotic event occurring before DNA fragmentation *(65)*. The mitochondrial membrane changes have, however, been principally attributed to the opening of a large conductance channel, known as the mitochondrial permeability transition (PT) pore (reviewed in ref. *66)*. This pore complex straddles the outer and inner mitochondrial membranes, containing several molecules and a voltage-dependent anion channel (VDAC). It is not clear whether this change in membrane potential may occur before the release of cytochrome *c*, or be a consequence of its release, but mitochondrial membrane changes occur early in apoptosis and PT pore function can be blocked by BCL-2 in vitro *(67)*.

Although the exact nature and function of these membrane changes is not entirely clear, it is possible that members of the BCL-2 family interact with each other on the mitochondrial membrane to influence the apoptotic process through the formation of different conduction channels.

Clinical Role of the BCL-2 Family

Inappropriate overexpression of *BCL-2* is implicated in oncogenesis, as seen in its role in B-cell follicular lymphoma *(68,69)*. The complete absence of *BCL-2* is compatible with normal animal development despite the importance of apoptosis in embryogenesis. *BCL-2* "knockout" mice develop normally through embryogenesis, although they display growth retardation and early postnatal mortality. Lymphocyte proliferation is initially normal, but later in life, massive lymphoid apoptosis occurs in the thymus and spleen. There are melanocyte, neuronal, and intestinal lesions, and the terminal event is renal failure from polycystic kidney disease *(70)*. *Bax*, on the other hand, being proapoptotic, might be expected to act as a tumor suppressor. It is seen to be mutated in human gastrointestinal cancers and leukemias *(71,72)*. Loss of bax has been seen to increase tumorigenicity in some systems *(73)*.

Investigating the role *BCL-2* in a clinical scenario is more difficult without clear understanding of its actions at a biological level. Protein expression can be detected by immunohistochemistry (IHC) strongly in lymphoid tissue and also in a wide variety of normal and malignant tissues. In lymphoma, as previously stated, the gene and its protein product are implicated in the development of the disease and appear to be a poor prognostic factor. In solid tumors, however, the expression of *BCL-2* often shows a relationship with good prognosis disease. In breast cancer, *BCL-2* is associated with other favorable factors, such as estrogen receptor (ER) expression *(74,75)*. The presence of *BCL-2* suggests good prognosis in non-small-cell lung cancer (NSCLC) *(76)*, but *BCL-2* has no prognostic value in colorectal cancer *(77,78)*. Favoring good prognosis might be contrary to what one might expect from a gene that inhibits apoptosis, thus potentially providing a survival advantage to tumor cells.

As an antiapoptotic gene, *BCL-2* could also be implicated in resistance to chemotherapy, as seen when overexpressed in acute leukemia *(79)*. However, studies in vivo in patients with breast and bowel cancer have not shown any predictive value for *BCL-2* in response or resistance to chemotherapy *(80,81)*. In the breast cancer study, the expression of *BCL-2* was correlated with a both a low apoptotic and proliferative score, suggesting its action is antiapoptotic. The presence of high *BCL-2* expression, as measured by immunohistochemistry, however, predicted for a *better* response to tamoxifen in ER+ metastatic breast cancer *(82)*. In breast cancer, there is clearly a link between *BCL-2* expression and ER; *BCL-2* acts differently in other tumors. *BCL-2* may interact with ER or there may be greater influence of other members of the BCL-2 family, such as bax. More studies are needed in tumors to ascertain the role and interactions of these proteins to gain clinical advantage. Important interactions of *BCL-2* include that with another important gene involved in cancer and apoptosis, *p53*.

p53-Mediated Apoptosis

p53 Protein and DNA Repair

Preserving genomic integrity by the repair or removal of damaged DNA is essential for cell survival. The persistence of genomic damage could potentially lead to neoplasia. There are many genes involved in damage recognition and DNA repair and the most studied of these is *p53*, the most frequently mutated gene seen in human cancer.

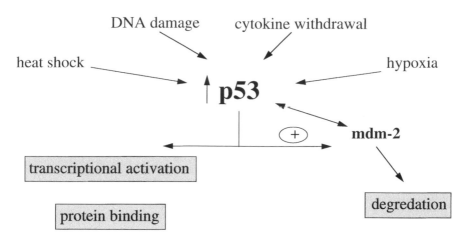

Fig. 3. Role of p53. p53 activation is triggered by a variety of stimuli. The link between stimuli and p53 may be mediated through kinases that phosphorylate latent p53 or may be mediated by interrupting the p53–mdm-2 interaction. This produces a negative feedback loop.

Mutation rates vary in different tumor types, occurring in 25–30% of breast carcinomas and up to 70% of poorly differentiated ovarian, colorectal, and head and neck tumors *(83)*. The gene is highly vulnerable to mutation; single base changes can produce a dysfunctional protein, and loss or disruption of a single allele can alter the phenotype despite a normal (wild-type) allele also being present.

The *p53* gene encodes a 393-amino-acid nuclear DNA-binding phosphoprotein. The protein acts mainly as a transcriptional regulator, but can also interact directly with cellular proteins. It is present in vivo in a biologically latent form. p53 activation is triggered by DNA damage, withdrawal of growth factors, hypoxia, and heat shock *(84)*. The link between the stimulus and p53 is possibly mediated through kinases that phosphorylate latent p53 *(85)* or perhaps by interruption of p53–mdm-2 interaction *(86)*. p53 is normally broken down rapidly by a ubiquitin-dependent proteosome pathway.This pathway is triggered by the binding of p53 to mdm-2, the production of which is stimulated by p53 itself, thus providing a negative feedback loop *(87)* (Fig. 3).

There are two outcomes of p53 activation: cell-cycle arrest and apoptosis. Cell-cycle arrest is at least partly mediated by the up-regulation of p21 (waf1–cip1), a cyclin-dependent kinase inhibitor (CKI) *(88)*. The mechanism by which p53 induces apoptosis is still unclear, but there have been several transcriptional targets of p53 identified that could provide the link to caspase activation.

One model of p53-mediated apoptosis has been proposed, after SAGE (sequential analysis of gene expression) analysis of more than 7000 transcripts induced after p53 activation in a human colorectal cell line. Fourteen transcripts including p21 were highly overexpressed, and others were named p53-induced genes (PIGs). Many of these were found to encode proteins involved in response to, or generation of, oxidative stress. It is known that after the transcriptional induction of redox-related genes, reactive oxygen species were formed that were seen to lead to oxidative damage to the mitochondria and triggering of the apoptotic cascade *(89)*.

p53 and bax

Another transcriptional target of p53 is bax, its expression being directly induced by binding of the p53 protein to sequences within its promoter region *(90)*. Induction of bax expression and down-regulation of BCL-2 have been seen in vitro after p53 activation leading to an altered BCL-2/bax ratio which may be important in encouraging apoptosis *(91)*. BCL-xl is capable of inhibiting p53-mediated apoptosis in certain breast carcinoma cell lines *(92)*. There is also evidence for transcriptional regulation of the "death receptor" group, FAS *(93)*, and DR5 *(94,95)*. Studies have shown that p53-induced apoptosis can occur in the absence of transcriptional activation *(96)*, indicating that p53 may act through direct binding to cellular proteins.

Cell Cycle Arrest or Apoptosis?

It is clear that the *p53*-dependent pathways leading to cell cycle arrest and apoptosis are distinct: the cell either undergoes cell cycle arrest *or* apoptosis after *p53* activation, rather than a period of cell-cycle arrest to allow for repair, which then can lead to apoptosis *(97)*. *p21*-deficient mice have impairment to cell-cycle arrest in response to DNA damage, but can undergo apoptosis *(98)*. The pathway after *p53* activation may be cell specific or it may be that each cell has the capacity to undergo cell-cycle arrest or apoptosis.

How and why a cell undergoes apoptosis rather than growth arrest in response to DNA damage is of great importance clinically. Most agents used in cancer treatment, such as irradiation and many chemotherapeutic agents, act by inducing DNA damage and have been shown to induce *p53*-mediated apoptosis *(99)*. The presence of *p53* mutations in many tumor types is associated with poor outcome, for example, in both node-negative *(100)* and node-positive breast cancer *(101)*. The poor outcome may be due to in part to chemoresistance. The ability to direct a cancer cell with wild-type *p53* down a pathway to apoptosis after a treatment could improve response rates and outcome, as could restoring wild-type activity. However, apoptosis occurs after treatments by *p53*-independent mechanisms that may also be defective. Thus, the route to apoptosis after treatment may be different depending on the treatment modality and tumor type being treated. The resistance mechanisms may therefore also vary. Inhibitors of *p53*-mediated apoptosis exist; BCL-2, for example can inhibit *p53*-mediated apoptosis but not *p53*-induced cell-cycle arrest *(102)*. The presence of *p53* mutations in cancer cells may not only impair the apoptotic response to treatment but also, through impairment of cell-cycle arrest, allow the cell to enter S phase with genomic damage.

Clinical Importance of p53

p53 Detection

Clinical studies examining the effect of *p53* in prognosis and outcome are numerous and at present use two methods to detect mutant *p53*: IHC, which is generally only sufficiently sensitive to detect stabilized dysfunctional protein, and DNA-based methods such as single-strand conformation polymorphism analysis (SSCP). Although there is generally a significant correlation between IHC- and DNA-based methods, there are some discrepancies, providing uncertainty in the interpretation of data *(103)*. Microarray technology is now available to test large numbers of samples for *p53* and other mutations, but at present is prohibitively expensive for routine use *(104)*. (Chapter 15 of this volume discusses the microarray technique.)

Clinical Outcome

Although the presence of mutated *p53* can lead to a poor outcome in patient cohorts, the individual prediction of response or identification of the phenotype of chemo- or radioresistant material may be more clinically useful. It is the tumor cells left after treatment that will have the potential to repopulate and ultimately cause death. If *p53* is important in apoptosis induced after DNA damaging agents, as it is believed to be, then treatment may lead to the selection of *p53*-mutated cells. In a study in patients with doxorubicin-treated locally advanced breast cancer, a significantly higher frequency of *p53* mutations were seen in those patients who progressed on treatment. These progressing patients had mutations affecting the same position on the *p53* gene, suggesting that different *p53* mutations may have different biological effects *(105)*.

There are some instances where the *presence* of wild-type *p53* could lead to a poor response to treatment. The presence of wild-type *p53* has been reported to decrease the cytotoxicity of paclitaxel, a tubulin-binding drug. This decrease could be attributed to a block in G_1 after treatment due to normal *p53* activation, thus preventing the cells from reaching G_2–M, where the tubulin binders act *(106)*. More recent work in ovarian and other tumor cell lines has shown very little difference in paclitaxel sensitivity between wild-type and mutant *p53* cells, although an increase in *p53* and downstream genes such as *bax* and *p21* were seen soon after paclitaxel treatment *(107)*. In a small clinical study, the presence of a *p53* mutation did not appear to alter the response to therapy *(108)*. In cell lines, there are clear differences in the response to different chemotherapeutic agents depending on the *p53* status *(109)*.

p53 Homologues

Further complications or potential explanations to the mechanisms of *p53*-induced apoptosis and its controls are emerging with the identification of *p53* homologues, *p73* and *ket (110)*. *p73* appears to have the ability to act like *p53* to induce growth inhibition and apoptosis *(111)*. More work is needed to evaluate the role of these homologues in vivo.

C-*myc*-Induced Apoptosis

C-myc Expression

C-*myc* is a proto-oncogene involved in normal cell growth. The protein product is expressed continually in cycling cells, increasing as the cell enters S phase, and expressed at very low levels in G_0 cells. However, its functions extend beyond cell proliferation and involve inhibition of terminal differentiation and apoptosis.

C-*myc* is inappropriately expressed in a wide range of human tumors. Deregulated c-*myc* is part of a multistep process of oncogenesis that involves mutations of other proto-oncogenes, such as *ras*. (For reviews of basic c-*myc* function, see refs. *112–114*). Several proteins are encoded for by the c-*myc* gene, two sometimes called c-myc1 and c-myc2. It has been suggested that differing forms may have slightly different functions *(115)*, which may explain the diverse actions this oncogene product has.

C-myc proteins have the ability to homodimerize or heterodimerize with other proteins. Most of the proteins involved share some sequence similarity but are coded for by separate genes. The main dimer for c-myc is a 160-amino-acid protein called Max. This protein appears to be relatively stable, in contrast to c-myc. Max/myc heterodimers are formed when both are present in preferences to myc homodimers, which are inactive. The binding of myc to max appears to be important for its physiological actions *(116)*.

It is unclear how *myc* induces apoptosis: in different situations overexpression and underexpression can lead to apoptosis *(117)*. In MCF-7 breast adenocarcinoma cells, treatment with doxorubicin caused a prolonged reduction in c-myc mRNA, paralleling DNA fragmentation and growth arrest, followed by loss of cells *(118)*. C-myc can cause apoptosis through various mechanisms so far discussed, for example, p53 *(119)* and FAS *(120)*, and can be inhibited by BCL-2 *(121)* (see review [*122*]). C-*myc* thus has wide-ranging actions, controlling cell proliferation as well as apoptosis and this might be manipulated to clinical advantage.

Conclusion

The field of apoptosis has expanded dramatically in recent years, as has the spectrum of human pathology in which it is involved. In cancer, loss of the normal relationship between apoptosis and proliferation may lead to the development of tumors and their growth. Induction of apoptosis is now thought to be the principal mechanism by which both radiotherapy and chemotherapeutic agents exert their actions. It is therefore fundamental to understand the apoptotic response to treatment and how differing expression of the regulatory molecules can influence that treatment response to enable us to maximize current treatments and find targets for new therapies.

References

1. Kerr JFR WA, Currie AR. Apoptosis: a basic biological phenomenon with wide ranging implications for tissue kinetics. *Br J Cancer.* 1972; 26:239–57.
2. Raff MC. Social controls on cell survival and cell death. *Nature.* 1992; 356:397–400.
3. Ellis RE, Yuan JY, Horvitz HR. Mechanisms and functions of cell death. *Annu Rev Cell Biol.* 1991; 7:663–98.
4. Ameisen JC, Estaquier J, Idziorek T, De Bels F. Programmed cell death and AIDS pathogenesis: significance and potential mechanisms. *Curr Top Microbial Immunol.* 1995; 200:195–211.
5. Dragunow M, MacGibbon GA, Lawlor P, et al. Apoptosis, neurotrophic factors and neurodegeneration. *Rev Neurosci.* 1997; 8:223–65.
6. Lipponen P, Aaltomaa S, Kosma VM, Syrjanen K. Apoptosis in breast cancer as related to histopathological characteristics and prognosis. *Eur J Cancer* 1994; 14:2068–73.
7. Wyllie AH KJ, Currie AR. Cell death: The significance of apoptosis. *Int Rev Cytol.* 1980; 68:251–304.
8. Wyllie AH. Glucocorticoid-induced thymocyte apoptosis is associated with endogenous endonuclease activation. *Nature* 1980; 284:555–6.
9. Oberhammer F, Wilson JW, Dive C, et al. Apoptotic death in epithelial cells: cleavage of DNA to 300 and/or 50 kb fragments prior to or in the absence of internucleosomal fragmentation. *EMBO J.* 1993; 12(9):3679–84.
10. Wijsman JH JR, Keijzer R, Van de Velde CJH, Cornelisse CJ, Vaj Dierendonck JH. A

new method to detect apoptosis in paraffin sections: in situ labelling of fragmented DNA. *J Histochem Cytochem.* 1993; 41:7–12.

11. Gavrieli Y SY, Ben-Sasson SA. Identification of programmed cell death in situ via specific labelling of nuclear DNA fragmentation. *J Cell Biol.* 1992; 119:493–501.

12. Mainwaring P, Ellis P, Detre S, Smith I, Dowsett M. Comparison of in situ methods to assess DNA cleavage in apoptotic cells in patients with breast cancer. *J Clin Pathol.* 1998; 51:34–37.

13. Gorcyzca W SY, Ben-Sasson SA. Identification of programmed cell death in situ via specific labelling of nuclear DNA fragmentation. *J Cell Biol.* 1992; 119:493–501.

14. Dowsett M, Detre S, Ormorod M, et al. Analysis and sorting of apoptotic cells from fine needle aspirates of human primary breast carcinomas. *Cytometry.* 1998; 32:291–300.

15. van Engeland M, Ramaekers FC, Schutte B, Reutelingsperger CP. A novel assay to measure loss of plasma membrane asymmetry during apoptosis of adherent cells in culture. *Cytometry.* 1996; 24:131–9.

16. Hengartner MO, Ellis RE, Horvitz HR. *Caenorhabditis elegans* gene *ced-9* protects cells from programmed cell death. *Nature* 1992; 356:494–9.

17. Alnemri ES, Livingston DJ, Nicolson DW, et al. Human ICE/CED-3 protease nomenclature. *Cell.* 1996; 87:171.

18. Hengartner MO, Horvitz HR. *C. elegans* cell survival gene *ced-9* encodes a functional homolog of the mammalian proto-oncogene *bcl-2. Cell.* 1994; 76:665–76.

19. Zou H, Henzel WJ, Liu X, Lutschg A, Wang X. Apaf-1, a human protein homologous to *C. elegans* CED-4, participates in cytochrome *c*-dependent activation of caspase-3. *Cell.* 1997; 90:405–13.

20. Yuan J, Shaham S, Ledoux S, Ellis HM, Horvitz HR. The *C. elegans* cell death gene *ced-3* encodes a protein similar to mammalian interleukin-1 β-converting enzyme. *Cell.* 1993; 75:641–52.

21. Miura M, Zhu H, Rotello R, Hartwieg EA, Yuan J. Induction of apoptosis in fibroblasts by IL-1 β-converting enzyme, a mammalian homology of the *C. elegans* cell death gene *ced-3. Cell.* 1993; 75:653–60.

22. Nicholson DW, Thornberry NA. Caspases: killer proteases. *Trends Biochem Sci.* 1997; 22:299–306.

23. Liu X, Kim CN, Yang J, Jemmerson R, Wang X. Induction of apoptotic program in cell-free extracts: requirement for dATP and cytochrome c. *Cell.* 1996; 86:147–57.

24. Yang J, Liu X, Bhalla K, et al. Prevention of apoptosis by Bcl-2: release of cytochrome *c* from mitochondria blocked. *Science.* 1997; 275:1129–32.

25. Zhivotovsky B, Orrenius S, Brustugun OT, Doskeland SO. Injected cytochrome *c* induces apoptosis. *Nature.* 1998; 391:449–50.

26. Li P, Nijhawan D, Budihardjo I, et al. Cytochrome *c* and dATP-dependent formation of Apaf-1/caspase-9 complex initiates an apoptotic protease cascade. *Cell.* 1997; 91:479–89.

27. Enari M, Sakahira H, Yokoyama H, Okawa K, Iwamatsu A, Nagata S. A caspase-activated DNase that degrades DNA during apoptosis, and its inhibitor ICAD. *Nature.* 1998; 391:43–50.

28. Sakahira H, Enari M, Nagata S. Cleavage of CAD inhibitor in CAD activation and DNA degradation during apoptosis. *Nature.* 1998; 391:96–9.

29. Tang DG, Li L, Zhu Z, Joshi B. Apoptosis in the absence of cytochrome *c* accumulation in the cytosol. *Biochem Biophys Res Commun.* 1998; 242:380–4.

30. Nagata S, Golstein P. The Fas death factor. *Science.* 1995; 267:1449–56.

31. Rouvier E, Luciani MF, Golstein P. Fas involvement in Ca$(^{2+})$-independent T cell-mediated cytotoxicity. *J Exp Med.* 1993; 177:195–200.

32. Boldin MP, Varfolomeev EE, Pancer Z, Mett IL, Camonis JH, Wallach D. A novel protein that interacts with the death domain of Fas/APO1 contains a sequence motif related to the death domain. *J Biol Chem.* 1995; 270:7795–8.

33. Srinivasula SM, Ahmad M, Fernandes Alnemri T, Litwack G, Alnemri ES. Molecular ordering of the Fas-apoptotic pathway: the Fas/APO-1 protease Mch5 is a CrmA-inhibitable protease that activates multiple Ced-3/ICE-like cysteine proteases. *Proc Natl Acad Sci USA.* 1996; 93:14486–91.

34. Hirata H, Takahashi A, Kobayashi S, et al. Caspases are activated in a branched protease cascade and control distinct downstream processes in Fas-induced apoptosis. *J Exp Med.* 1998; 187:587–600.

35. Bodmer JL, Burns K, Schneider P, et al. TRAMP, a novel apoptosis-mediating receptor with sequence homology to tumor necrosis factor receptor 1 and Fas(Apo-1/CD95). *Immunity.* 1997; 6:79–88.

36. Kitson J, Raven T, Jiang YP, et al. A death-domain-containing receptor that mediates apoptosis. *Nature.* 1996; 384:372–5.

37. Hsu H, Xiong J, Goeddel DV. The TNF receptor 1-associated protein TRADD signals cell death and NF-κ B activation. *Cell.* 1995; 81:495–504.

38. Boise LH, Thompson CB. Bcl-x(L) can inhibit apoptosis in cells that have undergone Fas-induced protease activation. *Proc Natl Acad Sci USA.* 1997; 94:3759–64.

39. Yang E, Korsmeyer SJ. Molecular thanatopsis: a discourse on the BCL2 family and cell death. *Blood.* 1996; 88:386–401.

40. Srinivasan A, Li F, Wong A. et al. Bcl-xL functions downstream of caspase-8 to inhibit Fas- and tumor necrosis factor receptor 1-induced apoptosis of MCF7 breast carcinoma cells. *J Biol Chem.* 1998; 273:4523–9.

41. Hellquist HB, Olejnicka B, Jadner M, Andersson T, Sederholm C. Fas receptor is expressed in human lung squamous cell carcinomas, whereas bcl-2 and apoptosis are not pronounced: a preliminary report. *Br J Cancer.* 1997; 76:175–9.

42. Owen Schaub LB, Radinsky R, Kruzel E, Berry K, Yonehara S. Anti-Fas on nonhematopoietic tumors: levels of Fas/APO-1 and bcl-2 are not predictive of biological responsiveness. *Cancer Res.* 1994; 54:1580–6.

43. Micheau O, Solary E, Hammann A, Martin F, Dimanche Boitrel MT. Sensitization of cancer cells treated with cytotoxic drugs to fas-mediated cytotoxicity. *J Natl Cancer Inst.* 1997; 89:783–9.

44. Hahne M, Rimoldi D, Schroter M, et al. Melanoma cell expression of Fas(Apo-1/CD95) ligand: implications for tumor immune escape. *Science.* 1996; 274:1363–6.

45. Thomas WD, Hersey P. CD4 T cells kill melanoma cells by mechanisms that are independent of Fas (CD95). *Int J Cancer.* 1998; 75:384–90.

46. Irmler M, Thome M, Hahne M, et al. Inhibition of death receptor signals by cellular FLIP. *Nature.* 1997; 388:190–5.

47. Tamiya S, Etoh K, Suzushima H, Takatsuki K, Matsuoka M. Mutation of *CD95 (Fas/Apo-1)* gene in adult T-cell leukemia cells. *Blood.* 1998; 91:3935–42.

48. Newmeyer DD, Farschon DM, Reed JC. Cell-free apoptosis in *Xenopus* egg extracts: inhibition by *Bcl-2* and requirement for an organelle fraction enriched in mitochondria. *Cell.* 1994; 79:353–64.

49. Tsujimoto Y, Cossman J, Jaffe E, Croce CM. Involvement of the *bcl-2* gene in human follicular lymphoma. *Science.* 1985; 228:1440–3.

50. Vaux DL, Cory S, Adams JM. *Bcl-2* gene promotes haemopoietic cell survival and cooperates with c-*myc* to immortalize pre-B cells. *Nature.* 1988; 335:440–2.

51. Hockenbery D, Nunez G, Milliman C, Schreiber RD, Korsmeyer SJ. Bcl-2 is an inner mitochondrial membrane protein that blocks programmed cell death. *Nature.* 1990; 348:334–6.

52. Chen Levy Z, Cleary ML. Membrane topology of the Bcl-2 proto-oncogenic protein demonstrated in vitro. *J Biol Chem.* 1990; 265:4929–33.

53. Chao DT, Korsmeyer SJ. BCL-2 family: regulators of cell death. *Annu Rev Immunol.* 1998; 16:395–419.

54. Boise LH, Gonzalez Garcia M, Postema CE, et al. *bcl-x,* a *bcl-2*-related gene that functions as a dominant regulator of apoptotic cell death. *Cell.* 1993; 74:597–608.

55. Chittenden T, Flemington C, Houghton AB, et al. A conserved domain in Bak, distinct from BH1 and BH2, mediates cell death and protein binding functions. *EMBO J.* 1995; 14:5589–96.

56. Boyd JM, Gallo GJ, Elangovan B, et al. Bik, a novel death-inducing protein shares a distinct sequence motif with Bcl-2 family proteins and interacts with viral and cellular survival-promoting proteins. *Oncogene.* 1995; 11:1921–8.

57. Oltvai ZN, Milliman CL, Korsmeyer SJ. Bcl-2 heterodimerizes in vivo with a conserved homolog, Bax, that accelerates programmed cell death. *Cell.* 1993; 74:609–19.

58. Yin XM, Oltvai ZN, Korsmeyer SJ. BH1 and BH2 domains of Bcl-2 are required for inhibition of apoptosis and heterodimerization with Bax. *Nature.* 1994; 369:321–3.

59. Haldar S, Jena N, Croce CM. Inactivation of Bcl-2 by phosphorylation. *Proc Natl Acad Sci USA.* 1995; 92:4507–11.

60. Muchmore SW, Sattler M, Liang H, et al. X-ray and NMR structure of human Bcl-xL, an inhibitor of programmed cell death. *Nature.* 1996; 381:335–41.

61. Minn AJ, Velez P, Schendel SL, et al. Bcl-x(L) forms an ion channel in synthetic lipid membranes. *Nature.* 1997; 385:353–7.

62. Schendel SL, Xie Z, Montal MO, Matsuyama S, Montal M, Reed JC. Channel formation by antiapoptotic protein Bcl-2. *Proc Natl Acad Sci USA.* 1997; 94:5113–8

63. Schlesinger PH, Gross A, Yin XM, et al. Comparison of the ion channel characteristics of proapoptotic BAX and antiapoptotic BCL-2. *Proc Natl Acad Sci USA.* 1997; 94:11357–62.

64. Antonsson B, Conti F, Cilavatta A, et al. Inhibition of Bax channel-forming activity by Bcl-2. *Science.* 1997; 277:370–2.

65. Petit PX, Lecoeur H, Zorn E, Dauguet C, Mignotte B, Gougeon ML. Alterations in mitochondrial structure and function are early events of dexamethasone-induced thymocyte apoptosis. *J Cell Biol.* 1995; 130:157–67

66. Hirsch T, Marzo I, Kroemer G. Role of the mitochondrial permeability transition pore in apoptosis. *Biosci Rep.* 1997; 17:67–76.

67. Zamzami N, Susin SA, Marchetti P, et al. Mitochondrial control of nuclear apoptosis. *J Exp Med.* 1996; 183:1533–44.

68. McDonnell TJ, Korsmeyer SJ. Progression from lymphoid hyperplasia to high-grade malignant lymphoma in mice transgenic for the t(14; 18). *Nature.* 1991; 349:254–6.

69. Korsmeyer SJ. Regulators of cell death. *Trends Genet.* 1995; 11:101–5.

70. Veis DJ, Sorenson CM, Shutter JR, Korsmeyer SJ. Bcl-2-deficient mice demonstrate fulminant lymphoid apoptosis, polycystic kidneys, and hypopigmented hair. *Cell.* 1993; 75:229–40.

71. Rampino N, Yamamoto H, Ionov Y, et al. Somatic frameshift mutations in the *BAX* gene in colon cancers of the microsatellite mutator phenotype. *Science.* 1997; 275:967–9.

72. Meijerink JP, Mensink EJ, Wang K, et al. Hematopoietic malignancies demonstrate loss-of-function mutations of *BAX. Blood.* 1998; 91:2991–7.

73. Yin C, Knudson CM, Korsmeyer SJ, Van Dyke T. *Bax* suppresses tumorigenesis and stimulates apoptosis in vivo. *Nature.* 1997; 385:637–40.

74. Leek RD, Kaklamanis L, Pezzella F, Gatter KC, Harris AL. *bcl-2* in normal human breast and carcinoma, association with oestrogen receptor-positive, epidermal growth factor receptor-negative tumours and in situ cancer. *Br J Cancer.* 1994; 69:135–9.

75. Silvestrini R, Veneroni S, Daidone MG, et al. The Bcl-2 protein: a prognostic indicator strongly related to p53 protein in lymph node-negative breast cancer patients. *J Natl Cancer Inst.* 1994; 86:499–504.

76. Pezzella F, Turley H, Kuzu I, et al. bcl-2 protein in non-small-cell lung carcinoma. *N Engl J Med.* 1993; 329:690–4.

77. Tollenaar RA, van Krieken JH, van Slooten HJ, et al. Immunohistochemical detection of p53 and Bcl-2 in colorectal carcinoma: no evidence for prognostic significance. *Br J Cancer.* 1998; 77:1842–7.

78. Kaklamanis L, Savage A, Whitehouse R, et al. Bcl-2 protein expression: association with p53 and prognosis in colorectal cancer. *Br J Cancer.* 1998; 77:1864–9.

79. Campos L, Rouault JP, Sabido O, et al. High expression of bcl-2 protein in acute myeloid leukemia cells is associated with poor response to chemotherapy. *Blood.* 1993; 81: 3091–6.

80. van Slooten HJ, Clahsen PC, van Dierendonck JH, et al. Expression of Bcl-2 in node-negative breast cancer is associated with various prognostic factors, but does not predict response to one course of perioperative chemotherapy. *Br J Cancer.* 1996; 74:78–85.

81. Schneider HJ, Sampson SA, Cunningham D, et al. Bcl-2 expression and response to chemotherapy in colorectal adenocarcinomas. *Br J Cancer.* 1997; 75:427–31.

82. Elledge RM, Green S, Howes L, et al. bcl-2, p53, and response to tamoxifen in estrogen receptor-positive metastatic breast cancer: a Southwest Oncology Group study. *J Clin Oncol.* 1997; 15:1916–22.

83. Soussi T, Legros Y, Lubin R, Ory K, Schlichtholz B. Multifactorial analysis of p53 alteration in human cancer: a review. *Int J Cancer.* 1994; 57:1–9.

84. Graeber TG, Peterson JF, Tsai M, Monica K, Fornace AJ Jr, Giaccia AJ. Hypoxia induces accumulation of p53 protein, but activation of a G1-phase checkpoint by low-oxygen conditions is independent of p53 status. *Mol Cell Biol.* 1994; 14:6264–77.

85. Jackson SP. The recognition of DNA damage. *Curr Opin Genet Dev.* 1996; 6:19–25.

86. Shieh SY, Ikeda M, Taya Y, Prives C. DNA damage-induced phosphorylation of p53 alleviates inhibition by MDM2. *Cell.* 1997; 91:325–34.

87. Midgley CA, Lane DP. p53 protein stability in tumour cells is not determined by mutation but is dependent on Mdm2 binding. *Oncogene.* 1997; 15:1179–89.

88. Hansen R, Oren M. p53; from inductive signal to cellular effect. *Curr Opin Genet Dev.* 1997; 7:46–51.

89. Polyak K, Xia Y, Zweier JL, Kinzler KW, Vogelstein B. A model for p53-induced apoptosis. *Nature.* 1997; 389:300–5.

90. Miyashita T, Reed JC. Tumor suppressor p53 is a direct transcriptional activator of the human *bax* gene. *Cell.* 1995; 80:293–9.

91. Selvakumaran M, Lin HK, Miyashita T, et al. Immediate early up-regulation of *bax* expression by p53 but not TGF β 1: a paradigm for distinct apoptotic pathways. *Oncogene.* 1994; 9:1791–8.

92. Schott AF, Apel IJ, Nunez G, Clarke MF. *Bcl-XL* protects cancer cells from p53-mediated apoptosis. *Oncogene.* 1995; 11:1389–94.

93. Owen Schaub LB, Zhang W, Cusack JC, et al. Wild-type human p53 and a temperature-sensitive mutant induce Fas/APO-1 expression. *Mol Cell Biol.* 1995; 15:3032–40.

94. Wu GS, Burns TF, McDonald ER, et al. KILLER/DR5 is a DNA damage-inducible p53-regulated death receptor gene. *Nat Genet.* 1997; 17:141–3.

95. Sheikh MS, Burns TF, Huang Y, et al. p53-dependent and -independent regulation of the death receptor *KILLER/DR5* gene expression in response to genotoxic stress and tumor necrosis factor α. *Cancer Res.* 1998; 58:1593–8.

96. Caelles C, Helmberg A, Karin M. *p53*-dependent apoptosis in the absence of transcriptional activation of *p53*-target genes. *Nature.* 1994; 370:220–3.

97. Attardi LD, Lowe SW, Brugarolas J, Jacks T. Transcriptional activation by p53, but not induction of the *p21* gene, is essential for oncogene-mediated apoptosis. *EMBO J.* 1996; 15:3693–701.

98. Brugarolas J, Chandrasekaran C, Gordon JI, Beach D, Jacks T, Hannon GJ. Radiation-induced cell cycle arrest compromised by p21 deficiency. *Nature.* 1995; 377:552–7.

99. Lowe SW, Schmitt EM, Smith SW, Osborne BA, Jacks T. p53 is required for radiation-induced apoptosis in mouse thymocytes. *Nature.* 1993; 362:847–9.

100. Elledge RM, Fuqua SA, Clark GM, Pujol P, Allred DC, McGuire WL. Prognostic significance of *p53* gene alterations in node-negative breast cancer. *Breast Cancer Res Treat.* 1993; 26:225–35.

101. Silvestrini R, Benini E, Veneroni S, et al. *p53* and *bcl-2* expression correlates with clinical outcome in a series of node-positive breast cancer patients. *J Clin Oncol.* 1996; 14:1604–10.

102. Chiou SK, Rao L, White E. Bcl-2 blocks p53-dependent apoptosis. *Mol Cell Biol.* 1994; 14:2556–63.

103. Silvestrini R. Re: the *p53* gene in breast cancer: prognostic value of complementary DNA sequencing versus immunohistochemistry. *J Natl Cancer Inst.* 1996; 88:1499–500.

104. Kononen J, Bubendorf L, Kallioniemi A, et al. Tissue microarrays for high-throughput molecular profiling of tumour specimens. *Nat Med.* 1998; 4:944–847.

105. Aas T, Borresen AL, Geisler S, et al. Specific *P53* mutations are associated with de novo resistance to doxorubicin in breast cancer patients. *Nat Med.* 1996; 2:811–4.

106. Wahl AF, Donaldson KL, Fairchild C, et al. Loss of normal *p53* function confers sensitization to Taxol by increasing G2/M arrest and apoptosis. *Nat Med.* 1996; 2:72–9.

107. Debernardis D, Sire EG, De Feudis P, et al. *p53* status does not affect sensitivity of human ovarian cancer cell lines to paclitaxel. *Cancer Res.* 1997; 57:870–4.

108. Smith-Sorensen B, Kaern J, Holm R, Dorum A, Trope C, Borresen Dale AL. Therapy effect of either paclitaxel or cyclophosphamide combination treatment in patients with epithelial ovarian cancer and relation to *TP53* gene status. *Br J Cancer.* 1998; 78:375–81.

109. O'Connor PM, Jackman J, Bae I, et al. Characterization of the *p53* tumor suppressor pathway in cell lines of the National Cancer Institute anticancer drug screen and correlations with the growth-inhibitory potency of 123 anticancer agents. *Cancer Res.* 1997; 57:4285–300.

110. Oren M. Lonely no more: *p53* finds its kin in a tumor suppressor haven. *Cell.* 1997; 90:829–32.

111. Jost CA, Marin MC, Kaelin WG Jr. *p73* is a human p53-related protein that can induce apoptosis. *Nature.* 1997; 389:191–4.

112. Spencer CA, Groudine M. Control of c-*myc* regulation in normal and neoplastic cells. *Adv Cancer Res.* 1991; 56:1–48.

113. Marcu KB, Bossone SA, Patel AJ. *myc* function and regulation. *Annu Rev Biochem.* 1992; 61:809–60.

114. Ryan KM, Birnie GD. *Myc* oncogenes: the enigmatic family. *Biochem J.* 1996; 314:713–21.

115. Hann SR, Dixit M, Sears RC, Sealy L. The alternatively initiated c-Myc proteins differen-

tially regulate transcription through a noncanonical DNA-binding site. *Genes Dev.* 1994; 8:2441–52.

116. Amati B, Brooks MW, Levy N, Littlewood TD, Evan GI, Land H. Oncogenic activity of the c-Myc protein requires dimerization with Max. *Cell.* 1993; 72:233–45.

117. Wood AC, Waters CM, Garner A, Hickman JA. Changes in c-*myc* expression and the kinetics of dexamethasone-induced programmed cell death (apoptosis) in human lymphoid leukaemia cells. *Br J Cancer.* 1994; 69:663–9.

118. Fornari FA Jr, Jarvis WD, Grant S, et al. Induction of differentiation and growth arrest associated with nascent (nonoligosomal) DNA fragmentation and reduced c-*myc* expression in MCF-7 human breast tumor cells after continuous exposure to a sublethal concentration of doxorubicin. *Cell Growth Different.* 1994; 5:723–33.

119. Hermeking H, Eick D. Mediation of c-Myc-induced apoptosis by p53. *Science.* 1994; 265:2091–3.

120. Hueber AO, Zornig M, Lyon D, Suda T, Nagata S, Evan GI. Requirement for the CD95 receptor-ligand pathway in c-Myc-induced apoptosis. *Science.* 1997; 278:1305–9.

121. Fanidi A, Harrington EA, Evan GI. Cooperative interaction between c-*myc* and *bcl-2* proto-oncogenes. *Nature.* 1992; 359:554–6.

122. Thompson EB. The many roles of c-Myc in apoptosis. *Annu Rev Physiol.* 1998; 60: 575–600.

10

DNA Repair Pathways

Mechanisms and Defects in the Maintenance of Genome Stability

Murray O. Robinson

Introduction

Nobel laureate Michael Bishop accurately described the etiology of cancer as "a malady of the genes" *(1)*. The ability to maintain the integrity of the genome is critical for preventing genetic alterations which, in turn, can both initiate and contribute to the multistep progression of cancer. DNA is susceptible to mutation either through errors introduced during replication, chemical or physical modification of the nucleotides, or changes in large-scale nucleic acid structures that serve to protect the integrity of chromosomes. To avoid genome instability, several highly conserved pathways have evolved across distantly related organisms to repair modifications in DNA, due to either replication error or DNA damage.

Previous chapters in this volume have discussed many aspects of molecular control of the cell cycle and how proto-oncogenes and oncogenes are involved in carcinogenesis. The goal of this chapter is to review the known pathways for DNA repair and the results of mutations in or loss of these pathways in humans. In addition, protection of genome integrity has been attributed to maintenance of telomeres, specialized structures at the ends of chromosomes *(2,3)*. Clinically relevant outcomes of mutation of these pathways are discussed, as are the potential for novel therapeutic intervention. Each of these topics spans a large area of research, much of which has been reviewed extensively. Appropriate references to the many excellent reviews are provided for further study.

DNA Repair Pathways

Preservation of an organism's genetic material is essential for its long-term viability. Accordingly, several highly conserved systems have evolved to monitor and repair defects in the DNA sequence. These systems include:

- mismatch excision repair, which primarily repairs errors made during replication *(4,5)* (Fig. 1);
- base excision repair, which primarily acts on spontaneous and chemically induced damage *(6)*;

From: *Principles of Molecular Oncology*
Edited by: M. H. Bronchud, M. A. Foote, W. P. Peters, and M. O. Robinson © Humana Press Inc., Totowa, NJ

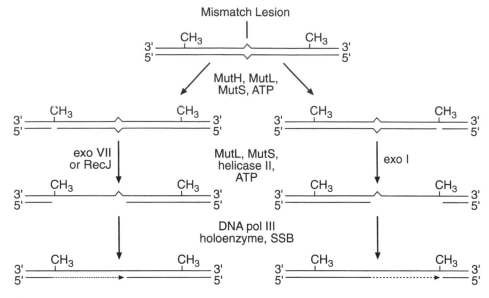

Fig. 1. Diagram of mismatch repair in prokaryotes. (Adapted from ref. *5*).

- nucleotide excision repair, which has been best characterized as a repair system for recognizing and repairing ultraviolet (UV) photoproduct damage *(6–8)*;
- O^6-methylguanine DNA methyltransferase (MGMT), an enzyme that directly reverses methylation adducts on DNA *(6)*; and
- double-strand break repair, which repairs damage done by agents such as ionizing radiation *(7)*.

Each of these systems is briefly outlined below, with special attention paid to the human genes and their potential for involvement in the cancer phenotype.

Mismatch Excision Repair

This system recognizes and repairs errors made during DNA replication, as well as some DNA-damaging agents. The identification of a mismatch repair (MMR) system originally came from the discovery of bacterial strains that exhibited dramatically increased mutation rates. These studies led to the elucidation of a mechanism in which misincorporated bases are recognized and corrected. The process of recognition and repair in bacteria has been reconstituted in vivo with mismatched hemimethylated DNA and over a dozen proteins *(4* and references therein). A mismatched nucleotide pair is recognized and bound by the protein MutS, which then recruits the MutL protein to the site. To determine which of the mispaired bases to correct, the system uses the methylation status of the DNA to choose which base to remove and repair. The parental strand of bacterial DNA is adenine methylated at GATC sites. This methylated base is recognized by the *Escherichia coli* endonuclease MutH which then cleaves the unmethylated DNA strand. The GATC sequence can be as much as a kilobase (kb) away from the mispaired site. Furthermore, the GATC can be either 3′ or 5′ to the lesion. The nicked segment is then removed using *UvrD* (helicase II), and *ExoI* (for nicks 3′ to the lesion) or *Exo*VII or *RecJ* (for nicks 5′ to the lesion). Single-strand binding protein and DNA *pol*III holoenzyme then facilitate resynthesis of the excised strand which is finally closed by DNA ligase.

The MMR system of bacteria has apparently been largely retained in eukaryotes, including both yeast and humans. The identification of functionally similar biochemical activities in human cells and the identification of a number of human genes that exhibit significant homology to the *E. coli* proteins provide good evidence of evolutionary conservation of this repair system. Humans exhibit several homologs to the bacterial mutS proteins. The mutS homolog MSH2 can bind to single mismatches as well as insertions and deletions of up to four nucleotides. MSH2 can form heterodimers with other mutS homologs hMSH3 (previously called MRP1) and hMSH6 (previously called GTBP). These two heterodimers exhibit overlapping, but distinct, specificity for various mismatches. The MutL function appears to be facilitated by heterodimers of MLH1 and PMS2 (reviewed in *5*). Loss and mutation of these human MMR genes leads to dramatic changes in mutation rates in human tumors, and is discussed later in this chapter.

Base Excision Repair

Base excision repair (BER) is a process of DNA repair that serves to correct spontaneous damage to the DNA (Fig. 2). As such, this repair system is responsible for DNA maintenance. Damage can come from either endogenous cellular activities such as *S*-adenosylmethionine, hydrolysis from free radical attack, or from exogenous DNA modifiers such as alkylating agents.

The process of BER begins with the recognition of the modified base and its subsequent cleavage by one of several glycosylases. ACH glycolase recognizes and cleaves specific modified bases. These enzymes cleave the *N*-glycosyl bond which links the base to the deoxyribose-phosphate backbone, releasing the modified base. The human UNG1 protein (uracil DNA glycosylase) serves to remove uracil bases from the DNA. Uracil bases arise commonly from the deamination of cytosine. UNG1 protein can also correct the incorporation of the chemotherapeutic agent 5-fluorouracil (5-FU). Other human DNA glycosylases include 3-methyladenine-DNA glycosylase and formamido-pyrimidine-DNA glycosylase. The latter enzyme, encoded by *fpg* in bacteria and *MMH1* in humans, is responsible for cleavage of 8-hydroxyguanine-modified bases (8oxoG). This base modification occurs readily in cells subjected to ionizing radiation and oxidative stress. The *E. coli* gene has been shown to function in mammalian cells to lower the frequency of mutations induced by γ-rays *(9)*.

After base removal, another enzymatic activity cleaves the phosphodiester backbone just 5′ to the apurinic or apyrimidic site. This protein, the AP endonuclease, is encoded by the *HAP1* gene in humans. The gene shares significant homology with the *E. coli* *Xth* gene, demonstrating once again that this pathway is evolutionarily conserved. AP endonuclease can also recognize spontaneously produced apurinic or apyrimidinic sites, which is significant, as it has been calculated that up 10,000 bases per cell undergo base cleavage each day *(10)*. After backbone cleavage, resynthesis and ligation occurs through one of at least two polymerase pathways. DNA polymerase-β is sufficient for repair of these lesions, as it possesses the ability to cleave the 5′-terminal deoxyribose phosphate in addition to its polymerase activity *(11)*.

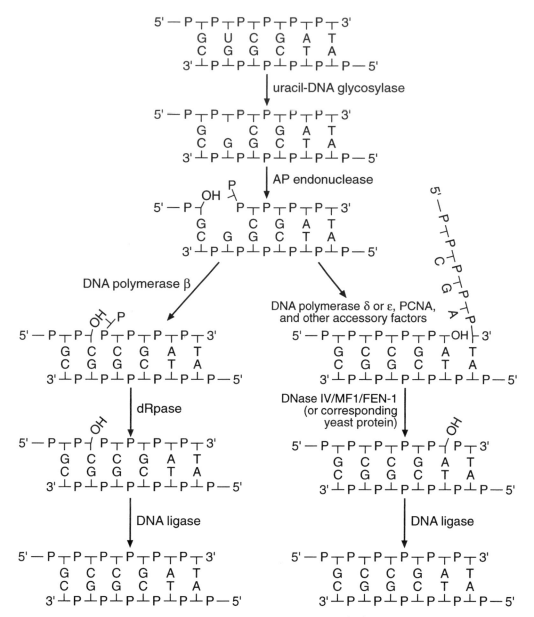

Fig. 2. Diagram of base excision repair. (Adapted from ref. *6*).

Nucleotide Excision Repair

The nucleotide excision repair (NER) system is essential to carry out the repair of UV photoproduct damage (Fig. 3). However, NER is probably a far more versatile repair system, as it appears to be able to recognize and correct all known covalent base modifications. In addition, NER is the only repair system capable of repairing bulky DNA modifications such as cisplatin–G adducts.

In humans, NER is not essential for survival. This is evidenced in the inherited disorder xeroderma pigmentosa (XP), in which NER can be completely deficient. This

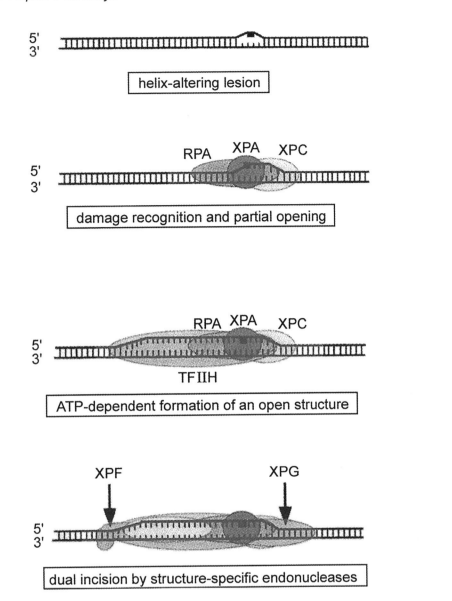

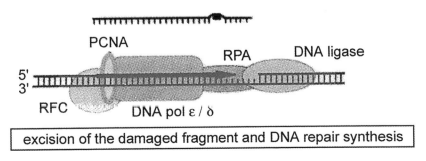

Fig. 3. Diagram of nucleotide excision repair. (Adapted from ref. 6).

disease contains seven complementation groups, A–G. These complementation groups correspond well with the specific loss of several corresponding genes critical for NER. In addition, studies in rodent cell lines have contributed to the identification of the *ERCC* (excision repair cross-complementing) genes. In yeast, studies of UV sensitivity led to mutants of the *Rad* class. The high homology to lower eukaryotes and the availability of the XP groups and the *ERCC* genes has led to rapid and extensive characterization of this pathway.

The classic lesions repaired by this pathway include UV photoproduct dimers. The two types typically observed are cyclobutane pyrimidine dimers (T–C, C–C, T–T, C–T), and pyrimidine/pyrimidone lesions. A model for the process of recognition and repair of these lesions is outlined below. The human XPA protein (Rad 14 in yeast) and the human damage DNA-binding (UV-DDB) protein can recognize and bind modified lesions. The XPA is known to form a complex with the single-strand DNA-binding protein RPA, which is also required for NER. This complex is thought to bind and partially open the DNA strand. Next, the DNA strand is unwound with proteins of the TFIIH complex. TFIIH is a component of the basal transcription machinery; the link between transcription and NER has led to much study on the effects of transcription on this process (transcription-coupled repair). Two components of the TFIIH complex are the XPB and XPD proteins. XPB and XPD possess helicase activity and are required to unwind the DNA near the lesion, setting up the excision reactions. Several nucleases carry out the excision of 25–32 base pairs (bps) of the damaged strand. The 5′ excision reaction is carried out by a complex between XPF and ERCC1 protein; the 3′ cleavage is performed by the XPG protein. The resultant single-stranded region is filled using DNA polymerase-δ or -ε, and finished using DNA ligase. Proliferating cell nuclear antigen (PCNA) is also required for resynthesis of the excised strand. This process has been reconstituted in vitro and requires approx 30 polypeptides: XPA, XPB (associated with XPD and TFIIH), XPC, XPF, XPG, RPA, DNA polymerase ε, RFC, PCNA, and DNA ligase *(12)*.

O[6] Methylguanine DNA Methyltransferase

Other enzymatic mechanisms also exist for repairing damaged DNA. One direct mechanism to reverse modifications is found in MGMT. MGMT is a suicide enzyme that covalent transfers the methyl group from methylated guanines to a cysteine residue on the protein. This mechanism is particularly effective at reversing simple alkylating agents (methyl halides and methylnitrosourea). Loss of MGMT function causes hyper-sensitivity to methylating agents. Subsequent resistance is achieved through the inactivation of MMR proteins. Such tolerant cells have a greatly increased mutational rate, so-called mutator phenotypes. Generation of mutator phenotypes in cells in vivo may contribute to oncogenic progression.

Double-Strand Break Repair

Double-strand breaks normally occur in normal cellular processes such as somatic recombination. However, double-strand breaks are also primary lesions in cells treated with ionizing radiation and oxidative stress. Relative to the systems discussed previously, much less is known about the mechanics of double-strand break repair, although several of the genes responsible for this activity have been identified in humans. The best studied is perhaps the DNA-PK heterotrimer, whose serine/threonine kinase function is activated by DNA binding. This gene is involved in genetic recombination in T cells and has been functionally linked to the murine severe combined immunodeficiency (SCID) mouse. Cell lines deficient in double-strand break repair have been shown to contain inactive DNA-PK. The heterotrimer consists of the enormous 450-kDa DNA–PK catalytic subunit and the Ku regulatory subunits, Kup70 and Kup86. The Ku subunits appear to be involved in stabilizing the DNA–DNA-PK interaction. DNA-PK is related to two other proteins involved in double-strand break repair, the product of the ataxia telangiectasia gene, *ATM*, and the related *ATR* gene product. DNA-PK, ATM, and ATR all appear to be members of a DNA-dependent protein kinase family. Work in yeast has identified several other members of the double-strand break repair pathway, including a complex of proteins encoded by the *mre11*, *rad 50*, and *XRS2* genes. Human homologs, *hmre11* and *hrad50*, have been cloned and have been shown to associate with double-strand breaks in mammalian cells. Another human gene found in this complex is the gene associated with Nijmegan breakage syndrome, *NBS1 (13,14)*. The encoded protein, nebrin, contains two motifs that have been previously associated with proteins involved in DNA repair: a forkhead-associated motif and a breast cancer C-terminus domain (BRCT). Based on the homologous complex in yeast, *NBS1* is suspected to function as the homolog of the yeast *XRS2* gene, yet the *NBS1* gene shares little sequence homology to the yeast *XRS2* gene.

Repair Defects in Cancer

Inherited Repair Syndromes

Several inherited human conditions exhibit both increased incidence of cancer and defects in DNA repair pathways. These conditions have been useful for establishing the relationship between DNA repair and cancer, and have provided insight into similar mutations in sporadic tumors.

Xeroderma Pigmentosa

This syndrome is characterized by light-induced skin lesions and a 1000-fold increase in the incidence of skin cancer. Patients with XP fall into seven complementation groups, A–G. As described previously, these complementation groups gave rise to the names of the XP proteins involved in NER. Other related syndromes that exhibit mutations in genes used by the NER system, but do not result in an increased cancer incidence, are Cockayne's syndrome (CS) and trichothiodystrophy (TTD). Patients with CS are photosensitive, and exhibit dwarfism and mental retardation. Two complementation groups of CS, CSA and CSB, encode proteins that interact with the p44 protein of the TFIIH complex. Other forms of CS have mutations in *XPB*, *XPD*, or *XPG* genes. Patients with TTD exhibit physical and mental retardation and UV sensitivity. Mutations in the XPB and XPD helicases have been identified in two complementation groups of TTD patients. It is hypothesized that the XP protein mutations in these syndromes primarily affect transcription and not DNA repair.

Ataxia Telangiectasia

As the name suggests, patients with ataxia telangiectasia (AT) exhibit a combination of neurological abnormalities, particularly difficulty with balance, and dilated blood vessels in the eyes and on the surface of the skin. In addition, patients usually have immune system abnormalities, causing recurrent infections, exhibit sensitivity to ionizing radiation, and display an increased incidence of cancer. This autosomal recessive disease is caused by mutations in the telangiectasia (*ATM*) gene, a DNA-dependent protein kinase. A role for *ATM* in double-strand break repair is hypothesized based on the phenotype of ATM mutants and its homology to the DNA-PK protein, described previously.

Nijmegan Breakage Syndrome

Long considered to be a variant of AT, Nijmegan breakage syndrome (NBS) is a rare autosomal recessive syndrome with characteristics very similar to those of AT. Patients exhibit chromosomal instability, developmental defects including growth and mental retardation, immune deficiency, and a predisposition to cancer, especially B-cell lymphomas (reviewed in *14*). The gene for this disorder, *NBS1*, was identified, demonstrating that NBS and AT are distinct genetic disorders. The protein encoded by the *NBS* gene has been shown to interact with other proteins implicated in double-strand DNA repair (*13*). The similarity between NBS and AT suggests that these distinct proteins function in similar or overlapping pathways.

Hereditary Nonpolyposis Colorectal Cancer

A fraction of human colorectal cancers is associated with a strong familial inheritance. This condition, hereditary nonpolyposis colorectal cancer (HNPCC) correlates with an increased incidence of colorectal carcinoma as well as a number of other tumor types. HNPCC is inherited as an autosomal dominant trait. Variations in diagnostic criteria for the disease led to various reports of its incidence in human populations, from as high as 1:200 to as low as 1:8000–15,000. The genes responsible for this condition were cloned and found to code for inactivating mutations in proteins involved in the human MMR pathway. Genetic mutations causing HNPCC have been identified in MSH2 and MLH1 (the majority), PMS1, and PMS2. The dominant inheritance pattern is due to frequent conversion of the wild-type gene leading to the loss of gene function. Tumors invariably exhibit somatic mutation or loss of heterozygosity (LOH) of the corresponding wild-type gene. Approximately 80% of HNPCC tumors feature unstable DNA sequences as assayed by microsatellite instability (MSI), which is presumed to be due to the loss of MMR function (discussed further later in this chapter).

Interestingly, HNPCC tumors have a reasonably good prognosis. It has been hypothesized that the increased mutation rate of HNPCC tumors can cause a number of genetic changes that are deleterious to the tumor.

Acquired Repair Defects—Microsatellite Instability

Evaluation of genomic structure in HNPCC tumor cell lines revealed the presence of somatic alteration of repeated DNA elements called microsatellites, termed MSI. The structure of these repeat elements can be readily assayed by polymerase chain reaction (PCR) fingerprinting of genomic DNA; the MSI phenotype is confirmed by observing changes in the banding pattern of microsatellites across clonal subsets of a population (*15,16*). This genetic instability is used a marker for defects in MMR function in tumor cells, and is presumed to result from the inability to resolve mismatched repeat sequences. The MSI phenotype initially observed in HNPCC tumors has also been observed in a significant percentage of sporadic tumors of many types, including roughly 15% of sporadic colorectal tumors, 67% of pancreatic tumors, 50% of squamous skin cell cancers, 45% of small-cell lung cancers, 18–39% of gastric tumors, 20% of endometrial tumors, 16% of ovarian tumors, and a lower incidence in several other tumor types including leukemias *(5,17–19)*. The MIS phenotype is considered to represent increased genome-wide mutation frequency. Several specific gene mutations have been studied in these mutator cells. For example, mutations of the type II transforming growth factor-β *(TGF-β)* receptor gene have been linked to the mutator phenotype *(20,21)*. Frameshift mutations were found in small repeat tracts of the gene, leading to the functional inactivation of the receptor. As *TGF-β* receptor has a tumor suppressor function, this mutation is oncogenic. A second gene that is frequently inactivated in MSI phenotype tumors is the proapoptotic *bax* gene. A tract of 8 Gs in the *bax* sequence has been shown to be sensitive to mutation in these tumor types *(22)*.

Gene mutations leading to MSI are the same as those associated with HNPCC (MSH2 and MLH1, PMS1, and PMS2). A few other mutations have been identified that cause particular defects in the pathway. A mutation in the GTBP protein is associated with a particular mononucleotide tract defect phenotype *(23)*. A nonsense mutation in the *PMS2* gene was shown to confer a dominant negative effect over the wild-type copy, causing a mutator phenotype *(24)*.

Telomerase, Telomere Maintenance, and Cancer

Organisms with linear chromosomes lose a small amount of DNA from the chromosome ends with each round of DNA replication. This is thought to result from an intrinsic inability of the DNA replication machinery to replicate the ends of DNA strands. This conundrum is referred to as the "end replication problem." To avoid this problem, and the subsequent loss of genetic material, most organisms, including all vertebrates examined, possess specialized structures at the chromosome ends called telomeres *(25–29)*. In vertebrates, this structure contains the simple sequence TTAGGG repeated in arrays of 100–10,000. These sequences are generated and maintained by a ribonucleoprotein enzyme termed "telomerase." Although evidence for the presence of this enzyme was available decades earlier, telomerase activity was first identified in the ciliate *Tetrahymena* in 1985 by Greider and Blackburn *(30)*. Once again, this process is highly conserved across distantly related species, so molecular and biochemical characterization in lower eukaryotes, as well as the advent of ever shorter telomeres (EST) databases, has greatly facilitated our understanding of telomerase in human cells.

The Telomere Hypothesis

Human cells do not proliferate indefinitely in culture. Hayflick discovered that cells in culture exhibit limited life-span dictated by the number of cell divisions, now referred to as the "Hayflick number" *(31)*. Fibroblasts in culture do not express telomerase and exhibit telomere shortening with increasing division number. Fibroblasts from young people will undergo more cell divisions and have longer telomeres than similar cells from older individuals. This led to the "telomere hypothesis," a notion that telomere length may represent a molecular clock that determines the life-span of a cell *(3,32)*.

As cancer cells are generally considered to be immortal, it was postulated that tumors required a mechanism to overcome telomeric loss.

Telomerase Activity in Human Tissue and Tumors

Telomerase activity in humans was demonstrated in 1989 *(33)*, and evidence of telomere shortening in tumors was also observed, but it was not until a sensitive assay was developed for this activity that a potential role for telomerase in tumors was revealed *(33)*.

Telomerase activity is present in approx 90% of human tumor samples examined *(34)*. In contrast, telomerase activity is absent from most normal adult tissues. Germ cells express abundant telomerase activity, and consequently maintain long telomeres. A number of tissues and specific cells have been shown to express some level of telomerase activity, although these levels are not sufficient to maintain telomere length. Bone marrow progenitor cells appear to be telomerase negative, yet will activate telomerase activity upon stimulation with cytokines (reviewed in *2*). However, careful studies of telomere length in blood cells demonstrated that telomere length still decreases with age. Lymphocytes also express low levels of telomerase activity, yet undergo telomere shortening. An exception has been reported in stimulated germinal B cells, which demonstrate high telomerase activity and telomere maintenance. It is likely that a number of proliferating cell populations will express telomerase activity; it is not clear whether this activity is required for the viability of these populations.

Human Telomerase Components

Telomerase RNA

The telomerase enzyme is a ribonucleoprotein in which the RNA component serves as a template for the addition of specific repeats onto the chromosome end. The first mammalian component of telomerase, the RNA, was identified through selection of RNAs containing the telomerase template region *(35,36)*. This RNA component is essential for telomerase activity in vitro and vivo. Deletion of the RNA component in mice results in the absence of telomerase activity *(37)* and is discussed further below.

TEP1

The ciliate *T. thermophila* has been a favorite organism for telomerase researchers owing to the massive numbers of chromosomes present during its replicative growth phase. This large number of chromosome ends necessitated high levels of telomerase activity, facilitating biochemical purification of the enzyme. Purification and cloning of two proteins from *Tetrahymena*, P80 and P95 *(38)*, enabled the identification of the first component from humans by homology *(39,40)*.

The human protein TEP1 is a homolog of the *Tetrahymena* P80 subunit, and both exhibit specific binding to the telomerase RNA. The human protein also contains a large WD domain, indicating a role for this protein as one subunit of a multiprotein complex. TEP1 is ubiquitously expressed and is not required for in vitro telomerase activity *(41,42)*; it role in telomerase activity and telomere maintenance in vivo awaits the characterization of TEP1 knockout mice.

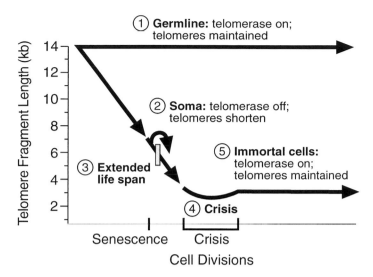

Fig. 4. Diagram of telomere status, telomerase activity, and immortalization of fibroblasts. (Adapted from ref. *27*).

TERT

Genetic screens in the yeast *Saccharomyces cerevisiae* led to the identification of the EST phenotype. Four complementation groups were identified, three of which are not required for telomerase activity in vitro *(43–45)*. Biochemical purification of telomerase activity from another ciliate, *Euplotes*, led to the identification of a protein p123, which exhibited high homology to the EST2 protein, the only *EST* gene required for in vitro telomerase activity. These homologs had distinct homology to reverse transcriptases, could bind telomerase RNA, and appeared to be the catalytic subunit of telomerase *(46)*.

The human homolog, hTERT, was rapidly identified by sequence similarity *(47–50)*. hTERT also contains motifs common to the reverse transcriptases; mutation of conserved residues will inactivate the function of the protein. hTERT expression is primarily limited to cells that exhibit telomerase activity, suggesting that hTERT is the limiting component for telomerase activity. hTERT forms a complex with TEP1 and the telomerase RNA, identifying it as an integral component of the telomerase complex. hTERT also appears to be the critical protein required for telomerase activity in primary fibroblasts, as expression of hTERT in those cells can confer telomerase activity, telomere lengthening, and extended life-span *(51,52)* (Fig. 4). Although telomerase activity can be reconstituted in vitro using the hTERT protein and the telomerase RNA *(53,54)*, it is likely that other proteins are required for functional telomerase activity in the cell.

Prospects for Telomerase Inhibition

Evidence from a number of studies argues that telomerase inhibition may provide an effective treatment for human malignancy. Telomere maintenance appears to be required for the long-term survival of unicellular organisms such as yeast and ciliates. In mammalian cells, there is a strong correlation between telomere length and replicative capacity. Moreover, activation of telomerase is sufficient for telomere extension and extended life-span of fibroblasts in culture, suggesting that telomerase activity can act to maintain telomere length. In addition, the strong correlation between telomerase activity and tumors suggests that telomerase may be required for telomere maintenance in most tumor cells.

Current data suggest that telomerase activity itself is not required for tumor cell growth, rather the essential trait is the continued maintenance of telomeres. Human cells in culture can divide many times without telomerase activity, yet proliferation ceases only when average telomere length becomes critically short *(55)*.

Human tumors and cell lines that lack telomerase activity have been reported *(56)* and mechanisms for alternate lengthening of telomeres have been postulated based on mechanisms discovered in yeast *(37)*. It is not known to what extent these mechanisms may be functioning in telomerase-positive tumor cells. In addition, mice lacking the gene for the telomerase RNA component possess no telomerase activity, yet are viable for up to six generations *(37)*. Cell lines have been derived from these mice that are competent to form tumors in nude mice.

With the recent identification of the molecular components of the telomerase complex, the requirement for telomerase activity in tumor cells can now be directly addressed using molecular genetic techniques. If telomerase is indeed important for tumor cell viability, the catalytic subunit, hTERT, may provide a tractable target for the development of small molecule inhibitors.

References

1. Bishop JM. Molecular themes in oncogenesis. *Cell.* 1991; 64:235–48.
2. Greider CW. Telomeres and senescence: the history, the experiment, the future. *Curr Biol.* 1998; 8:178–81.
3. Harley CB. Telomere loss: mitotic clock or genetic time bomb? *Mutat Res.* 1991; 256: 271–82.
4. Kolodner RD. Mismatch repair: mechanisms and relationship to cancer susceptibility. *Trends Biochem Sci.* 1995; 20:397–401.
5. Modrich P, Lahue R. Mismatch repair in replication fidelity, genetic recombination, and cancer biology. *Annu Rev Biochem.* 1996; 65:101–33.
6. Wood RD. DNA repair in eukaryotes. *Annu Rev Biochem.* 1996; 65:135–67.
7. Sancar A. DNA repair in humans. *Annu Rev Genet.* 1995; 29:69–105.
8. Tornaletti S, Pfeifer GP. UV damage and repair mechanisms in mammalian cells. *Bioessays.* 1996; 18:221–8.
9. Laval F. Expression of the *E. coli fpg* gene in mammalian cells reduces the mutagenicity of γ-rays. *Nucleic Acids Res.* 1994; 22:4943–6.
10. Barzilay G, Hickson I. Structure and function of apurinic/apyrimidinic endonucleases. *Bioessays.* 1995; 17:713–9.
11. Matsumoto Y, Kim K. Excision of deoxyribose phosphate residues by DNA polymerase beta during DNA repair. *Science.* 1995; 269:699–702.
12. Aboussekhra A, Biggerstaff M, Shivji MK, et al. Mammalian DNA nucleotide excision repair reconstituted with purified protein components. *Cell.* 1995; 80:859–68.
13. Carney JP, Maser RS, Olivares H, et al. The hMre11/hRad50 protein complex and Nijmegen

breakage syndrome: linkage of double-strand break repair to the cellular DNA damage response. *Cell.* 1998; 93:477–86.

14. Varon R, Vissinga C, Platzer M, et al. Nibrin, a novel DNA double-strand break repair protein, is mutated in Nijmegen breakage syndrome. *Cell.* 1998; 93:467–76.

15. Shiloh Y. Ataxia-telangiectasia and the Nijmegen breakage syndrome: related disorders but genes apart. *Annu Rev Genet.* 1997; 31:635–62.

16. de la Chapelle A, Peltomaki P. Genetics of hereditary colon cancer. *Annu Rev Genet.* 1995; 29:329–48.

17. Ionov Y, Peinado MA, Malkhosyan S, Shibata D, Perucho M. Ubiquitous somatic mutations in simple repeated sequences reveal a new mechanism for colonic carcinogenesis. *Nature.* 1993; 363:558–61.

18. Baccichet A, Benachenhou N, Couture F, Leclerc JM, Sinnett D. Microsatellite instability in childhood T cell acute lymphoblastic leukemia. *Leukemia.* 1997; 11:797–802.

19. Eshleman JR, Markowitz SD. Microsatellite instability in inherited and sporadic neoplasms. *Curr Opin Oncol.* 1995; 7:83–9.

20. Gartenhaus RB. Microsatellite instability in hematologic malignancies. *Leuk Lymphoma.* 1997; 25:455–61.

21. Benson JR, Wells K. Microsatellite instability and a TGF β receptor: clues to a growth control pathway. *Bioessays.* 1995; 17:1009–12.

22. Markowitz S, Wang J, Myeroff L, et al. Inactivation of the type II TGF-β receptor in colon cancer cells with microsatellite instability. *Science.* 1995; 268:1336–8.

23. Rampino N, Yamamoto H, Ionov Y, et al. Somatic frameshift mutations in the *BAX* gene in colon cancers of the microsatellite mutator phenotype. *Science.* 1997; 275:967–9.

24. Papadopoulos N, Nicolaides NC, Liu B, et al. Mutations of GTBP in genetically unstable cells. *Science.* 1995; 268:1915–7.

25. Nicolaides NC, Littman SJ, Modrich P, Kinzler KW, Vogelstein B. A naturally occurring *hPMS2* mutation can confer a dominant negative mutator phenotype. *Mol Cell Biol.* 1998; 18:1635–41.

26. Autexier C, Greider CW. Telomerase and cancer: revisiting the telomere hypothesis. *Trends Biochem Sci.* 1996; 21:387–91.

27. Greider CW. Telomerase activity, cell proliferation, and cancer. *Proc Natl Acad Sci USA* 1998; 95:90–2.

28. Greider CW. Telomere length regulation. *Annu Rev Biochem.* 1996; 65:337–65.

29. Harley CB, Sherwood SW. Telomerase, checkpoints and cancer. *Cancer Surv.* 1997; 29:263–84.

30. Greider CW, Blackburn EH. Identification of a specific telomere terminal transferase activity in *Tetrahymena* extracts. *Cell.* 1985; 43:405–13.

31. Hayflick L. The limited in vitro lifetime of human diploid strains. *Exp Cell Res* 1961; 25:614–36.

32. Harley CB, Futcher AB, Greider CW. Telomeres shorten during ageing of human fibroblasts. *Nature.* 1990; 345:458–60.

33. Morin GB. The human telomere terminal transferase enzyme is a ribonucleoprotein that synthesizes TTAGGG repeats. *Cell.* 1989; 59:521–29.

34. Kim NW, Piatyszek MA, Prowse KR, et al. Specific association of human telomerase activity with immortal cells and cancer. *Science.* 1994; 266:2011–5.

35. Shay JW, Bacchetti S. A survey of telomerase activity in human cancer. *Eur J Cancer.* 1997; 33:787–91.

36. Blasco MA, Funk W, Villeponteau B, Greider CW. Functional characterization and developmental regulation of mouse telomerase RNA. *Science.* 1995; 269:1267–70.

37. Feng J, Funk WD, Wang SS, et al. The RNA component of human telomerase. *Science.* 1995; 269:1236–41.

38. Blasco MA, Lee HW, Hande MP, et al. Telomere shortening and tumor formation by mouse cells lacking telomerase RNA. *Cell.* 1997; 91:25–34.

39. Collins K, Kobayashi R, Greider CW. Purification of *Tetrahymena* telomerase and cloning of genes encoding the two protein components of the enzyme. *Cell.* 1995; 81:677–86.

40. Harrington L, McPhail T, Mar V, et al. A mammalian telomerase-associated protein. *Science.* 1997; 275:973–77.

41. Nakamura TM, Morin GB, Chapman KB, et al. Telomerase catalytic subunit homologs from fission yeast and human. *Science.* 1997; 277:955–9.

42. Beattie TL, Zhou W, Robinson MO, Harrington L. Reconstitution of human telomerase activity in vitro. *Curr Biol.* 1998; 8:177–80.

43. Weinrich SL, Pruzan R, Ma L, et al. Reconstitution of human telomerase with the template RNA component hTR and the catalytic protein subunit hTRT. *Nat Genet.* 1997; 17:498–502.

44. Lendvay TS, Morris DK, Sah J, Balasubramanian B, Lundblad V. Senescence mutants of *Saccharomyces cerevisiae* with a defect in telomere replication identify three additional *EST* genes. *Genetics.* 1996; 144:1399–412.

45. Lingner J, Cech TR, Hughes TR, Lundblad V. Three ever shorter telomere (EST) genes are dispensable for in vitro yeast telomerase activity. *Proc Natl Acad Sci USA* 1997; 94:11190–5.

46. Lundblad V, Blackburn EH. RNA-dependent polymerase motifs in EST1: tentative identification of a protein component of an essential yeast telomerase. *Cell.* 1990; 60:529–30.

47. Lingner J, Hughes TR, Shevchenko A, Mann M, Lundblad V, Cech TR. Reverse transcriptase motifs in the catalytic subunit of telomerase. *Science.* 1997; 276:561–7.

48. Harrington L, Zhou W, McPhail T, et al. Human telomerase contains evolutionarily conserved catalytic and structural subunits. *Genes Dev.* 1997; 11:3109–15.

49. Kilian A, Bowtell DD, Abud HE, et al. Isolation of a candidate human telomerase catalytic subunit gene, which reveals complex splicing patterns in different cell types. *Hum Mol Genet.* 1997; 6:2011–9.

50. Meyerson M, Counter CM, Eaton EN, et al. hEST2, the putative human telomerase catalytic subunit gene, is up-regulated in tumor cells and during immortalization. *Cell.* 1997; 90: 785–95.

51. Nakayama J, Saito M, Nakamura H, Matsuura A, Ishikawa F. TLP1: a gene encoding a protein component of mammalian telomerase is a novel member of WD repeats family. *Cell.* 1997; 88:875–84.

52. Bodnar AG, Ouellette M, Frolkis M, et al. Extension of life-span by introduction of telomerase into normal human cells. *Science.* 1998; 279:349–52.

53. Vaziri H, Benchimol S. Reconstitution of telomerase activity in normal human cells leads to elongation of telomeres and extended replicative life span. *Curr Biol* 1998; 8:279–82.

54. Counter CM, Avilion AA, LeFeuvre CE, et al. Telomere shortening associated with chromosome instability is arrested in immortal cells which express telomerase activity. *EMBO J.* 1992; 11:1921–9.

55. Bryan TM, Reddel RR. Telomere dynamics and telomerase activity in in vitro immortalised human cells. *Eur J Cancer.* 1997; 33:767–73.

56. Lundblad V. The end replication problem: more than one solution. *Nat Med.* 1997; 3:1198–9.

11

Angiogenesis Switch Pathways

Jaume Piulats and Francesc Mitjans

Introduction

The ravages of cancer still seem to be far from being eradicated. This has led the scientific community to search for new approaches that could be used as therapeutic strategies. One of the most promising pharmacological interventions that has been proposed is the control of tumor neovascularization. The pioneering works of Folkman's group in the 1970s *(1–3)* established that solid tumors arc dependent on angiogenesis; this opened a new basis for therapy of cancer *(4,5)*.

The aim of this chapter is to provide a comprehensive and updated review of the current knowledge on tumor neovascularization mechanisms and of the current therapeutic approaches based on angiogenesis control.

Angiogenesis may be defined as the formation of new blood vessels from the existing vascular bed *(6)*, whereas the term *vasculogenesis* defines the development of the vasculature from structures in the early embryo *(7)*. Angiogenesis is a complex process mainly carried out by the extracellular matrix (ECM) and endothelial cells (EC), and is regulated by angiogenic factors: inducers and inhibitors. Physiological angiogenesis can be found in wound healing or in endometrium vascularization during the menstrual cycle. However, the sophisticated machinery of neovascularization is also an important component of many pathological processes such as cancer, atherosclerosis, psoriasis, diabetic retinopathy, and endometriosis. This chapter concentrates on the mechanisms that direct the switch to the angiogenic phenotype of tumors. Intimate knowledge of angiogenesis pathways in cancer can, alternatively, offer two advantages: the opportunity to establish the potential prognostic relevance of tumor angiogenesis in the evaluation of cancer disease, and the chance to discover new pharmaceutical targets for therapy of malignant neoplasia.

The angiogenesis switch pathways seem to be related, with a balance between positive and negative regulators of angiogenesis *(8)*. Among the positive angiogenic factors, is the important vascular endothelial growth factor (VEGF) (also known as vascular permeability factor, VPF), which fulfills the criteria of a "direct-acting" angiogenesis growth factor *(9)*; the main endogenous negative regulators are angiostatin *(10)* and thrombospondin *(11,12)*. Angiostatin is an angiogenesis inhibitor produced by the primary tumor that mediates the suppression of angiogenesis in its metastases *(8)*. This

From: *Principles of Molecular Oncology*
Edited by: M. H. Bronchud, M. A. Foote, W. P. Peters, and M. O. Robinson © Humana Press Inc., Totowa, NJ

role of angiostatin has demonstrated the influence of solid tumors on metastases *(10)*. A second negative regulator is thrombospondin, which seems to be up-regulated by wild-type *p53* and down-regulated during the switch to the angiogenic phenotype *(13,14)*. Folkman has proposed that the primary tumor producing both angiogenic stimulators and inhibitors could direct the evolution of the tumor depending on the blood levels of these mediators *(8)*.

This apparent simplicity masks more complex processes in which many additional factors are involved. The roles of vitronectin receptor (integrin αvβ3) and proteolytic enzymes (e.g., metalloproteinases) are emphasized in defining the angiogenesis pathways, owing to their pivotal role in the design of new therapeutic strategies *(15)*.

Although the antiangiogenic approach should be considered as an adjuvant therapy, clinical trials completed with many different compounds have not shown significant effects on tumor regression *(7)*. Nevertheless, a new wave of inhibitors is now being developed. A more immediate clinical application is the assessment of tumor angiogenesis as a prognostic marker in malignant neoplasia.

All these topics are reviewed in this chapter in an attempt to explain the complex phenomenon of tumor angiogenesis to the experimental and clinical oncologist. The next few years will be crucial for determining the practical application of pharmacological intervention to angiogenesis in the control of malignant growth.

Mechanisms of Tumor Neovascularization

It is now well established that a tumor is unable to grow larger than about 1 mm^3 without developing a new blood supply. Neovascularization is thus controlled by tumor cells, which may secrete angiogenic factors to attract ECs. The activated ECs, in turn, may also produce paracrine growth factors for the tumor. This crosstalk between tumor cells and ECs is one of the major features in angiogenesis. The second feature is the delicate equilibrium between the endogenous inducers and inhibitors of neovascularization (Fig. 1). Normal cells secrete low amounts of inducers and high amounts of inhibitors. However, when progressing to malignancy, the tumor cells tip this balance to an angiogenic phenotype.

Tumor Angiogenic Switch

The essential role of angiogenesis in tumor progression and metastasis and the balance between positive and negative regulatory factors lead to the idea of an angiogenic "switch" that is activated in tumor angiogenesis. Cells may switch to an angiogenic phenotype during progression toward tumorigenicity and this switch often takes place early, before tumorigenicity. In vivo switches develop angiogenesis in a graded fashion through several stages. In melanoma, for instance, a significant increase in vessel counts is first observed in the progression from benign to dysplastic nevi. A further increase in vessel counts from radial to vertical melanoma has been correlated with greater risk of recurrence, metastasis, and death. Similarly, angiogenesis in breast carcinoma is first noted in ductal carcinomas *in situ* (CIS), the angiogenic CIS being the stage before invasive carcinomas. In addition, transgenic mouse models have allowed researchers to study and define the angiogenic switch in early stages of tumor development preceding the appearance of solid tumors *(16,17)*. All of this suggests that activation of angiogenesis, the switching on, is a discrete event in tumor development.

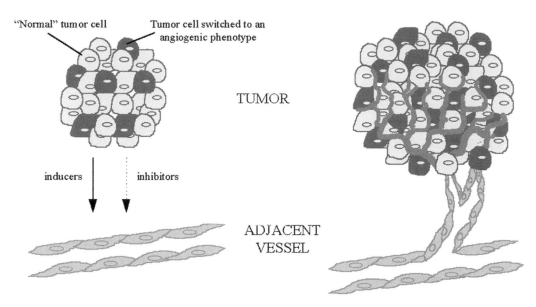

Fig. 1. Angiogenic switch. Some cells in the developing tumor switch to an angiogenic phenotype. The angiogenic cascade starts with the initiation phase in which angiogenic factors are released by tumor and accessory cells. The balance between the endogenous inducers and inhibitors is a key feature in angiogenesis. Endothelial cells, in response to angiogenic factors, proliferate and invade the stroma toward the tumor mass. During this step integrins and proteolytic enzymes play a capital role. Later phases lead to differentiation of the newly formed capillaries to mature vessels. The crosstalk between tumor and endothelial cells is the second key feature in angiogenesis.

Thus, it seems clear that changes in the balance between positive and negative signals mediate the angiogenic switch. A net balance of inhibitors over activators would maintain the switch in the "off" position, whereas a shift to an excess of activating stimuli would turn angiogenesis to the "on" position.

Endothelial Cells: Key Component in Angiogenesis

Most of the tumor vessels arise from the sprouting of new vessels from preexisting ones and are thus derived from normal, nonmalignant host cells. Although they are composed of normal cells, vessels elicited by tumors are frequently distinct from those in adjacent normal tissue: vessels elicted by tumors are leaky and abnormal in size and shape. ECs appear to be fenestrated; they also increase cell-adhesion molecules such as E-selectin *(18)* and specific integrins such as $\alpha v\beta 3$ *(19)*, essential for their viability during growth. It has been shown that microcapillary ECs from different organs exhibit a differential display of cell receptors, making it possible to target them by specific peptide sequences *(20)*. Activated ECs also release a variety of growth factors, such as basic fibroblast growth factor (bFGF), platelet-derived growth factor (PDGF), and insulin-like growth factor (IGF-1), that can both maintain EC activation and act as paracrine stimulators of tumor cells. They are also capable of producing a variety of factors that may inhibit tumor cell growth, such as interleukin (IL)-6, to which early-stage melanomas have been shown to be sensitive but to which late-stage melanomas are often resistant *(21,22)*.

It may be considered that angiogenesis generally occurs in at least three differentiated steps: induction–initiation, proliferation–invasion, and maturation–remodeling (Fig. 1). In the first stage, angiogenic inducers, such as growth factors or cytokines, are released both by the tumor cells themselves and by the accessory cells recruited to the site. These factors stimulate vascular-cell proliferation and invasion, thereby promoting blood vessel growth toward the tumor mass. One important result associated with cell invasion is that changes in the cell-adhesion molecules enable ECs to interact with the surrounding stroma wherever the EC is proliferating and invading. In turn, the adhesion molecule-mediated signaling ensures continued cell survival, proliferation, and invasion. Later phases of angiogenesis involve a halt in proliferation, cell differentiation, and both tubular structure and lumen formation leading to blood circulation. The basal lamina is modified and the newly formed blood vessel is surrounded by differentiated pericytes and smooth muscle cells *(22)*.

Inducers of Angiogenesis

A number of both in vitro and in vivo bioassays have been developed to mimic the complex process of angiogenesis, especially two in vitro assays in which either EC proliferation or EC migration is studied. Both assays are often complemented by the use of an in vivo assay, such as implants into the normally avascular cornea of rabbits or rodents, referred to as the corneal pocket assay. Using these assays, a number of inducers of angiogenesis have been identified, and these are briefly reviewed in this section.

Vascular Endothelial Growth Factor

VEGF can be considered as one of the capital angiogenic factors as it is the first factor produced during embryogenesis to control both vasculogenesis and angiogenesis *(23)*. Moreover, it is the only growth factor described to date whose −/− mice are not viable *(24,25)*. VEGF was first identified by its ability to elicit vascular permeability. Subsequently this factor was shown to be a mitogen for ECs and it has been described as a potent inducer of angiogenesis in vivo *(26)*. Three related endothelial growth factors, VEGF-B, VEGF-C, and VEGF-D, have also been identified *(27–29)*. VEGF is induced by hypoxia and hypoglycemia and binds to three specific receptors of the tyrosine kinase family (flk, flt-1, and flt-4) which may be up-regulated on tumor ECs *(30)*. In addition, the VEGF/VEGFR system is highly specific: although VEGF may be expressed by a number of cells, its receptors are expressed mainly by ECs. VEGF may be stored in the ECM as a heparin-binding protein bound to heparin sulfate proteoglycans. When angiogenesis is required, VEGF may be released from the ECM *(31)* or may be newly produced because its expression is often up-regulated in many tumor cells. Indeed, some oncogenes, such as mutated *ras*, have been found to transcriptionally activate the expression of VEGF *(32)*.

Fibroblast Growth Factors

Having at least nine forms, FGF constitutes a family of growth factors characterized by high-affinity binding to heparin; basic and acidic FGF forms have been most widely studied. They are unusual in that they lack the signal sequence for secretion; however, both may be released from cells in certain conditions. Both acidic and basic FGF bind receptors on ECs that are transmembrane tyrosine kinases, and are thus coupled through the signal-transduction cascade. There are at least four FGF receptors (FGFR1–4) that are widely expressed *(33)*. Like receptors, FGFs are also expressed in a number of tissues including tumors and ECs *(34)*. FGFs possess an extremely strong affinity for heparin and then they are sequestered in the ECM until proteolytic enzymes degrade ECM during angiogenesis. FGF is a potent mitogen and chemotactic factor for ECs. It also induces formation of capillary-like structures *(35)* and has shown angiogenic activities in vivo.

Transforming Growth Factor-β

TGF-β is a homodimeric polypeptide secreted in a biologically inactive, latent form. This form may be activated in vitro by heat, acidification, and proteases *(36)* providing a regulatory mechanism. TGF-β, similarly to tumor necrosis factor-α (TNF-α), affects ECs in two ways. It inhibits ECs in vitro but stimulates angiogenesis in vivo *(37)*. It has been proposed that TGF-β induces angiogenesis by an indirect mechanism: it is highly chemotactic for monocytes and other accessory cells that, in turn, release angiogenic factors that are mitogenic for ECs *(38)*. TGF-β and its receptors are expressed in many tissues but it seems that the differences in the response to TGF-β are attributable to differences in the surface expression of TGF-β receptors.

Tumor Necrosis Factor-α

TNF-α, a secreted protein synthesized primarily by activated macrophages and by some tumor cells *(39)*, was first described as causing solid tumor necrosis and regression. As described previously, TNF-α, like TGF-β, has paradoxical angiogenic activity. In vitro, TNF-α has an antiproliferative effect on ECs, whereas in vivo, it induces angiogenesis. However, the angiogenic activity in vivo is, in turn, also dual. When used at low concentrations, TNF-α induces angiogenesis: both vessel growth and EC proliferation. At high concentrations, TNF-α inhibits angiogenesis. Some authors *(40)* also suggested that the mode of delivery of TNF-α to ECs may play a role in their response.

Platelet-Derived Endothelial Growth Factor and Thymidine Phosphorylase

PDGF was first described in platelets as a new angiogenic factor. However, PDGF is not a mitogen for ECs, so the name is inappropriate *(41)*. When cloned and sequenced, the gene for human thymidine phosphorylase matched that of PDGF. Since then, many authors have described thymidine phosphorylase as an angiogenic enzyme. It is now known that the angiogenic molecule is not the enzyme by itself but rather the product of thymidine phosphorylase action on thymidine: 2-deoxy-D-ribose is mainly responsible for the angiogenic activity *(41)*. PDGF/thymidine phosphorylase is a particularly intriguing molecule to study: first, it is an angiogenic enzyme and not a classic growth factor; and second, its expression is exceptionally high in most solid tumors compared with expression in normal tissues.

Transforming Growth Factor-α and Epidermal Growth Factor

TGF-α and epidermal growth factor (EGF) share 40% homology and both bind to EGFR. TNF-α is expressed in macrophages and some tumor cells and, like EGF, it stimulates the proliferation of ECs in vitro. Both factors induce migration in vitro and capillary-like tube formation and angiogenesis in vivo *(42)*, although EGF is less potent.

Other Angiogenic Compounds

Finally, a number of other angiogenic molecules have been described, but in most cases the mechanism of action is not completely known or understood, or appears to be indirect. Angiogenin, for instance, a protein of the pancreatic ribonuclease family, is angiogenic in vivo but not in vitro *(43)*. ILs also play a role in inducing angiogenesis: IL-8 has been shown to potently stimulate angiogenesis *(44)*. Even some prostaglandins *(45)* and nicotinamide *(46)* have been reported to have angiogenic activity.

Cell-Adhesion Molecules and Angiogenesis

It is well established that cell-adhesion receptors mediate processes of cell adhesion, proliferation, migration, and invasion involved in the cascade of angiogenesis. As described earlier, angiogenesis not only depends on growth factors, but is also influenced by cell-adhesion molecules.

There are at least four different families of cell-adhesion receptors, classified depending on their biochemical and structural characteristics: the selectins, the immunoglobulin (IG) supergene family, the cadherins, and the integrins. Members of selectins, transmembrane receptors that mediate interaction to sialylated glycans, include P-selectin, L-selectin, and E-selectin. Furthermore, both P-selectin and E-selectin may also be expressed in a soluble form. P-selectin and E-selectin are up-regulated in ECs after exposure to inflammatory agents such as TNF-α, lipopolysaccharide (LPS), and IL-1β *(18)*. E-selectin is also expressed in proliferating ECs of the childhood hemangiomas (benign tumors composed of ECs). Supporting a possible functional role for E-selectin in angiogenesis, Koch and colleagues *(47)* have demonstrated that soluble E-selectin, although unable to induce EC proliferation in vitro, stimulated EC migration in vitro and angiogenesis in vivo. Nevertheless, E-selectin and P-selectin knockout mice showed no defects in blood vessel formation *(48)*.

Studies also implicate members of the Ig supergene family in angiogenic processes. These cell-adhesion molecules share the characteristic repetitive extracellular Ig-like domains and mediate heterophilic cell–cell adhesion *(49)*. Members of the family are ICAM-1, ICAM-2, ICAM-3, VCAM-1, and PECAM. Similarly to selectins, VCAM-1 and ICAM-1 can also be expressed as soluble forms. Whereas ICAM-2 and PECAM are highly expressed in both resting and activated ECs, ICAM-1 and VCAM-1 are up-regulated after stimulation with inflammatory cytokines such as IL-1, TNF-α, and interferon-γ (IFN-γ). ICAM-3 is highly expressed in tumor ECs but not in sites of inflammation *(50)*. However, as happens with selectins, there is only one member of Ig supergene family that could be clearly involved in angiogenesis. Soluble VCAM-1 is able to induce EC migration in vitro and angiogenesis in vivo *(47)* although, like soluble E-selectin, it is unable to induce EC proliferation *(47)*.

The cadherin family of cell–cell adhesion molecules, composed of E-cadherin, P-cadherin, L-cadherin, and VE-cadherin, are transmembrane proteins that mediate homophilic cell–cell adhesion in a calcium-dependent manner. Although there is no conclusive evidence involving cadherins in angiogenesis, low expression of N-cadherin has been described in ECs, and VE-cadherin has been shown to be specific for ECs *(51)*. Yet, cadherins could play a role in different stages of angiogenesis, as has been suggested *(52)*. The loss of cadherins, for instance, might promote increased invasion of activated ECs as shown for invasive tumor cells.

Integrins are heterodimeric transmembrane cell–ECM adhesion receptors composed of a β chain noncovalently associated with an α chain. At least 15 different α-subunits and 8 β-subunits have been identified that can combine to yield at least 20 different integrins. These combinations, in turn, define their cellular and adhesive specificities. Integrins predominantly mediate cell–ECM interactions, although some members may intervene in cell–cell adhesive events. Ligands for integrins include fibronectin, collagen, laminin, vitronectin, thrombospondin, fibrinogen, and others. Importantly, several integrins recognize the tripeptide sequence of Arg–Gly–Asp (RGD) within the ligands. In recent years, a growing body of evidence has suggested a critical role for integrin receptors in the regulation of angiogenesis and vascular development. For example, the ECM molecules that are ligands for integrins are abundant in the surrounding vascular matrix and subendothelial basement membrane of blood vessels. This situation leads to inevitable changes in the integrin repertoire of new vessels, thus providing evidence of the importance of integrins in angiogenesis. ECs express members of the β1, β3, and β5 subfamilies, and stimulation of these cells with bFGF in vitro causes increased expression of β1 and β3 integrins. In vitro experiments have also demonstrated the involvement of α6β1 (laminin receptor) in endothelial cord formation but not in capillary lumen formation, which seems to need the participation of α2β1 integrin *(53)*. Recently, α1β1 and α2β1 integrins have been involved in angiogenesis through an up-regulation promoted by VEGF *(54)*. Notwithstanding, integrin function during blood vessel formation in vivo has been studied most extensively for αvβ3.

The integrin αvβ3, also named the vitronectin receptor (VNR), is minimally expressed in quiescent blood vessels, but it is highly up-regulated after stimulation by either angiogenic growth factors or tumors *(19)*. Enenstein and colleagues reported that αv integrins were highly expressed on the tips of sprouting angiogenic blood vessels *(55)*. In vitro, both antibodies (Abs) against αv, β3, and αvβ3 and synthetic RGD-containing peptides affected microvessel outgrowth from rat aorta rings embedded in fibrin gels *(56–58)* and endothelial cord formation *(59,60)*. Furthermore, Abs and cyclic-RGD peptides, used in vivo as antagonists of αvβ3, blocked angiogenesis induced by cytokines and solid human tumors in several models, such as the chick chorioallantoic membrane (CAM) *(61)*, rabbit cornea *(62)*, mouse retina *(63)*, nude mice *(64)*, and human skin–severe combined immunodeficiency (SCID) mouse chimeras *(65)*.

Role of the Vitronectin Receptor in Angiogenesis

Integrin αvβ3 (VNR) can be considered as the most promiscuous member of the integrin family. It may recognize any of the following ligands: vitronectin, fibronectin, fibrinogen, laminin, collagen, von Willebrand's factor, osteopontin, thrombospontin, tenascin, adenovirus pentone base, bone sialoprotein, and MMP2, as well as other RGD-containing proteins. This feature confers to any αvβ3 expressing cell the ability to adhere to, migrate on, and respond to almost any environment it may encounter *(66)*. As noted previously, VNR has low expression in normal tissues but is up-regulated in activated ECs. In addition, αvβ3 is also expressed in some invasive tumors such as late-stage glioblastomas *(67)* and malignant melanomas *(68)*. Interestingly, αvβ3 overexpression has been well correlated with the degree of malignancy and invasion in melanomas. Although normal melanocytes and nevi, as well as noninvasive radial growth phase (RGP) melanomas, are negative for αvβ3 expression, both invasive vertical growth phase (VGP) and metastatic melanomas are highly positive *(69)*. Indeed, this differential expression has been proposed as a prognostic factor *(70)*. Furthermore, other authors have studied, on the basis of experimental models, the use of the integrin αvβ3 as a therapeutic target in melanoma lesions *(71,72)* (Fig. 2).

The highly restricted αvβ3 expression and its up-regulation during neovascularization suggests that it may have a functional role in angiogenesis. Thus, antagonists of αvβ3 (both monoclonal antibodies [mAbs] and cyclic RGD-containing peptides) prevented blood vessel formation in a number of in vitro and in vivo models of angiogenesis *(19,59–65)*. Interestingly, a related integrin, αvβ5, is also involved in angiogenesis. In an elegant study using the rabbit corneal model, Friedlander and colleagues *(62)* showed that antagonists of αvβ3 integrin inhibited angiogenesis induced by βFGF, but had little if any effect on VEGF-induced angiogenesis. In contrast, antagonists of αvβ3 integrin were able to block VEGF-induced but not bFGF-induced, angiogenesis. Most importantly, antagonists of αv integrins inhibited both cytokine-induced and tumor-induced angiogenesis. These findings define two distinct pathways leading to angiogenesis depending on the particular αv integrin involved. Studies have elucidated the possible mechanisms by which αvβ3 antagonists inhibit angiogenesis. Both mAbs and cyclic-RGD peptides selectively induce programmed cell death (apoptosis) in angiogenically activated ECs in vivo. First, Montgomery and co-workers showed that αvβ3 provides survival signals when it interacts with denatured collagen *(73)*. Subsequent studies demonstrated that systemic administration of αvβ3 antagonists promotes apoptosis in developing, but not in resting, blood vessels *(61,74)*. Much more recently our studies proved that αv antagonists also induce apoptosis in growing αvβ3 positive human melanomas independently of their antiangiogenic activity *(75)*. All these results support the hypothesis of a key role of the αvβ3 integrin in angiogenesis. However, there are at least two controversial situations that reveal the need of further investigations in this field. Patients with Glanzmann thrombasthenia lack the β3 subunit and are defective for αvβ3 integrin. Therefore, although they have normal blood vessels, their wound repair function is severely compromised *(76)*. Such patients might develop blood vessels by an alternative mechanism involving αvβ5 integrin. Second, some αv knockout mice not only survive a short time after birth but also have normal blood vessels in most organs (lungs, for instance) *(77)*. Nevertheless, these animals develop cerebral hemorrhage, thus suggesting abnormalities in brain blood vessel development. This differential behavior may be explained by the fact that vessels of tissues of mesodermal origin (lungs) are formed by vasculogenesis (which does not depend on αvβ3) while vessels of tissues of endodermal origin (brain) are formed by angiogenesis (which does depend on αvβ3) *(22)*.

Proteases

Angiogenesis is not only regulated by the action of growth factors and cell-adhesion molecules but is also influenced by many other molecules. Among them, enzymes that degrade the ECM provide a suitable environment for EC migration through the adjacent stroma. There are at least three main families of proteolytic enzymes that could play

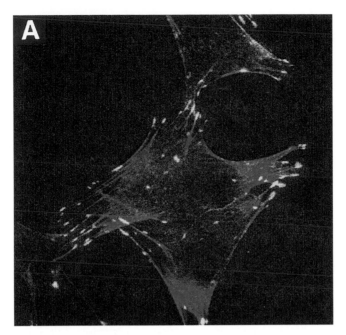

Fig. 2(a). Confocal image of human melanoma cells stained with the anti-αv integrin mAb 17E6. Secondary Ab is FITC-labeled and actin is visualized using Phalloidine-TRICT. Note the focal contact staining with 17E6. For further information *see text* and ref. *71*.

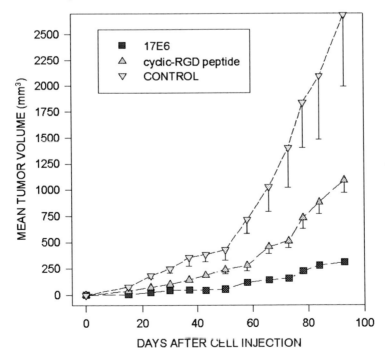

Fig. 2(b). M21 human melanoma cells were subcutaneously injected on nude mice. Therapeutic drugs were mAb 17E6 and cyclic-RGD peptide. mAb 17E6 was administered at days 0, 32, 39, 46, and 53. Peptide was injected daily. For further details *see text* and refs. *71* and *75*.

a role in angiogenesis and tumor progression: the serine proteases (including urokinase plasminogen activator, uPA), the matrix metalloproteases (MMPs), and the cysteine proteases (cathepsins B and L) *(78)*. Expression of uPA receptor (uPAR) on ECs, for instance, is increased by tumor-cell-conditioned medium *(79)* and VEGF *(80)*. In addition, uPAR in conjunction with integrins *(81)* could direct proteolysis at the leading edge of migrating ECs. uPAR up regulation thus is a pivotal feature in angiogenic processes. Furthermore, antagonists of uPAR showed antiangiogenic activity both in vitro and in vivo *(82)*, although uPA knockout mice have normal angiogenesis *(83)*. uPA could also be indirectly involved in angiogenesis regulation. Studies from Folkman's laboratory showed that a fragment of plasminogen (angiostatin) acts as an endogenous inhibitor of angiogenesis *(10)*. Other workers have suggested that either uPA *(84)*, macrophage metalloelastase *(85)*, pancreas elastase, or even metalloproteinases *(86)* could be the enzymes responsible for the generation of angiostatin.

MMPs form a family of zinc-dependent endopeptidases with a broad spectrum of activity and are secreted as inactive zymogens *(78)*. They may be classified as collagenases, gelatinases, and stromelysins depending on their substrate specificity. MMP overexpression may be detected in tumor tissue or in adjacent stroma but not in surrounding normal tissue *(87,88)*. Similarly, in vitro MMP overexpression in ECs was described after bFGF or TNF-α stimulation *(89)*. Both natural inhibitors, known as tissue inhibitors of MMP (TIMP), and synthetic inhibitors of MMP have been described as potential antiangiogenic and antimetastatic drugs. TIMP were active in blocking lung colonization by tumor cells and angiogenesis in vivo. The MMP inhibitor batimastat was able to inhibit angiogenesis *(90)* as well as tumor growth *(91)* in experimental models. Recently, MMP2 has been colocalized with $\alpha v \beta 3$ in activated ECs in vivo *(92)*, supporting the importance of both molecules in angiogenesis. Recently, a new family of MMP, in which members exhibit a transmembrane domain, has been discovered. These membrane-type MMPs (MT-MMPs) are able to bind inactive gelatinases, such as MMP2, mediating their activation and focusing on the proteolytic activity *(93)*.

Inhibitors of Angiogenesis

A variety of molecules produced by normal mammalian cells can inhibit angiogenesis, but they represent only about one-quarter of all known inhibitors. Most inhibitors produced by mammalian cells are effective in the form in which they are secreted (e.g., thrombospondin) but some are proteolytic products of the extracellular cleavage of molecules that are angiogenically inactive when intact: examples are angiostatin *(10)* and endostatin *(94)*. Others are synthetic compounds with antiangiogenic activity in one or many angiogenesis models. Of the approx 200 compounds with antiangiogenic activity described to date, the most representative are discussed. Additional information can be obtained in recent reviews *(95,96)*.

The amount of thrombospondin, an ECM component, is lower in human breast cell lines than in control or in immortal rat tracheal epithelial cells compared with primary cells. Thrombospondin is also down-regulated when normal human fibroblasts immortalize as a result of loss of p53. In those cases, the decrease in thrombospondin shifts the phenotype of the cells from antiangiogenic to angiogenic *(97)*. As thrombospondin can also inhibit in vivo angiogenesis, it may be considered as an angiogenesis inhibitor.

Folkman's group discovered two new endogenous angiogenesis inhibitors, namely angiostatin and endostatin. They belong to a new family of antiangiogenic agents produced from the cleavage of natural nonangiogenic molecules. The first to be described was angiostatin *(10)*. It is derived from plasminogen, and the fragment, not the whole plasminogen, has an antiproliferative effect on ECs in vitro, blockades neovascularization in vivo, and prevents the growth of primary tumor as well as metastases *(10,98)*. Interestingly, angiostatin has no detectable direct effect on tumor cells. Although a number of researchers have investigated the mechanism by which the primary tumor produces angiostatin from plasminogen *(84–86)*, the mechanism of action of angiostatin remains unknown. The second molecule is endostatin, a proteolytic fragment of collagen XVIII *(94)*. Endostatin has similar activity to angiostatin: it may block endothelial proliferation in vitro as well as primary tumor growth. Again, tumor cells were not directly affected by the compound.

Many other molecules have been proposed as antiangiogenic and they are currently under active investigation or even in clinical trials. IFN-γ, for instance, was shown to inhibit both EC proliferation and angiogenesis in vitro. Furthermore it had a dramatic effect in the treatment of hemangioendotheliomas. It is assumed to function through modulation of the FGFR. Another class of newly discovered angiogenesis inhibitors derived from fumagillin, an antibiotic purified from fungal cultures, inhibit EC proliferation in vitro. To avoid toxic effects of the parent compound, AGM-1470/TNP-470, a synthetic analog with enhanced antiangiogenic activity, has been synthesized *(99)* and is being tested in clinical trials. Protamine, a cationic protein derived from sperm, was also shown to be a specific inhibitor of angiogenesis, probably by interfering with growth factors. Platelet factor-IV, released from platelets during aggregation, is able to inhibit the growth of solid tumors when used as a recombinant protein. A series of corticosteroids tested in a number of animal models in conjunction with heparin showed effective antiangiogenic activity. They have been termed "angiostatic steroids." Some inhibitors of the signal transduction from the angiogenic factor receptors, such as genistein or herbimycin, are also being investigated as angiogenic inhibitors *(100)*. Even additional natural compounds, such as extracts from avascular tissues, have been proved to be antiangiogenic. Moses and co-workers, for instance, identified an inhibitor of neovascularization from cartilage *(101)*.

Prognostic Value of Angiogenesis

As early as 1972, Folkman et al. *(102)* developed a microscopic angiogenesis grading system with which to quantify the tumor angiogenesis. The goal was to establish an objective method for measuring the tumor vasculature and its relationship with the clinical parameters of the disease. This entailed the search for a useful angiogenic index, not only for its prognostic value, but also for its ability to stratify patients for therapy *(103)*. The first results obtained by several groups showed a high level of variation related with the sample selection and interobserver and intraobserver variation, due to the limited experience in vessel counting and the specificity of the marker used. These limitations delayed the achievement of their goal. Nevertheless, 20 yr later it was demonstrated in breast cancer that microvessel density was an independent prognostic marker for both relapse-free and overall survival. These studies were done using factor VIII to identify the endothelium and established criteria for microvessel assessment *(103–106)*.

Because the reproducibility of the method is poor, several improvements have been proposed. Fox et al. *(107)* proposed a counting system using a microscope eyepiece grid. Other groups are testing more sensitive endothelial markers, such as CD31 or CD34. Kawaguchi et al. *(108)* examined the correlation between tumor angiogenesis and prognosis of lung adenocarcinoma (T1NOMO) using a mAb to CD31, and they showed that microvessel count may be a major prognostic factor and a useful tool to predict recurrence in patients with lung adenocarcinoma. CD34 has also been used successfully on samples from patients with ovarian cancer *(109)*, gastric carcinomas *(110)*, and malignant mesotheliomas *(111)*.

Vermeulen et al. *(112)* proposed the standardization of angiogenic quantification to reduce interlaboratory variability and to confirm the prognostic value of intramural microvessel density (IMD) in solid tumors. This study proposed a detailed standard immunostaining (CD-31 marker) method for IMD assessment and predicted the increased role of serum levels of angiogenic factors (βFGF, VEGF) as markers of tumor progression. Moreover, new specific markers for activated endothelium (e.g., Abs to endoglin [CD105] and integrins) are being studied to verify whether the ratio of activated/quiescent ECs could add prognostic information to IMD assessment.

Other investigators have demonstrated the positive correlation between the tumor neovascularization assessed by immunohistochemical (IHC) staining with anti-CD31 Ab and VEGF mRNA expression in breast tumors *(113)*. Further studies have shown the direct relationship between VEGF expression and tumor angiogenesis in cervical intraepithelial neoplasia and head and neck squamous cell carcinoma (HNSCC) *(114,115)*. These reports are consistent with previous studies that reported the association of VEGF expression with early relapse in bladder carcinomas and its use as an independent prognostic marker in breast carcinomas *(116,117)*.

Despite the discrepancies observed in the literature, owing mainly to the criteria used for microvessel counting, the results seem to demonstrate a significant correlation between high tumor neovascularization and a reduction in patient survival. The definitive angiogenic index may turn out to be a multiparametric factor instead of a single histological measure of microvessel density in tumor tissue.

Therapeutic Approaches

As described previously, angiogenesis is a complex multistep process in which many potential key points might be susceptible to therapeutic intervention. Our current knowledge on the paracrine interaction between tumor and ECs allows us to define specific targets for therapy. These include endothelial mitogens released by tumor cells; tumor growth factors secreted by ECs; proteases released by both populations for degrading the local stroma; and the pivotal role of some integrins, such as αvβ3 and αvβ5, in EC proliferation and migration. Finally, the natural endogenous angiogenesis inhibitors all contribute to neovascularization and are, therefore, potential targets for pharmacological modulation.

The theoretical advantages of antiangiogenic therapy would include the expected low toxicity of the specific antiangiogenic agents due to the slow turnover rate of the ECs in normal tissues compared with the turnover of cells involved in tumor angiogenesis; the

Table 1
Antiangiogenic Therapy

Strategy	Agents
Inhibition of EC proliferation / migration	TNP-470, angiostatin, endostatin linomide, genistein, IFNs, suramin, Abs against angiogenic growth factors or their receptors, thrombospondin, angiostatic steroids
Inhibition of proteolytic enzymes	TIMPS, metalloproteinase inhibitors (batimastat, marimastat), cartilage-derived inhibitors, plasminogen activator inhibitors, minocycline, tetracycline
Inhibition of cell tube formation and induction of apoptosis	$\alpha v \beta 3$ integrin antagonists: vitaxin, 17E6, cyclic-RGD peptides, mimetics, IFNs, angiostatin, endostatin

For further information see text and ref. *15.*

reduction of the risk of developing drug resistance because of the stability of the EC genome; and the dual effect of the therapy when the target chosen is expressed by both tumor cells and ECs (e.g., MMP, $\alpha v \beta 3$ expression on melanoma and ECs).

The current preclinical and clinical research can be summarized: inhibition of EC proliferation/migration; inhibition of the proteolytic enzymes involved in the ECM degradation; and inhibition of cell tube formation and induction of apoptosis. Table 1 summarizes these approaches and the agents involved. For a detailed review of the antiangiogenic compounds, see the recent review of Kuiper et al. *(118).*

Inhibition of Endothelial Cell Proliferation/Migration

The most important representatives of the inhibition of EC proliferation and migration are TNP-470 and carboxyamidotriazole (CAI). TNP-470 is an analog of fumagillin, a naturally occurring antibiotic produced by the fungus *Aspergillus fumigatus*. The antiproliferative mechanism of TNP-470 in EC is unknown, but it appears to affect the late G_1 phase of the cell cycle, inducing an arrest by a potential inactivation of cyclin-dependent kinases (CDK), which phosphorylate the retinoblastoma (Rb) protein. TNP-470 has been tested in phase 1 trials in patients with refractory solid tumors and in AIDS (acquired immunodeficiency syndrome) patients with Kaposi's sarcoma. Phase 2 trials in a variety of tumors and phase 3 trials in pancreatic cancer are currently underway *(119).* Recently, it has been shown that TNP-470 up-regulates the expression of prostate-specific antigen (PSA) in patients with androgen-independent prostate cancer, making clinical use of this marker a problem *(120).* Carboxyamidotriazole (CAI) inhibits the influx of calcium into cells and inhibits tumor growth and angiogenesis. At present, this compound is being tested in phase 1 trials *(121).*

Since VEGF emerged as a key growth factor in angiogenesis, several therapeutic approaches have attempted to inhibit angiogenesis by blocking either VEGF, VEGFR, or the signaling induced by VEGF–VEGFR interaction. Thus, high-affinity mAbs against VEGF were used in models of tumor growth in vivo. Such Abs were found to exert a potent inhibitory effect on the growth of at least three different human tumor cell lines in vivo *(122)* without affecting the growth of the tumor cells in vitro. Further studies showed the efficacy of this strategy in distinct in vivo models *(123,124)*. Similar therapeutic approaches were conducted by Millauer and co-workers, who focused on the receptor instead of the growth factor *(125)*. In an elegant study, dominant negative receptors (flk-1) were delivered to the endothelium by retrovirus, to inhibit the growth of glioblastoma multiforme and other tumors in vivo *(125,126)*. However, while the VEGF therapeutic approach seems to be effective, the FGF approach is not as clear. Abs to FGF or its receptors showed confusing results *(127)*, indicating that further studies are needed. Finally, suramin, a polyanion that disrupts binding of FGFs to their receptors, has also been used in murine models with promising results, and is being studied in phase 1 trials *(128)*.

This approach could also include the known endogenous inhibitors of angiogenesis, such as angiostatin and endostatin, although they are not yet available for clinical research. These compounds not only inhibit angiogenesis, but also maintain sustained dormancy of tumors and metastasis by means of an increase in the apoptotic rate in tumor cells *(129,130)*. Importantly, experimental antiangiogenic therapy using endostatin revealed no acquired drug resistance *(131)* in contrast to standard chemotherapy. This work has caused new expectancies, and concerns for an antiangiogenic therapy in cancer have increased since its publication. Folkman's group has proposed a novel antiangiogenic gene therapy with either angiostatin, endostatin, or a fusion protein of both molecules *(132,133)*. Again, the antiangiogenic therapy showed antitumor effects through the maintenance of the dormant status in micrometastasis *(132)*. Although it is thought that angiostatin and endostatin will be used in clinical trials soon, nothing is known about the possible effect of these endogenous compounds in humans. Nevertheless, angiostatin and endostatin have achieved some of the more promising preclinical data in the field of antiangiogenic therapy.

Inhibition of the Proteolytic Enzymes

Proteinase inhibitors can block proteolytic activity of both activated ECs and migrating tumor cells. Both natural inhibitors (TIMP) and synthetic inhibitors of MMP have been described as potential antiangiogenic, as well as antimetastatic, drugs. However, the most exciting progress has been made in the field of synthetic inhibitors of MMP.

The first generation of synthetic MMP inhibitors is represented by the compounds known as galardin and batismastat *(90)*. Both agents showed a poor oral bioavailability, but batismastat was entered into phase 1 clinical trials using the intraperitoneal route in patients with malignant ascites, or the intrapleural route in patients with malignant pleural effusions. A new generation of orally active MMP inhibitors includes the compound marimastat, which has already been tested in phase 2 clinical trials with 232 patients *(134)*. The oral bioavailability is very good and the main side effects observed were myalgias and arthralgias of unknown origin. At present, several phase 2 and 3 trials are underway *(135)*.

Inhibition of Cell Tube Formation and Induction of Apoptosis

A third approach aims to disrupt the vessel formation and to induce EC apoptosis. The main agents for this mechanism of action are the inhibitors of $\alpha v \beta 3$ integrin. Antagonists of $\alpha v \beta 3$ prevent blood vessel formation in a number of in vitro and in

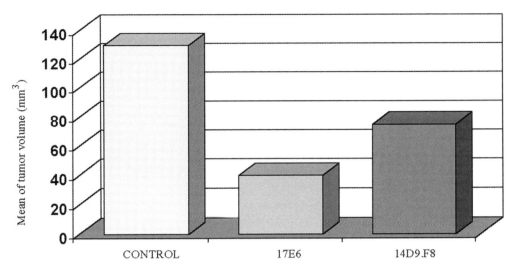

Fig. 3. Normal human skin was grafted onto SCID mice. After wound healing, M21-L human melanoma cells (negative for αvβ3) were intradermically injected into the human dermis. Therapeutic drugs were mAbs 17E6 and 14D9.F8 (anti-αv). For further details *see text* and refs. *71* and *75*.

vivo models of angiogenesis *(19,56,65)*. This angiogenesis blockade also results in tumor-growth modulation and, eventually, in a regression of preexisting αvβ3-negative human tumors *(61,64)*. Moreover, owing to the lack of expression of αvβ3 in quiescent vasculature, the antagonists do not affect normal blood vessels and are unlikely to cause toxic or side effects. Most of these studies were done using either a mAb directed to the αvβ3 heterodimer, LM609 *(65)*; a mAb directed to the αv subunit, 17E6 *(71,75, and our unpublished observations)* and thus recognizing both αvβ3 and αvβ 5 *(62)*; or cyclic pentapeptides or heptapeptides containing the adhesive RGD sequence *(63)*. In particular, the use of low-molecular-weight molecules such as cyclic-RGD peptides is of great interest both because of the relative ease with which they reach the tumor vessels and because they are synthetic compounds with low production cost.

Some investigators have followed a mixed approach to obtain novel antagonists of the VNR. Using phage display technology, several groups have created libraries of single-chain Abs with loops containing heptapeptides *(136,137)*. In this way, highly active new sequences were identified. Furthermore, those constructions, when tested in vivo, were targeted to the tumor blood vessels *(20)*. LM609 has been humanized (vitaxin) and clinical trials are ongoing *(118)*. Our group has developed the aforementioned anti-αv 17E6 mAb as well as cyclic-RGD peptides, which have shown a potent inhibition of both αvβ3 and αvβ 5 targets *(71,75,138)* (Fig. 3). The preclinical research done on both compounds has confirmed their effectiveness as antiangiogenic agents. The cyclic-RGD peptide was scheduled to enter phase 1 trials during 1998, but meanwhile, a new generation of synthetic mimetics are currently being investigated.

Conclusion

The progression to malignancy and the establishment of metastasis clearly depends on the induction of neovascularization. In other words, cells in a developing tumor

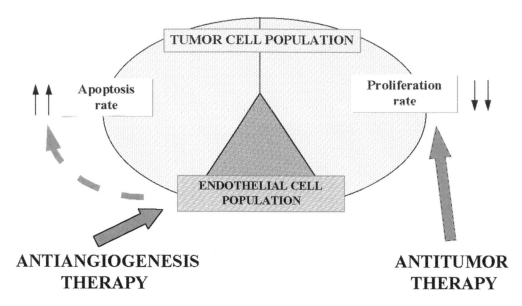

Fig. 4. Model of combined therapy. Within a tumor two compartments may be distinguished: the tumor cell population and the EC population. An antitumor therapy (affecting the proliferative rate of tumor cells) combined with an antiangiogenic therapy (affecting both the EC population and the apoptosis rate of the tumor cell population; *see text*) would lead to a more effective anticancer global therapy. (Modified from ref. *141*.)

will progress only if they acquire the angiogenic phenotype necessary to attract the new vessels on which their survival depends. This chapter reviewed the distinct pathways involved in such a process, referred as the angiogenic switch. One key step is undoubtedly the delicate balance between natural inducers and inhibitors of angiogenesis. The tipping of this balance toward one or the other side would favor the inhibition of angiogenesis or the promotion of neovascularization. Current antiangiogenesis research is engaged in the pursuit of novel, potent inhibitors that may lead to new therapeutic drugs for cancer treatment.

The preliminary clinical research with the first generation of antiangiogenic agents may establish whether this approach can soon lead to an adjuvant treatment for controlling residual cancer. Antiangiogenic therapy would enhance the action of the classic cytotoxic chemotherapy in patients with cancer due to the action on the two cell compartments within a tumor: endothelial and tumor cell populations *(139,140)* (Fig. 4). Therefore, this approach may mimic the endogenous inhibitors of angiogenesis, such as angiostatin, maintaining tumor dormancy. Consequently, this therapy could facilitate a strategy useful in the treatment of cancer in a similar way to the treatment of diabetes and AIDS.

Note Added in Proof

During the production of this book, there have been important findings and advances in the field of tumor angiogenesis. Just as a note, a Medline search within the last year generated around a quarter of the total (10 years) references containing the word angiogenesis. Such a large amount of information would itself fill a new chapter on angiogenesis and, of course, this is far beyond the scope of this section. Here, we will summarize and update the latest important findings in the field of tumor angiogenesis. As antiangiogenesis therapy is our main goal, we focused only on work that could be translated to therapy approaches. This, by no means, indicates a lack of appreciation for the rest of the topics.

Previous work has already suggested a role of cyclooxigenases (COX) in angiogenesis *(142,143)*. However, a step in the definition of new potential targets has been the identification of thomboxane A2 (a COX-2 product) as a critical intermediary of angiogenesis *(144)*. Thus, the antithrombotic agents acquire a new protagonism as putative antiangiogenic drugs.

One of the recently elucidated ligand/receptor systems involved in angiogenesis is the angiopoietins and the transmembrane endothelial receptor tyrosine kinase Tie2 *(145)*. In this way, it is important to note the significant tumor growth inhibition achieved in mice models by means of adenoviral delivery of a recombinant Tie2 receptor *(146)*. Similar results in terms of tumor growth inhibition in vivo were obtained by other authors *(147)*. This time, an ex vivo gene therapy method was used to transfect cells with a soluble form of Flt-1, a receptor for VEGF. Those experiments also put tumor angiogenesis as an important goal for gene therapy *(148,149)*. Also some of the new and most exciting antiangiogenic molecules, angiostatin *(150)* and endostatin *(151)*, have been used in vivo in antiangiogenic gene therapy experiments *(148,152)*. Furthermore, work with those two proteins begins to elucidate the mechanism by which they act as antiangiogenic compounds *(153,154)*. Angiostatin, for instance, has been shown to bind ATP synthase on the surface of human ECs *(155)*. Moreover, it seems that angiostatin is not selectively acting in endothelial cells since it also binds smooth muscle cells blocking their proliferation and migration in vitro *(156)*. However, one of the most intriguing results indicates that tumor cells themselves could form their own blood vessels by a mechanism called vasculogenic mimicry, just molding tumor cells into vascular channels *(157)*. This opens the door to new unsuspected *antiangiogenic* therapies.

Acknowledgments

We appreciate the helpful comments and criticisms of this manuscript by Dr. Angels Fabra and Dr. Simon Goodman. We also wish to thank all the members of our laboratory for their fruitful comments and especially C. Calvis for her experimental work. We thank Susanna Castel from Serveis Cientifico-Tecnics (University of Barcelona) for her assistance in confocal microscopy. The authors also thank Robin Rycroft for his expert editorial help.

References

1. Folkman J, Long DM, Becker FF. Growth and metastasis of tumors in organ culture. *Cancer.* 1963; 16:453–67.
2. Gimbrone MA Jr, Leapman S, Cotran RS, Folkman J. Tumor angiogenesis: iris neovascularization at a distance from experimental intraocular tumours. *J Natl Cancer Inst.* 1973; 50:219–28.

3. Gimbrone MA Jr, Leapman SB, Cotran RS, Folkman J. Tumor dormancy in vivo by prevention of neovascularization. *J Exp Med.* 1972; 136:261–76.

4. Folkman J. Anti-angiogenesis: new concept for therapy of solid tumors. *Ann Surg.* 1972; 175:409–16.

5. Folkman J. What is the evidence that tumors are angiogenesis dependent? *J Natl Cancer Inst.* 1990; 82:4–6.

6. Fox B, Gather CK, Harris LA. Tumour angiogenesis. *J Pathol.* 1996; 179:232–7.

7. Bicknell R, Lewis CE, Ferrara N. *Tumor Angiogenesis*, Oxford University Press, Oxford, New York, 1997.

8. Folkman J. New perspectives in clinical oncology from angiogenesis research. *Eur J Cancer.* 1996; 14:2534–9.

9. Rak J, Kerbel RS. Treating cancer by inhibiting angiogenesis: new hopes and potential pitfalls. *Cancer and Metastasis Reviews.* 1996; 15:231–6.

10. O'Reilly MS, Holmgren L, Shing Y, et al. Angiostatin: a novel angiogenesis inhibitor that mediates the suppression of metastases by a Lewis lung carcinoma. *Cell.* 1994, 79:315–28.

11. Good DJ, Polverini PJ, Rastinejad F, et al. A tumor suppressor-dependent inhibitor of angiogenesis is immunologically and functionally indistinguishable from a fragment of thrombospondin. *Proc Natl Acad Sci USA.* 1990; 87:6624–8.

12. DiPietro LA. Thrombospondin as a regulator of angiogenesis. *EXS.* 1997; 79:295–314.

13. Rastinejad F, Polverini P, Bouck NP. Regulation of the activity of a new inhibitor of angiogenesis by a cancer suppressor gene. *Cell.* 1989; 56:345–55.

14. Dameron KM, Volpert OV, Tainsky MA, Bouck N. Control of angiogenesis in fibroblasts by p53 regulation of thrombospondin-1. *Science.* 1994; 265:1582–4.

15. Gasparini G. Angiogenesis research up to 1996. A commentary on the state of art and suggestions for future studies. *Eur J Cancer.* 1996; 32A:2379–85.

16. Hanahan D, Christofori G, Naik P, Arbeit J. Transgenic mouse models of tumour angiogenesis: the angiogenic switch, its molecular controls, and prospects for preclinical therapeutic models. *Eur J Cancer.* 1996; 32A(14):2386–93.

17. Hanahan D, Folkman J. Patterns and emerging mechanisms of the angiogenic switch during tumorigenesis. *Cell.* 1996; 86(3):353–64.

18. Gotsch U, Jager U, Dominis M, Vestweber D. Expression of P-selectin on endothelial cells is upregulated by LPS and TNF-α in vivo. *Cell Adhes Commun.* 1994; 2:7–14.

19. Brooks PC, Clark RA, Cheresh DA. Requirement of vascular integrin $\alpha v\beta 3$ for angiogenesis. *Science.* 1994; 264:569–71.

20. Pasqualini R, Koivunen E, Ruoslahti E. αv integrins as receptors for tumor targeting by circulating ligands. *Nat Biotechnol.* 1997; 15:542–6.

21. Rak JW, Hegmann EJ, Lu C, Kerbel RS. Progressive loss of sensitivity to endothclium-derived growth inhibitors expressed by human melanoma cells during disease progression. *J Cell Physiol.* 1994; 159:245–55.

22. Risau W. Mechanisms of angiogenesis. *Nature.* 1997; 386:671–4.

23. Jakeman LB, Armanini M, Phillips HS, Ferrara N. Developmental expression of binding sites and messenger ribonucleic acid for vascular endothelial growth factor suggests a role for this protein in vasculogenesis and angiogenesis. *Endocrinology* 1993; 133:848–59.

24. Carmeliet P, Schoonjans L, Kieckens L, et al. Physiological consequences of loss of plasminogen activator gene function in mice. *Nature.* 1994; 368:419–24.

25. Ferrara N, Carver-Moore K, Chen H, et al. Heterozygous embryonic lethality induced by targeted inactivation of the *VEGF* gene. *Nature.* 1996; 380:439–42.

26. Senger DR, Van de Water L, Brown LF, et al. Vascular permeability factor (VPF, VEGF) in tumor biology. *Cancer Metastas Rev.* 1993; 12:303–24.

27. Olofsson B, Pajusola K, Kaipainen A, et al. Vascular endothelial growth factor B, a novel growth factor for endothelial cells. *Proc Natl Acad Sci USA.* 1996; 93:2576–81.

28. Joukov V, Pajusola K, Kaipainen A, et al. A novel vascular endothelial growth factor, VEGF-C, is a ligand for the Flt4 (VEGFR-3) and KDR (VEGFR-2) receptor tyrosine kinases. *EMBO J.* 1996; 15:290–8.

29. Achen MG, Jeltsch M, Kukk E, et al. Vascular endothelial growth factor D (VEGF-D) is a ligand for the tyrosine kinases VEGF receptor 2 (Flk1) and VEGF receptor 3 (Flt4). *Proc Natl Acad Sci USA.* 1998; 95:548–53.

30. Brown LF, Berse B, Jackman RW, et al. Expression of vascular permeability factor (vascular endothelial growth factor) and its receptors in breast cancer. *Hum Pathol.* 1995; 26:86–91.

31. Park JE, Keller GA, Ferrara N. The vascular endothelial growth factor (VEGF) isoforms: differential deposition into the subepithelial extracellular matrix and bioactivity of extracellular matrix-bound VEGF. *Mol Biol Cell* 1993; 4:1317–26.

32. Rak J, Mitsuhashi Y, Bayko L, et al. Mutant *ras* oncogenes upregulate VEGF/VPF expression: implications for induction and inhibition of tumor angiogenesis. *Cancer Res.* 1995; 55:4575–80.

33. Friesel RE, Maciag T. Molecular mechanisms of angiogenesis: fibroblast growth factor signal transduction. *FASEB J.* 1995; 9:919–25.

34. Yu ZX, Biro S, Fu YM, et al. Localization of basic fibroblast growth factor in bovine endothelial cells: immunohistochemical and biochemical studies. *Exp Cell Res.* 1993; 204:247–59.

35. Montesano R, Vassalli JD, Baird A, Guillemin R, Orci L. Basic fibroblast growth factor induces angiogenesis in vitro. *Proc Natl Acad Sci USA.* 1986; 83:7297–301.

36. Sporn MB, Roberts AB, Wakefield LM, de Crombrugghe B. Some recent advances in the chemistry and biology of transforming growth factor-β. *J Cell Biol.* 1987; 105:1039–45.

37. Leibovich SJ, Polverini PJ, Shepard HM, Wiseman DM, Shively V, Nuseir N. Macrophage-induced angiogenesis is mediated by tumour necrosis factor-α. *Nature.* 1987; 329:630–2.

38. Wahl SM; Hunt DA; Wakefield LM; et al. Transforming growth factor type β induces monocyte chemotaxis and growth factor production. *Proc Natl Acad Sci USA.* 1987; 84: 5788–92.

39. Sherry B, Cerami A. Cachectin/tumor necrosis factor exerts endocrine, paracrine, and autocrine control of inflammatory responses. *J Cell Biol.* 1988; 107:1269–77.

40. Leibovich SJ. (1995) Role of cytokines in the process of tumor angiogenesis. *In Human cytokines: their role in cell disease and therapy* (ed. B.B. Aggarwal and R.K. Puri) 539–64. Blackwell *Science.* Oxford.

41. Moghaddam A. et al. (1997) Thymidine phosphorylase / platelet endothelial cell derived growth factor: an angiogenic enzyme. In: *Tumor angiogenesis* (ed: R. Bicknell, C.E. Lewis and N. Ferrara) 251–260, Oxford University Press.

42. Schreiber AB, Winkler ME, Derynck R. Transforming growth factor-α: a more potent angiogenic mediator than epidermal growth factor. *Science.* 1986; 232:1250–3.

43. Bikfalvi A. Significance of angiogenesis in tumour progression and metastasis. *Eur J Cancer.* 1995; 31A:1101–4.

44. Desbaillets I, Diserens AC, Tribolet N, Hamou MF, Van Meir EG. Upregulation of interleukin 8 by oxygen-deprived cells in glioblastoma suggests a role in leukocyte activation, chemotaxis, and angiogenesis. *J Exp Med.* 1997; 186:1201–12.

45. Gullino PM. Prostaglandins and gangliosides of tumor microenvironment: their role in angiogenesis. *Acta Oncol.* 1995; 34:439–41.
46. Kull FC Jr, Brent DA, Parikh I, Cuatrecasas P. Chemical identification of a tumor-derived angiogenic factor. *Science.* 1987; 236:843–5.
47. Koch AE, Halloran MM, Haskell CJ, Shah MR, Polverini PJ. Angiogenesis mediated by soluble forms of E-selectin and vascular cell adhesion molecule–1. *Nature.* 1995; 376:517–9.
48. Frenette PS, Mayadas TN, Rayburn H, Hynes RO, Wagner DD. Susceptibility to infection and altered hematopoiesis in mice deficient in both P- and E-selectins. *Cell.* 1996; 84:563–74.
49. Stad RK, Buurman WA. Current views on structure and function of endothelial adhesion molecules. *Cell Adhes Commun.* 1994; 2:261–8.
50. Patey N, Vazeux R, Canioni D, Potter T, Gallatin WM, et al. Intercellular adhesion molecule–3 on endothelial cells. Expression in tumors but not in inflammatory responses. *Am J Pathol.* 1996; 148:465–72.
51. Dejana E, Corada M, Lampugnani MG. Endothelial cell-to-cell junctions. *FASEB J.* 1995; 9:910–8.
52. Brooks PC. Cell adhesion molecules in angiogenesis. *Cancer Metastasis Rev.* 1996; 15:187–94.
53. Davis GE, Camarillo CW. An $\alpha2\beta1$ integrin-dependent pinocytic mechanism involving intracellular vacuole formation and coalescence regulates capillary lumen and tube formation in three-dimensional collagen matrix. *Exp Cell Res.* 1996; 224:39–51.
54. Senger DR, Claffey KP, Benes JE, Perruzzi CA, Sergiou AP, Detmar M. Angiogenesis promoted by vascular endothelial growth factor: regulation through $\alpha1\beta1$ and $\alpha2\beta1$ integrins. *Proc Natl Acad Sci USA* 1997; 94:13612–17.
55. Enenstein J, Kramer RH. Confocal microscopic analysis of integrin expression on the microvasculature and its sprouts in the neonatal foreskin. *J Invest Dermatol.* 1994; 103:381–6.
56. Nicosia RF, Bonanno E. Inhibition of angiogenesis in vitro by Arg-Gly-Asp-containing synthetic peptide. *Am J Pathol.* 199; 138:829–33.
57. Goodman SL, Diefenbach B, Sutter A, et al. Highly selective cyclic-RGD peptides block αv integrins and inhibit angiogenesis and tumor growth. Keystone Symposium 1996.
58. Sutter A, Goodman S, Jonczyk A, et al. Cyclic RGD peptides with high selectivity for αv integrins as potent inhibitors of angiogenesis and tumor growth. Gordon Conferences. 1995.
59. Davis CM, Danehower SC, Laurenza A, Molony JL. Identification of a role of the vitronectin receptor and protein kinase C in the induction of endothelial cell vascular formation. *J Cell Biochem.* 1993; 51:206–18.
60. Gamble JR, Matthias LJ, Meyer G, et al. Regulation of in vitro capillary tube formation by anti-integrin antibodies. *J Cell Biol.* 1993; 121:931–43.
61. Brooks PC; Montgomery AM; Rosenfeld M; et al. Integrin αvβ3 antagonists promote tumor regression by inducing apoptosis of angiogenic blood vessels. *Cell.* 1994; 79: 1157–64.
62. Friedlander M, Brooks PC, Shaffer RW, Kincaid CM, Varner JA, Cheresh DA. Definition of two angiogenic pathways by distinct αv integrins. *Science.* 1995; 270:1500–2.
63. Hammes HP, Brownlee M, Jonczyk A, Sutter A, Preissner KT. Subcutaneous injection of a cyclic peptide antagonist of vitronectin receptor-type integrins inhibits retinal neovascularization. *Nat Med.* 1996; 2:529–33.
64. Möhler T, et al. An antiangiogenic cyclic peptide antagonist of integrin αvβ3 / αvβ5 inhibits tumor growth in nude mice and human skin. (1999) in preparation.

65. Brooks PC, Stromblad S, Klemke R, Visscher D, Sarkar FH, Cheresh DA. Antiintegrin αvβ3 blocks human breast cancer growth and angiogenesis in human skin. *J Clin Invest.* 1995; 96:1815–22.

66. Varner JA. The role of vascular cell integrins αvβ3 and αvβ5 in angiogenesis. In: *Regulation of angiogenesis*, (1997), 361–90. Eds. Goldberg, I. D. and Rosen, E. M. Birkhäuser Verlag. Basel.

67. Gladson CL, Cheresh DA. Glioblastoma expression of vitronectin and the α v β 3 integrin. Adhesion mechanism for transformed glial cells. *J Clin Invest.* 199; 88:1924–32.

68. Albelda SM, Mette SA, Elder DE, et al. Integrin distribution in malignant melanoma: association of the β3 subunit with tumor progression. *Cancer Res.* 1990; 50:6757–64.

69. Danen EH, Ten Berge PJ, Van Muijen GN, Van'tHof-Grootenboer AE, Brocker EB, Ruiter DJ. Emergence of α5β1 fibronectin- and αvβ3 vitronectin-receptor expression in melanocytic tumour progression. *Histopathology.* 1994; 24:249–56.

70. Natali PG, Hamby CV, Felding-Habermann B, et al. Clinical significance of α(v)β3 integrin and intercellular adhesion molecule–1 expression in cutaneous malignant melanoma lesions. *Cancer Res.* 1997; 57:1554–60.

71. Mitjans F, Sander D, Adan J, et al. An anti-αv-integrin antibody that blocks integrin function inhibits the development of a human melanoma in nude mice. *J Cell Sci.* 1995; 108:2825–38.

72. Marshall JF, Rutherford DC, McCartney AC, Mitjans F, Goodman SL, Hart IR. αvβ1 is a receptor for vitronectin and fibrinogen, and acts with α5β1 to mediate spreading on fibronectin. *J Cell Sci.* 1995; 108:1227–38.

73. Montgomery AM, Reisfeld RA, Cheresh DA. Integrin αvβ3 rescues melanoma cells from apoptosis in three-dimensional dermal collagen. *Proc Natl Acad Sci USA.* 1994; 91:8856–60.

74. Stromblad S, Becker JC, Yebra M, Brooks PC, Cheresh DA. Suppression of p53 activity and p21WAF1/CIP1 expression by vascular cell integrin αvβ3 during angiogenesis. *J Clin Invest.* 1996; 98:426–33.

75. Peticlerc E, Stromblad S, von Schalscha TL, Mitjans F, Piulats J, Montgomery AM, Cheresh DA, Brooks PC. Integrin alpha(v)beta3 promotes M21 melanoma growth in human skin by regulating tumor cell survival. *Cancer Res.* 1999; 59(11):2724–30.

76. Nurden AT, Caen JP. An abnormal platelet glycoprotein pattern in three cases of Glanzmann's thrombasthenia. *Br J Haematol.* 1974; 28:253–60.

77. Bader BL, Raybrun H, Hynes RO. Targeted disruption of the mouse av integrin gene. In *Integrins and signalling events in cell biology and disease. Keystone Symposium*, (1996) abstract 401.

78. Meyer T, Hart I. Mechanisms of tumor metastasis. *Eur J Cancer.* 1998; 34:214–21.

79. Seghezzi G, Marelli R, Mandriota SJ, Nolli ML, Mazzieri R, Mignatti P. Tumor cell-conditioned medium stimulates expression of the urokinase receptor in vascular endothelial cells. *J Cell Physiol.* 1996; 169:300–8.

80. Mandriota SJ, Seghezzi G, Vassalli JD, et al. Vascular endothelial growth factor increases urokinase receptor expression in vascular endothelial cells. *J Biol Chem.* 1995; 270:9709–16.

81. Xue W, Mizukami I, Todd RF, Petty IIR. Urokinase-type plasminogen activator receptors associate with β1 and β3 integrins of fibrosarcoma cells: dependence on extracellular matrix components. *Cancer Res.* 1997; 57:1682–9.

82. Min HY, Doyle LV, Vitt CR, Zandonella CL, et al. Urokinase receptor antagonists inhibit angiogenesis and primary tumor growth in syngeneic mice. *Cancer Res.* 1996; 56:2428–33.

83. Carmeliet P, Schoonjans L, Kieckens L, et al. Physiological consequences of loss of plasminogen activator gene function in mice. *Nature.* 1994; 368:419–24.

84. Gately S, Twardowski P, Stack MS, et al. The mechanism of cancer-mediated conversion of plasminogen to the angiogenesis inhibitor angiostatin. *Proc Natl Acad Sci USA.* 1997; 94:10868–72.

85. Dong Z, Kumar R, Yang X, Fidler IJ. Macrophage-derived metalloelastase is responsible for the generation of angiostatin in Lewis lung carcinoma. *Cell.* 1997; 88:801–10.

86. Patterson BC, Sang QA. Angiostatin-converting enzyme activities of human matrilysin (MMP–7) and gelatinase B/type IV collagenase (MMP–9). *J Biol Chem.* 1997; 272:28823–5.

87. Yoshimoto M, Itoh F, Yamamoto H, Hinoda Y, Imai K, Yachi A. Expression of MMP–7(PUMP–1) mRNA in human colorectal cancers. *Int J Cancer.* 1993; 54:614–8.

88. Davies B, Miles DW, Happerfield LC, et al. Activity of type IV collagenases in benign and malignant breast disease. *Br J Cancer.* 1993; 67:1126–31.

89. Cornelius LA, Nehring LC, Roby JD, Parks WC, Welgus HG. Human dermal microvascular endothelial cells produce matrix metalloproteinases in response to angiogenic factors and migration. *J Invest Dermatol.* 1995; 105:170–6.

90. Taraboletti G, Garofalo A, Belotti D, et al. Inhibition of angiogenesis and murine hemangioma growth by batimastat, a synthetic inhibitor of matrix metalloproteinases. *J Natl Cancer Inst.* 1995; 87:293–8.

91. Wang X, Fu X, Brown PD, Crimmin MJ, Hoffman RM. Matrix metalloproteinase inhibitor BB–94 (batimastat) inhibits human colon tumor growth and spread in a patient-like orthotopic model in nude mice. *Cancer Res.* 1994; 54:4726–8.

92. Brooks PC, Stromblad S, Sanders LC, et al. Localization of matrix metalloproteinase MMP–2 to the surface of invasive cells by interaction with integrin $\alpha v \beta 3$. *Cell.* 1996; 85:683–93.

93. Tokuraku M, Sato H, Murakami S, Okada Y, Watanabe Y, Seiki M. Activation of the precursor of gelatinase A/72 kDa type IV collagenase/MMP–2 in lung carcinomas correlates with the expression of membrane-type matrix metalloproteinase (MT-MMP) and with lymph node metastasis. *Int J Cancer.* 1995; 64:355–9.

94. O'Reilly MS, Boehm T, Shing Y, et al. Endostatin: an endogenous inhibitor of angiogenesis and tumor growth. *Cell.* 1997; 88:277–85.

95. Auerbach W, Auerbach R. Angiogenesis inhibition: a review. *Pharmacol Ther.* 1994; 63:265–311.

96. Bicknell R, Harris AL. Mechanisms and therapeutic implications of angiogenesis. *Curr Opin Oncol.* 1996; 8:60–5.

97. Bouck N, Stellmach V, Hsu SC. How tumors become angiogenic. *Adv Cancer Res.* 1996; 69:135–74.

98. Folkman J. Angiogenesis in cancer, vascular, rheumatoid and other disease. *Nat Med.* 1995; 1:27–31.

99. Yamaoka M, Yamamoto T, Masaki T, Ikeyama S, Sudo K, Fujita T. Inhibition of tumor growth and metastasis of rodent tumors by the angiogenesis inhibitor O-(chloroacetyl-carbamoyl)fumagillol (TNP–470; AGM–1470). *Cancer Res.* 1993; 53:262–7.

100. Fotsis T, Pepper M, Adlercreutz H, et al. Genistein, a dietary-derived inhibitor of in vitro angiogenesis. *Proc Natl Acad Sci USA.* 1993; 90:2690–4.

101. Moses MA, Sudhalter J, Langer R. Identification of an inhibitor of neovascularization from cartilage. *Science.* 1990; 248:1408–10.

102. Brem S, Cotran R, Folkman J. Tumor angiogenesis: a quantitative method for histologic grading. *J Natl Cancer Inst.* 1972; 48:347–56.

103. Fox SB. Tumour angiogenesis and prognosis. *Histopathology.* 1997; 30:294–301.

104. Weidner N, Semple JP, Welch WR, Folkman J. Tumor angiogenesis and metastasis—correlation in invasive breast carcinoma. *N Engl J Med.* 1991; 324:1–8.

105. Weidner N, Folkman J, Pozza F, et al. Tumour angiogenesis a new significant and independent prognostic indicator in early stage breast carcinoma. *J Natl Cancer Inst.* 1992; 84:1875–7.

106. Bosari S, Lee AK, DeLellis RA, Wiley BD, Heatley GJ, Silverman M. Microvessel quantitation and prognosis in invasive breast carcinoma. *Hum Pathol.* 1992; 23(7):755–61.

107. Fox SB, Leek RD, Weekes MP, Whitehouse RM, Gatter KC, Harris AL. Quantitation and prognostic value of breast cancer angiogenesis: Comparison of microvessel density, Chalkley count, and computer image analysis. *J Pathol.* 1995; 177:275–83.

108. Kawaguchi T, Yamamoto S, Kudoh S, Soto K, Wakasa K, Sakurai M. Tumor angiogenesis as a major prognostic factor in stage I lung adenocarcinoma. *Anticancer Res.* 1997; 17:3743–6.

109. Heinburg S, Ochler MK, Kristen P, Papadopoulos T, Caffier H. The endothelial marker CD34 in the assessment of tumour vascularization in ovarian cancer. *Anticancer Res 1997.* 17:3149–51.

110. Tanigawa N, Amaya H, Matsumura M, Shimomatsuya T. Association of tumour vasculature with tumour progression and overall survival of patients with non-early gastric carcinomas. *Br J Cancer.* 1997; 75:566–71.

111. Kumar-Singh S, Vermeulen PB, Weyler J, et al. Evaluation of tumour angiogenesis as a prognostic marker in malignant mesothelioma. *J Pathol.* 1997; 182:211–6.

112. Vermeulen PB, Gasparini G, Fox SB, et al. Quantification of angiogenesis in solid human tumours: an international consensus on the methodology and criteria of evaluation. *Eur J Cancer.* 1996; 32A:2474–84.

113. Anan K, Morisaki T, Katano M, et al. Preoperative assessment of tumour angiogenesis by vascular endothelial growth factor mRNA expression in homogeneate samples of breast carcinoma: fine-needle aspirates vs resection samples. *J Surg Oncol.* 1997; 66:257–63.

114. Dobbs SP, Hewett PW, Johnson IR, Carmichael J, Murray JC. Angiogenesis is associated with vascular endothelial growth factor expression in cervical intraepithelial neoplasia. *Br J Cancer.* 1997; 76:1410–5.

115. Eisma RJ, Spiro JD, Krentzer DL. Vascular endothelial growth factor expression in head and neck squamous cell carcinoma. *Am J Surg.* 1997; 174:513–7.

116. O'Brien T, Cranston D, Fuggle S, Bicknell R, Harris AL. Different angiogenic pathways characterize superficial and invasive bladder cancer. *Cancer Res.* 1995; 55:510–3.

117. Toi M, Hoshina S, Takayanagi T, Tominaga T. Association of vascular endothelial growth factor expression with tumour angiogenesis and with early relapse in primary breast cancer. *Jpn J Cancer Res.* 1994; 85:1045–9.

118. Kuiper RA, Schellens JH, Blijham GH, Beijnen JH, Voest EE. Clinical research on antiangiogenic therapy. *Pharmacol Res.* 1998: 37:1–16.

119. Welles L, Saville MW, Lietzau J, Pluda JM, Wyvill KM, Feuerstein I, Figg WD, Lush R, Odom J, Wilson WH, Ajardo MT, Humphrey RW, Feigal E, Tuck D, Steinberg SM, Broder S, Yarchoan R. Phase II trial with dose titration of paclitaxel for the therapy of human immunodeficiency virus-associated Kaposi's sarcoma. *J Clin Oncol.* 1998; 16(3):1112–21.

120. Dixon SC, Horti J, Logothetis C, et al. TNP–470 up regulates the expression of prostate specific antigen (abstract 298). *Proc Am Assoc Cancer Res.* 1998; 39:44.

121. Berlin J, Tutsch KD, Hutson P, Cleary J, Rago RP, Arzoomanian RZ, Alberti D, Feierabend C, Wilding G. Phase I clinical and pharmacokinetic study of oral carboxyamidotriazole, a signal transduction inhibitor. *J Clin Oncol.* 1997; 15(2):781–9.

122. Kim KJ, Li B, Winer J, et al. Inhibition of vascular endothelial growth factor-induced angiogenesis suppresses tumour growth in vivo. *Nature.* 1993; 362:841–4.
123. Melnyk O, Shuman MA, Kim KJ. Vascular endothelial growth factor promotes tumor dissemination by a mechanism distinct from its effect on primary tumor growth. *Cancer Res.* 1996; 56:921–4.
124. Borgstrom P, Hillan KJ, Sriramarao P, Ferrara N. Complete inhibition of angiogenesis and growth of microtumors by anti-vascular endothelial growth factor neutralizing antibody: novel concepts of angiostatic therapy from intravital videomicroscopy. *Cancer Res.* 1996; 56:4032–9.
125. Millauer B, Shawver LK, Plate KH, Risau W, Ullrich A. Glioblastoma growth inhibited in vivo by a dominant-negative Flk–1 mutant. *Nature.* 1994; 367:576–9.
126. Millauer B, Longhi MP, Plate KH, et al. Dominant-negative inhibition of Flk–1 suppresses the growth of many tumor types in vivo. *Cancer Res.* 1996; 56:1615–20.
127. Coppola G, Atlas-White M, Katsahambas S, et al. Effect of intraperitoneally, intravenously and intralesionally administered monoclonal anti-β-FGF antibodies on rat chondrosarcoma tumor vascularization and growth. *Anticancer Res.* 1997; 17:2033–9.
128. Kobayashi K, Vokes EE, Vogelzang NJ, Janisch L, Soliven B, Ratain MJ. Phase I study of suramin administered by intermittent infusion without adaptive control to cancer patients: update of two expanded dose levels near the maximally tolerated dose. *J Clin Oncol.* 1996; 14(9):2622–3.
129. O'Reilly MS, Holmgren L, Chen C, Folkman J. Angiostatin induces and sustains dormancy of human primary tumors in mice. *Nat Med.* 1996;2:689–92.
130. Holmgren L, O'Reilly MS, Folkman J. Dormancy of micrometastases: balanced proliferation and apoptosis in the presence of angiogenesis suppression. *Nat Med.* 1995;1:149–53.
131. Boehm T, Folkman J, Browder T, O'Reilly MS. Antiangiogenic therapy of experimental cancer does not induce acquired drug resistance. *Nature.* 1997; 390:404–7.
132. Cao Y, O'Reilly MS, Marshall B, Flynn E, Ji RW, Folkman J. Expression of angiostatin cDNA in a murine fibrosarcoma suppresses primary tumor growth and produces long-term dormancy of metastases. *J Clin Invest.* 1998; 101:1055–63.
133. Bachelot T, Pawliuk R, Treilleux I, et al. Retrovirus-mediated gene transfer of an Angiostatin-Endostatin fusion protein with enhanced anti-tumor properties in vivo (abstract 1856). *Proc. Amer. Assoc. Cancer Res.* 1998; 39:1856–7.
134. Gore M, A'Hern R, Stankiewicz M, Slevin M. Tumour marker levels during marimastat therapy. *Lancet.* 1996; 348(9022):263–4.
135. Twardowski P, Gradishar WJ. Clinical trials of antiangiogenic agents. *Curr Opin Oncol.* 1997; 9:584–9.
136. Koivunen E, Wang B, Ruoslahti E. Isolation of a highly specific ligand for the α5β1 integrin from a phage display library. *J Cell Biol.* 1994; 124:373–80.
137. Rosell E, Kraft S, Recacha C, et al. Obtención de ligandos específicos para moléculas de adhesión a partir de una genoteca de heptapéptidos al azar. *Inmunología* 1997; 16:30 (abstract A6.96).
138. Möhler T, Brooks PC, Mitjans F, Jonczyk A, Goodman S, Cheresh DA. Antagonists of integrin αvβ3 / αvβ5: an anti-angiogenic strategy for the treatment of cancer (abstract 656). *Proc Amer Assoc Cancer Res.* 1998; 39:97.
139. Teicher BA, Holden SA, Ara G, et al. Potentiation of cytotoxic cancer therapies by TNP–470 alone and with other anti-angiogenic agents. *Int J Cancer.* 1994; 57:920–5.
140. Folkman J. Tumor angiogenesis and tissue factor. *Nat Med.* 1996; 2:167–8.
141. Folkman J. Addressing tumor blood vessels. *Nat Biotechnol.* 1997; 15(6):510.

142. Tsujii M, Kawano S, Tsuji S, Sawaoka H, Hori M, DuBois RN. Cyclooxygenase regulates angiogenesis induced by colon cancer cells. *Cell*. 1998; 93(5):705–16.

143. Chiarugi V, Magnelli L, Gallo O. Cox-2, iNOS and p53 as play-makers of tumor angiogenesis (review). *Int J Mol Med*. 1998; 2(6):715–9.

144. Daniel TO, Liu HL, Morrow JD, Crews BC, Marnett LJ. Thromboxane A2 is a mediator of cyclooxygenase-2-dependent endothelial migration and angiogenesis. *Cancer Res*. 1999; 59:4574–7.

145. Davis S, Yancopoulos GD. The angiopoietins: Yin and Yang in angiogenesis. *Curr Top Microbiol Immunol*. 1999; 237:173–85.

146. Lin P, Buxton JA, Acheson A, Radziejewski C, Maisonpierre PC, Yancopoulos GD, Channon KM, Hale LP, Dewhirst MW, George SE, Peters KG. Antiangiogenic gene therapy targeting the endothelium-specific receptor tyrosine kinase Tie2. *Proc Natl Acad Sci USA*. 1998; 95(15):8829–34.

147. Goldman CK, Kendall RL, Cabrera G, Soroceanu L, Heike Y, Gillespie GY, Siegal GP, Mao X, Bett AJ, Huckle WR, Thomas KA, Curiel DT. Paracrine expression of a native soluble vascular endothelial growth factor receptor inhibits tumor growth, metastasis, and mortality rate. *Proc Natl Acad Sci USA*. 1998; 95(15):8795–800.

148. Chen QR, Kumar D, Stass SA, Mixson AJ. Liposomes complexed to plasmids encoding angiostatin and endostatin inhibit breast cancer in nude mice. *Cancer Res*. 1999; 59(14): 3308–12.

149. Liu Y, Thor A, Shtivelman E, Cao Y, Tu G, Heath TD, Debs RJ. Systemic gene delivery expands the repertoire of effective antiangiogenic agents. *J Biol Chem*. 1999; 274(19): 13338–44.

150. Cao Y. Therapeutic potentials of angiostatin in the treatment of cancer. *Haematologica*. 1999; 84(7):643–50.

151. John H, Preissner KT, Forssmann WG, Standker L. Novel glycosylated forms of human plasma endostatin and circulating endostatin-related fragments of collagen XV. *Biochemistry*. 1999; 38(32):10217–24.

152. Blezinger P, Wang J, Gondo M, Quezada A, Mehrens D, French M, Singhal A, Sullivan S, Rolland A, Ralston R, Min W. Systemic inhibition of tumor growth and tumor metastases by intramuscular administration of the endostatin gene. *Nat Biotechnol*. 1999; 17(4):343–8.

153. Cao Y. Endogenous angiogenesis inhibitors: angiostatin, endostatin, and other proteolytic fragments. *Prog Mol Subcell Biol*. 1998; 20:161–76.

154. Bergers G, Javaherian K, Lo KM, Folkman J, Hanahan D. Effects of angiogenesis inhibitors on multistage carcinogenesis in mice. *Science* 1999; 284(5415):808–12.

155. Moser TL, Stack MS, Asplin I, Enghild JJ, Hojrup P, Everitt L, Hubchak S, Schnaper HW, Pizzo SV. Angiostatin binds ATP synthase on the surface of human endothelial cells. *Proc Natl Acad Sci USA*. 1999; 96(6):2811–6.

156. Walter JJ, Sane DC. Angiostatin binds to smooth muscle cells in the coronary artery and inhibits smooth muscle cell proliferation and migration in vitro. *Arterioscler Thromb Vasc Biol*. 1999; 19(9):2041–8.

157. Maniotis AJ, Folberg R, Hess A, Seftor EA, Gardner LM, Pe'er J, Trent JM, Meltzer PS, Hendrix MJ. Vascular channel formation by human melanoma cells in vivo and in vitro: vasculogenic mimicry. *Am J Pathol*. 1999; 155(3):739–52.

12

Invasion and Metastasis

Maria Rosa Bani and Raffaella Giavazzi

The previous chapter discussed how tumor cells provide for a blood supply. This chapter discusses another aspect of tumor growth, that of metastasis.

Metastasis: The Spread of Tumors

Metastases are the main cause of cancer deaths. A tumor is said to be "benign" when it remains localized and is therefore generally amenable to local surgical removal and survival of the patient. "Malignant" is a term applied to a neoplasm that can invade and destroy adjacent structures and/or spread to distant sites, transferring the disease from one organ to another not directly connected with it. Approximately 30% of newly diagnosed patients with solid tumors (excluding skin cancer other than melanomas) have detectable metastases. An additional 20% have occult metastases at the time of diagnosis (1). Dissemination is a major factor in people's fear of neoplastic disease; in fact it strongly prejudices, if not precludes, the possibility of cure. It is therefore obvious that no achievement would yield greater benefit for patients than the development of strategies aimed at controlling metastasis.

Malignant neoplasms disseminate by one of three pathways: by seeding within body cavities, by lymphatic spread, or by hematogenous spread (2). Seeding of cancers occurs when neoplasms invade a natural body cavity. An example of this mode of dissemination is ovarian carcinoma. This cancer has the ability to reimplant itself elsewhere in the peritoneal cavity, a property apparently distinct from its capacity to invade, the reimplanted tumors widely cover the surfaces but often do not invade the parenchyma of the abdominal organs. Carcinomas typically spread through the lymphatic system, whereas sarcomas favor the hematogenous route. However, given the numerous interconnections between lymphatic and vascular systems, all forms of cancer may disseminate by both routes (1–3). In some cases, the cancer cells may traverse the lymph nodes to ultimately reach the vascular compartment. The blood-borne cells follow the venous flow draining the site of neoplasm (the arteries are much less penetrable than the veins [2]). Because all the portal-area drainage flows to the liver and all caval blood flows to the lungs, it is not surprising that the liver and lungs are

From: *Principles of Molecular Oncology*
Edited by: M. H. Bronchud, M. A. Foote, W. P. Peters, and M. O. Robinson © Humana Press Inc., Totowa, NJ

the most frequently involved secondary sites. Anatomical drainage does not fully explain the systemic distribution of metastases in specific organs. For example, muscle is well vascularized and kidney receives up to 25% of cardiac blood output, yet those organs are rarely the sites of secondary deposits *(1,4,5)*. This led Paget in 1989 to propose that the tropism of metastasis is the consequence of the interaction of tumor cells (the seeds) with a favorable organ environment (the soil) *(6)*. All the above observations reinforce the notion that tumor dissemination is an enormously complex process whose outcome depends upon numerous interactions between the cancer cell and host cells *(4,5)*, which ultimately is highly inefficient *(7)*. It is very important to realize that the metastatic process is highly dynamic and intertwined. It is possible to summarize some major steps in the process which may either operate concurrently or evolve from one step into another without interruption. After tumor growth at the primary site, tumor cells must:

- detach from the solid mass;
- invade the surrounding normal tissues;
- intravasate into vascular channels;
- survive, either as a single cell or as a clump, in the circulation;
- stop in the capillary bed of the new site;
- extravasate through the vessels wall;
- infiltrate the surrounding host tissue compartment;
- grow as a solid mass in the newly colonized organ;
- start the process all over again.

The metastatic cascade is illustrated in Fig. 1.

During the entire process, the tumor cells must elude immunosurveillance mechanisms *(8,9)*, lose responsiveness to the normal growth controls *(10)*, and promote angiogenesis *(11,12)*. Of particular clinical impact is the concept that the growth of solid tumors, beyond the size of approx 1–2 mm, is largely dependent on the formation of new blood vessels (angiogenesis). Neovascularization is in itself an important requisite for the release of tumor cells from the primary tumor in the circulation, but also plays an important role in controlling the expansion of the metastatic foci in the secondary sites. The relevance of angiogenesis in tumor progression and metastasis as well as the molecular mechanisms that regulate this process are discussed in another chapter of this book (Chapter 11).

It is generally believed that malignant progression involves genetic alterations, accumulation of which leads to permanent phenotypic changes associated with the development of full-blown malignancy *(13)*. Genomic instability generates heterogeneity resulting in clones with new phenotypes; unknown microevolutionary selection pressures will then allow the progressive selection of clones with enhanced malignant potential *(14–16)*. Such continuous emerging of cell populations with different abilities to invade and form metastasis represent a major obstacle to therapy.

The information acquired from basic studies of the genetic alterations associated with tumor progression toward malignancy can be exploited to improve risk assessment, hereditary predisposition, early diagnosis, better prognosis, and therapeutic targets and, thus, treatment of human cancer.

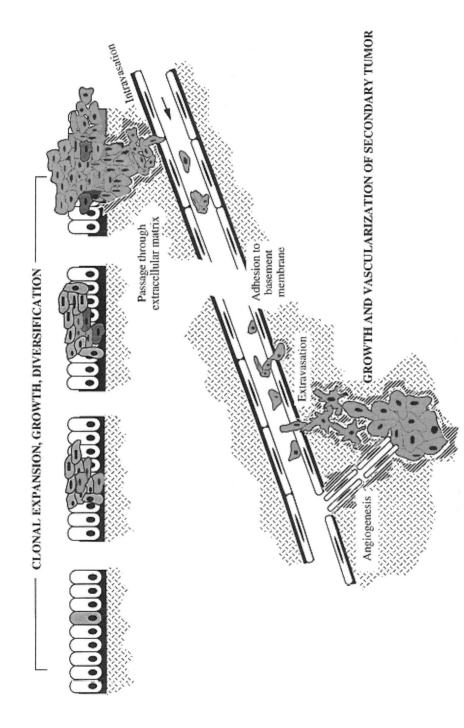

CLONAL EXPANSION, GROWTH, DIVERSIFICATION

Intravasation

Passage through extracellular matrix

Adhesion to basement membrane

Extravasation

Angiogenesis

GROWTH AND VASCULARIZATION OF SECONDARY TUMOR

Fig. 1. Schematic of the metastatic cascade.

299

Molecular Genetics of Metastasis

Three classes of genes are the principal target of genetic alterations:

- Oncogenes, whose action is considered dominant because, upon activation, they act despite the presence of their normal counterpart allele
- Tumor suppressor genes, whose effect can take place only if both alleles are inactivated
- DNA repair genes which affect the ability to repair nonlethal damage in other genes, including oncogenes and tumor suppressor genes.

The loss of tumor suppressor genes (TSGs) and/or activation of oncogenes has been consistently associated with malignancy *(17,18)*; however, it remains to be defined which of the biological properties typically associated with advanced stages of the disease are causative, strictly associated, and/or simply coregulated with malignancy. Moreover, to increase the potential to relate any molecular alteration to clinical behavior and response to therapy, development in the techniques of molecular analysis should aim at being applicable to a large range of clinical material, such as cytological preparations and fixed tissue specimens.

Genetic control of the metastatic phenotype has been addressed by DNA-transfer experiments, showing that metastatic ability could indeed have a genetic basis. However, any hope for a metastasis-specific "dominant/gain of function" gene was lost when transfer of high-molecular-weight DNA failed to identify any candidate gene. Transfection with a variety of single oncogenes (e.g., *ras, src, E1a*), while demonstrating the possibility of inducing metastatic competence in some recipient cells, showed that in some cell types the malignant phenotype was either not affected or was inhibited by the forced gene expression *(19)*. In addition, the ability to switch on the metastatic process in the "permissive" cells indicated that a multitude of downstream-regulated genes were activated and contributed to the metastatic behavior of the cells *(19)*. These observations suggest that in certain recipient cells, the failure to induce metastasis despite the expression of the oncogene may reflect some deficiencies in the activation of the necessary downstream effector genes.

More recent approaches, such as searching for metastasis genes by comparing cDNA from metastatic and nonmetastatic cells, have implicated "loss of function" genes (e.g., *nm23, KAI1, KiSS-1*) as the major players in metastatic behavior, as their forced reexpression in certain tumor cell types indeed suppressed metastasis formation in animal models.

nm23

nm23, originally found by differential screening of cDNA libraries constructed from metastatic and nonmetastatic clones isolated from K-1735 murine melanoma, is highly expressed in nonmetastatic cells *(20)*. It was later shown to behave as a metastasis suppressor gene in the same murine melanoma model *(21)* and in a human breast carcinoma model in nude mice *(22)*. Unfortunately, the role and the function of *nm23* still remain unclear *(23)*. It displays sequence homology with nucleoside diphosphate (NDP) kinase and it shows NDP kinase activity *(24)*. It may participate in signal transduction involving serine residues autophosphorylation *(25)*. It might also act as a transcription factor, as suggested by the analysis of the motifs present in its sequence *(24)*. The expression of the two human homologues *nm23-H1* and *nm23-H2*, located on chromosome 17, has been shown to correlate inversely with the malignancy (metastatic potential) of some, but not all, human tumors *(23)*.

KAI1

KAI1, known as "kang ai" (Chinese for "anticancer"), has been cloned and shown to map on human chromosome 11p11.2–13 *(26)*. It is expressed in normal human prostate, but expression has been detected at a very low level in five human prostate cancer cell lines derived from metastatic lesions. After the gene was transferred into a highly metastatic rat prostate cancer cell line, *KAI1*-expressing cells showed reduced metastatic capability whereas their growth as primary tumor was not affected *(26)*. Reduction in KAI1 protein expression was consistent with the progression of human prostate cancer in immunohistochemical (IHC) analysis of patient specimens *(27)*. The observed down-regulation did not involve mutations or allelic losses of the gene. KAI1 protein is located on the plasma membrane of normal prostate epithelial cells *(27)* and it is identical to the glycoprotein encoded by the *CD82* gene, a type III integral membrane. Although its precise function is unknown, the localization and the analysis of the deduced protein sequence suggest that it might be involved in cell–cell and/or cell-ECM interactions. It was reported that *KAI1/CD82* down-regulation is associated with poor prognosis in patients with non-small-cell lung cancer (NSCLC) *(28)*.

KiSS-1

KiSS-1 was isolated from malignant melanoma cells by way of a subtraction hybridization strategy in which metastatic C8161 cells and their nonmetastatic derivative, obtained by the introduction of one intact copy of human chromosome 6, were compared *(29)*. *KiSS-1* maps on human chromosome 1q32–q41, suggesting that it might be a downstream effector of gene(s) on chromosome 6. Its function remains unknown but the deduced amino-acid sequence suggests that *KiSS-1* encodes for a protein with a putative SH3 ligand domain *(29)*. Such a motif is frequently found in proteins involved in signal-transduction pathways. Transfection of *KiSS-1* in melanoma and breast cancer human cell lines resulted in the reduced ability of the transfectants to colonize the lung of nude mice without altering their tumorigenicity *(29–31)*.

The usefulness of these metastasis genes in predicting disease outcome is, at present, uncertain. Despite their proven ability to suppress metastasis of some recipient cells in in vivo experimental models, it is unlikely that they will represent the universally implicated metastasis suppressor gene. In interfering with the single event, a necessary step of a complex mechanism, the whole biological program may be blocked. Vice versa, it is not possible to evocate the whole process by simulating that single event.

Because it appears that each discrete step of the metastatic process is regulated by changes in different genes, we expect that the strongest candidate genes for predicting metastasis are those encoding for cell-adhesion molecules, receptors, degradative enzymatic activities, chemotactic factors, angiogenic factors, and for molecules involved in the most diverse pathways that allow the maintenance of the tumor-cell metabolism despite a variety of microenvironmental signals. Given that the (un)coordinate expression of multiple genes contributes to metastasis, it cannot be excluded that their (de)regulation might even occur in a tissue-specific manner. It is therefore not surprising that different patterns of gene expression/regulation will from time to time come into play even if it appears that a series of defined phenotypic features and biological abilities are necessary in any given tumor type.

Phenotypes of Metastatic Cells: Adhesion, Invasion, and Motility

The mechanisms regulating malignant dissemination (the behavior of the tumor cell and the features of host–tumor cell interactions) can be paralleled to those involved in physiological processes such as wound healing, inflammation, tissue regeneration and remodeling, trophoblast implantation, mammary gland involution, and embryonic morphogenesis. This suggests that the differences between normal processes and the pathogenic nature of tumor spread involve, by way of tumor cells, the use of physiological mechanisms in a deregulated manner. These observations have provided insights into the identification of molecules and mechanisms involved in tumor dissemination. Key events include changes in cellular adhesion; production of proteolytic enzymes capable of degrading ECM; and secretion of a variety of molecules able to activate stromal cells, endothelial cells (ECs), and tumor cells themselves.

Adhesion

There is evidence that adhesion plays an important role in tumor progression and metastasis and that molecules mediating the deregulated adhesion events contribute essentially to malignancy.

Cadherins

The initial step in the metastatic cascade is the detachment of cells from the primary tumor mass, suggesting that cell cohesiveness in malignant tumors is not as strong as it is in benign tumors, thus making cells more readily detachable from the primary mass. Such reduced cohesiveness is thought to correlate with a down-regulation of active homotypic cell-adhesion molecules. For example, in epithelial tumors, cell–cell attachment is mediated essentially by E-cadherin, which normally mediates adhesion of epithelial cells through adherens junctions. The extracellular part of E-cadherin is responsible for calcium-dependent homophilic interaction with neighboring cells, whereas the cytoplasmic part interconnects with the actin cytoskeleton through intracellular proteins known as catenins *(32)*. The cadherins are a family of transmembrane glycoproteins that mediate homotypic intercellular adhesion, playing a key role during morphogenesis and in the maintenance of the differentiated phenotype. Deregulated function of E-cadherin has been correlated with invasiveness. The addition of antibodies (Abs) against E-cadherin to differentiated kidney epithelial cells conferred them a fibroblastic morphology and the ability to invade both collagen gel and embryonal tissues *(33)*. Using human carcinoma cell lines, invasiveness could be inhibited by E-cadherin expression and reinduced by neutralizing Abs against E-cadherin *(34)*. It has been shown that expression of E-cadherin in a human breast carcinoma cell line, spontaneously metastasizing to the lung of nude mice, reduced the metastatic ability of the cells *(35)*. Accordingly, in a transgenic mouse model of pancreatic β-cell carcinogenesis, it was shown that loss of E-cadherin expression coincided with transition from well-differentiated adenoma to invasive carcinoma. When E-cadherin expression was maintained in β cells, the tumor progression arrested at the adenoma stage, whereas forced expression of a dominant negative form of E-cadherin induced tumor-cell invasion and metastasis *(36)*. Interestingly, it has also been shown that tamoxifen treatment suppressed the invasive phenotype and restored E-cadherin expression of a human breast cancer cell line *(37)*, an effect that might shed light on some of the antimetastatic effects of this drug. These experimental results are accompanied by a number of IHC studies, in which loss or reduction of E-cadherin expression correlated with the clinical stage in a broad range of malignancies including cancer of the head and neck, lung, breast, prostate, esophagus, stomach, bladder, pancreas, and colorectum *(38)*. In gastric carcinoma, the loss of protein expression was shown to correlate with allelic loss and frequent somatic allelic inactivation of the gene *(39)*. However, the reduction in E-cadherin protein is not the only reason for the loss of cohesiveness. In this respect, changes in catenin expression can also lead to loss of cadherin functions. In some studies, the loss of function of components of the E-cadherin/catenin complex has been correlated with reduced survival and poor prognosis *(40)*. The product of the adenomatous polyposis coli (APC) suppressor gene, mutated in many tumors, binds to catenins, suggesting that catenins might play roles other than simply modulating cell adhesion *(41)*. In a recent series of reports, Armadillo-type catenins have been shown to interact with transcription factors of the LEF-1/TCF (lymphoid enhancer factor/T-cell factor) family and mediate signaling of the wnt/wingless pathway to the cell nucleus *(42–46)*. Normally the APC protein, along with GSK-3β (glycogen synthase kinase), binds and modulates the degradation of β-catenin, thus regulating the cellular level of this catenin. In cells where APC is mutated, the level of free β-catenin increases and, by binding LEF-1/TCF, drives gene expression. Moreover, the β-catenin/LEF-1 signaling pathway can also be activated by mutation in β-catenin *(45)*. Consequently, the influence of the cadherin/catenin complex on tumor progression and metastasis might be double: modulation of homophilic cell adhesion on one side and direct signaling to the nucleus on the other. Furthermore, it has been shown that abrogation of E-cadherin function leads to the up-regulation of urokinase plasminogen activator (uPA), a matrix degrading enzyme *(47)*, suggesting a possible signaling pathway connecting adhesion and proteolytic degradation. Because the penetration of the surrounding tissues/ stroma, particularly basement membrane, is a hallmark of invasion by malignant cells, it is tempting to speculate that such a process might be initiated by deregulation of a particular type of adhesion event.

Integrins

As described previously, the deadhesion mechanism as a consequence of down-regulation of specific molecules contributes to metastasis because of the higher propensity of tumor cells to detach from the primary site. Other alterations may also take place in the adhesive events occurring between the released tumor cell and ECM, so that the neoplastic cell is then able to gain access to the underlying substrates. During malignant dissemination, cells are required to cross many tissue barriers, and they must therefore penetrate a variety of ECMs. For example, to initiate the metastatic process, a carcinoma cell must first penetrate the epithelial basement membrane and then invade the interstitial stroma. For distant metastases, both intravasation and extravasation require passage through the capillary walls and the invasion of the subendothelial basement membranes. The first step in the invasion of the basement membranes involves adhesion to the matrix. Attachment to specific glycoproteins of ECM is mediated through tumor-cell receptors of both integrin and nonintegrin variety.

Integrins are a large class of widely expressed $\alpha\beta$ heterodimeric receptors with broad specificity and great importance in cell–substrate interactions. Such cell-surface proteins are transmembrane molecules able to transduce signals *(18)* and influence diverse functions such as migration, differentiation, and apoptosis *(49,50)*. Signals can be transmitted from the outside to the inside of cells in response to ligand binding, thus affecting gene transcription; or from the inside to the outside of the cells modulating both the binding affinity and the density of receptors. Integrins are believed to create the structural link between components of ECM and the cytoskeleton by binding to talin, vinculin, and actin microfilaments. Thus their function is an important determinant of cell shape *(51)*. At least 14 α and 8 β subunits have been identified, which noncovalently associate to produce more than 20 different integrins *(48)*. Ligand specificity is determined largely by the subunit composition. Individual receptors can bind to more than one type of ligand and ligands can be recognized by more than one integrin. The $\beta1$ subfamily contains eight heterodimers (VLA-1 to VLA-8) that serve as receptors for ECM components such as laminin (VLA-1, -2, -3, -6) collagen (VLA-1, -2, -3), and fibronectin (VLA-3, -4, -5). One of the members, VLA-4 ($\alpha4\beta1$), also functions as a heterophilic cell–cell adhesion molecule by recognizing the immunoglobulin vascular cell adhesion molecule-1 (VCAM-1). Because VLA-4 is implicated in normal leukocyte traffic, it is thought that tumor cells expressing VLA-4 may use this receptor for hematogenous dissemination. The $\beta3$ cytoadhesion subfamily consists of two members: $\alpha v\beta3$ that serves as receptor for vitronectin, von Willebrand factor, fibrinogen, thrombospondin, and osteopontin; and the platelet $\alpha IIb\beta3$ complex that serves as receptor for fibrinogen, fibronectin, vitronectin, and von Willebrand factor. Other integrins serving as receptors for fibronectin are $\alpha v\beta1$, $\alpha v\beta5$, and $\alpha v\beta6$, where $\alpha v\beta5$ binds also vitronectin. The $\beta2$ integrins have three members, LFA-1 ($\alpha L\beta2$), Mac-1 ($\alpha M\beta2$), and p150/95 ($\alpha X\beta2$), whose expression is primarily restricted to leukocytes. They mediate cell–cell interaction by binding to intercellular adhesion molecules (ICAMs) whereas additional soluble ligands are fibrinogen and complement protein fragments.

The relationship between individual integrin expression and tumor progression appears to be complex, probably because integrins may be required not only for tumor-cell migration and adherence but also for the infiltrative behavior of cytotoxic effector cells. Moreover, it is possible that cell–matrix adhesion has dual roles: it may be required for cell locomotion in certain cases whereas it may impose constraints on motility in others.

Analysis of the adhesion molecules of the integrin superfamily on lymphocytes migrating into metastatic tissues indicates no specific expression of individual $\beta1$ or $\beta2$ integrins *(52)* whereas differences in integrin expression between normal and malignant tissues have been documented for many tissue types. A reduction in protein expression or changes in cellular distribution of a variety of integrins including $\alpha1\beta1$, $\alpha2\beta1$, $\alpha3\beta1$, $\alpha6\beta1$, $\alpha v\beta1$, and $\alpha v\beta5$ has been found. A consistent pattern has emerged from histological studies showing the main involvement of laminin and collagen receptors and it has been observed in breast *(53,54)*, pancreas *(55,56)*, colon *(57,58)*, and lung cancers *(59)*, and melanoma *(60)*. These observations suggest that the loss of attachment to the basement membrane, which is composed mainly of laminin and collagen IV, is an important event in favoring tumor development. Conversely, not all tumors manifest a generalized down-regulation of integrin expression. Elevated expression of both integrins of the cytoadhesion family, αIIbβ3 *(61,62)* and αvβ3 *(63,64)*, has been demonstrated in melanoma progression. Moreover, in cutaneous malignant melanoma, expression of α4β1 was negatively associated with the length of disease-free interval and the overall survival time *(65)*. Interestingly, reduced amounts of α6β4 were observed in primary breast cancer and pleural metastases, whereas a higher level of expression was observed in lymph node metastasis *(66)*. The latter observation raises two possible scenarios: either in different organs there is a selection allowing only a specific subset of cells to transit/arrest, or the different tissue microenvironments modulate the expression of integrins by the tumor cells.

Much experimental evidence supports the role of integrins in modulating metastasis. Results from several studies examining the effects of integrin overexpression support the observations acquired from naturally occurring cancers, with integrins being down-regulated in the more advanced/progressed stages of the diseases *(67,68)*. Conversely, other investigators have shown that the adhesive interactions mediated by integrins are necessary requirements for metastasis formation. In a human breast cancer cell line, experimental metastasis were inhibited by a monoclonal antibody (mAb) against the α5β1 fibronectin receptor. Similarly, inoculation of nude mice with a polymeric form of fibronectin inhibited the subsequent formation of metastasis by melanoma, osteosarcoma, and colon carcinoma cell lines *(69,70)*. The latter is in agreement with a previous study in which coinjection of a peptide containing the recognition site for many integrins (the Arg-Gly-Asp [RGD]-binding motif) inhibited the formation of experimental lung metastasis in syngeneic mice by B16 murine melanoma cells *(71)*. In our laboratory, we have investigated the involvement of α4β1 expressed by human melanoma cells in the augmentation of experimental metastasis induced by the inflammatory cytokines interleukin (IL)-1 and tumor necrosis factor (TNF)-α. Only melanoma cells expressing α4β1 were able to produce more lung colonies in cytokine-treated mice *(72)*. Treatment of tumor cells with mAbs against α4β1 inhibited this augmentation *(72)*. As discussed in another section of this chapter, melanoma cells expressing α4β1 integrin recognize VCAM-1 expressed on activated ECs *(73)*: the adhesion of VLA-4-positive cells was abolished by treating tumor cells with Abs to VLA-4 or by treating ECs with anti-VCAM-1 Abs *(72,74)*. These observations suggest that VLA-4/VCAM-1 is the major adhesion pathway for melanoma adhesion to activate ECs and it is probably responsible for the increase in metastases induced by cytokines.

Paradoxically integrins appear to be down-regulated in the more advanced/progressed stages of the disease, yet they are important in facilitating the occurrence of metastasis. IHC analysis of integrin expression in clinical specimens should be interpreted with caution, first, because Abs that can detect integrins on fixed tissue sections do not give information about the functionality of such molecules; and second, because the function of integrins cannot be inferred from their expression alone. More importantly, the adhesiveness mediated by integrins can be rapidly modulated by the cell on which they are expressed, without affecting the level of expression. It has been shown that integrin-dependent migration is affected by three variables: substratum ligand density, level of integrin expression, and integrin-ligand binding affinity *(75)*. These parameters might have profound influence upon the behavior of different tumor types. Clearly the nature of the substrate will vary according to anatomical locations and both integrin expression and ligand-binding affinity can be modulated by local cytokines *(76)*.

Immunoglobulins and Selectins

Conversely to cadherins and integrins, up-regulation of certain adhesion molecules has been shown to correlate with a higher potentiality of the tumor cells to metastasize. Molecules such as those of the immunoglobulin (Ig) superfamily and/or the selectin family, involved in several cell–cell heterophilic interactions, including the adherence of tumor cells to the endothelium, may play a determinant role in malignant transformation and progression to metastatic disease.

The Ig superfamily consists of molecules that share the same basic architecture of the Igs. A few members of this family have been implicated in tumor metastasis *(77)*. ICAM-1 was first identified as a ligand for LFA-1 (αLβ2 integrin) but later found to bind Mac-1 (αMβ2 integrin) as well. ICAM-1 is expressed on various types of squamous cell carcinomas and melanomas. Particularly, ICAM-1 has been shown to be a marker of progression in malignant cutaneous melanoma *(78,79)*. It is possible to consider that, since ICAM-1 binds to β2 integrins expressed on circulating leukocytes, an indirect interaction with leukocytes may mediate binding between tumor cell and endothelium allowing for enhanced extravasation. A circulating form of ICAM-1 has been found in patients with cancer *(80–82)* and increased levels were associated with advanced disease and poor outcome in Hodgkin disease (HD) *(83)* and malignant melanoma *(84)*. It remains to be determined whether the increased level merely reflects a greater tumor burden or contributes to the progression of malignancies.

VCAM-1 is a ligand for VLA-4 (α4β1 integrin). It is constitutively expressed on bone marrow stromal cells and, for this reason, it has been hypothesized to be partly responsible for the retention of leukemia cells in the marrow and the bone marrow lymphoma metastasis *(85)*. The existence of a circulating form of VCAM-1 has been reported and increased amounts have been found in patients with cancer *(81)*. Studies of VCAM-1, which is a potential endothelial ligand for cytotoxic effector lymphocytes, have shown lost expression on blood vessels within melanoma metastasis in an experimental model and within a carcinoma metastasis in the lung of a patient *(86)*. These observations suggest that tumor cells may escape host defense by preventing the effector cells extravasation, thus implying that adhesion molecules may have a role in mediating cytotoxic immune response during the metastatic process.

The homophilic neural cell adhesion molecule (NCAM) is expressed in small-cell lung carcinomas (SCLCs) and its circulating form has been proposed as a potential marker for this type of cancer *(87)*. It is also frequently expressed in bile duct cancer and a correlation has been found between NCAM expression and perineural invasion of this type of neoplasia *(88)*. This correlation suggests the possible existence of a mechanism used by tumor cells to recognize the same molecule expressed on neural cells.

The neural adhesion molecule L1 (NgCAM) is expressed on some lymphomas where, in contrast to other members of the Ig family, the metastatic ability correlated negatively with its expression *(89)*. Because L1 mediates homophilic cell–cell interaction, it is tempting to speculate that the loss of such an adhesion pathway, as shown for cadherins, could be an important step for the spreading of certain tumor types.

A transmembrane protein product with sequence similarity to the neural cell-adhesion family of molecules is encoded by the *DCC* (deleted in colorectal carcinoma) gene, mapping on chromosome 18q21.1. Allelic losses affecting 18q were detected in most primary colorectal carcinomas and IHC analysis showed that the expression of *DCC* product was markedly reduced or absent in most colorectal cancers. Moreover, the data accumulated support *DCC* inactivation in many tumor types *(90)*. Although ligands and/or receptors for *DCC* have not been identified, the loss of function of this gene may affect cell–cell as well as cell–substrate interactions and it is likely that *DCC* may function in specific signaling processes. Further studies will be necessary to determine its role in the metastatic process.

Also pertaining to the Ig superfamily is the clinically useful marker of early or recurrent colorectal cancer known as carcinoembryonic antigen (CEA). CEA has been shown to function as a homophilic adhesion molecule in colon carcinoma cells *(91)*; however, it is not known how the deregulation of this molecule leads to the spread of tumor cell to distant sites.

Selectins are a family of transmembrane glycoproteins initially identified on platelets, endothelium, and leukocytes (P-, E-, and L-selectin, respectively) that mediate adhesive interactions in inflammation *(92)*. Selectins have calcium-dependent, lectin-like domains at their extracellular extremities that enable them to bind carbohydrate ligands. The role of carbohydrates and lectins in metastases has been recognized for several years. In this regard, changes in the cell-surface carbohydrates profile have been associated with the malignant phenotype and the endogenous lectins can select for metastatic properties *(93)*. The carbohydrate derivative sialyl-Lewis^X (sLe^X) and its isomer sialyl-Lewis^a (sLe^a) have been found on several different carcinomas. Such cells have been found to adhere to activated endothelium and form metastasis in experimental models *(94)*. Furthermore, increased expression of sialyl-Le^X has been shown to correlate with the clinical stage and the overall survival of patients with colorectal cancer *(95)*.

Other Molecules

Several other adhesive interactions and adhesive molecules, including CD44 and Lu-ECAM-1, have been implicated in metastatic spread *(96)*. The CD44 hyaluronic acid receptor, originally described as a lymphocyte homing receptor, was found to be expressed as different isoforms on metastatic murine tumors *(97)*. The expression of CD44 isoforms has subsequently been demonstrated in malignant human tumors; however, their relevance as markers of metastasis and their role in tumor dissemination is uncertain.

The fact that adhesion mechanisms are critical events in many steps of the metastatic process might mean that there are ways to interfere with tumor spread, and thus there is the possibility to control metastasis. Moreover, the assessment of adhesion molecule expression and of individual levels of soluble receptors may facilitate diagnosis and increase prognostic accuracy by helping to define subgroups of patients at different risk of developing metastasis.

Interestingly, recent studies propose the involvement of cell–cell adhesion mechanisms in the resistance of solid tumors to anticancer drug treatments *(98)*. For example, hyaluronidase treatment was not only able to inhibit increased intercellular adhesion in three-dimensional EMT-6 spheroid culture, but it was also able to sensitize the cells to anticancer agents both in vitro and in vivo. These observations suggest the possibility of using antiadhesive agents as chemosensitizer in combination with conventional chemotherapeutic approaches.

Interaction with Endothelial Cells

The arrest of tumor cells in the capillary bed of secondary organs is a necessary step preceding the extravasation of metastatic cells. Preferential adhesion of metastatic tumor cells to vascular ECs of certain tissues has been demonstrated in experimental tumors, some of which can be explained by organ-specific adhesion molecules expressed by vascular ECs *(99,100)*. It is well known that vascular changes can easily influence the interaction of tumor cells with endothelium and thus the whole metastatic process. For example, the formation of platelet-fibrin thrombi influences the arrest of tumor cells *(101,102)* and the release of chemotactic factors from the vascular wall has been shown to induce tumor cell motility *(103,104)*. ECM components may affect EC recognition structures responsible for tumor–EC interactions *(105)*. Furthermore, disseminating tumor cells might, through the direct or indirect release of cytokines, modify their capacity to interact and arrest *(106)*. Inflammatory cytokines stimulate leukocyte adhesion on ECs and this is mediated by the induction or increased expression of multiple adhesion molecules *(107)*. In vivo studies from our laboratory and others have shown an increase in the number of experimental metastasis in mice receiving IL-1 or TNF *(108,109)*. Cancer cells and leukocytes share several adhesion molecules and the mechanisms proposed for lymphocyte migration appear to play a role in the extravasation of metastatic cells *(110–112)*. The adhesion molecules on ECs mainly responsible for this response are E-selectin, VCAM-1, and ICAM-1. In this regard, the enhanced binding of colon-related carcinomas to cytokine-activated ECs is mainly mediated by E-selectin *(110,113)* and, as described above, sLe^x and sLe^a (ligands recognized by selectins) contribute to tumor-cell arrest in secondary organs *(114)*. At variance, VCAM-1 on activated ECs mainly binds melanoma and sarcoma cells *(72,73)*.

We investigated the interaction of human tumor cells with cultured ECs under dynamic flow conditions, using a parallel-plate laminar-flow chamber. Tumor cells studied under these conditions adhered to IL-1-activated ECs with different adhesion patterns. For example, several types of carcinoma cells adhered to ECs preceded by rolling, whereas melanomas and osteosarcomas adhered firmly, without rolling *(115)*. E-selectin mediated the dynamic interaction of colon carcinoma cells *(115,116)*, whereas the firm adhesion of melanoma cells was partly blocked by anti-VCAM-1 Abs *(115)*. Therefore, the understanding of the dynamic interactions between tumor cells and ECs may have important implications in the patterns of tumor metastasis formation.

Invasion

During the metastatic process, the cells must pass through structural barriers. ECM and basement membrane barriers must be breached for cells to intravasate and extravasate. Moreover, within the tissue at either the primary or secondary sites and as the tumor mass expands in size, ECMs appear to require degradation. These observations suggest that tumor cells that have acquired the ability to degrade the components of basement membranes might be able to traverse them more readily. As a consequence, they may have enhanced ability to form distant metastasis. Alternatively, some of the required proteolytic activities may be derived from tumor-associated host tissues including adjacent stromal components and infiltrating immune cells. A wide range of proteolytic enzymes might contribute to this process. Many of them have been shown to increase the invasiveness of cells in experimental settings or to have prognostic implications when identified in tumor samples *(117)*. There are four main families of proteolytic enzymes that are candidates for facilitating tumor cell invasion and metastasis and thus thought to be involved in tumor malignancy *(117,118)*:

- the serine proteases which include uPA, elastase, plasmin, and cathepsin G;
- the cysteine proteases which include cathepsin B and L;
- the aspartic proteases which include cathepsin D;
- the matrix metalloproteinases (MMPs) which comprise the gelatinases, the interstitial collagenases, the stromelysins, and matrilysin.

The regulation of enzymatic activity is complex and it is balanced between the local concentration of the enzymes themselves and their endogenous activators and inhibitors. The production and the secretion of any of them could be affected during malignant progression and dissemination.

Metalloproteinases and Their Inhibitors

MMPs are a family of secreted or transmembrane protein with an optimum pH for activity in the physiological range. They are active against virtually all the ECM and basement membrane components. In particular, this family comprises the only enzymes capable of cleaving and denaturing fibrillar collagen. Currently, 16 members have been identified. They share a conserved metal-binding site in the catalytic domain, responsible for ligating Zn^{2+}, which is essential for catalytic functions. Moreover, a distinct conserved sequence in the pro-region is responsible for maintaining the latency of the zymogen, thus introducing an additional regulation at the level of proteolytic activation. There are three major subgroups of MMPs, identified by their substrate preferences:

- the collagenases (comprised of interstitial collagenase, neutrophil collagenase, and collagenase-3) active against the native, fibrillar forms of collagen I, II, and III;
- the stromelysins (including stromelysin-1, -2, -3, and matrilysin) which degrade preferentially proteoglycans and glycoproteins;
- the gelatinases (consisting of gelatinase A and B) particularly potent in the degradation of nonfibrillar and denatured collagens (gelatin).

The recently identified membrane-type MMPs (MT-MMPs) are membrane-bound proteinases involved in the activation of the other MMPs *(118,119)*. MMP activity has been demonstrated to be highly regulated at many levels. mRNA for most family members is transcriptionally modulated by biological agents such as growth factors, hormones, inflammatory cytokines, and oncogenes *(120–122)*. There is also evidence for posttranscriptional/translational regulation, for example, by alteration of mRNA stability *(123,124)*. Posttranslational regulation occurs by storage in secretory granules and by activation of the secreted latent form *(125)*. Proteinase cascade involving other MMPs and other enzyme classes (e.g., plasmin, trypsin) have been implicated in MMP activation. The active enzyme MMPs are susceptible to inhibition by endogenous inhibitors such as the general serum proteinase inhibitor α_2-macroglobulin and a family of specific inhibitors: the tissue inhibitors of metalloproteinases (TIMPs) whose own expression is also influenced by local cytokines and growth factors. Currently four members of the TIMP family have been identified. They have the MMP-inhibitory activity in common, but differ in the expression patterns and associations with latent MMP (TIMP-1 associates with pro-gel B and is expressed mainly in ovary and bone; TIMP-2 associates with pro-gel A and is mainly expressed in placenta; TIMP-3 associates with ECMs and is expressed mainly in kidney and brain; and TIMP-4 is expressed mainly in the heart and its association with other MMPs has not yet been determined). TIMPs inhibit metalloproteinase activity by forming a complex with active MMPs, but they do not distinguish effectively between the individual family members (118,126). Thus, during physiological events, the enzymatic activities of these molecules are tightly regulated. In malignant progression and dissemination, the disruption of such a regulation may contribute to the increase of tissue destruction and invasion, a hallmark of malignancy.

The first piece of evidence implicating the importance of MMPs in the metastatic process was the finding that metastatic tumor cells expressed more type IV collagenase activity than their nonmetastatic counterparts (127). The enzymes responsible for the degradation of collagen IV, a major structural component of the basement membrane, are now recognized to be either gelatinase A (72 kDa type IV collagenase, MMP-2) or gelatinase B (92 kDa type IV collagenase, MMP-9). A study comparing the production of MMP-9 in cell lines isolated from human melanoma lesion at different stages of disease progression showed that the enhanced or *de novo* MMP-9 production was associated with advanced melanomas (128). Extensive literature reports the association of MMP and TIMP family members with tumor progression (118,119,126,129). IHC studies in tissue sections have shown positive staining for MMP which was limited to tumor cells in some cases and to stromal tissues in others. Furthermore, "hot spots" of gelatinase activity have been observed at the tumor–stroma interface. Such findings suggest that the host tissue might be an integral part of the MMP profile in malignant disease.

As mentioned earlier, the activity of both MMPs and TIMPs can be influenced, often differentially, by factors such as transforming growth factor-β (TGF-β) and basic-fibroblast growth factor (b-FGF) which are released from ECMs during their degradation. This phenomenon may amplify the degradative process and emphasize the dynamic nature of the tumor spread and stress the importance of the microenvironment. An important contribution of the "host" is the formation of new vasculature necessary for a tumor to grow beyond 1–2 millimeters. MMPs appear to be involved in the formation of the new vessels by mediating the remodeling of ECM that must accompany new capillary growth.

Given all this, inhibitors of matrix metalloproteinases (MMPIs) might be of therapeutic value in the treatment of metastatic disease, first by preventing tumor local invasion and second by inhibiting tumor angiogenesis (130). Studies with MMPIs have shown their ability to inhibit the degradation of ECM in vitro by tumor cells (131,132). In experimental tumor models in vivo, MMPI treatment caused inhibition of tumor growth and of the metastatic spread in rodent and human tumor models (131–134). The possibility of using MMPI as a therapeutic strategy is currently being explored in clinical trials.

MMPs are not the only proteolytic contributor in tumor progression, and it should be noted that interactions between members of other classes of proteolytic enzymes might provide additional levels of complexity and regulation.

Urokinase Plasminogen Activator and Its Receptor

uPA is secreted as inactive precursor pro-uPA and binds its GPI (glycosyl-phosphatidyl-inositol)-linked membrane receptor (uPAR). Upon binding, membrane-bound plasmin cleaves uPA, originating an active enzyme able to catalyze the conversion of plasminogen into plasmin. Plasmin can either directly degrade proteins or activate zymogens, mainly of the MMPs family. The activity of uPA is modulated by inhibitors such as the plasminogen–activator–inhibitor (PAI) family and the protease nexin-1. The uPA/uPAR system plays a key role in many physiological processes including embryogenesis, angiogenesis, and wound healing. Evidence exists that this system is important in tumor spread. IHC studies showed that components of this system were localized both at the invasive front of the tumor and in the stromal tissue *(135)*, once again suggesting the complexity of interactions existing between tumor and host during the invasive process. In breast cancer, the relapse rate correlated positively with the expression level of uPA within the tumor *(136)* as well as in the tissue stroma *(137)*. Furthermore, a high uPA level was also linked to a worse prognosis in patients with breast *(138)*, colorectal *(139)*, and gastric *(140)* cancers. Experimental studies have indicated that the ability of tumor cells to invade and metastasize could be decreased by interfering with the uPA/uPAR system, thus offering some prospects for therapeutic intervention *(141)*.

Motility

The role of tumor cell motility in invasion is not completely known nor has it been fully demonstrated, but it is quite clear that tumor cells are capable of active movements through tissues. Individual or small aggregates of tumor cells are found physically separated from the main tumor mass. Tumor cells in tissue culture can move randomly (chemokinesis) or directionally toward attractants. Motility can occur by either chemotaxis or haptotaxis, depending on whether the attractant(s) is soluble or substrate bound. In this regard, motility factors are thought to play an essential role in the migration processes at various levels of the metastatic cascade, for example, infiltration of the cells into adjacent tissues, migration through the vessel wall into the circulation, and subsequent extravasation into secondary sites. A variety of agents have been shown to modulate the motile response of tumor cells in vitro, including growth factors, components of ECM, hyaluronians, host-derived scatter factors, and tumor-secreted factors. This variety of stimuli could give cells multiple opportunities to move across different microenvironments during the metastatic process.

Recently, autotaxin (ATX), a potent new cytokine with a molecular mass of 125 kDa, has been purified from the conditioned medium of a human melanoma cell line *(142)*. ATX was shown to be active in stimulating both chemotactic and chemokinetic responses in the ATX-producing cells as well as other tumor cells *(143)*. It is likely that ATX stimulates the cell through G-protein-linked cell-surface receptor, as the motile response is abolished when cells are treated with pertussin toxin. By using the cDNA sequence from the melanoma-derived ATX, another autotoxin, which shows

94% homology by analysis of the deduced amino-acid sequence, was cloned from a human teratocarcinoma cell line *(144)*. Together these findings suggest that the autocrine production of motility factors by tumor cells could play a major role in the local invasive behavior of the metastatic cell. The existence and the extent of possible correlations between such production and infiltrative behavior remains to be determined. However, the prospect inhibiting the invasive process by blocking the production of and/or the response to motility factors cannot be excluded.

How the motility factors, which are known to be produced or to act upon tumor cells, regulate cell movement is not completely understood. The transduction of signals after ligand–receptor coupling is likely to be important in the modulation of cell locomotion. Moreover, signaling systems may be dissimilar in different cell types and they may also express dissimilar receptors. For example, the binding of ATX to its receptor is followed by events mediated by G-protein *(142)* whereas hepatocyte growth factor (HGF)/scatter factor (SF) operate through tyrosine kinase *(145)*, both probably controlling important aspects of cell activities.

HGF was discovered as a mitogen for hepatocytes and was later shown to be identical to SF *(146)*, a mesenchymal cell-derived cytokine that dissociated cohesive sheets of epithelium into individual cells (scatter activity) *(147)*. The ability to dissociate epithelia might affect adhesion molecules. HGF–SF has been demonstrated to alter the tyrosine phosphorylation of the cadherin-associated β-catenin *(147)*, which may in turn impair cadherin adhesive functions. HGF–SF also stimulates directed cell migration and promotes invasion *(146,147)*. In this regard, HGF/SF has been shown to up-regulate the expression of both uPA and uPAR *(149)*, suggesting its potential ability to activate cellular programs for the invading cell, for example, modulating focal degradation of ECM. HGF/SF is overexpressed in tumors. High levels of HGF/SF in primary breast cancers correlate with poor prognosis and were shown to be a strong predictor of relapse *(150)*. HGF/SF is the ligand for a transmembrane tyrosine kinase (HGF-R) encoded by the c-*Met* protooncogene, linking cell movement with a known transforming oncogene *(151)*.

The relevance of ECM proteins in the metastatic process has also been demonstrated to govern motility. The use of ECM proteins (e.g., laminin, fibronectin, type IV collagen, thrombospondin) in motility assays showed their ability to stimulate both chemotaxis and haptotaxis. Chemotaxis and haptotaxis to the same ECM protein appear to generate motility signals through different signal-transduction pathways. When cells are treated with pertussin toxin, the chemotactic response to laminin is diminished and the response to type IV collagen is abolished. In contrast, haptotaxic response to the same proteins was unaffected *(152)*. Interestingly, studies with thrombospondin identified distinct chemotaxis-promoting and haptotaxis-promoting domains on the same molecule *(153)*.

Conclusions

Metastasis is a complex process in which the eventual outcome is the result of a number of interactions between tumor cells and the host. Several compounds derived from knowledge of this process are under investigation in preclinical and clinical settings. The apparent redundancy of the mechanisms involved in the metastatic process might imply the use of more than one therapeutic intervention in blocking metastasis spread and growth. A better understanding of the molecular basis is necessary to identify novel and selective targets for therapy.

Acknowledgments

The support of Italian Association for Cancer Research (AIRC) is greatly acknowledged. We would like to thank Maria Pirocchi for her secretarial assistance.

References

1. Kumar V, Cotran RS, Robbins SL. Neoplasia. In: *Basic Pathology*, 6th edit. (Kumar V, Cotran RS, Robbins SL, eds.), WB Saunders, Philadelphia, 1997, pp. 132–74.
2. Hart IR, Saini A. Biology of tumour metastasis. *Lancet.* 1992; 339:1453–7.
3. Fidler IJ, Gersten DM, Hart IR. The biology of cancer invasion and metastasis. *Adv Cancer Res.* 1978; 28:149–250.
4. Liotta LA, Stetler-Stevenson WG. Principles of molecular cell biology of cancer: cancer metastasis. In: *Cancer: Principles and Practice of Oncology*, 4th edit. (DeVita VT, Hellman S, Rosemberg SA, eds.), Lippincott, Philadelphia, 1993, pp. 134–9.
5. Fidler IJ. 7th Jan Waldenstrom Lecture: The biology of human cancer metastasis. *Acta Oncol.* 1991; 30:668–75.
6. Paget S. The distribution of secondary growths in cancer of the breast. *Lancet.* 1989; 1:571–3.
7. Weiss L. Metastatic inefficiency. *Adv Cancer Res.* 1990; 54:159–211.
8. Roth C, Rochlitz C, Kourilsky P. Immune response against tumors. *Adv Immunol.* 1994; 57:281–351.
9. Henderson RA, Finn OJ. Human tumor antigens are ready to fly. *Adv Immunol.* 1996; 62:217–56.
10. Kerbel RS. Expression of multi-cytokine resistance and multi-growth factor independence in advance stage metastatic cancer—malignant melanoma as a paradigm. *Am J Pathol.* 1992; 141:519–24.
11. Folkman J. Clinical applications of research on angiogenesis. *N Engl J Med.* 1995; 333:1757–63.
12. Holmgren L, O'Reilly MS, Folkman J. Dormancy of micrometastases: balanced proliferation and apoptosis in the presence of angiogenesis suppression. *Nat Med.* 1995; 1:149–53.
13. Fearon ER, Vogelstein B. A genetic model for colorectal tumorigenesis. *Cell.* 1990; 61:759–67.
14. Nowell PC. The clonal evolution of tumor cell populations. *Science.* 1976; 194:23–28.
15. Waghorne C, Thomas M, Lagarde A, Kerbel RS, Breitman ML. Genetic evidence for progressive selection and overgrowth of primary tumors by metastatic cell subpopulations. *Cancer Res.* 1988; 48:6109–114.
16. Bani MR, Rak J, Adachi D, et al. Multiple features of advanced melanoma recapitulated in tumorigenic variants of early stage (radial growth phase) human melanoma cell lines: evidence for a dominant phenotype. *Cancer Res.* 1996; 56:3075–86.
17. Bishop JM. Molecular themes in oncogenesis. *Cell.* 1991; 64:235–48.
18. Weinberg RA. Prospects for cancer genetics. *Cancer Surveys.* 1997; 25:3–12.
19. Chambers AF, Tuck AB. *Ras*-responsive genes and tumor metastasis. *Crit Rev Oncogene* 1993; 4:95–114.
20. Steeg PS, Bevilacqua G, Kopper L, et al. Evidence for a novel gene associated with low tumor metastatic potential. *J Natl Cancer Inst.* 1988; 80:200–4.

21. Leone A, Flatow U, King CR, et al. Reduced tumor incidence, metastatic potential, and cytokine responsiveness of *nm23*-transfected melanoma cells. *Cell.* 1991; 65:25–35.

22. Leone A, Flatow U, Van Houtte K, Steeg PS. Transfection of human *nm23–H1* into the human MDA-MB-435 breast carcinoma cell line: effects on tumor metastatic potential, colonization and enzymatic activity. *Oncogene.* 1993; 8:2325–33.

23. MacDonald NJ, De La Rosa A, Steeg PS. The potential roles of *nm23* in cancer metastasis and cellular differentiation. *Eur J Cancer.* 1995; 31A:1096–1100.

24. Golden A, Benedict M, Shearn A, et al. Nucleoside diphosphate kinases, *nm23*, and tumor metastasis: possible biochemical mechanisms. *Cancer Treat Rev.* 1992; 63:345–58.

25. MacDonald NJ, De La Rosa A, Benedict MA, et al. A serine phosphorylation of *Nm23*, and not its nucleoside diphosphate kinase activity, correlates with suppression of tumor metastatic potential. *J Biol Chem.* 1994; 268:25780–9.

26. Dong JT, Lamb PW, Rinker-Shaeffer CW, et al. *KAI1*, a metastasis suppressor gene for prostate cancer on human chromosome 11p11.2. *Science.* 1995; 268:884–6.

27. Dong JT, Suzuki H, Pin SS, et al. Downregulation of the *KAI1* metastasis suppressor gene during the progression of human prostatic cancer infrequently involves gene mutation of allelic loss. *Cancer Res.* 1996; 56:4387–90.

28. Adachi M, Taki T, Ieki Y, Huang CL, Higashiyama M, Miyake M. Correlation of *KAI1/CD82* gene expression with good prognosis in patients with non-small cell lung cancer. *Cancer Res.* 1996; 56:1751–5.

29. Lee JH, Miele ME, Hicks DJ, et al. *KiSS-1*, a novel human malignant melanoma metastasis-suppressor gene. *J Natl Cancer Inst.* 1996b; 88:1731–7.

30. Lee JH, Welch DR. Suppression of metastasis in human breast carcinoma MDA-MB-435 cells after transfection with the metastasis suppressor gene, *KiSS-1*. *Cancer Res.* 1997; 57:2384–7.

31. Lee JH, Welch DR. Identification of highly expressed genes in metastasis-suppressed chromosome 6/human malignant melanoma hybrid cells using subtractive hybridization and differential display. *Int J Cancer.* 1997; 71:1035–44.

32. Hulsken J, Birchmeier W, Behrens J. E-cadherin and APC compete for the interaction with β-catenin and cytoskeleton. *J Cell Biol.* 1994; 127:2061–9.

33. Behrens J, Mareel MM, Van Roy FM, Birchmeier W. Dissecting tumor cell invasion: epithelial cells acquire invasive properties after the loss of uvomorulin-mediated cell–cell adhesion. *J Cell Biol.* 1989; 108:2435–47.

34. Frixen UH, Behrens J, Sachs M, et al. E-cadherin-mediated cell–cell adhesion prevents invasiveness of human carcinoma cells. *J Cell Biol.* 1991; 113:173–85.

35. Meiners S, Brinkmann V, Naundorf H, Birchmeier W. Role of morphogenetic factors in metastasis of mammary carcinoma cells. *Oncogene.* 1998; 16:9–20.

36. Perl AK, Wilgenbus P, Dahl U, Semb H, Christofori G. A causal role for E-cadherin in the transition from adenoma to carcinoma. *Nature.* 1998; 392:190–3.

37. Bracke ME, Charlier C, Bruyneel EA, Labit C, Mareel MM, Castronovo V. Tamoxifen restores the E-cadherin function in human breast cancer MCF-7/6 cells and suppresses their invasive phenotype. *Cancer Res.* 1994; 54:4607–9.

38. Birchmeier W, Behrens J. Cadherin expression in carcinomas: role in the formation of cell junctions and the prevention of invasiveness. *Biochim Biophys Acta Biomembr.* 1994; 1198:11–26.

39. Becker KF, Hofler H. Frequent somatic allelic inactivation of the E-cadherin gene in gastric carcinomas. *J Natl Cancer Inst.* 1995; 87:1082–4.

40. Nakanishi Y, Ochiai A, Akimoto S, et al. Expression of E-cadherin, α-catenin, β-catenin

and plakoglobin in esophageal carcinomas and its prognostic significance: immunohisto-chemical analysis of 96 lesions. *Oncology*. 1997; 54:158–65.

41. Su LK, Vogelstein B, Kinzler KW. Association of the APC tumor suppressor protein with catenins. *Science*. 1993; 262:1734–7.

42. Behrens J, von Kries JP, Kuhl M, et al. Functional interaction of β-catenin with the transcription factor LEF-1. *Nature*. 1996; 382:638–42.

43. Molenaar M, van de Wetering M, Oosterwegel M, et al. XTcf-3 transcription factor mediates β-catenin-induced axis formation in *Xenopus* embryos. *Cell*. 1996; 86:391–9.

44. Korinek V, Barker N, Morin PJ, et al. Constitutive transcriptional activation by a β-catenin-Tcf complex in APC-/- colon carcinoma. *Science*. 1997; 275:1784–7.

45. Morin PJ, Sparks AB, Korinek V, et al. Activation of β-catenin-Tcf signaling in colon cancer by mutations in β-catenin or APC. *Science*. 1997; 275:1787–90.

46. Rubinfeld B, Robbins P, El-Gamil M, Albert I, Porfiri E, Polakis P. Stabilization of β-catenin by genetic defects in melanoma cell lines. *Science*. 1997; 275:1790–2.

47. Frixen UH, Nagamine Y. Stimulation of urokinase-type plasminogen activator expression by blockage of E-cadherin-dependent cell–cell adhesion. *Cancer Res*. 1993; 53:3618–23.

48. Hynes RO. Integrins: versatility, modulation, and signaling in cell adhesion. *Cell*. 1992; 69:11–25.

49. Brooks PC, Montegomery AM, Rosenfeld M, et al. Integrin αvβ3 antagonists promote tumor regression by inducing apoptosis of angiogenic blood vessels. *Cell*. 1994; 79:1157–64.

50. Cheresh DA, Mecham RP. *Integrins: Molecular and Biological Responses to the Extracellular Matrix*. Academic Press, London, 1994.

51. Horwitz A, Duggan K, Buck C, Beckerle MC, Burridge K. Interaction of plasma membrane fibronectin receptor with talin: a transmembrane linkage. *Nature*. 1986; 320:531–3.

52. Garia-Barcina M, Bidaurrazaga I, Neaud V, et al. Variations in the expression of cell-adhesion molecules on liver-associated lymphocytes and peripheral-blood lymphocytes in patients with and without liver metastasis. *Int J Cancer*. 1995; 61:475–9.

53. Koukoulis GK, Virtanen I, Korhonen M, Laitinen L, Quaranta V, Gould VE. Immunohisto-chemical localization of integrins in the normal, hyperplastic and neoplastic breast. Correlations with their functions as receptors and cell adhesion molecules. *Am J Pathol*. 1991; 139:787–99.

54. Gui GPH, Wells CA, Yeomans P, Jordan SE, Vinson GP, Carpenter R. Integrin expression in breast cancer cytology: a novel predictor of axillary metastasis. *Eur J Surg Oncol*. 1996; 22:254–8.

55. Hall PA, Coates P, Lemoine NR, Horton MA. Characterisation of integrin chains in normal and neoplastic human pancreas. *J Pathol*. 1991; 165:33–41.

56. Weinel RJ, Rosendahl A, Pinschmidt E, Kisker O, Simon B, Santoso S. The α 6-integrin receptor in pancreatic carcinoma. *Gastroenterology*. 1995; 108:523–32.

57. Koretz K, Schlag P, Boumsell L, Moller P. Expression of VLA-α 2, VLA-α 6 and VLA-β 1 chains in normal mucosa and adenomas of the colon, and in colon carcinomas and their liver metastases. *Am J Pathol*. 1991; 138:741–750.

58. Lindmark G, Gerdin B, Pahlman L, Glimelius B, Gehlsen K, Rubin K. Interconnection of integrins α 2 and α 3 and structure of the basal membrane in colorectal cancer: relation to survival. *Eur J Surg Oncol*. 1993; 19:50–60.

59. Roussel E, Gingras MC, Ro JY, Branch C, Roth JA. Loss of α1 β1 and reduced expression of other β 1 integrins and CAM in lung adenocarcinoma compared with pneumocytes. *J Surg Oncol*. 1994; 56:198–208.

60. Natali PG, Nicotra MR, Cavaliere R, Giannarelli D, Bigotti A. Tumor progression in human malignant melanoma is associated with changes in α 6/β 1 laminin receptor. *Int J Cancer.* 1991; 49:168–72.

61. McGregor BC, McGregor JL, Weiss LM, et al. Presence of cytoadhesions (IIb-IIIa-like glycoproteins) on human metastatic melanomas but not on benign melanocytes. *Am J Clin Pathol.* 1989; 92:495–9.

62. Nicrodzik ML, Kleptish A, Karpatkin S. Role of platelets, thrombin, integrin IIb-IIIa, fibronectin and von Willebrand factor on tumor adhesion in vitro and metastasis in vivo. *Thromb Haemostas.* 1995; 74:282–90.

63. Albelda SM, Mette SA, Elder DE, et al. Integrin distribution in malignant melanoma: association of the β 3 subunit with tumor progression. *Cancer Res.* 1990; 50:6757–64.

64. Danen EH, Jansen KF, Van Kraats AA, Cornelissen IM, Ruiter DJ, Van Muijen GN. α v-integrins in human melanoma: gain of α v β 3 and loss of α v β 5 are related to tumor progression in situ but not to metastic capacity of cell lines in nude mice. *Int J Cancer.* 1995; 61:491–6.

65. Schadendorf D, Heidel J, Gawlik C, Suter L, Czarnetzki BM. Association with clinical outcome of expression of VLA-4 in primary cutaneous malignant melanoma as well as P-selectin and E-selectin on intratumoral vessels. *J Natl Cancer Inst.* 1995; 87: 366–371.

66. Natali PG, Nicotra MR, Botti C, Mottolese M, Bigotti A, Segatto O. Changes in expression of α 6/β 4 integrin heterodimer in primary and metastatic breast cancer. *Br J Cancer.* 1992; 66:318–22.

67. Giancotti FG, Ruoslahti E. Elevated levels of the α5β1 fibronectin receptor suppress the transformed phenotype of Chinese hamster ovary cells. *Cell.* 1990; 60:849–59.

68. Zutter MM, Santoro SA, Staatz WD, Tsung YL. Re-expression of the α 2 β 1 integrin abrogates the malignant phenotype of breast carcinoma cells. *Proc Natl Acad Sci USA.* 1995; 92:7411–5.

69. Akiyama SK, Olden K, Yamada KM. Fibronectin and integrins in invasion and metastasis. *Cancer and Metastasis Reviews.* 1995; 14:173–89.

70. Pasqualini R, Bourdoulous S, Koivunen E, et al. A polymeric form of fibronectin has antimetastatic effects against multiple tumour types. *Nat Med.* 1996; 2:1197–1203.

71. Humphries MJ, Olden K, Yamada KM. A synthetic peptide from fibronectin inhibits experimental metastasis of murine melanoma cells. *Science.* 1986; 233:467–70.

72. Garofalo A, Chirivi RGS, Foglieni C, et al. Involvement of the very late antigen 4 integrin on melanoma in interleukin-1-augmented experimental metastases. *Cancer Res.* 1995; 55:414–9.

73. Martin-Padura I, Mortarini R, Lauri D, et al. Heterogeneity in human melanoma cell adhesion to cytokine activated endothelial cells correlates with VLA-4 expression. *Cancer Res.* 1991; 51:2239–41.

74. Mould AP, Askari JA, Craig SE, Garratt AN, Clements J, Humphries MJ. Integrin α 4 β 1-mediated melanoma cell adhesion and migration on vascular cell adhesion molecule-1 (VCAM-1) and the alternatively spliced IIICS region fibronectin. *J Biol Chem.* 1994; 269:27224–30.

75. Palecek SP, Loftus JC, Ginsberg MH, Lauffenburger DA, Horwitz AF. Integrin-ligand binding properties govern cell migration speed through cell-substratum adhesiveness. *Nature.* 1997; 385:537–40.

76. Kim LT, Yamada KM. The regulation of expression of integrin receptors. *Proc Soc Exp Biol Med.* 1997; 214:123–31.

77. Johnson JP. Cell adhesion molecules of the immunoglobulin supergene family and their

role in malignant transformation and progression to metastatic disease. *Cancer Met Rev.* 1991; 10:11–22.

78. Johnson JP, Stade BG, Holzmann B, Schwable W, Riethmuller G. De novo expression of intercellular-adhesion molecule 1 in melanoma correlates with increased risk of metastasis. *Proc Natl Acad Sci USA.* 1989; 86:641–4.

79. Natali P, Nicotra MR, Cavaliere R, et al. Differential expression of intercellular adhesion molecule 1 in primary and metastatic melanoma lesions. *Cancer Res.* 1990; 50:1271–8.

80. Tsujisaki M, Imai K, Hirata H, et al. Detection of circulating intercellular adhesion molecules-1 antigen in malignant diseases. *Clin Exp Immunol.* 1991; 85:3–8.

81. Banks RE, Gearing AJ, Hemingway IK, Norfolk DR, Perren TJ, Selby PJ. Circulating intercellular adhesion molecule-1 (ICAM-1), E-selectin and vascular cell adhesion molecule-1 (VCAM-1) in human malignancies. *Br J Cancer.* 1993; 68:122–4.

82. Giavazzi R, Chirivi RG, Garofalo A, et al. Soluble intercellular adhesion molecule 1 is released by human melanoma cells and is associated with tumor growth in nude mice. *Cancer Res.* 1992; 52:2628–30.

83. Gruss HJ, Dolken G, Brach MA, Mertelsmann R, Herrmann F. Serum levels of circulating ICAM-1 are increased in Hodgkin's disease. *Leukemia.* 1993; 7:1245–9.

84. Harning R, Mainolfi E, Bystryn JC, Henn M, Merluzzi VJ, Rothlein R. Serum levels of circulating intercellular adhesion molecule 1 in human malignant melanoma. *Cancer Res.* 1991; 51:5003–5.

85. Juneja HS, Schmalsteig FC, Lee S, Chen J. Vascular cell adhesion molecule-1 and VLA-4 are obligatory adhesion proteins in the heterotypic adherence between human leukemia/lymphoma cells and marrow stromal cells. *Exp Hematol.* 1993; 21:444–450.

86. Piali L, Fichtel A, Terpe HJ, Imhof BA, Gisler RH. Endothelial vascular cell adhesion molecule 1 expression is suppressed by melanoma and carcinoma. *J Exp Med.* 1995; 181:811–6.

87. Jacques G, Auerbach B, Pritsch M, Wolf M, Madry N, Havemann K. Evaluation of serum neural cell adhesion molecule as a new tumor marker in small cell lung cancer. *Cancer.* 1993; 72:418–25.

88. Seki H, Tanaka J, Sato Y, Kato Y, Umezawa A, Koyama K. Neural cell adhesion molecule (NCAM) and perineural invasion in bile duct cancer. *J Surg Oncol.* 1993; 53:78–83.

89. Kowitz A, Kadmon G, Verschueren H, et al. Expression of L1 cell adhesion molecule is associated with lymphoma growth and metastasis. *Clin Exp Metastas.* 1993; 11:419–29.

90. Cho KR, Fearon ER. DCC: Linking tumour suppressor genes and altered cell surface interactions in cancer? *Eur J Cancer.* 1995; 31A:1055–60.

91. Benchimol S, Fuks A, Jothy S, Beauchemin N, Shirota K, Stanners CP. Carcinoembryonic antigen, a human tumor marker, functions as an intercellular adhesion molecule. *Cell.* 1989; 57:327–34.

92. McEver RP. Selectins: novel receptors that mediate leukocyte adhesion during inflammation. *Thromb Haemost.* 1991; 65:223–8.

93. Raz A, Lotan R. Endogenous galactoside-binding lectins: a new class of functional tumor cell surface molecules related to metastasis. *Cancer Metastas. Rev.* 1987; 6:433–52.

94. Giavazzi R. Cytokine-mediated tumor-endothelial cell interaction in metastasis. In: *Current Topics in Microbiology and Immunology; Attempts to Understand Metastasis Formation II: Regulatory Factors* (Günthert U, Birchmeier W, eds.), Springer-Verlag, Berlin, 1996, pp. 13–30.

95. Nakamori S, Kameyama M, Imaoka S, et al. Increased expression of sialyl Lewis^x antigen correlates with poor survival in patients with colorectal carcinoma: clinicopathological and immunohistochemical study. *Cancer Res.* 1993; 53:3632–7.

96. Hart IR, Hogg N. *Cell Adhesion and Cancer.* Cold Spring Harbor Laboratory Press, Cold Spring Harbor, New York, 1995.

97. Gunthert U, Hofmann M, Rudy W, et al. A new variant of glycoprotein CD44 confer metastatic potential to rat carcinoma cells. *Cell.* 1991; 65:13–24.

98. St Croix B, Kerbel RS. Cell adhesion and drug resistance in cancer. *Curr Opin Oncol.* 1997; 9:549–56.

99. Nicolson GL. Organ specificity of tumor metastasis: role of preferential adhesion, invasion and growth of malignant cells at specific secondary sites. *Cancer Metastas Rev.* 1988; 7:143–88.

100. Pauli BU, Augustin-Voss HG, el-Sabban ME, Johnson RC, Hammer DA. Organ-preferences of metastasis. The role of endothelial cell adhesion molecules. *Cancer Metastas Rev.* 1990; 9:175–89.

101. Gasic GJ. Role of plasma, platelets, and endothelial cells in tumor metastasis. *Cancer Metastas Rev.* 1984; 3:99–114.

102. Weiss L, Orr FW, Honn KV. Interactions between cancer cells and the microvasculature: a rate-regulator for metastasis. *Clin Exp Metastas.* 1989; 7:127–67.

103. Orr FW, Buchanan MR, Tron VA, Guy D, Lauri D, Sauder DN. Chemotactic activity of endothelial cell-derived interleukin 1 for human tumor cells. *Cancer Res.* 1988; 48:6758–63.

104. Wang JM, Taraboletti G, Matsushima K, Van Damme J, Mantovani A. Induction of haptotactic migration of melanoma cells by neutrophil activating protein/interleukin-8. *Biochem Biophys Res Commun.* 1990; 169:165–70.

105. Pauli BU, Lee CL. Organ preference of metastasis. The role of organ-specifically modulated endothelial cells. *Lab Invest.* 1988; 58:379–87.

106. Giavazzi R, Bani MR. The metastatic process: involvement of cytokines. *Forum: Trends Exp Clin Med.* 1992; 2:57–65.

107. Osborn L. Leukocyte adhesion to endothelium in inflammation. *Cell.* 1990; 62:3–6.

108. Bani MR, Garofalo A, Scanziani E, Giavazzi R. Effect of interleukin-1-β on metastasis formation in different tumor systems. *J Natl Cancer Inst.* 1991; 83:119–23.

109. Giavazzi R, Garofalo A, Bani MR, et al. Interleukin 1-induced augmentation of experimental metastases from a human melanoma in nude mice. *Cancer Res.* 1990; 50:4771–5.

110. Chirivi RG, Nicoletti MI, Remuzzi A, Giavazzi R. Cytokines and cell adhesion molecules in tumor-endothelial cell interaction and metastasis. *Cell Adhes Commun.* 1994; 2:219–24.

111. Bevilacqua MP. Endothelial-leukocyte adhesion molecules. *Annu Rev Immunol.* 1993; 11:767–804.

112. Dejana E, Bertocchi F, Bortolami MC, et al. Interleukin 1 promotes tumor cell adhesion to cultured human endothelial cells. *J Clin Invest.* 1988; 82:1466–70.

113. Lauri D, Needham L, Martin-Padura I, Dejana E. Tumor cell adhesion to endothelial cells: endothelial leukocyte adhesion molecule-1 as an inducible adhesive receptor specific for colon carcinoma cells. *J Natl Cancer Inst.* 1991; 83:1321–4.

114. Dejana E, Martin-Padura I, Lauri D, Bernasconi S, Bani MR, Garofalo A, Giavazzi R, Magnani J, Mantovani A, Menard S. Endothelial leukocyte adhesion molecule-1 dependent adhesion of colon carcinoma cells to vascular endothelium is inhibited by an antibody to Lewis fucosylated type I carbohydrate chain. *Lab Invest.* 1992; 66:324–30.

115. Giavazzi R, Foppolo M, Dossi R, Remuzzi A. Rolling and adhesion of human tumor cells on vascular endothelium under physiological flow conditions. *J Clin Invest.* 1993; 92:3038–44.

116. Tozeren A, Kleinman HK, Grant DS, Morales D, Mercurio AM, Byers SW. E-selectin-

mediated dynamic interactions of breast- and colon-cancer cells with endothelial-cell monolayers. *Int J Cancer.* 1995; 60:426–31.

117. Duffy MJ. Proteases as prognostic markers in cancer. *Clin Cancer Res.* 1996; 2: 613–8.

118. DeClerck YA, Imren S, Montgomery AM, et al. Proteases and protease inhibitors in tumor progression. In: *Advances in Experimental Medicine and Biology: Chemistry and Biology of Serpins.* (Church FC, Cunningham DD, Ginsburg D, et al., eds.), Plenum Press, New York, 1997, pp. 89–97.

119. MacDougall JR, Matrisian LM. Contributions of tumor and stromal matrix metallo-proteinases to tumor progression, invasion and metastasis. *Cancer Metastas Rev.* 1995; 14:351–62.

120. Matrisian LM, Leroy P, Ruhlmann C, Gesnel MC, Breathnach R. Isolation of the oncogene and epidermal growth factor-induced transin gene: complex control in rat fibroblasts. *Mol Cell Biol.* 1986; 6:1679–86.

121. Matrisian LM, Hogan BL. Growth factor-regulated proteases and extracellular matrix remodeling during mammalian development. *Curr Top Dev Biol.* 1990; 24:219–59.

122. Mauviel A. Cytokine regulation of metalloproteinase gene expression. *J Cell Biochem.* 1993; 53:288–95.

123. Overall CM, Wrana JL, Sodek J. Transcriptional and post-transcriptional regulation of 72-kDa gelatinase/type IV collagenase by transforming growth factor-β1 in human fibroblasts: comparison with collagenase and tissue inhibitor of matrix metalloproteinase gene expression. *J Biol Chem.* 1991; 266:14064–71.

124. Delany AM, Brinckerhoff CE. Post-transcriptional regulation of collagenase and stromely-sin gene expression by epidermal growth factor and dexamethasone in cultured human fibroblasts. *J Cell Biochem.* 1992; 50:400–10.

125. Springman EB, Angleton EL, Birkedal-Hansen H, Van Wart HE. Multiple modes of activation of latent human fibroblast collagenase: evidence for the role of Cys73 active-site zinc complex in latency and a 'cysteine switch' mechanism for activation. *Proc Natl Acad Sci USA.* 1990; 87:364–8.

126. Wojtowicz-Praga SM, Dickson RB, Hawkins MJ. Matrix metalloproteinase inhibitors. *Invest New Drugs.* 1997; 15:61–75.

127. Liotta LA, Tryggvason K, Garbisa S, Hart I, Foltz CM, Shafie S. Metastatic potential correlates with enzymatic degradation of basement membrane collagen. *Nature.* 1980; 284:67–68.

128. MacDougall JR, Bani MR, Lin Y, Rak J, Kerbel RS. The 92-kDa gelatinase B is expressed by advanced stage melanoma cells: suppression by somatic cell hybridization with early stage melanoma cells. *Cancer Res.* 1995; 55:4174–81.

129. Chambers AF, Matrisian LM. Changing views of the role of matrix metalloproteinases in metastasis. *J Natl Cancer Inst.* 1997; 89:1260–70.

130. Brown PD, Giavazzi R. Matrix metalloproteinases inhibition: a review of anti-tumor activity. *Ann Oncol.* 1995; 6:967–74.

131. Chirivi R, Garofalo A, Crimmin MJ, et al. Inhibition of the metastatic spread and growth of B16-BL6 murine melanoma by a synthetic matrix metalloproteinase inhibitor. *Int J Cancer.* 1994; 58:460–4.

132. Taraboletti G, Garofalo A, Belotti D, et al. Inhibition of angiogenesis and murine hemangi-oma growth by batimastat, a synthetic inhibitor of matrix metalloproteinases. *J Natl Cancer Inst.* 1995; 87:293–8.

133. Davies B, Brown PD, East N, Crimmin MJ, Balkwill FR. A synthetic matrix metalloprotei-

nase inhibitor decreases tumor burden and prolongs survival of mice bearing human ovarian carcinoma xenografts. *Cancer Res.* 1993; 53:2087–91.

134. Giavazzi R, Garofalo A, Ferri C, et al. Batimastat, a synthetic inhibitor of matrix metalloproteinases, potentiates the antitumor activity of cisplatin in ovarian carcinoma xenografts. *Clin Cancer Res.* 1998; 4:985–92.

135. Pyke C, Kristensen P, Ralfkiaer E, et al. Urokinase-type plasminogen activator is expressed in stromal cells and its receptor in cancer cells at invasive foci in human colon adenocarcinomas. *Am J Pathol.* 1991; 138:1059–67.

136. Janicke F, Schmitt M, Hafter R, et al. Urokinase-type plasminogen activator (u-PA) antigen is a predictor of early relapse in breast cancer. *Fibrinolysis.* 1990; 4:69–78.

137. Kim SJ, Shiba E, Taguchi T, et al. Urokinase type plasminogen activator receptor is a novel prognostic factor in breast cancer. *Anticancer Res.* 1997; 17:1373–8.

138. Duggan C, Maguire T, McDermott E, et al. Urokinase plasminogen activator and urokinase plasminogen activator receptor in breast cancer. *Int J Cancer.* 1995; 61:597–600.

139. Ganesh S, Sier CF, Griffioen G, et al. Prognostic relevance of plasminogen activators and their inhibitors in colorectal cancer. *Cancer Res.* 1994; 54:4065–71.

140. Nekarda H, Schmitt M, Ulm K, et al. Prognostic impact of urokinase-type plasminogen activator and its inhibitor PAI-1 in completely resected gastric cancer. *Cancer Res.* 1994; 54:2900–7.

141. Fazioli F, Blasi F. Urokinase-type plasminogen activator and its receptor: new targets for anti-metastatic therapy? *Trends Pharmacol Sci.* 1994; 15:25–29.

142. Stracke ML, Krutzsch HC, Unsworth EJ, et al. Identification, purification, and partial sequence analysis of autotaxin, a novel motility-stimulating protein. *J Biol Chem.* 1992; 267:2524–9.

143. Kohn EC, Francis EA, Liotta LA, Schiffmann E. Heterogeneity of the motility responses in malignant tumor cells: a biological basis for the diversity and homing of metastatic cells. *Int J Cancer.* 1990; 46:287–92.

144. Lee HY, Murata J, Clair T, et al. Cloning, chromosomal localization, and tissue expression of autotaxin from human teratocarcinoma cells. *Biochem Biophys Res Commun.* 1996; 218:714–9.

145. Boyer B, Valles AM, Thiery JP. Model systems of carcinoma cell dispersion. *Curr Top Microbiol Immunol.* 1996; 213:179–94.

146. Bhargava M, Joseph A, Knesel J, et al. Scatter factor and hepatocyte growth factor: activities, properties, and mechanism. *Cell Growth Different.* 1992; 3:11–20.

147. Stoker M, Gherardi E, Perryman M, Gray J. Scatter factor is a fibroblast-derived modulator of epithelial cell mobility. *Nature.* 1987; 327:239–42.

148. Shibamoto S, Hayakawa M, Takeuchi K, et al. Tyrosine phosphorylation of β-catenin and plakoglobin enhanced by hepatocyte growth factor and epidermal growth factor in human carcinoma cells. *Cell Adhes Commun.* 1994; 1:295–305.

149. Pepper MS, Matsumoto K, Nakamura T, Orci L, Montesano R. Hepatocyte growth factor increases urokinase-type plasminogen activator (u-PA) and u-PA receptor expression in Madin–Darby canine kidney epithelial cells. *J Biol Chem.* 1992; 267:20493–6.

150. Yamashita J, Ogawa M, Yamashita S, et al. Immunoreactive hepatocyte growth factor is a strong and independent predictor of recurrence and survival in human breast cancer. *Cancer Res.* 1994; 54:1630–3.

151. Rosen EM, Knesel J, Goldberg ID. Scatter factor and its relationship to hepatocyte growth factor and met. *Cell Growth Different.* 1991; 2:603–7.

152. Aznavoorian S, Stracke ML, Krutzsch H, Schiffmann E, Liotta LA. Signal transduction for chemotaxis and haptotaxis by matrix molecules in tumor cells. *J Cell Biol.* 1990; 110:1427–38.

153. Taraboletti G, Roberts DD, Liotta LA. Thrombospondin-induced tumor cell migration: haptotaxis and chemotaxis are mediated by different domains. *J Cell Biol.* 1987; 105:2409–15.

13

Molecular Pathways of Drug Resistance

Christos Tolis, Carlos G. Ferreira, Herbert M. Pinedo, and Giuseppe Giaccone

Introduction

Resistance to cytotoxic chemotherapy is a frequent clinical problem in patients with cancer that leads to their ineffective treatment. Although important progress has been made in oncology in recent years, most tumors respond only temporarily to the current drugs.

Tumor resistance to chemotherapy can be classified into intrinsic (or *de novo*) and acquired. The former refers to resistance present at diagnosis (i.e., tumors fail to respond to first-line chemotherapy); tumors such as pancreatic cancer, malignant melanoma, renal cancer, and colon cancer are all in this category. Acquired drug resistance is common in tumors such as breast cancer, small-cell lung cancer (SCLC), and ovarian cancer. These tumors initially are highly responsive to anticancer therapy, but upon tumor recurrence they exhibit an entirely different phenotype when exposed to the same drugs. They resist both the previously used drugs and new compounds with different structures and mechanisms of action. This phenomenon is called multidrug resistance (MDR).

It is unclear whether the underlying mechanisms are the same in *de novo* and acquired types of drug resistance. Several factors probably affect the development of drug resistance, and a number of these may coexist. The factors involved in clinical drug resistance can be grouped into pharmacologic and cellular factors. Pharmacologic factors (Table 1) include conditions that influence adequate drug exposure at the tumor cell. Cellular factors (Table 1) that mediate drug resistance are those that affect the concentration of active drug at the target sites. These resistance mechanisms were discovered in preclinical models. Additional questions remain regarding the role of these mechanisms in a patient's response to cancer chemotherapy.

Multidrug Resistance Mediated by Altered Drug Accumulation

Decreased intracellular drug accumulation is one of the most common mechanisms of drug resistance. Drug accumulation can result from a decreased influx of cytotoxic agent caused by defects in the transport system (e.g., methotrexate [MTX] and nitrogen mustard resistance) *(1)*. More frequently, however, reduced uptake results from

From: *Principles of Molecular Oncology*
Edited by: M. H. Bronchud, M. A. Foote, W. P. Peters, and M. O. Robinson © Humana Press Inc., Totowa, NJ

Table 1
Mechanisms of Resistance to Chemotherapy

1. Pharmacological factors
   Low drug dose
   Inappropriate infusion rate
   Inadequate route of delivery
   Drug metabolism

2. Cellular factors
   Altered intracellular drug accumulation due to overexpression of transport proteins (e.g., Pgp, MRP)
   Altered expression of metabolic and detoxification processes (e.g., glutathione-*S*-transferase [GST])
   Decreased drug sensitivity due to altered drug–target complexes either due to increased amounts of drug targets or mutations of these targets (e.g., DNA topoisomerases)
   Alteration in signaling pathways (e.g., *erb-B2, ras*)
   Increased repair of drug-induced damage (e.g., O^6-alkylguanine-DNA-alkyltransferase [MGMT])
   Alterations in drug-induced apoptosis (e.g., *p53, bcl-2*)

enhanced drug efflux or altered intracellular trafficking of the drugs; examples are MDR due to overexpression of permeability glycoprotein (Pgp) and MDR-related protein (MRP). MDR has been studied extensively in the laboratory, using cultured cell lines as model systems. Drug-resistant cell lines are derived in the laboratory by increasing exposure to a single chemotherapeutic agent in a stepwise manner, but these cells ultimately become cross-resistant to many structurally and functionally unrelated compounds to which they have never been exposed.

P-Glycoprotein-mediated Multidrug Resistance

Pgp was discovered more than 20 yr ago *(2)* and is the most extensively studied marker in MDR cells. Pgp is a 170-kDa integral plasma membrane glycoprotein that belongs to the ABC (ATP-binding cassette) superfamily of membrane proteins. Other members of this family are the ring 4/11 peptide transporter of the human major histocompatibility complex (MHC), the cystic fibrosis transmembrane receptor (CFTR) protein defective in cystic fibrosis patients, the sulfonyluria receptor (SUR) *(3)*, and ItpgpA, a *Leishmania* protein that confers resistance to arsenic and antimony-centered oxyanions *(4)*. These proteins use energy derived from ATP hydrolysis to export many drugs from the cytosol to the extracellular matrix (ECM) against a concentration gradient. The cloning and sequencing of cDNAs encoding this protein revealed that Pgp is encoded by small gene families. Pgp is linked on the long arm of chromosome 7 *(5)*, with two members in humans (MDR1, MDR2/3) and three in rodents (mdr1, mdr2, mdr3) *(6)*. Immunohistochemical (IHC) localization studies have demonstrated that Pgp is present primarily in the plasma membrane at the cell surface of MDR cells *(7)*. However, small amounts of Pgp also have been associated with the organelles involved in the processing of glycosylated integral membrane proteins (e.g., endoplasmic

Table 2
Agents that Interact with P-glycoprotein

Anthracyclines	*Other*
Daunorubicin	Topotecan
Doxorubicin	Mitomycin C
	Mitoxantrone
Vinca alkaloids	Actinomycin D
Vincristine	Plicamycin
Vinblastine	Ethidium Bromide
	Mitramycin
Taxanes	Colchicine
Paclitaxel	
Docetaxel	
Epipodophyllotoxins	
Etoposide	
Teniposide	

reticulum [ER] and Golgi apparatus). Gene transfer experiments have shown that only MDR1 cells express the MDR phenotype *(8),* and overexpression of the MDR2/3 glycoprotein is not involved in cellular drug resistance. The deduced amino-acid sequence of Pgp predicts the presence of two pairs of six transmembrane domains and two ATP-binding sites. Photoaffinity labeling experiments have demonstrated direct binding of drugs to Pgp and active transport *(9,10)* (Table 2).

MDR1 also is expressed in abundance in several normal tissues. Studies have demonstrated that, in human adults, high amounts of MDR1 mRNA are expressed in the adrenal glands, kidney, liver, pancreatic ductules, jejunum, ileum, and colon; intermediate amounts are expressed in the pregnant uterus, capillary endothelium of the blood–brain barrier, and the testes; and low amounts are expressed in several other tissues *(11,12).* Although the physiologic role of Pgp is unclear, the role probably includes secretion of natural and metabolic toxins into the bile, intestinal lumen, or protection of anatomic sites as drug sanctuaries (e.g., central nervous system, pregnant uterus, testes) *(13).* Thus, Pgp evolved to transport a variety of toxic and natural products and coincidentally acquired the ability to transport drugs with recognizable structures. Tumors derived from cell types intrinsically expressing Pgp (e.g., hepatomas) frequently are resistant to virtually all chemotherapeutic agents, presumably because these tumors exhibit increased expression of Pgp.

In human malignancies, large amounts of MDR1 expression have been detected in adult acute myelogenous leukemia (AML), chronic lymphocytic leukemia (CLL), and multiple myeloma. Studies on these malignancies indicated an association between Pgp expression and decreased remission or resistance to therapy with agents that are substrates for Pgp *(14,15).* Solid tumors, originating from tissues that normally express high levels of Pgp (including colon, kidney, liver, and pancreas) also frequently express high levels of MDR1 transcript *(16,17).* In pediatric sarcoma and neuroblastoma, overexpression of Pgp has been correlated with decreased disease-free and overall survival *(18,19).* In other untreated tumors, MDR1 expression is low (breast, non-small-cell lung cancer [NSCLC], SCLC, melanoma, Wilms' tumor), but their clinical response is variable indicating that mechanisms other than MDR may be important *(20,21).* Overall, despite numerous studies, conclusions have disagreed with respect to the proportion of patients with significant levels of MDR1 tumor cells. Disagreement results in part from the lack of a universal standard for quantifying expression. Use of different methodologies make comparison of studies difficult *(22).*

Given the compelling experimental and clinical evidence supporting the important role of Pgp in MDR, research has focused on developing strategies to reverse or prevent MDR in human malignancies. Several agents can partially or completely reverse drug accumulation defects in MDR cells, including calcium channel blockers (e.g., verapamil, nifedipine, bepridril), calmodulin inhibitors (e.g., phenothiazines), immunosuppressive agents (e.g., cyclosporine A), or derivatives (i.e., PSC-833) and many others *(23–27).* The mechanism(s) by which these drugs reverse MDR is incompletely understood, but direct interactions between these agents and Pgp is believed to interfere with antineoplastic drug efflux activity. Interpretation of the results of MDR reversal trials may be difficult because multiple-resistance mechanisms are coexpressed in a given tumor sample; effective Pgp modulators must bind Pgp with sufficient specificity to yield a reasonable therapeutic index; and treatment with Pgp inhibitors alters the pharmacokinetics of anticancer drugs and thereby causes increased toxicity associated with those drugs.

Another approach to reverse the MDR phenotype may be the use of antisense oligodeoxynucleotides (ODN). Antisense ODNs can form complementary double-helix structures with their target mRNAs and inhibit their translation *(28).* Different ODN sequences were designed to target *MDR1* gene expression. Some reports have demonstrated that the use of different delivery systems can inhibit 40–50% of Pgp expression *(29,30).* This approach certainly merits further investigation, although appropriate delivery systems have not been developed yet.

Multidrug Resistance-Associated Protein

MDR also has been described in cell lines and tumors that are independent of Pgp overexpression. MRP was identified from the parental drug-sensitive SCLC line H69 after stepwise exposure to doxorubicin. The *MRP* gene was subsequently cloned *(31,32)* and found to be localized on chromosome 16p13.1. It encodes a 190-kDa integral transmembrane glycoprotein found in the plasma membrane and endomembrane structures *(33).* Subsequently, MRP has been identified in non-Pgp-MDR cell lines from various tumors types, including cancers of the breast, prostate, NSCLC, fibrosarcomas, and leukemias *(34–38).* In some cell lines, coexpression of Pgp and MRP also has been observed *(39,40).* MRP, like Pgp, belongs to the ABC superfamily of transmembrane proteins, but their structure similarly is limited largely to the conserved ATP-binding domains *(41).* MRP1 is the first identified member of a family of homologue genes that encodes for multispecific organic anion transporter (MOAT) proteins, which also includes MRP2, MRP3, MRP4, and MRP5 *(42).* A member of this family is the cMOAT (*MRP2*) gene (located on chromosome 10q24), which is overexpressed in the liver and cisplatin-resistant tumor cell lines *(43)* and is implicated in the transport of bilirubin–anion conjugates. Transfection experiments of MRP1 into drug-sensitive cell lines induced the MDR phenotype *(44).* The MDR phenotypes due to Pgp and MRP1

Table 3
Multidrug Resistance-Associated Substrates

Doxorubicin	Estradiol
Daunorubicin	Bilirubin
Etoposide	Bile salts
Vincristine	Leukotriene, LTC4
Melphalan	

are similar, conveying cross-resistance to anthracyclines, epipodophyllotoxins, and *Vinca* alkaloids, but resistance to colchicine, taxane, and mitoxantrone is significantly lower in MRP1-expressing cells (Table 3) *(45)*. MRP also confers resistance to certain antimonial and arsenical oxyanions, a property not associated with overexpression of Pgp *(46)*. MRP could not be demonstrated to actively transport chemotherapeutic agents such as vincristine, daunorubicin, or etoposide *(47,48)*. In contrast, it is well established that MRP can actively transport a wide variety of structurally diverse conjugated organic anions, such as the cysteinyl leukotriene LTC4 and glutathione (GSH) conjugates of aflatoxin B_1, prostaglandin A_2, ethacrynic acid, and conjugates of bile salts and hormones *(49,50)*. Evidence in tumor cells does not indicate that conjugation to GSH or other endogenous small molecules (e.g., glucoronic acid) is an important pathway for biotransformation of chemotherapeutic agents to which MRP confers resistance *(51)*. A recent study demonstrated that MRP can actively cotransport GSH and unmodifed vincristine and that these compounds probably interact, either with the LTC4-binding site on the protein or with a mutually exclusive site *(52)*.

Interestingly, these experiments showed that MRP contributes to drug efflux at the plasma membrane and also is involved in sequestration of drugs in cytoplasmic vesicles, thereby providing another means of protection to cellular targets *(44)*. Another difference between Pgp and MRP1 is that MRP1 primarily transports GSH conjugates, whereas Pgp transports unmodified compounds *(53)*.

The tissue distribution of mRNA for MRP indicates that the highest levels of expression are in testes, skeletal muscle, heart, kidney, and lung. Lower levels are also detected in brain, spleen, liver, intestine, and hematopoietic cells *(54,55)*. The physiological function(s) of MRP in these tissues is not known. Human malignancies that express MRP include leukemias (acute lymphoblastic leukemia [ALL], AML, CLL) and solid tumors (lung and neuroblastoma) *(15,56,57)*. The significance of MRP expression in the clinical resistance of human cancers is still unproven although some studies suggest such a role *(57–59)*.

TAP

TAP, another member of the ABC superfamily, is involved in cytoplasmic transport. TAP plays a significant role in the presentation of MHC I-restricted antigen (Ag), by trafficking peptide Ags across the ER *(60,61)*. These transporters, encoded by two genes (*TAP-1* and *TAP-2*), also can transport cytotoxic drugs. Transfection of the *TAP-1* and *TAP-2* genes into TAP-deficient cell lines confers a 2.5-fold resistance to etoposide, vincristine, and doxorubicin *(62)*. However, the role of TAP in clinical MDR is unproven.

Lung-Resistance Protein

When a cytotoxic drug enters the cell, it must be directed to the site of action, frequently the nucleus. Besides ABC transporters, other molecules exist that contribute to diverting the drugs from their intracellular targets and thereby confer MDR.

Scheper et al. described a 100-kDa vesicular protein, which they called lung-resistance protein (LRP). Subsequently it was recognized that LRP is the human major vault protein *(63,64)*. Vaults are complex ribonucleoprotein particles that are primarily located in the cytoplasm but also present in the nuclear membrane and nuclear pore complex (NPC) *(65,66)*. Their function is largely unknown, but vaults may mediate the bidirectional transport of various substrates between the nucleus and the cytoplasm *(66)*. LRP is widely distributed in normal human tumors *(67)*. High LRP expression has been observed in the epithelium of the bronchi and digestive tract and in keratinocytes, adrenal cortex, and macrophages. Lower levels of expression were detected in the proximal tubules of the kidney, transitional urothelium, ductal pancreatic cells, and germ cells. Tissues with high LRP expression (e.g., epithelim of the bronchi and digestive tract) and macrophages also display increased levels of other drug resistance proteins, such as Pgp and MRP *(11)*. The LRP-associated MDR phenotype is broad and includes drugs that are substrates of Pgp and MRP (i.e., doxorubicin and vincristine), and some nonclassic MDR-related drugs (e.g., cisplatin, carboplatin, and melphalan) *(68)*. In the panel of 61 cell lines used at the National Cancer Institute (NCI) for screening of new anticancer drugs and in 174 tumor specimens derived from 27 tumor types, LRP expression was demonstrated in 78% and 63% of cases, respectively. Frequently, MRP was expressed at comparable levels, whereas Pgp was detected at relatively low levels in the same samples *(67,68)*. Clinical studies on childhood ALL, AML, and ovarian carcinoma suggested that LRP is a clinically relevant marker of drug resistance *(69,70)*. However, in a study on lung cancer, expression was not predictive for response to chemotherapy, although strikingly different was the expression of LRP in NSCLC vs SCLC (60% vs 5%), respectively *(71)*.

Multidrug Resistance Mediated by Altered Drug Detoxification

Another important pathway exists for acquiring drug resistance to many chemotherapeutic agents: tumor cells can potentially alter their capacity to detoxify and/or sequester drugs, rendering them inactive. One mechanism is mediated by the glutathione/glutathione-*S*-transferase (GSH/GST) detoxification system. GSH tripeptide (γ-glutamyl-cysteine-glycine) is an important intracellular antioxidant and the most abundant nonprotein thiol in the cell.

As a group, substrates for conjugation to GSH are electrophilic. The cysteinyl group of GSH spontaneously reacts at physiologic pH with the electrophilic metabolites of alkylating agents and cisplatin. GSH alone could be a significant detoxification agent, but it does not appear to work alone. Instead, cytosolic isoenzymes that belong to a multigene family GSTs cooperate with GSH to detoxify many agents. GSTs catalyze the conjugation of reduced GSHs to a wide range of electrophilic compounds, making these compounds less toxic against cellular targets and more readily excretable.

This family of GSTs comprises at least four classes of isoenzymes, designated a, m, p, and q. These enzymes exist as monomers, but their catalytic activity requires

Table 4
GSH or GST Substrates

Cyclophosphamide	Doxorubicin
Chlorambucil	Bleomycin
Melphalan	Cisplatin
Nitrogen mustard	Carboplatin
Phosphoramide mustard	Acrolein
BCNU	Ethacrynic acid
Thiotepa	

homo- or heterodimerization. Each of these GST isoenzymes has a different substrate specificity, but a degree of overlap in substrate range is evident. Most DNA-alkylating agents are characterized by their electrophilicity and are substrates of GSTs. Table 4 lists some compounds that are GSH/GST substrates.

Most evidence supporting the role of GST in drug resistance comes from the overexpression in cell lines made resistant to certain chemotherapeutic agents. The strongest evidence, however, derives from transfection experiments, in which GST transfected into *Saccharomyces cerevisiae* and Chinese hamster ovary (CHO) cells increased their resistance to chlorambucil, doxorubicin, cisplatin, and carboplatin 2- to 16-fold.

After GSH conjugates have been formed, several transport systems remove them from the cell. An Na^+-dependent transporter was described *(72)* that is localized in the basolateral membrane of the kidney and intestine. Another Na^+-independent GSH transporter has been localized in intestine and liver cells *(73)*. An efflux system, initially named GSH-xenobiotic (GSH-x) pump, has been implicated in the excretion of GSH conjugates. This pump may be an ATP-dependent transporter that is similar to the above described MRP protein *(74)*.

Significantly increased amounts of GSH and GST compared with normal tissues have been observed in 58/60 tumor cell lines used by the NCI for drug screening and in human tumors (i.e., leukemias, ovarian, breast, lung, bladder, and colorectal cancers). Increased intracellular levels of these enzymes convey resistance to drugs that conjugate with GSH.

The intracellular concentrations of GSH and GST are critical for drug detoxification, so agents that interfere with GSH biosynthesis or GST activity have been investigated as potential modifiers of drug resistance. Promising results have been obtained with buthionine sulfoxamine (BSO), sulfasalazine, and ethacrynic acid *(75,76)*. GSH/GST-induced MDR can be circumvented by designing prodrugs that are activated by these enzymes *(78)*.

Multidrug Resistance Mediated by Altered Drug Targets

DNA topoisomerases are nuclear enzymes that catalyze the formation of transient single- or double-stranded DNA breaks, facilitate the passage of DNA strands through these breaks, and assist in the rejoining of DNA strands *(79)*. Topoisomerases are critical for DNA replication, transcription, chromosome segregation, and DNA recombination. Two major types of topoisomerases are present in all cells: type I (topo I) catalyzes single-stranded DNA breaks and type II (topo II) cuts double-stranded DNA.

In mammalian cells, two isoenzymes of topoisomerase II exist: topo IIα and topo IIβ. These proteins are encoded by two genes, localized on 17q21–23 and 3q, respectively, and are differentially expressed through the cell cycle. Topo IIα is expressed preferentially in S-phase, whereas topo IIβ is expressed throughout the cell cycle with no significant difference between proliferating and nonproliferating cells *(80)*.

Topoisomerases are primary targets of many commonly used anticancer drugs (e.g., anthracyclines, epipodophyllotoxins, and aminoacridines [topo II] and camptothecin derivatives [topo I]). Topoisomerase-interacting drugs exert their cytotoxicity by stabilizing the otherwise transient DNA–topoisomerase complex (cleavable complex). Stabilization subsequently leads to double-strand breaks in the DNA and is followed by cell-cycle arrest, DNA repair, or apoptosis. Another class of topoisomerase inhibitors that includes merbarone and the bis-2,6-dioxopiperazine group (ICRF193, ICRF187, ICRF159, MST16) does not stabilize such complexes but instead either prevents binding of the enzyme to DNA or blocks another step in the topo II catalytic activity.

Resistance to topoisomerase inhibitors has been investigated thoroughly using cell lines resistant to topo I or topo II inhibitors. Many topo II inhibitors also are substrates for the membrane transporters responsible for classical MDR (Pgp or MRP). However, the pattern of resistance to topo II poisons differs in some important aspects from classical MDR: resistance to these drugs usually is not associated with drug transport defect or Pgp overexpression, unless multiple mechanisms of drug resistance coexist; cells that display resistance to topo II inhibitors usually are sensitive to antimicrotubule agents (i.e., *Vinca* alkaloids and taxanes), which are involved in classical MDR; and resistance to topo II poisons are related to qualitative and quantitative changes in enzyme activity in resistant cells.

Several mechanisms of resistance to topoisomerase inhibitors have been identified in cell lines. Transcriptional downregulation of *topo I* and *topo II* gene expression can contribute to reduced levels of the enzymes in drug-resistant cell lines. A direct relationship between the cytotoxicity of topo inhibitors and topo levels has been shown in several model systems, thereby suggesting that drug resistance results from reduction in nuclear topo enzyme *(81–83)*. This relationship has been observed with topo I and topo IIα and less clearly with topo IIβ.

The cellular content of topo I and topo IIα is proliferation dependent. Resting cells typically express low topo IIα levels and increased drug resistance *(84)*. Treatment with topo II inhibitors results in the accumulation of cells in G_2/M-phase, whereas topo I inhibitors arrest cells in S-phase, suggesting that these inhibitor compounds are cell-cycle specific. Thus, in rapidly dividing cells, regulation of cell-cycle progression may be a more important factor for topoisomerase inhibitors than their actual levels of expression.

In some mammalian cells, resistance to topoisomerase inhibitors was associated with mutations in the *topo IIα* gene *(85,86)*. These mutations appear to cluster in hotspot regions and lead to amino-acid substitutions near the active tyrosine or in the ATP-binding domain. These substitutions change the catalytic or DNA cleavage activity of topo IIα and disrupt the formation of complexes. This change correlates well with drug resistance in vitro. The relevance for clinical drug resistance of *topo IIα* gene mutations remains unknown. Mutations also occur in the *topo I* gene of drug-resistant cells, resulting in reduced topo I activity *(87)*.

Other qualitative changes in topo II activity and structure have been identified in cell lines selected for drug resistance to topoisomerase inhibitors: hypophosphorylation of topo IIα accounts for decreased DNA cleavage and contributes to the drug-resistant phenotypes; decreased quantity of topo IIα associated with the nuclear matrix contributes to the resistance phenotype; and cytoplasmic or membrane structures may be responsible for altered topo II activity *(88–90)*.

Resistance to Antimetabolites

For the past 30 yr, antimetabolites have been the mainstay of treatment for patients with various solid tumors and hematologic malignancies. Antimetabolites are similar to normal intermediates of cellular metabolism, and their cytotoxic profile stems from their ability to interfere with or inhibit key enzymatic steps of nucleic acid metabolism. Mechanisms of resistance to antimetabolites can be described using the paradigm of three well-known compounds: the antifolate methotrexate (MTX); the fluoropyrimidine, 5-fluorouracil (5-FU); and cytosine arabinoside (cytarabine, Ara-C).

The antifolate MTX displays significant antitumor activity against human tumors (e.g., acute leukemias, breast cancer, head and neck cancer, and osteosarcoma), emphasizing its clinical importance. Cellular uptake of MTX is mediated by the reduced folate–MTX carrier system *(91)*. Once inside the cell, MTX is polyglutamylated by the enzyme folylpolyglutamate synthase. The formed polyglutamates and MTX inhibit dihydrofolate reductase (DHFR), an enzyme that converts dihydrofolate (FH_2) to tetrahydrofolate (FH_4). Depletion of FH_4 inhibits thymidylate (TMP) synthesis and subsequently DNA synthesis. MTX polyglutamates also inhibit purine biosynthesis directly or indirectly by inhibiting FH_4 formation. Resistance to MTX may result from changes in drug transport, polyglutamylation, elevated levels of the target enzymes for antifolates (e.g., DHFR and thymidylate synthase), or breakdown of MTX polyglutamates.

Reduced influx can result from a decrease in the expression or function of the reduced folate carrier *(92,93)*. Increased enzyme activity almost invariably results from *DHFR* gene amplification. Resistance to MTX in human cell lines exposed to increasing concentrations of MTX has been associated with increased synthesis of DHFR and a proportional increase in *DHFR* gene copies *(94)*. Amplification of the *DHFR* gene is the second most common mechanism of acquired resistance to MTX, occurring in 20–30% of patients with ALL in relapse *(95)*. Acquired resistance to MTX also may result from decreased intracellular concentrations of polyglutamylated forms of MTX caused by increased activity of the enzyme folylpolyglutamyl hydrolase, which induces MTX-polyglutamate breakdown *(96)*. Mutations in *DHFR* leading to decreased binding of MTX and its polyglutamates to the enzyme also have been described in tumors *(97)*.

The pyrimidine-based 5-FU has been used for decades to treat gastrointestinal (GI) tumors, breast cancer, head and neck cancer, and other tumor types. However, >80% of patients have tumors with intrinsic resistance to 5-FU. The best-characterized mechanism of fluoropyrimidine cytotoxicity involves inhibition of thymidylate synthase (TS) by 5-fluoro-2′-deoxyuridine monophosphate (FdUMP). Incorporation of the metabolite 5-fluorouridine triphosphate (FUTP) into RNA also has been correlated with 5-FU cytotoxicity.

Resistance to 5-FU can be caused by multiple factors. Transport deficiencies are the major mode of resistance for many drugs, but not for 5-FU. Cellular transport of 5-FU is very rapid and does not limit its cytotoxic effect *(98)*. Significant evidence has accumulated to support the theory that insufficient inhibition of TS by FdUMP is a major resistance mechanism *(99,100)*. The physiologic function of TS is to catalyze the conversion of dUMP to dTMP. Inhibition of FdUMP is mediated by the formation of a covalent ternary complex between FdUMP, TS, and CH_2-tetrahydrofolate. The stability of this ternary complex is highly dependent on the availability of CH_2-tetrahydrofolate *(101)*.

Alterations in enzymes involved in fluoropyrimidine metabolism, particularly those associated with conversion of 5-FU to FdUMP may confer resistance to 5-FU *(102)*. Also, changes in TS levels or its affinity for FdUMP have been associated with 5-FU resistance *(103)*.

Strategies to improve 5-FU activity include prolonged or continuous exposure to the drug or coadministration with 5-FU of the reduced folate leucovorin. The efficacy of this combination stems from leucovorin-independent increases in intracellular CH_2-THF, the cofactor that stabilizes the FdUMP-TS complex *(104,105)*.

Ara-C is an important analogue of deoxycytidine, an effective treatment of acute leukemias. Membrane transport of Ara-C at micromolar concentrations is mediated by facilitated diffusion *(106)*; at higher concentrations, the drug enters the cell by passive diffusion *(107)*. Inside the cell, a series of kinases activates Ara-C to its active metabolite, Ara-CTP. Ara-CTP, a substrate and inhibitor of DNA polymerase, is incorporated into nascent DNA, where it causes premature chain termination and ultimately cell death by apoptosis *(108)*. The cytotoxic form Ara-CTP or its precursors (Ara-CMP and Ara-CDP) can be catabolized by phosphatases or inactivated by deaminases. Cells are very sensitive to Ara-C during S-phase, during which DNA synthesis is active, although activity also occurs in other phases of the cell cycle *(109)*.

Several mechanisms of resistance to Ara-C have been described. Cell-cycle distribution of neoplastic cells may confer resistance, especially if cells are quiescent and fail to enter S-phase during the treatment interval. Deficiency of deoxycytidine kinase has been shown in cell lines, but alterations either at the enzyme or the genomic level occur infrequently in patients. In one report, mutations present in cell lines were present in blast cells of patients with AML *(110)*. Deamination may decrease antitumor activity as demonstrated in leukemic cells, when the ratio between deaminase and kinase was considered. In responding patients, the deaminase/kinase ratio was low; in nonresponders it was high *(111,112)*.

Drug Resistance and DNA Repair

The long-term existence of one species may improve with genetic changes and recombination, but the survival of the individual certainly requires genetic stability. To maintain genetic stability, cells use an extremely precise mechanism to replicate DNA during mitosis and a complex machinery to repair the many random lesions that occur continuously in the DNA. DNA repair is the collective name of the group of processes that can correct these lesions. For this reason they can be considered a multifaceted process, in which particular types of DNA damage are repaired through damage-specific pathways, allowing for some overlapping *(113)*.

Many anticancer drugs (e.g., platinum compounds, alkylating agents, and nitrosureas) cause direct damage to the structural integrity of the DNA, leading to the formation

Table 5
Mechanisms of DNA Repair and Drug Resistance

Mechanism of repair	Drugs affected	Drugs potentially affected
O^6-Alkyltransferase	Nitrosureas	Simple alkylating agents
Base excision repair (BER)	Simple alkylating agents	Anthracyclines; anthracenediones
Nucleotide excision repair (NER)	Platinum compounds	—
Mismatch repair (MMR)	—	Platinum compounds; simple alkylating agents

of lesions called bifunctional adducts. The mechanism by which these adducts lead to cell death remains unclear, but evidence suggests that cytotoxic levels of cisplatin, for example, can lead to apoptosis *(114)*. Two sequences of events after drug-DNA binding can be envisaged: direct drug-induced DNA damage triggers cell death through apoptosis or other mechanisms; or, on the other hand, the adducts themselves might not suffice, and the cell-death process would be launched only after DNA breaks are established during attempts to replicate the DNA damaged by anticancer drugs during mitosis. Whatever the mechanism that results from the action of DNA-damaging agents, any substantial increase in the repair of DNA lesions can possibly generate drug resistance, as less chemotherapy-induced cell death will consequently occur *(115)*.

To understand the biochemical mechanisms of DNA repair and the potential mechanisms resulting from them, an understanding of how drugs bind to and damage the DNA is required. Platinum compounds, for instance, react readily with the N-7 position of purines to form various monofunctional and bifunctional DNA adducts. The intrastrand adducts have been proposed as the lesion responsible for the cytotoxic effect of platinum compounds *(116,117)*. Alkylating agents bind most frequently to the N-7 position of guanine but also can bind the O-6 and N-1 positions, depending on the chemical structure of the nonreactive portion of the drug molecule *(118,119)*.

Nitrosureas bind to the O-6 position of the guanine in the DNA either by crosslinking *(120)* or covalent bonding of a methyl group *(121)*. The pathways of DNA repair involved in the correction of DNA lesions induced by chemotherapy agents are determined by the type of DNA lesion produced by the agents and can be divided in four groups: O^6-alkyltransferase, base excision repair (BER), nucleotide excision repair (NER), and mismatch repair (MMR) (Table 5).

O^6 Alkyltransferase

This type of DNA repair activity is specific for O-6-alkylation damage, which is induced mainly by nitrosureas. The enzyme O^6-alkyltransferase was discovered in 1980 and subsequently shown to remove adducts from the O-6 position of guanine, thereby repairing the damage and allowing the cell to survive *(122,123)*. Cells with large amounts of this enzyme (MER$^+$) were found more resistant to nitrosureas than the ones with low amounts (MER$^-$) *(124)*. Removal of the monoadducts produced by nitrosureas, done by the enzyme O^6-alkyltransferase, was confirmed as an important mechanism of resistance to these compounds and triggered interest in the development of clinically effective inhibitors or modulators of this enzyme *(125–128)*. The use of streptozotocin to occupy and block the alkyltransferase before the administration of another nitrosurea is an example of this approach.

Base Excision Repair

BER is the process involved in correcting DNA base damage produced by ionizing radiation and simple alkylating agents *(129)*. In this process, DNA glycosilases excise altered bases, leading to the appearance of an apurinic or apyrimidic (AP) site in cellular DNA; subsequently DNA polymerase and DNA ligase filled the gap. Recent data provide evidence for two branches in the BER pathway, known as "short patch" and "long patch" *(130,131)*. The "short patch" process involves the repair of one isolated AP site; the more complex "long patch" process deals with up to six bases and involves proliferating cell nuclear antigen (PCNA) and DNase IV in addition to the machinery used in the "short patch" branch *(131)*.

According to Reed *(113)*, the frequency with which chemotherapeutic agents, especially simple alkylating agents, induce AP sites is unclear but must be relatively common. In theory, oxidative agents (e.g., anthracyclines and anthracenediones) also may induce this kind of damage and trigger BER activity. The clinical relevance, if any, of the BER pathway in the determination of resistance to chemotherapeutic agents has not been addressed.

Nucleotide Excision Repair

NER, a more complex mechanism of repair, can remove DNA lesions in the form of 27–29 oligonucleotides. In theory, NER can remove almost any type of DNA damage that produces a large change in the DNA double helix (e.g., pyrimidine dimers caused by ultraviolet [UV] light, large hydrocarbonate lesions, and platinum–DNA adducts) *(132)*. Rather than search for specific base changes, NER scans the DNA for distortions in the double helix. NER, a multienzymatic system, can be divided roughly into two complexes that perform complementary functions: the excision and the helicase complex *(113)*. Whether other protein complexes are involved is unclear. A defective NER system is responsible for the genetic disease xeroderma pigmentosum (XP), a condition in which pyrimidine dimers accumulate in the cells exposed to sunlight and lead to skin lesions and skin cancer.

Platinum compounds, because of the bulky DNA lesions they induce, are the prototype of drugs to be studied in relation to the role of the NER system in drug resistance. In fact, resistance to platinum compounds is multifactorial, including altered drug transport, drug inactivation, increased platinum tolerance, and DNA repair *(133)*. However, evidence from in vitro studies suggests that, at least for low levels of resistance (<20-fold), DNA repair may be the most important factor in determining cisplatin resistance *(134–137)*.

Among the components of the NER complex, *ERCC1* (excision repair cross-complementary group 1) *(138)* may be the leading gene *(139)*. In fact, most of the data that correlate NER with cisplatin resistance are based on *ERCC1* mRNA levels *(140,141)*. Analyzing tissue samples from 28 patients with ovarian cancer pretreatment, Dabholkar et al. *(140)* observed that samples from patients who were clinically resistant to chemotherapy had higher levels of *ERCC1* mRNA than samples obtained from individuals clinically sensitive to therapy. Metzger et al. *(141)* obtained similar findings in patients with gastric cancer.

The NER complex has a possible relation with *p53* transcription control and apoptosis. The *p53* gene interacts with NER and modulates the helicase complex, as demonstrated by the ability of *p53* to bind to transcription factor IIH (TFIIH)-associated components, including XPD and XPB *(142,143)*. In addition, the TFIIH components XPB and XPD are components of the *p53*-mediated apoptosis pathway *(144)*. The significance and relevance of the interactions between DNA repair, *p53,* and apoptosis to drug resistance are still unclear but deserve further investigation, because they can provide a broader insight into the determinants of drug sensitivity and resistance.

Mismatch Repair

This pathway, also called mismatch proofreading system, differs from most DNA repair mechanisms by not depending on the recognition of abnormal nucleotides in the DNA. Alternatively, it recognizes slight alterations that result from the misfit between structurally normal noncomplementary bases. In other words, it recognizes mismatches between normal bases that breach the pairing rules proposed by Watson and Crick. According to these rules, bases A and G on one strand should pair with bases T and C, respectively, on the other. Mutations in the genes involved in the MMR system are responsible for a major hereditary form of colon cancer *(145),* hereditary nonpolyposis colorectal cancer (HNPCC).

Some evidence indicates that MMR might be involved in the recognition of lesions other than conventional mispairs *(146),* so a role for this pathway in drug resistance has been proposed. The relationship between cisplatin resistance and MMR was studied in colon and ovarian cancer, but the study results are inconclusive. Apart from possible involvement in the repair of some alkylator-induced lesions and a conceivable secondary contribution to the cisplatin resistance phenotype, MMR may play a small role in the direct repair of drug-induced DNA damage *(113)*. Recent evidence, however, points toward a role of the MMR system in the connection between DNA damage and apoptosis *(147)*. Additional studies are needed to define the mechanism through which this interaction occurs and its relevance.

Apoptosis Inhibition as a Mechanism of Broad Drug Resistance

For many years, the action of anticancer drugs was attributed to a general cellular toxicity, which consequently would lead to a block in cell proliferation. Recently, cumulative evidence has suggested that antineoplastic agents exert at least part of their biologic effect by launching a common death pathway in target cells, a pathway known as programmed cell death or apoptosis *(148–150)*. (Chapters 6 and 9 of this book discuss other aspects of apoptosis.)

Apoptosis is the process of orderly and genetically regulated cell death that occurs largely under physiologic conditions. Apoptosis is responsible for normal tissue homeostasis *(151,152)* achieved through a balance in cell death and cell proliferation. As a consequence, deregulation of the apoptotic pathways may favor cancer formation by providing tumor cells with a survival advantage compared with their normal counterparts. In addition, since essentially all anticancer drugs kill tumor cells by apoptosis, alterations in the apoptotic pathways potentially can lead to a broad-spectrum drug resistance, irrespective of chemotherapeutic drug class or intracellular target. Among the genes implicated in the regulation of the apoptotic process, *p53,* the *bcl-2* family, and c-*myc,* have been studied extensively in their relation with sensitivity/resistance to chemotherapy and will be discussed.

p53

The *p53* gene, a 53-kDa nuclear phosphoprotein, is the product of a 20-kilobase (kb) gene localized on the short arm of human chromosome 17 at position 17p13.1 *(153,154).* The *p53* gene has 11 exons. The first exon is located 8 to 10 kbs away from the second exon and is noncoding. The product of the *p53* tumor suppressor gene (TSG) functions as a transcription factor. The p53 protein binds to double-stranded DNA and transactivates or represses downstream genes through its transactivation domain in the N-terminus of the molecule, which recognizes and binds to a specific DNA-consensus sequence in the promoter region of p53-responsive genes *(153).* Two classes of *p53* binding sites have been identified, suggesting a mechanism for target-gene selectivity by *p53 (155).*

The main physiologic functions of *p53* are cell-cycle regulation at the G_1/S and G_2/M checkpoints, induction of apoptosis, and stabilization of the genome. Each function is an indispensable gatekeeping device of cellular homeostasis; alterations of the *p53* gene may play a central role in the multistep carcinogenesis process and in the prognosis and response to therapy of a variety of tumors.

Cell Cycle Arrest and p53

Wild-type *p53* is present in minute quantities in normal cells and has a rapid turnover rate on the order of minutes. The *p53* gene can be induced by a variety of environmental stimuli, including ionizing radiation, UV light, hypoxia, and hyperthermia as well as growth-factor deprivation and DNA damage induced by various cytotoxic agents. After a genotoxic insult, such as exposure to antineoplastic agents, cells can either undergo a *p53*-dependent G_0/G_1 phase cell-cycle arrest, followed by DNA repair or apoptosis *(156,157).* The best characterized action of *p53* in cell cycle is the arrest in G_0/G_1 phase. This arrest is mediated by the induction of the wild-type-*p53*-activated fragment (*WAF1*) gene (also named *CIP1* or *p21*), which codes for a cyclin-dependent kinase (CDK) inhibitor. Increased amounts of *p21* result in underphosphorylation of the retinoblastoma (Rb) protein, which in turn sequesters the E2F transcription factor required for producing the DNA-synthesis machinery. Thus, the cell cycle is blocked before the S-phase. Recent evidence suggests that *p53* also may induce G_0/G_1 arrest in a *p21*-independent manner and involve the Siah family of proteins *(158).* In addition, *p53* also plays a role in the transition of cells through the G_2/M boundary of the cell cycle *(159,160).*

Apoptosis and p53

Two possibilities for apoptosis have been described after DNA damage and *p53* accumulation: in some experimental systems *p53*-dependent sequence-specific transactivation (SST) induction of the expression of downstream genes was essential for apoptosis; in others, SST was not required for *p53*-mediated apoptosis, and programmed cell death occurred in the absence of *de novo* RNA or protein synthesis *(161,162).*

When SST is concerned, a number of *p53* target genes have been studied in relation to apoptosis. Among these genes, the apoptosis-promoting factor *Bax* has the *p53* recognition motif in its promoter. Under normal conditions *Bax* and *Bcl-2* form hetero-dimers and maintain homeostasis. The *p53* gene induces the expression of *Bax* and shifts the balance with *Bcl-2* in favor of *Bax,* initiating the apoptotic pathway *(163).* Yet, the wild-type *p53* product also can inhibit *Bcl-2* expression through its interaction with a *p53*-dependent negative response element in the *Bcl-2* gene *(164,165).* Human *Bcl-2* expression can completely prevent *p53*-mediated apoptosis and divert the activity of *p53* from induction of apoptosis to induction of growth arrest at multiple points in the cell cycle. The ability of *Bcl-2* to bypass *p53*-mediated induction of apoptosis may contribute to its oncogenic and antiapoptotic activity *(166).* An alternative model for *p53*-induced apoptosis has been proposed that involves transcriptional induction of redox-related genes, formation of reactive oxygen species (ROS), and oxidative degrada-tion of mitochondrial components, leading to programmed cell death *(167).*

Another pathway of *p53*-dependent apoptosis is activation of the CD95 (Fas/Apo-1)–CD95 ligand system. CD95 is the transcriptional target of *p53,* and *p53* can induce CD95 expression on the cell surface of tumor cells *(168).* In addition, *p53* activation may lead to apoptosis by allowing redistribution of cytoplasmatic death receptors to the cell membrane *(169).*

In the case of SST-independent apoptosis, *p53* forms protein–protein complexes with cellular proteins involved in DNA synthesis (e.g., replicating protein Ag), DNA repair (RPA, XPB, and topoisomerase 1), and apoptosis (XPB and XPD). These protein–protein interactions between p53 and the TFIIH complex provide an interesting model for a connection between DNA repair and apoptosis *(143).* The cellular context, and probably the apoptotic stimulus, will determine whether p53 can induce apoptosis independently of its transcription-transactivation function.

The *p53* gene is inactive in most tumors as a result of inactivation by mutations. Most *p53* mutations are missense mutations (approx 85%), deletions or insertions (approx 8%), nonsense mutations (6%), or other mutations (e.g., frameshift mutations), and 0.8% are silent mutations that do not result in any amino-acid changes. Most *p53* mutations occur in the highly conserved core domain of the gene, within exons 5–9 *(170);* however, many *p53* mutations lie outside the core domain of the gene and frequently are missed when neglecting to screen the entire coding domain of the gene (exons 2–11) *(171).* Mutations in the *p53* gene often result in the production of a p53 protein with increased stability and this leads to the presence of positive p53 IHC staining of mutant cells. In contrast, cells containing wild-type *p53* generally do not stain owing to the relatively short half-life of the wild-type p53 protein *(172).* The *p53* gene mutations cause altered DNA binding and reduced transactivation of p53-dependent genes *(173).* Apart from inactivation by mutations, p53 can become inactive through interactions with its physiologic counterpart, called mdm2 (mouse double minute 2), or with viral proteins (e.g., the adenovirus EIA or the E7 proteins) *(63,174,175).*

Acting as a mediator of apoptosis, *p53* could mediate the chemosensitivity to antican-cer agents. Alternatively, by inducing cell-cycle arrest and favoring DNA repair, *p53* has the potential to increase cell resistance to drugs that induce DNA damage. The analysis of current preclinical and clinical data provides evidence to support both scenarios.

Preclinical Data

The experiments describing the role of *p53*-induced apoptosis in modulating cytotoxicity of anticancer agents for the first time suggest p53 as a mediator of broad chemosensitivity *(176,177)*. Other groups also have emphasized the necessity of a p53 functional protein for chemotherapy-launched apoptosis, suggesting that its inactivation potential would lead to a *p53*-associated broad resistance *(178–181)*. As an example, the restoration of wild-type *p53* function in HL-60 cells increased sensitivity to multiple drugs (i.e., 5-FU, FdUrd, cisplatin, VP-16), although this increase in chemosensitivity varied among the different compounds *(178)*. In addition, wild-type *p53* potentiated the cytotoxicity of 5-FU in colon cancer cell lines *(181)*. The cell lines of the NCI anticancer drug screen, which harbors the mutant *p53* sequence, tended to exhibit less growth inhibition than cell lines with wild-type *p53* when treated with most clinically used anticancer agents, including DNA-crosslinking agents, antimetabolites, and topoisomerases I and II inhibitors *(179,180)*. However, with antimitotic agents (e.g., paclitaxel, *Vinca* alkaloids), growth-inhibitory activity was independent of *p53* status. This contrast in dependence on *p53* status between compounds with different mechanisms of action also occurred in ovarian cancer cell lines that showed reduced sensitivity to cisplatin after inactivation of the *p53* gene and no change in the pattern of chemosensitivity to camptothecin and paclitaxel *(182)*.

If *p53* prevalent function is determined by the cellular context, then cell-cycle arrest and DNA repair may be the major *p53*-mediated event after drug exposure. In this alternative pathway, *p53* would provide both time (G_1 arrest) and tools (activation of GADD45 and interaction with the TFIIH protein complex) to reverse drug-induced DNA damage. A study demonstrated that the inactivation of *p53* enhanced sensitivity to multiple chemotherapeutic agents (i.e., cisplatin, carboplatin, melphalan, nitrogen mustard) *(183)*. Exploring the relations between *p53* and its transcriptional activated factors, p21 induced after DNA damage protected wild-type *p53* cells from doxorubicin cytotoxicity *(184)*. In addition, the use of a temperature-sensitive *p53* mutant provided evidence that nonfunctional *p53* induces much stronger sensitization to drug cytotoxicity than the wild-type protein *(185)*.

Conflicts in the results of the in vitro data are even more pronounced when antimitotic agents, especially paclitaxel, are considered. In addition to the studies mentioned *(179,182,183)*, the presence of a functional p53 was not a determinant of cytotoxicity induced by paclitaxel in ovarian cell lines, although an increase in its level and activation of the transcription of the p53-downstream genes *p21, GADD45,* and *Bax* was observed after drug exposure *(186)*. The disruption of the *p53* gene also did not markedly affect the sensitivity of Burkitt's lymphoma (BL) and lymphoblastoid cell lines to the actions of vincristine and paclitaxel *(187)*. However, human ovarian teratocarcinoma cells presenting *p53* disruption after transfection with HPV16 E6 became 100 times more resistant to paclitaxel (among other drugs) compared with the parental wild-type *p53* cell line *(188)*. Nonetheless, in two studies performed in models in which human foreskin fibroblasts were used instead of established laboratory tumor cell lines, an increased sensitization to paclitaxel was found after *p53* functional disruption *(189)*. An explanation for the findings of the last two studies could be that, owing to the recently demonstrated *p53* involvement in spindle cell checkpoint at mitosis *(190)*, the loss or disruption of p53-tubulin surveillance might potentiate paclitaxel-induced microtubule polymerization and consequently its cytotoxicity. The use of different experimental models hampers at this point the possibility to draw definite conclusions on the role of *p53* status in the cytotoxicity of antimitotic agents, as significant differences are found between different cellular models.

Clinical Data

Attempts have been made to correlate *p53* status and chemosensitivity in clinical studies *(191–210)*. A combination of finding that wild-type *p53* status is more common in the chemosensitive than in the chemoresistant cancers, promising initial preclinical data *(176,177)*, and the results from some IHC studies correlating *p53* status and treatment outcome *(205,206,208)* generated the understanding that loss of wild-type *p53* function is associated with failure to respond to chemotherapy. Unfortunately, the more recent reports, published for most frequent solid tumors, contain very contradictory data about the relation between *p53* status and chemosensitivity in cancer patients. These studies have been based mainly on two major approaches: IHC staining that detects predominantly the stabilized form of the p53 protein (presumed to be mutant) and single-strand conformational polymorphism (SSCP), a nucleic acid-based screening for mutations of the *p53* gene. The most relevant studies performed in solid tumors are summarized in Table 6.

Some pitfalls associated with the clinical studies could explain their contradictory results. Initially, most of these studies were based on IHC, and the accumulation or overexpression of *p53* was considered to be the mutant form. The series contained great variations regarding the p53 antibody (Ab) used (target at similar but not identical epitopes), methods for Ag retrieval, different material used (frozen versus fixed sections), and cutoff points established for positivity, including or not including a grading score. Furthermore, most Abs used recognize both wild-type and mutant protein. However, up to 30% of the overexpressed protein can actually have wild-type conformation *(179)*, and increase in the levels may result from posttranslation mechanisms such as protein–protein interactions. On the other hand, negative staining, considered as wild-type *p53* in some of these studies, can represent a subcellular redistribution of the mutant protein leading to levels below the established cutoff values. Although SSCP associated with sequencing can identify whether the *p53* gene is mutant or wild-type, it is impossible to assure, although very likely, that a *p53* mutation will act as a transdominant mutation in p53-heterozygous tumors. In vitro studies have suggested a gene-dose effect (i.e., wild-type *p53* function may not be completely abolished in a p53-heterozygous context). Moreover, SSCP may yield false-negative results when used in samples extracted from paraffin-embedded material, because of the focal positivity of p53 *(211)*. Another important point to consider is that the interpretation of the relation between *p53* status and chemosensitivity in these clinical studies may be hampered by most participating patients being treated with combination chemotherapy regimens.

Summing up the data about *p53* and response to chemotherapy, some important points must be considered. The widespread belief that wild-type *p53* would favor response to chemotherapy and mutant *p53* would lead invariably to chemoresistance is not straightforward. The real role of *p53* in determinating sensitivity/resistance to chemotherapy cannot yet be settled.

Table 6
Major Studies that Correlate p53 Overexpression by IHC
or p53 Mutation by Molecular Analysis with Response to Chemotherapy

Studies	Number of patients	Assay for p53 Analysis	Treatment	Response to chemotherapy
Breast cancer				
Bergh et al. *(191)*	312	PCR/Seq	Adjuvant	Decreased
Clahsen et al. *(195)*	441	IHC	Adjuvant	Decreased
Degeorges et al. *(196)*	282	IHC	Neoadjuvant	Unaltered
Elledge et al. *(198)*	564	IHC	Adjuvant	Unaltered
Jacquemier et al. *(199)*	81	IHC	Adjuvant	Unaltered
Linn et al. *(201)*	40	IHC	Neoadjuvant	Unaltered
Makris et al. *(202)*	57	IHC	Neoadjuvant	Unaltered
Stal et al. *(208)*	139	IHC	Adjuvant	Decreased
Ovarian cancer				
Buttita et al. *(194)*	68	IHC and SSCP	CT for stage III and IV	Decreased
Di Leo et al. *(197)*	72	IHC	CT for stage III and IV	Unaltered
Renninson et al. *(209)*	50	IHC and PCR	CT for stage III and IV	Unaltered
Righetti et al. *(204)*	33	IHC and SSCP	CT for stage III and IV	Decreased
Sorenson et al. *(207)*	45	PCR/Seq	CT for stage III and IV	Unaltered
Lung cancer				
Kawasaki et al. *(210)*	111 (NSCLC)	IHC	CT stage III and IV	Decreased
Kawasaki et al. *(210)*	64 (SCLC)	IHC	CT	Unaltered
Rosell et al. *(205)*	62 (NSCLC)	PCR/SSCP	CT stage III and IV	Decreased
Rusch et al. *(206)*	52 (NSCLC)	IHC	Neoadjuvant stage III	Decreased
Gastrointestinal				
Boku et al. *(192)*	39	IHC	CT for advanced disease	Decreased
Brett et al. *(193)*	59	IHC	CT for advanced disease	Decreased
Lenz et al. *(200)*	36	IHC and PCR/Seq	CT for advanced disease	Decreased
Paradiso et al. *(203)*	71	IHC	CT for advanced disease	Unaltered

IHC, immunohistochemistry; SSCP, single-strand conformation polymorphism; PCR/seq, polymerase chain reaction followed by direct DNA sequencing; CT, chemotherapy.

Table 7
Bcl-2-Related Genes

Antiapoptotic death antagonistics	Apoptotic death agonistics
Bcl-2	Bax
Bcl-X$_L$	Bcl-X$_S$
Bcl-w	Bak
Mcl-1	Bad
A1	Bid

Bcl-2 *Family*

The *Bcl-2* gene originally described at the chromosomal breakpoint of t(14;18)-bearing B-cell lymphomas *(212)*. The first evidence for the biologic function of *Bcl-2* was obtained in in vitro experiments in which enforced expression of *Bcl-2* led to long-term survival of interleukin (IL)-dependent hematopoietic cell lines after growth-factor deprivation *(213–215)*. In fact, these experiments provided evidence that *Bcl-2* promotes cell survival, but not proliferation, and suggested that these two processes are indeed under distinct genetic control. In subsequent experiments with *Bcl-2*-deficient mice to investigate the physiologic role of *Bcl-2,* these animals showed progressive immunodeficiency caused by a premature death of their normally long-lived peripheral lymphocytes *(216)*. These findings indicate that *Bcl-2* has a crucial physiologic role in maintaining the viability of important cells that are meant to be long lived. Recent reports also suggest that *Bcl-2* has a role in cell-cycle regulation, because its overexpression causes both a delay in the reentry of quiescent G$_0$ cells into the cell cycle upon stimulation *(217),* and promotes exit of cells into G$_0$ under conditions of stress. The physiologic consequences of the *Bcl-2* effect on the cell-cycle control remains unclear, however.

The *Bcl-2* gene is localized on the mitochondrial outer membrane, nuclear membrane, and ER *(218)*. Insertion of *Bcl-2* into membranes is essential for *Bcl-2* to regulate apoptosis *(215)*. The first evidence for a role of *Bcl-2* in drug resistance was mainly provided by experiments with transgenic mice. Within a given cell type, overexpression of *Bcl-2* dramatically increased resistance to a broad range of cytotoxic conditions, including exposure to anticancer drugs *(219,220)*. These results form the basis for two important concepts regarding the role of *Bcl-2* in apoptosis: *Bcl-2* stands out among the gene products involved in apoptosis on account of its ability to protect from apoptosis induced by various stimuli; *Bcl-2* antagonizes the common effector machinery for different signaling pathways to apoptosis *(221)*. Despite the broad spectrum of apoptosis inhibition provided by *Bcl-2*, the existence of *Bcl-2*-insensitive pathways has been recognized *(222)*.

Some proteins that are structurally related to Bcl-2, the Bcl-2 protein family, recently have been described *(223)*. Family members are either pro- or antiapoptotic (Table 7) and differ in their tissue-activation-dependent expression patterns and structural features.

The first Bcl-2 homologue identified was Bax, which is 45% homologous to Bcl-2 *(224)*. In overexpression models, Bax committed cells to apoptosis and could antagonize the antiapoptotic effect of Bcl-2. The interaction between Bcl-2 and Bax, and the other Bcl-2-related proteins, occurs through conserved regions in the molecules called BH-domains, which confer on the proteins the ability to form hetero- and homodimers.

A model of a death agonist-antagonist rheostat has been proposed *(223)* in which the ratio of death antagonists (i.e., Bcl-2, Bcl-XI, Bcl-w, Mcl-1, A1) to agonists (i.e., Bax, Bak, Bcl-Xs, Bad, Bid) determines the fate of cells after an apoptotic signal. Competitive dimerization between selective pairs of agonists and antagonists would mediate the death–life rheostat. Determinants of the ratio of Bcl-2 family members are scarcely understood, but it is known that the product of the *p53* gene can alter the ratio between Bax and Bcl-2. The p53 protein can, through transcriptional regulation, increase Bax levels and decrease *Bcl-2* expression *(163–165)*. As an example, in a proposed model in follicular lymphomas, the ratio of Bax to Bcl-2 is envisioned as controlling the relative sensitivity of the cells to chemotherapy-induced apoptosis. When Bcl-2 level exceeds that of Bax, the cells are less likely to die. Conversely, if Bax level exceeds that of Bcl-2, apoptosis is induced *(220)*. Despite progress in understanding interactions among Bcl-2 members, current data cannot address which dimers are the real regulators of apoptosis. Another point to consider is the existence of posttranslational modifications of Bcl-2. Phosphorylation of Bcl-2 induced by anticancer drugs that act on the microtubules (e.g., taxanes and *Vinca* alkaloids) can neutralize the antiapoptotic function of Bcl-2 and lead to cell death *(225)*.

The role of *Bcl-2* family genes in chemoresistance has been investigated extensively in in vitro systems, animal models, and clinical studies. Initial in vitro data provided evidence of the role of *Bcl-2* family alterations in determining resistance to various chemotherapeutic agents (i.e., Ara-C, MTX, doxorubicin, Taxol®, VP-16, cisplatin, fludarabine, vincristine) *(220)*. Subsequently, animal studies provided partial evidence in support of a role of *Bcl-2* in regulating in vivo drug resistance *(226)*. Mice that received *Bcl-2* virus-transduced bone marrow cells had less myelosuppression in response to VP-16 than did the control animals *(227)*. In the last 10 yr, clinical studies analyzing *Bcl-2* expression and correlation with patient outcome have been published. High levels and aberrant patterns of *Bcl-2* expression have been observed in various hematologic malignancies and solid tumors *(219)*.

Correlative studies performed by IHC and molecular approaches (SSCP, polymerase chain reaction [PCR], and Southern blotting) have shown contradictory results in hematologic malignancies and some solid tumors. Two studies of patients with non-Hodgkin lymphomas (NHL) presenting diffuse histology showed a correlation between *Bcl-2* gene rearrangements and shorter disease-free survival or failure to achieve complete response (CR) *(228,229)*. In contrast, in six other studies, *Bcl-2* status was neither of prognostic significance nor predictive of response to chemotherapy (230–234). In patients with AML, a correlation was observed between high percentage of *Bcl-2*-positive cells and failure to achieve complete response (CR) *(235)*.

In one series of patients with adenocarcinoma of the prostate, *Bcl-2*-positive staining was correlated with failure to respond to antiandrogen therapy *(236)*. Similar results were found in 38 patients with SCLC in whom *Bcl-2* expression was a predictor of response to chemotherapy *(237)*. Two studies suggested an unexpected trend of a higher response to endocrine therapy when breast tumors were positive for *Bcl-2* immunostaining. Two other studies correlating response to chemotherapy and *Bcl-2* status in breast cancer had contradictory results. Bonetti et al. *(238)* suggest a correlation between *Bcl-2* positivity and poor response to chemotherapy, whereas van Slooten et al. *(239)* found no such correlation in the analysis of 441 patients.

Definitive conclusions about these correlative studies cannot be drawn on account of the contradictory study results. Possible reasons for the inconsistent results include small sample size, nonuniform treatment of patients, and technical problems, all of which complicate the interpretation of the results *(220)*.

c-myc

The c-*myc* oncogene plays an important role in the cell cycle progression. Its transcription product, a protein, targets DNA and acts mainly to form heterodimers with another protein, max *(240)*. During the G_1 phase of the cell cycle, *myc* expression seems to be under the control of the tumor suppressor gene *Rb*. Upon interactions with cyclins or viral antigens, *Rb* releases E2F, which activates the *myc* promoter P1/P2 *(241)*.

c-*myc* can bypass the *p53*-induced G_1 arrest and antagonize cyclin D1 action; however, this bypass occurs in an illegitimate manner. By generating an excessive proliferating signal, c-*myc* produces a paradoxical effect that leads to apoptosis and may influence the response to chemotherapy *(242)*.

Some clinical studies have addressed c-*myc* as a predictor of response to chemotherapy. In patients with advanced tumors of the upper respiratory and digestive tract, higher c-*myc* expression correlated with a better response to chemotherapy *(243)*. These results are in line with a study in patients with head and neck tumors, in which c-*myc* overexpression also was associated with a better response to chemotherapy *(244)*.

Concluding Remarks

Drug resistance is a common problem seen by physicians treating patients with cancer. Progress has been made, but most tumors respond only temporarily to existing cytotoxic drugs. It is hoped that further study will lead to the development of new modalities that will decrease the rate of drug resistance.

Acknowledgment

Christos Tolis is an ESMO Fellow, and Carlos G. Ferreira is supported by a grant from CAPES-Brasil.

References

1. Sirotnak FM, Moccio DM, Young CW. Increased accumulation of methotrexate by murine tumor cells in vitro in the presence of probenecid which is mediated by a preferential inhibition of efflux. *Cancer Res.* 1981; 41:966–76.
2. Juliano RL, Ling V. A surface glycoprotein modulating drug permeability in Chinese hamster ovary cell mutants. *Biochim Biophys Acta.* 1976; 455:152–62.
3. Aguilar-Bryan L, Nichols CG, Wechsler SW, et al. Cloning of the β cell high-affinity sulfonylurea receptor: a regulator of insulin secretion. *Science.* 1995; 268:423–6.
4. Papadopoulou B, Roy G, Dey S, Rosen BP, Ouellette M. Contribution of the *Leishmania*

P-glycoprotein-related gene *ItpgpA* to oxyanion resistance. *J Biol Chem.* 1994; 269:11980–6.

5. Ling V. Multidrug resistance: molecular mechanisms and clinical relevance. *Cancer Chemother Pharmacol.* 1997; 40(Suppl):S3–S8.

6. Chen CJ, Chin JE, Ueda K, et al. Internal duplication and homology with bacterial transport proteins in the *mdr1* (P-glycoprotein) gene from multidrug-resistant human cells. *Cell.* 1986; 47:381–9.

7. Willingham MC, Richerd ND, Cornwell MM, et al. Immunocytochemical localization of P170 at the plasma membrane of multidrug-resistant human cells. *J Histochem Cytochem.* 1987; 35:1451–6.

8. Ueda K, Cardarelli C, Gottesman MM, Pastan I. Expression of a full-length cDNA for the human "MDR1" gene confers resistance to colchicine, doxorubicin, and vinblastine. *Proc Natl Acad Sci USA.* 1987; 84:3004–8.

9. Safa AR, Glover CJ, Meyers MB, Biedler JL, Felsted RL. Vinblastine photoaffinity labeling of a high molecular weight surface membrane glycoprotein specific for multidrug-resistant cells. *J Biol Chem.* 1986; 261:6137–40.

10. Schlemmer SR, Yang CH, Sirotnak FM. Functional modulation of multidrug resistance-related P-glycoprotein by Ca^{2+}-calmodulin. *J Biol Chem.* 1995; 270:11040–2.

11. Cordon-Cardo C, O'Brien JP, Boccia J, Casals D, Bertino JR, Melamed MR. Expression of the multidrug resistance gene product (P-glycoprotein) in human normal and tumor tissues. *J Histochem Cytochem.* 1990; 38:1277–87.

12. Fojo AT, Ueda K, Slamon DJ, Poplack DG, Gottesman MM, Pastan I. Expression of a multidrug-resistance gene in human tumors and tissues. *Proc Natl Acad Sci USA.* 1987; 84:265–9.

13. Cordon-Cardo C, O'Brien JP, Casals D, et al. Multidrug-resistance gene (P-glycoprotein) is expressed by endothelial cells at blood–brain barrier sites. *Proc Natl Acad Sci USA.* 1989; 86:695–8.

14. Leith CP, Kopecky KJ, Godwin J, et al. Acute myeloid leukemia in the elderly: assessment of multidrug resistance (MDR1) and cytogenetics distinguishes biologic subgroups with remarkably distinct responses to standard chemotherapy. A Southwest Oncology Group study. *Blood.* 1997; 89:3323–9.

15. Willman CL. The prognostic significance of the expression and function of multidrug resistance transporter proteins in acute myeloid leukemia: studies of the Southwest Oncology Group Leukemia Research Program. *Semin Hematol.* 1997; 34:25–33.

16. Bosch I, Croop J. P-glycoprotein multidrug resistance and cancer. *Biochim Biophys Acta.* 1996; 1288:F37–F54.

17. Goldstein LJ, Galski H, Fojo A, et al. Expression of a multidrug resistance gene in human cancers. *J Natl Cancer Inst.* 1989; 81:116–24.

18. Chan HS, Thorner PS, Haddad G, Ling V. Immunohistochemical deletion of P-glycoprotein: prognostic correlation in soft tissue sarcoma of childhood. *J Clin Oncol.* 1990; 8:689–704.

19. Chan HS, Haddad G, Thorner PS, et al. P-glycoprotein expression as a predictor of the outcome of therapy for neuroblastoma. *N Engl J Med.* 1991; 325:1608–14.

20. Lai SL, Goldstein LJ, Gottesman MM, et al. *MDR1* gene expression in lung cancer. *J Natl Cancer Inst* 1989; 81:1144–50.

21. Savaraj N, Wu CJ, Xu R, et al. Multidrug-resistant gene expression in small-cell lung cancer. *Am J Clin Oncol.* 1997; 20:398–403.

22. Beck WT, Grogan TM, Willman CL, et al. Methods to detect P-glycoprotein-associated

multidrug resistance in patients' tumors: consensus recommendations. *Cancer Res.* 1996; 56:3010–20.

23. Dalton WS, Crowley JJ, Salmon SS, et al. A phase III randomized study of oral verapamil as a chemosensitizer to reverse drug resistance in patients with refractory myeloma. A Southwest Oncology Group study. *Cancer.* 1995; 75:815–20.

24. Naito M, Tsuruo T. New multidrug-resistance-reversing drugs, MS-209 and SDZ PSC 833. *Cancer Chemother Pharmacol.* 1997; 40(Suppl):S20–S24.

25. Shrivastava P, Hanibuchi M, Yano S, Parajuli P, Tsuruo T, Sone S. Circumvention of multidrug resistance by a quinoline derivative, MS-209, in multidrug-resistant human small-cell lung cancer cells and its synergistic interaction with cyclosporin A or verapamil. *Cancer Chemother Pharmacol.* 1998; 42:483–90.

26. Smith AJ, Mayer U, Schinkel AH, Borst P. Availability of PSC833, a substrate and inhibitor of P-glycoproteins, in various concentrations of serum. *J Natl Cancer Inst.* 1998; 90:1161–6.

27. Wishart GC, Bissett D, Paul J, et al. Quinidine as a resistance modulator of epirubicin in advanced breast cancer: mature results of a placebo-controlled randomized trial. *J Clin Oncol.* 1994; 12:1771–7.

28. Wagner RW. The state of the art in antisense research. *Nat Med.* 1995; 1:1116–8.

29. Cucco C, Calabretta B. In vitro and in vivo reversal of multidrug resistance in a human leukemia-resistant cell line by mdr1 antisense oligodeoxynucleotides. *Cancer Res.* 1996; 56:4332–7.

30. Hanchett LA, Baker RM, Dolnick BJ. Subclonal heterogeneity of the multidrug resistance phenotype in a cell line expressing MDR1 RNA. *Somat Cell Mol Genet.* 1994; 20:463–80.

31. Cole SP, Bhardwaj G, Gerlach JH, et al. Overexpression of a transporter gene in a multidrug-resistant human lung cancer cell line. *Science.* 1992; 258:1650–4.

32. Mirski SE, Gerlach JH, Cole SP. Multidrug resistance in a human small cell lung cancer cell line selected in Adriamycin®. *Cancer Res.* 1987; 47:2594–8.

33. Krishnamachary N, Center MS. The *MRP* gene associated with a non-P-glycoprotein multidrug resistance encodes a 190-kDa membrane bound glycoprotein. *Cancer Res.* 1993; 53:3658–61.

34. Barrand MA, Heppell-Parton AC, Wright KA, Rabbitts PH, Twentyman PR. A 190-kilodalton protein overexpressed in non-P-glycoprotein-containing multidrug-resistant cells and its relationship to the MRP gene. *J Natl Cancer Inst.* 1994; 86:110–7.

35. Schneider E, Horton JK, Yang CH, Nakagawa M, Cowan KH. Multidrug resistance-associated protein gene overexpression and reduced drug sensitivity of topoisomerase II in a human breast carcinoma MCF7 cell line selected for etoposide resistance. *Cancer Res.* 1994; 54:152–8.

36. Slapak CA, Fracasso PM, Martell RL, Toppmeyer DL, Lecerf JM, Levy SB. Overexpression of the multidrug resistance-associated protein (*MRP*) gene in vincristine but not doxorubicin-selected multidrug-resistant murine erythroleukemia cells. *Cancer Res.* 1994; 54:5607–13.

37. Slovak ML, Ho JP, Bhardwaj G, Kurz EU, Deeley RG, Cole SP. Localization of a novel multidrug resistance-associated gene in the HT1080/DR4 and H69AR human tumor cell lines. *Cancer Res.* 1993; 53:3221–5

38. Tasaki Y, Nakagawa M, Ogata J, et al. Reversal by a dihydropyridine derivative of non-P-glycoprotein-mediated multidrug resistance in etoposide-resistant human prostatic cancer cell line. *J Urol.* 1995; 154:1210–6.

39. Hasegawa S, Abe T, Naito S, et al. Expression of multidrug resistance-associated protein

(MRP), MDR1, and DNA topoisomerase II in human multidrug-resistant bladder cancer cell lines. *Br J Cancer.* 1995; 71:907–13.

40. Slapak CA, Mizunuma N, Kufe DW. Expression of the multidrug resistance associated protein and P-glycoprotein in doxorubicin-selected human myeloid leukemia cells. *Blood.* 1994; 84:3113–21.

41. Cole SP, Sparks KE, Fraser K. et al. Pharmacological characterization of multidrug resistant MRP-transfected human tumor cells. *Cancer Res.* 1994; 54:5902–10.

42. Kool M, deHaas M, Scheffer GL, et al. Analysis of expression of cMOAT (*MRP2*), *MRP3, MRP4,* and *MRP5,* homologues of the multidrug resistance-associated protein gene (*MRP1*), in human cancer cell lines. *Cancer Res.* 1997; 57:3537–47.

43. Taniguchi K, Wada M, Kohno K, et al. A human canalicular multispecific organic anion transporter (cMOAT) gene is overexpressed in cisplatin-resistant human cancer cell lines with decreased drug accumulation. *Cancer Res.* 1996; 56:4124–9.

44. Breuninger LM, Paul S, Gaughan K, et al. Expression of multidrug resistance-associated protein in NIH/3T3 cells confers multidrug resistance associated with increased drug efflux and altered intracellular drug distribution. *Cancer Res.* 1995; 55:5342–7.

45. Lautier D, Canitrot Y, Deeley RG, Cole SP. Multidrug resistance mediated by the multidrug resistance protein (*MRP*) gene. *Biochem Pharmacol.* 1996; 52:967–77.

46. Zaman GJ, Flens MJ, vanLeusden MR, et al. The human multidrug resistance-associated protein MRP is a plasma membrane drug-efflux pump. *Proc Natl Acad Sci USA.* 1994; 91:8822–6.

47. Heijn M, Hooijberg JH, Scheffer GL, Szabo G, Westerhoff HV, Lankelma J. Anthracyclines modulate multidrug resistance protein (MRP) mediated organic anion transport. *Biochim Biophys Acta.* 1997; 1326:12–22.

48. Muller M, Meijer C, Zaman GJ, et al. Overexpression of the gene encoding the multidrug resistance-associated protein results in increased ATP-dependent glutathione S-conjugate transport. *Proc Natl Acad Sci USA.* 1994; 91:13033–7.

49. Evers R, Cnubben NH, Wijnholds J, van Deetmer L, van Bladeren PJ, Borst P. Transport of glutathione prostaglandin A conjugates by the multidrug resistance protein 1. *FEBS Lett.* 1997; 419:112–6.

50. Zaman GJ, Cnubben NH, van Bladeren PJ, Evers R, Borst P. Transport of the glutathione conjugate of ethacrynic acid by the human multidrug resistance protein MRP. *FEBS Lett.* 1996; 391:126–30.

51. Tew KD. Glutathione-associated enzymes in anticancer drug resistance. *Cancer Res.* 1994; 54:4313–20.

52. Loe DW, Deeley RG, Cole SP. Characterization of vincristine transport by the M(r) 190,000 multidrug resistance protein (MRP): evidence for cotransport with reduced glutathione. *Cancer Res.* 1998; 58:5130–6.

53. Keppler D, Leier I, Jedlitschky G. Transport of glutathione conjugates and glucuronides by the multidrug resistance proteins MRP1 and MRP2. *Biol Chem.* 1997; 378:787–91.

54. Kruh GD, Gaughan KT, Godwin A, Chan A. Expression pattern of MRP in human tissues and adult solid tumor cell lines. *J Natl Cancer Inst.* 1995; 87:1256–8.

55. Zaman GJ, Versantvoort CH, Smit JJ, et al. Analysis of the expression of *MRP,* the gene for a new putative transmembrane drug transporter, in human multidrug resistant lung cancer cell lines. *Cancer Res.* 1993; 53:1747–50.

56. Broxterman HJ, Giaccone G, Lankelma J. Multidrug resistance proteins and other drug transport-related resistance to natural product agents. *Curr Opin Oncol.* 1995; 7:532–40.

57. Berger W, Hauptmann E, Elbling L, Vefterlein M, Kokoschka EM, Micksche M. Possible

role of the multidrug resistance-associated protein (MRP) in chemoresistance of human melanoma cells. *Int J Cancer.* 1997; 71:108–115.

58. Norris MD, Bordow SB, Marshall GM, Haber PS, Cohn SL, Haber M. Expression of the gene for multidrug-resistance-associated protein and outcome in patients with neuroblastoma. *N Engl J Med.* 1996; 334:231–8.

59. Zhou DC, Zittoun R, Marie JP. Expression of multidrug resistance-associated protein (MRP) and multidrug resistance (*MDR1*) genes in acute myeloid leukemia. *Leukemia.* 1995; 9:1661–6.

60. Elliott T. How does TAP associate with MHC class I molecules? *Immunol Today.* 1997; 18:375–9.

61. Neefjes JJ, Momburg F, Hammerling GJ. Selective and ATP-dependent translocation of peptides by the MHC-encoded transporter. *Science.* 1993; 261:769–71.

62. Izquierdo MA, Neefjes JJ, Mathari AE, Flens MJ, Scheffer GL, Scheper RJ. Overexpression of the ABC transporter TAP in multidrug-resistant human cancer cell lines. *Br J Cancer.* 1996; 74:1961–7.

63. Scheffner M, Werness BA, Huibregtse JM, Levine AJ, Howley PM. The E6 oncoprotein encoded by human papillomavirus types 16 and 18 promotes the degradation of p53. *Cell.* 1990; 63:1129–36.

64. Scheper RJ, Broxterman HJ, Scheffer GL, et al. Overexpression of a M(r) 110,000 vesicular protein in non-P-glycoprotein-mediated multidrug resistance. *Cancer Res.* 1993; 53:1475–9.

65. Chugani DC, Kedersha NL, Rome LH. Vault immunofluorescence in the brain: new insights regarding the origin of microglia. *J Neurosci.* 1991; 11:256–68.

66. Chugani DC, Rome LH, Kedersha NL. Evidence that vault ribonucleoprotein particles localize to the nuclear pore complex. *J Cell Sci.* 1993; 106:23–29.

67. Izquierdo MA, Scheffer GL, Flens MJ, et al. Broad distribution of the multidrug resistance-related vault lung resistance protein in normal human tissues and tumors. *Am J Pathol.* 1996; 148:877–87.

68. Izquierdo MA, Shoemaker RH, Flens MJ, et al. Overlapping phenotypes of multidrug resistance among panels of human cancer-cell lines. *Int J Cancer.* 1996; 65:230–7.

69. Izquierdo MA, van der Zee AG, Vermorken JB, et al. Drug resistance-associated marker Lrp for prediction of response to chemotherapy and prognoses in advanced ovarian carcinoma. *J Natl Cancer Inst.* 1995; 87:1230–7.

70. den Boer ML, Pieters R, Kazemier KM, et al. Relationship between major vault protein/lung resistance protein, multidrug resistance-associated protein, P-glycoprotein expression, and drug resistance in childhood leukemia. *Blood.* 1998; 91:2092–8.

71. Dingemans AM, van Ark-Ofte J, van der Valk P, et al. Expression of the human major vault protein LRP in human lung cancer samples and normal lung tissues. *Ann Oncol.* 1996; 7:625–30.

72. Lash LH, Jones DP. Renal glutathione transport. Characteristics of the sodium-dependent system in the basal-lateral membrane. *J Biol Chem.* 1984; 259:14508–14.

73. Hinchman CA, Truong AT, Ballatori N. Hepatic uptake of intact glutathione S-conjugate, inhibition by organic anions, and sinusoidal catabolism. *Am J Physiol.* 1993; 265:G547–54.

74. Loe DW, Stewart RK, Massey TE, Deeley RG, Cole SP. ATP-dependent transport of aflatoxin B1 and its glutathione conjugates by the product of the multidrug resistance protein (*MRP*) gene. *Mol Pharmacol.* 1997; 51:1034–41.

75. Gupta V, Jani JP, Jacobs S, et al. Activity of melphalan in combination with the glutathione transferase inhibitor sulfasalazine. *Cancer Chemother Pharmacol.* 1995; 36:13–19.

76. Prezioso JA, FitzGerald GB, Wick MM. Melanoma cytotoxicity of buthionine sulfoximine (BSO) alone and in combination with 3,4-dihydroxybenzylamine and melphalan. *J Invest Dermatol.* 1992; 99:289–93.

77. O'Dwyer PJ, LaCreta F, Nash S, et al. Phase I study of thiotepa in combination with the glutathione transferase inhibitor ethacrynic acid. *Cancer Res.* 1991; 51:6059–65.

78. Lyttle MH, Hocker MD, Hui HC, et al. Isozyme-specific glutathione-*S*-transferase inhibitors: design and synthesis. *J Med Chem.* 1994; 37:189–94.

79. Wang JC. DNA topoisomerases: why so many? *J Biol Chem.* 1991; 266:6659–62.

80. Hwang J, Hwong CL. Cellular regulation of mammalian DNA topoisomerases. *Adv Pharmacol.* 1994; 29A:167–89.

81. Kapoor R, Slade DL, Fujimori A, Pommier Y, Harker WG. Altered topoisomerase I expression in two subclones of human CEM leukemia selected for resistance to camptothecin. *Oncol Res.* 1995; 7:83–95.

82. Kaufmann SH, McLaughlin SJ, Kastan MB, Liu LF, Karp JE, Burke PJ. Topoisomerase II levels during granulocytic maturation in vitro and in vivo. *Cancer Res.* 1991; 51:3534–43.

83. Potmesil M, Hsiang YH, Liu LF, et al. Resistance of human leukemic and normal lymphocytes to drug-induced DNA cleavage and low levels of DNA topoisomerase II. *Cancer Res.* 1988; 48:3537–43.

84. Sullivan DM, Latham MD, Ross WE. Proliferation-dependent topoisomerase II content as a determinant of antineoplastic drug action in human, mouse, and Chinese hamster ovary cells. *Cancer Res.* 1987; 47:3973–9.

85. Campain JA, Gottesman MM, Pastan I. A novel mutant topoisomerase II α present in VP-16-resistant human melanoma cell lines has a deletion of alanine 429. *Biochemistry.* 1994; 33:11327–32.

86. Beck WT, Danks MK, Wolverton JS, et al. Resistance of mammalian tumor cells to inhibitors of DNA topoisomerase II. *Adv Pharmacol.* 1994; 29B:145–69.

87. Fujimori A, Harker WG, Kohlhagen G, Hoki Y, Pommier Y. Mutation at the catalytic site of topoisomerase I in CEM/C2, a human leukemia cell line resistant to camptothecin. *Cancer Res.* 1995; 55:1339–46.

88. Campain JA, Padmanabhan R, Hwang J, Gottesman MM, Pastan I. Characterization of an unusual mutant of human melanoma cells resistant to anticancer drugs that inhibit topoisomerase II. *J Cell Physiol.* 1993; 155:414–25.

89. Ganapathi R, Constantinou A, Kamath N, Dubyak G, Grabowski D, Krivacic K. Rersistance to etoposide in human leukemia HL-60 cells: reduction in drug-induced DNA cleavage associated with hypophosphorylation of topoisomerase II phosphopeptides. *Mol Pharmacol.* 1996; 50:243–8.

90. Ritke MK, Murray NR, Allan WP, Fields AP, Yalowich JC. Hypophosphorylation of topoisomerase II in etoposide (VP-16)-resistant human leukemia K562 cells associated with reduced levels of β II protein kinase C. *Mol Pharmacol.* 1995; 48:798–805.

91. Henderson GB, Tsuji JM, Kumar HP. Transport of folate compounds by leukemic cells. Evidence for a single influx carrier for methotrexate, 5-methyltetrahydrofolate, and folate in CCRF-CEM human lymphoblasts. *Biochem Pharmacol.* 1987; 36:3007–14.

92. Moscow JA, Gong M, He R, et al. Isolation of a gene encoding a human reduced folate carrier (RFC1) and analysis of its expression in transport-deficient, methotrexate-resistant human breast cancer cells. *Cancer Res.* 1995; 55:3790–4.

93. Wong SC, Proefke SA, Bhushan A, Matherly LH. Isolation of human cDNAs that restore methotrexate sensitivity and reduced folate carrier activity in methotrexate transport-defective Chinese hamster ovary cells. *J Biol Chem.* 1995; 270:17468–75.

94. Stark GR, Debatisse M, Giulotto E, Wahl GM. Recent progress in understanding mechanisms of mammalian DNA amplification. *Cell.* 1989; 57:901–8.

95. Matherly LH, Taub JW, Ravindranath Y, et al. Elevated dihydrofolate reductase and impaired methotrexate transport as elements in methotrexate resistance in childhood acute lymphoblastic leukemia. *Blood.* 1995; 85:500–9.

96. Rhee MS, Wang Y, Nair MG, Galivan J. Acquisition of resistance to antifolates caused by enhanced γ-glutamyl hydrolase activity. *Cancer Res.* 1993; 53:2227–30.

97. Schweitzer BI, Dicker AP, Bertino JR. Dihydrofolate reductase as a therapeutic target. *FASEB J.* 1990; 4:2441–52.

98. Domin BA, Mahony WB, Zimmerman TP. Transport of 5-fluorouracil and uracil into human erythrocytes. *Biochem Pharmacol.* 1993; 46:503–10.

99. Spears CP, Gustavsson BG, Berne M, Frosing R, Bernstein L, Hayes AA. Mechanisms of innate resistance to thymidylate synthase inhibition after 5-fluorouracil. *Cancer Res.* 1988; 48:5894–900.

100. Peters GJ, van der Wilt CL, van Groeningen CJ, Smid K, Meijer S, Pinedo HM. Thymidylate synthase inhibition after administration of fluorouracil with or without leucovorin in colon cancer patients: implications for treatment with fluorouracil. *J Clin Oncol.* 1994; 12:2035–42.

101. van der Wilt CL, Pinedo HM, de Jong M, Peters GJ. Effect of folate diastereoisomers on the binding of 5-fluoro-2′-deoxyuridine-5′-monophosphate to thymidylate synthase. *Biochem Pharmacol.* 1993; 45:1177–9.

102. Bapat AR, Zarow C, Danenberg PV. Human leukemic cells resistant to 5-fluoro-2′-deoxyuridine contain a thymidylate synthetase with lower affinity for nucleotides. *J Biol Chem.* 1983; 258:4130–6.

103. Jenh CH, Geyer PK, Baskin F, Johnson LF. Thymidylate synthase gene amplification in fluorodeoxyuridine-resistant mouse cell lines. *Mol Pharmacol.* 1985; 28:80–85.

104. Peters GJ, van Groeningen CJ. Clinical relevance of biochemical modulation of 5-fluorouracil. *Ann Oncol.* 1991; 2:469–80.

105. Pinedo HM, Peters GF. Fluorouracil: biochemistry and pharmacology. *J Clin Oncol.* 1988; 6:1653–64.

106. Sirotnak FM, Barrueco JR. Membrane transport and the antineoplastic action of nucleoside analogues. *Cancer Metastas Rev.* 1987; 6:459–80.

107. Capizzi RL, Yang JL, Rathmell JP, et al. Dose-related pharmacologic effects of high-dose ara-C and its self-potentiation. *Semin Oncol.* 1985; 12:65–74.

108. Ross DD, Cuddy DP, Cohen N, Hensley DR. Mechanistic implications of alterations in HL-60 cell nascent DNA after exposure to 1-β-D-arabinofuranosylcytosine. *Cancer Chemother Pharmacol.* 1992; 31:61–70.

109. Drenthe-Schonk AM, Holdrinet RS, van Egmond J, Wessels JM, Haanen C. Cytokinetic changes after cytosine arabinoside in acute non-lymphocyte leukemia. *Leuk Res.* 1981; 5:89–96.

110. Flasshove M, Strumberg D, Ayscue L, et al. Structural analysis of the deoxycytidine kinase gene in patients with acute myeloid leukemia and resistance to cytosine arabinoside. *Leukemia.* 1994; 8:780–5.

111. Fridland A, Verhoef V. Mechanism for ara CTP catabolism in human leukemic cells and effect of deaminase inhibitors on this process. *Semin Oncol.* 1987; 14:262–8.

112. Kreis W, Lesser M, Budman DR, et al. Phenotypic analysis of 1-β-D-arabinofuranosylcytosine deamination in patients treated with high doses and correlation with response. *Cancer Chemother Pharmacol.* 1992; 30:126–30.

113. Reed E. Platinum-DNA adduct, nucleotide excision repair and platinum based anti-cancer chemotherapy. *Cancer Treat Rev.* 1998; 24:331–44.

114. Barry MA, Behnke CA, Eastman A. Activation of programmed cell death (apoptosis) by cisplatin, other anticancer drugs, toxins and hyperthermia. *Biochem Pharmacol.* 1990; 40:2353–62.

115. Heiger-Bernays WJ, Essigmann JM, Lippard SJ. Effect of the antitumor drug *cis*-diammine-dichloroplatinum(II) and related platinum complexes on eukaryotic DNA replication. *Biochemistry* 1990; 29:8461–6.

116. Ewig RA, Kohn KW. DNA damage and repair in mouse leukemia L1210 cells treated with nitrogen mustard. 1,3-bis(2-chloroethyl)-1-nitrosourea, and other nitrosoureas. *Cancer Res.* 1977; 37:2114–22.

117. Sherman SE, Gibson D, Wang AH, Lippard SJ. X-ray structure of the major adduct of the anticancer drug cisplatin with DNA: cis-[Pt(NH$_3$)2(d(pGpG))]. *Science.* 1985; 230:412–7.

118. Hartley JA, Gibson NW. DNA damage and cytotoxicity of 2-chloroethyl (methylsulfonyl)-methanesulfonate (NSC 338947) produced in human colon carcinoma cells with or without methylating agent pretreatment. *Cancer Res.* 1986; 46:3871–5.

119. Hurley LH, Reynolds VL, Swenson DH, Petzold GL, Scahill TA. Reaction of the antitumor antibiotic CC-1065 with DNA: structure of a DNA adduct with DNA sequence specificity. *Science.* 1984; 226:843–4.

120. Kohn KW. Interstrand cross-linking of DNA by 1,3-bis(2-chloroethyl)-1 nitrosourea and other 1-(2-haloethyl)-1-nitrosoureas. *Cancer Res.* 1977; 37:1450–4.

121. Bennett RA, Pegg AE. Alklylation of DNA in rat tissues following administration of streptozotocin. *Cancer Res.* 1981; 41:2786–90.

122. Gonzaga PE, Brent TP. Affinity purification and characterization of human O^6-alkylguanine-DNA alkyltransferase complexed with BCNU-treated, synthetic oligonucleotide. *Nucleic Acids Res.* 1989; 17:6581–90.

123. Ludlum DB. DNA alkylation by the haloethylnitrosoureas: nature of modifications produced and their enzymatic repair or removal. *Mutat Res.* 1990; 233:117–26.

124. Wu ZN, Chan CL, Eastman A, Bresnick E. Expression of human O^6-methylguanine-DNA methyltransferase in a DNA excision repair-deficient Chinese hamster ovary cell line and its response to certain alkylating agents. *Cancer Res.* 1992; 52:32–35.

125. Chae MY, McDougall MG, Dolan ME, Swenn K, Pegg AE, Moschel RC. Substituted O^6-benzylguanine derivatives and their inactivation of human O^6-alkylguanine-DNA alkyltransferase. *J Med Chem.* 1994; 37:342–7.

126. Dolan ME, Moschel RC, Pegg AE. Depletion of mammalian O^6-alkylguanine-DNA alkyltransferase activity by O^6-benzylguanine provides a means to evaluate the role of this protein in protection against carcinogenic and therapeutic alkylating agents. *Proc Natl Acad Sci USA.* 1990; 87:5368–72.

127. McCormick JE, McElhinney RS. Nitrosoureas from chemist to physician: classification and recent approaches to drug design. *Eur J Cancer.* 1990; 26:207–21.

128. Pegg AE. Mammalian O^6-alkylguanine-DNA alkyltransferase: regulation and importance in response to alkylating carcinogenic and therapeutic agents. *Cancer Res.* 1990; 50:6119–29.

129. Seeberg E, Eide L, Bjoras M. The base excision repair pathway. *Trends Biochem Sci.* 1995; 20:391–7.

130. Frosina G, Fortini P, Rossi O, et al. Two pathways for base excision repair in mammalian cells. *J Biol Chem.* 1996; 271:9573–8.

131. Klungland A, Lindahl T. Second pathway for completion of human DNA base excision-

repair: reconstitution with purified proteins and requirement for DNase IV (FEN1). *EMBO J.* 1997; 16:3341–8.

132. Sancar A, Sancar GB. DNA repair enzymes. *Annu Rev Biochem.* 1988; 57:29–67.

133. Perez RP, Hamilton TC, Ozols RF, Young RC. Mechanisms and modulation of resistance to chemotherapy in ovarian cancer. *Cancer.* 1993; 71:1571–80.

134. Dabholkar M, Parker R, Reed E. Determinants of cisplatin sensitivity in non-malignant non-drug-selected human T cell lines. *Mutat Res.* 1992; 274:45–56.

135. Dabholkar M, Bradshaw L, Parker RJ, et al. Cisplatin-DNA damage and repair in peripheral blood leukocytes in vivo and in vitro. *Environ Health Perspect.* 1992; 98:53–59.

136. Godwin AK, Meister A, O'Dwyer PJ, Huang CS, Hamilton TC, Anderson ME. High resistance to cisplatin in human ovarian cancer cell lines is associated with marked increase of glutathione synthesis. *Proc Natl Acad Sci USA* 1992; 89:3070–74.

137. Parker RJ, Eastman A, Bostick-Bruton F, Reed E. Acquired cisplatin resistance in human ovarian cancer cells is associated with enhanced repair of cisplatin-DNA lesions and reduced drug accumulation. *J Clin Invest.* 1991; 87:772–777.

138. van Duin M, de Wit J, Odijk H, et al. Molecular characterization of the human excision repair gene ERCC-1: cDNA cloning and amino acid homology with the yeast DNA repair gene RAD10. *Cell.* 1986; 44:913–23.

139. Lee KB, Parker RJ, Bohr V, Cornelison T, Reed E. Cisplatin sensitivity/resistance in UV repair-deficient Chinese hamster ovary cells of complementation groups 1 and 3. *Carcinogenesis.* 1993; 14:2177–80.

140. Dabholkar M, Vionnet J, Bostick-Bruton F, Yu JJ, Reed E. Messenger RNA levels of XPAC and ERCC1 in ovarian cancer tissue correlate with response to platinum-based chemotherapy. *J Clin Invest.* 1994; 94:703–8.

141. Metzger R, Leichman CG, Danenberg KD, et al. ERCC1 mRNA levels complement thymidylate synthase mRNA levels in predicting response and survival for gastric cancer patients receiving combination cisplatin and fluorouracil chemotherapy. *J Clin Oncol.* 1998; 16:309–16.

142. Leveillard T, Andera L, Bissonnette N, et al. Functional interactions between p53 and the TFIIH complex are affected by tumour-associated mutations. *EMBO J.* 1996; 15:1615–24.

143. Wang XW, Yeh H, Schaeffer L, et al. p53 modulation of TFIIH-associated nucleotide excision repair activity. *Nat Genet.* 1995; 10:188–95.

144. Wang XW, Vermeulen W, Coursen JD, et al. The XPB and XPD DNA helicases are components of the p53-mediated apoptosis pathway. *Genes Dev.* 1996; 10:1219–32.

145. Modrich P. Mismatch repair, genetic stability, and cancer. *Science.* 1994; 266:1959–60.

146. Goldmacher VS, Cuzick RA Jr, Thilly WG. Isolation and partial characterization of human cell mutants differing in sensitivity to killing and mutation by methylnitrosourea and *N*-methyl-*N'*-nitro-*N*-nitrosoguanidine. *J Biol Chem.* 1986; 261:12462–71.

147. Drummond JT, Anthoney A, Brown R, Modrich P. Cisplatin and Adriamycin® resistance are associated with MutLα and mismatch repair deficiency in an ovarian tumor cell line. *J Biol Chem.* 1996; 271:19645–8.

148. Dive C, Hickman JA. Drug-target interactions: only the first step in the commitment to a programmed cell death? *Br J Cancer.* 1991; 64:192–6.

149. Fisher DE. Apoptosis in cancer therapy: crossing the threshold. *Cell.* 1994; 78:539–42.

150. Quillet-Mary A, Mansat V, Duchayne E, et al. Daunorubicin-induced internucleosomal DNA fragmentation in acute myeloid cell lines. *Leukemia.* 1996; 10:417–25.

151. Kerr JF, Wyllie AH, Currie AR. Apoptosis: a basic biological phenomenon with wide-ranging implications in tissue kinetics. *Br J Cancer.* 1972; 26:239–57.

152. Wyllie AH, Kerr JF, Currie AR. Cell death: the significance of apoptosis. *Int Rev Cytol.* 1980; 68:251–306.

153. Lane DP. p53 and human cancers. *Br Med Bull.* 1994; 50:582–99.

154. Linzer DI, Levine AJ. Characterization of a 54K dalton cellular SV40 tumor antigen present in SV40-transformed cells and uninfected embryonal carcinoma cells. *Cell.* 1979; 17:43–52.

155. Resnick-Silverman L, St. Clair S, Maurer M, Zhao K, Manfredi JJ. Identification of a novel class of genomic DNA-binding sites suggests a mechanism for selectivity in target gene activation by the tumor suppressor protein p53. *Genes Dev.* 1998; 12:2102–7.

156. Di Leonardo A, Linke SP, Clarkin K, Wahl GM. DNA damage triggers a prolonged p53-dependent G_1 arrest and long-term induction of Cip1 in normal human fibroblasts. *Genes Dev.* 1994; 8:2540–51.

157. Linke SP, Clarkin KC, Wahl GM. p53 mediates permanent arrest over multiple cell cycles in response to γ-irradiation. *Cancer Res.* 1997; 57:1171–9.

158. Shivakumar CV, Brown DR, Deb S, Deb SP. Wild-type human p53 transactivates the human proliferating cell nuclear antigen promoter. *Mol Cell Biol.* 1995; 15:6785–93.

159. Agarwal ML, Agarwal A, Taylor WR, Stark GR. p53 controls both the G_2M and the G_1 cell cycle checkpoints and mediates reversible growth arrest in human fibroblasts. *Proc Natl Acad Sci USA* 1995; 92:8493–7.

160. Stewart N, Hicks GG, Paraskevas F, Mowat M. Evidence for a second cell cycle block at G_2/M by p53. *Oncogene.* 1995; 10:109–15.

161. Attardi LD, Lowe SW, Brugarolas J, Jacks T. Transcriptional activation by *p53,* but not induction of the *p21* gene, is essential for oncogene-mediated apoptosis. *EMBO J.* 1996; 15:3693–3701.

162. Caelles C, Helmberg A, Karin M. *p53*-dependent apoptosis in the absence of transcriptional activation of *p53*-target genes. *Nature.* 1994; 370:220–3.

163. Miyashita T, Reed JC. Tumor suppressor *p53* is a direct transcriptional activator of the human bax gene. *Cell.* 1995; 80:293–9.

164. Miyashita T, Krajewski S, Krajewska M, et al. Tumor suppressor *p53* is a regulator of bcl-2 and bax gene expression in vitro and in vivo. *Oncogene.* 1994; 9:1799–1805.

165. Miyashita T, Harigai M, Hanada M, Reed JC. Identification of a *p53*-dependent negative response element in the bcl-2 gene. *Cancer Res.* 1994; 54:3131–5.

166. Chiou SK, Rao L, White E. *Bcl-2* blocks *p53*-dependent apoptosis. *Mol Cell Biol.* 1994; 14:2556–63.

167. Polyak K, Xia Y, Zweier JL, Kinzler KW, Vogelstein B. A model for *p53*-induced apoptosis. *Nature.* 1997; 389:300–5.

168. Owen-Schaub LB, van Golen KL, Hill LL, Price JE. Fas and Fas ligand interactions suppress melanoma lung metastasis. *J Exp Med.* 1998; 188:1717–23.

169. Bennett M, Macdonald K, Chan SW, Luzio JP, Simari R, Weissberg P. Cell surface trafficking of Fas: a rapid mechanism of *p53*-mediated apoptosis. *Science.* 1998; 282:290–3.

170. Hollstein M, Sidransky D, Vogelstein B, Harris CC. *p53* mutations in human cancers. *Science.* 1991; 253:49–53.

171. Casey G, Lopez ME, Ramos JC, et al. DNA sequence analysis of exons 2 through 11 and immunohistochemical staining are required to detect all known p53 alterations in human malignancies. *Oncogene.* 1996; 13:1971–81.

172. Iggo R, Gatter K, Bartek J, Lane D, Harris AL. Increased expression of mutant forms of *p53* oncogene in primary lung cancer. *Lancet.* 1990; 335:675–9.

173. Unger T, Nau MM, Segal S, Minna JD. p53: a transdominant regulator of transcription

whose function is ablated by mutations occurring in human cancer. *EMBO J.* 1992; 11:1383–90.

174. Demers GW, Halbert CL, Galloway DA. Elevated wild-type p53 protein levels in human epithelial cell lines immortalized by the human papillomavirus type 16 E7 gene. *Virology.* 1994; 198:169–74.

175. Yew PR, Berk AJ. Inhibition of *p53* transactivation required for transformation by adenovirus early 1β protein. *Nature.* 1992; 357:82–85.

176. Lowe SW, Ruley HE, Jacks T, Housman DE. *p53*-dependent apoptosis modulates the cytotoxicity of anticancer agents. *Cell.* 1993; 74:957–67.

177. Lowe SW, Bodis S, McClatchey A, et al. *p53* status and the efficacy of cancer therapy in vivo. *Science.* 1994; 266:807–810.

178. Ju JF, Banerjee D, Lenz HJ, et al. Restoration of wild-type *p53* activity in *p53*-null HL-60 cells confers multidrug sensitivity. *Clin Cancer Res.* 1998; 4:1315–22.

179. O'Connor PM, Jackman J, Bae I, et al. Characterization of the *p53* tumor suppressor pathway in cell lines of the National Cancer Institute anticancer drug screen and correlations with the growth-inhibitory potency of 123 anticancer agents. *Cancer Res.* 1997; 57:4285–4300.

180. Weinstein JN, Myers TG, O'Connor PM, et al. An information-intensive approach to the molecular pharmacology of cancer. *Science.* 1997; 275:343–9.

181. Yang B, Eshleman JR, Berger NA, Markowitz SD. Wild-type p53 protein potentiates cytotoxicity of therapeutic agents in human colon cancer cells. *Clin Cancer Res.* 1996; 2:1649–57.

182. Vasey PA, Jones NA, Jenkins S, Dive C, Brown R. Cisplatin, camptothecin, and taxol sensitivities of cells with *p53*-associated multidrug resistance. *Mol Pharmacol.* 1996; 50:1536–40.

183. Hawkins DS, Demers GW, Galloway DA. Inactivation of *p53* enhances sensitivity to multiple chemotherapeutic agents. *Cancer Res.* 1996; 56:892–8.

184. Vikhanskaya F, D'Incalci M, Broggini M. Decreased cytotoxic effects of doxorubicin in a human ovarian cancer-cell line expressing wild-type *p53* and *WAF1/CIP1* genes. *Int J Cancer.* 1995; 61:397–401.

185. Trepel M, Scheding S, Groscurth P, et al. A new look at the role of *p53* in leukemia cell sensitivity to chemotherapy. *Leukemia.* 1997; 11:1842–9.

186. Debernardis D, Sire EG, De Feudis P, et al. *p53* status does not affect sensitivity of human ovarian cancer cell lines to paclitaxel. *Cancer Res.* 1997; 57:870–4.

187. Fan S, Cherney B, Reinhold W, Rucker K, O'Connor PM. Disruption of *p53* function in immortalized human cells does not affect survival or apoptosis after Taxol or vincristine treatment. *Clin Cancer Res.* 1998; 4:1047–54.

188. Wu GS, El-Diery WS. *p53* and chemosensitivity. *Nat Med.* 1996; 2:255–6.

189. Wahl AF, Donaldson KL, Fairchild C, et al. Loss of normal *p53* function confers sensitization to Taxol by increasing G_2/M arrest and apoptosis. *Nat Med.* 1996; 2:72–79.

190. Cross SM, Sanchez CA, Morgan CA, et al. A *p53*-dependent mouse spindle checkpoint. *Science.* 1995; 267:1353–6.

191. Bergh J, Norberg T, Sjoegren S, Lindgren A, Holmberg L. Complete sequencing of the *p53* gene provides prognostic information in breast cancer patients, particularly in relation to adjuvant systemic therapy and radiotherapy. *Nat Med.* 1995; 1:1029–34.

192. Boku N, Chin K, Hosokawa K, et al. Biological markers as a predictor for response and prognosis of unrresectable gastric cancer patients treated with 5-fluorouracil and *cis*-platinum. *Clin Cancer Res.* 1998; 4:1469–74.

193. Brett MC, Pickard M, Green B, et al. p53 protein overexpression and response to biomodu-lated 5-fluorouracil chemotherapy in patients with advanced colorectal cancer. *Eur J Surg Oncol.* 1996; 22:182–5.

194. Buttitta F, Marchetti A, Gadducci A, et al. p53 alterations are predictive of chemoresistance and aggressiveness in ovarian carcinomas: a molecular and immunohistochemical study. *Br J Cancer.* 1997; 75:230–5.

195. Clahsen PC, van de Velde CJ, Duval C, et al. p53 protein accumulation and response to adjuvant chemotherapy in premenopausal women with node-negative early breast cancer. *J Clin Oncol.* 1998; 16:470–9.

196. Degeorges A, de Roquancourt A, Extra JM, et al. Is p53 a protein that predicts the response to chemotherapy in node negative breast cancer? *Breast Cancer Res Treat.* 1998; 47:47–55.

197. Di Leo A, Bajetta E, Biganzoli L, et al. An I.T.M.O. group study on second-line treatment in advanced epithelial ovarian cancer: an attempt to identify clinical and biological factors determining prognosis. *Eur J Cancer.* 1995; 31A:2248–54.

198. Elledge RM, Gray R, Monsour E, et al. Accumulation of p53 protein as a possible predictor of response to adjuvant combination chemotherapy with cyclophosphamide, methotrexate, fluorouracil, and prednisone for breast cancer. *J Natl Cancer Inst.* 1995; 87:1254–6.

199. Jacquemier J, Penault-Llorca F, Viens P, et al. Breast cancer response to adjuvant chemo-therapy in correlation with *erbB2* and *p53* expression. *Anticancer Res.* 1994; 14:2773–8.

200. Lenz HJ, Hayashi K, Salonga D, et al. *p53* point mutations and thymidylate synthase messenger RNA levels in disseminated colorectal cancer: an analysis of response and survival. *Clin Cancer Res.* 1998; 4:1243–50.

201. Linn SC, Pinedo HM, van Ark-Otte J, et al. Expression of drug resistance proteins in breast cancer, in relation to chemotherapy. *Int J Cancer.* 1997; 71:787–95.

202. Makris A, Powles TJ, Dowsett M, Allred C. p53 protein overexpression and chemosensitiv-ity in breast cancer. *Lancet* 1995; 345:1181–2.

203. Paradiso A, Rabinovich M, Vallejo C, et al. p53 and PCNA expression in advanced colorectal cancer: response to chemotherapy and long-term prognosis. *Int J Cancer.* 1996; 69:437–41.

204. Righetti SC, Delia-Torre TG, Pilotti S, et al. A comparative study of *p53* gene mutations, protein accumulation, and response to cisplatin-based chemotherapy in advanced ovarian carcinoma. *Cancer Res.* 1996; 56:689–93.

205. Rosell R, Gonzalez-Larriba JL, Alberola V, et al. Single-agent paclitaxel by 3-hour infusion in the treatment of non-small cell lung cancer: links between *p53* and K-*ras* gene status and chemosensitivity. *Semin Oncol.* 1995; 22:12–18.

206. Rusch V, Klimstra D, Venkatraman E, et al. Aberrant *p53* expression predicts clinical resistance to cisplatin-based chemotherapy in locally advanced non-small cell lung cancer. *Cancer Res.* 1995; 55:5038–42.

207. Smith-Sorensen B, Kaern J, Holm R, Dorum A, Trope C, Borresen-Dale AL. Therapy effect of either paclitaxel or cyclophosphamide combination treatment in patients with epithelial ovarian cancer and relation to *TP53* gene status. *Br J Cancer.* 1998; 78:375–81.

208. Stal O, Stenmark-Askmalm M, Wingren S, et al. *p53* expression and the result of adjuvant therapy of breast cancer. *Acta Oncol.* 1995; 34:767–70.

209. Renninson J, Baker BW, McGown AT, et al. Immunohistochemical detection of mutant p53 protein in epithelial ovarian cancer using polyclonal antibody CMI: correlation with histopathology and clinical features. *Br J Cancer.* 1994; 69:609–12.

210. Kawasaki M, Nakanishi Y, Kuwano K, Yatsunami J, Takayama K, Hara N. The utility of p53 immunostaining of transbronchial biopsy specimens of lung cancer: *p53* overexpression

predicts poor prognosis and chemoresistance in advanced non-small cell lung cancer. *Clin Cancer Res.* 1997; 3:1195–1200.

211. Apolinario RM, van der Valk P, de Jong JS, et al. Prognostic value of the expression of p53, bcl-2, and bax oncoproteins, and neovascularization in patients with radically resected non-small-cell lung cancer. *J Clin Oncol.* 1997; 15:2456–66.

212. Tsujimoto Y, Croce CM. Analysis of the structure, transcripts, and protein products of bcl-2, the gene involved in human follicular lymphoma. *Proc Natl Acad Sci USA.* 1986; 83:5214–8.

213. Nunez G, London L, Hockenbery D, Alexander M, McKearn JP, Korsmeyer SJ. Deregulated *Bcl-2* gene expression selectively prolongs survival of growth factor-deprived hemopoietic cell lines. *J Immunol.* 1990; 144:3602–10.

214. Vaux DL, Cory S, Adams JM. *Bcl-2* gene promotes haemopoietic cell survival and cooperates with c-*myc* to immortalize pre-B cells. *Nature.* 1988; 335:440–2.

215. Hockenbery D, Nunez G, Milliman C, Schreiber RD, Korsmeyer SJ. Bcl-2 is an inner mitochondrial membrane protein that blocks programmed cell death. *Nature.* 1990; 348:334–6.

216. Matsuzaki Y, Nakayama K, Nakayama K, et al. Role of bcl-2 in the development of lymphoid cells from the hematopoietic stem cell. *Blood.* 1997; 89:853–862.

217. Uhlmann EJ, D'Sa-Eipper C, Subramanian T, Wagner AJ, Hay N, Chinnadurai G. Deletion of a nonconserved region of Bcl-2 confers a novel gain of function: suppression of apoptosis with concomitant cell proliferation. *Cancer Res.* 1996; 56:2506–9.

218. Krajewski S, Tanaka S, Takayama S, Schibler MJ, Fenton W, Reed JC. Investigation of the subcellular distribution of the bcl-2 oncoprotein: residence in the nuclear envelope, endoplasmic reticulum, and outer mitochondrial membranes. *Cancer Res.* 1993; 53:4701–14.

219. Reed JC. Bcl-2 and the regulation of programmed cell death. *J Cell Biol.* 1994; 124:1–6.

220. Reed JC. Bcl-2: prevention of apoptosis as a mechanism of drug resistance. *Hematol Oncol Clin North Am.* 1995; 9:451–73.

221. Strasser A, Huang DC, Vaux DL. The role of the *bcl-2/ced-9* gene family in cancer and general implications of defects in cell death control for tumourigenesis and resistance to chemotherapy. *Biochim Biophys Acta.* 1997; 1333:F151–78.

222. Allsopp TE, Wyatt S, Paterson HF, Davies AM. The proto-oncogene *bcl-2* can selectively rescue neurotrophic factor-dependent neurons from apoptosis. *Cell.* 1993; 73:295–307.

223. Kroemer G. The proto-oncogene *Bcl-2* and its role in regulating apoptosis. *Nat Med.* 1997; 3:614–20.

224. Brown R. The bcl-2 family of proteins. *Br Med Bull.* 1997; 53:466–77.

225. Haldar S, Chintapalli J, Croce CM. Taxol induces bcl-2 phosphorylation and death of prostate cancer cells. *Cancer Res.* 1996; 56:1253–5.

226. Siegel RM, Katsumata M, Miyashita T, Louie DC, Greene MI, Reed JC. Inhibition of thymocyte apoptosis and negative antigenic selection of *bcl-2* transgenic mice. *Proc Natl Acad Sci USA.* 1992; 89:7003–7.

227. Kondo S, Yin D, Morimura T, Oda Y, Kikuchi H, Takeuchi J. Transfection with a *bcl-2* expression vector protects transplanted bone marrow from chemotherapy-induced myelosuppression. *Cancer Res* 1994; 54:2928–33.

228. Offit K, Koduru PR, Hollis R, et al. 18q21 rearrangement in diffuse large cell lymphoma: incidence and clinical significance. *Br J Haematol.* 1989; 72:178–83.

229. Yunis JJ, Mayer MG, Arnesen MA, Aeppli DP, Oken MM, Frizzera G. *bcl-2* and other genomic alterations in the prognosis of large-cell lymphoma. *N Engl J Med.* 1989; 320:1047–54.

230. Pezzella F, Jones M, Ralfkiaer E, Ersboll J, Gatter KC, Mason DY. Evaluation of bcl-2 protein expression and 14;18 translocation as prognostic markers in follicular lymphoma. *Br J Cancer.* 1992; 65:87–89.

231. Jacobson JO, Wilkes BM, Kwaiatkowski DJ, Medeiros LJ, Aisenberg AC, Harris NL. *bcl-2* rearrangements in de novo diffuse large cell lymphoma. Association with distinctive clinical features. *Cancer.* 1993; 72:231–6.

232. Piris MA, Pezzella F, Martinez-Montero JC, et al. *p53* and *bcl-2* expression in high-grade B-cell lymphomas: correlation with survival time. *Br J Cancer.* 1994; 69:337–41.

233. Romaguera JE, Pugh W, Luthra R, Goodacre A, Cabanillas F. The clinical relevance of t(14;18)/BCL-2 rearrangement and DEL 6q in diffuse large cell lymphoma and immunoblastic lymphoma. *Ann Oncol.* 1993; 4:51–54.

234. Wilson WH, Teruya-Feldstein J, Fest T, et al. Relationship of *p53, bcl-2,* and tumor proliferation to clinical drug resistance in non-Hodgkin's lymphomas. *Blood.* 1997; 89: 601–9.

235. Campos L, Rouault JP, Sabido O, et al. High expression of bcl-2 protein in acute myeloid leukemia cells is associated with poor response to chemotherapy. *Blood.* 1993; 81:3091–6.

236. McDonnell TJ, Troncoso P, Brisbay SM, et al. Expression of the protooncogene *bcl-2* in the prostate and its association with emergence of androgen-independent prostate cancer. *Cancer Res.* 1992; 52:6940–4.

237. Takayama K, Ogata K, Nakanishi Y, Yatsunami J, Kawasaki M, Hara N. *Bcl-2* expression as a predictor of chemosensitivities and survival in small cell lung cancer. *Cancer J Sci Am.* 1996; 2:212.

238. Bonetti A, Zaninelli M, Leone R, et al. *bcl-2* but not *p53* expression is associated with resistance to chemotherapy in advanced breast cancer. *Clin Cancer Res.* 1998; 4:2331–2336.

239. van Slooten HJ, Clahsen PC, van Dierendonck JH, et al. Expression of *Bcl-2* in node-negative breast cancer is associated with various prognostic factors, but does not predict response to one course of perioperative chemotherapy. *Br J Cancer.* 1996; 74:78–85.

240. Amati B, Dalton S, Brooks MW, Littlewood TD, Evan GI, Land H. Transcriptional activation by the human c-Myc oncoprotein in yeast requires interaction with Max. *Nature.* 1992; 359:423–6.

241. Oswald F, Lovec H, Moeroey T, Lipp M. E2F-dependent regulation of human MYC: trans-activation by cyclins D1 and A overrides tumour suppressor protein functions. *Oncogene.* 1994; 9:2029–36.

242. Chiarugi V, Ruggiero M. Role of three cancer "master genes" *p53, bc12* and c-*myc* on the apoptotic process. *Tumori.* 1996; 82:205–9.

243. Reyt E, Lavieille JP, Brambilla E, Barra Y, Riva C. [Expression of oncogenes C-*myc*, C- and N-*ras* in advanced cancers of the upper respiratory and digestive tracts. Correlation with tumor clinical response to chemotherapy]. *Ann Otolaryngol Chir Cervicofac.* 1993; 110:310–5.

244. Riva C, Lavieille JP, Reyt E, Brambilla E, Lunardi J, Brambilla C. Differential c-*myc*, c-*jun*, c-*raf* and *p53* expression in squamous cell carcinoma of the head and neck: implication in drug and radioresistance. *Eur J Cancer B Oral Oncol.* 1995; 31B:384–91.

III

FUTURE DIRECTIONS

14

Antitumor Immunity as Therapy for Human Cancer

Angelo A. Cardoso

Introduction

Over the past few decades, an enormous body of knowledge has emerged concerning the mechanisms implicated in the structural and functional organization of the immune system; the development of tumors; and the manipulation of cells, proteins, and genetic material. Included in the remarkable progress is the comprehension of the requirements for the initiation and execution of T cell-mediated immunity; the clarification of the pathways of antigen (Ag) processing and presentation; the identification and characterization of tumor Ags; and understanding of the principles of organization, regulation, and synthesis of molecular structures. In parallel, major technological strides have been made, resulting in the routine practice of formerly impossible manipulation, multiplication, and modification of cells, molecules, and genes.

Progress has been particularly impressive in the area of tumor immunology and has led to intense efforts to develop strategies of immune intervention to treat human cancer. In this chapter, our present knowledge of the mechanisms involved in the initiation and modulation of T cell-mediated immunity and the processing and presentation of Ags, and the impact of this valuable information on studies attempting to understand tumor immunity and the development of novel immunotherapeutic approaches are discussed.

Activation of Naive T Cells: Productive Immunity vs Anergy

For the generation of T cell-mediated immunity, T cells must receive signals from specialized cells, the antigen-presenting cells (APCs), which lead to the clonal expansion of Ag-specific T cells. The priming, expansion, and functional maturation of T cells are regulated by both intimate cell–cell interactions and signals delivered by soluble molecules.

The Two-Signal Model

The actual paradigm for the induction of a T cell-mediated immune response was originally proposed by Bretscher and Cohn (1) and later elaborated by Schwartz (2,3). This model postulates that T cells must receive two signaling events delivered by APCs (Fig. 1):

From: *Principles of Molecular Oncology*
Edited by: M. H. Bronchud, M. A. Foote, W. P. Peters, and M. O. Robinson © Humana Press Inc., Totowa, NJ

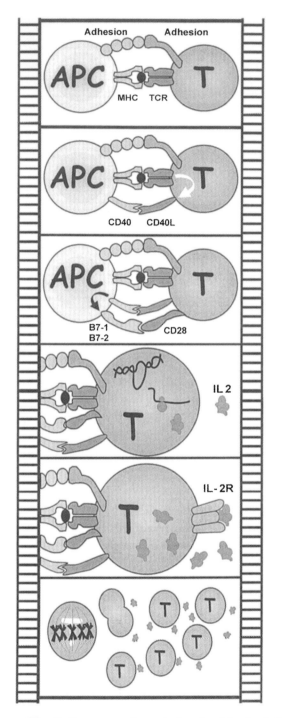

Recognition of the peptide-MHC complex by a suitable TCR. This interaction constitutes the cognitive signal, which is MHC-restricted and confers antigen (Ag) specificity.

This interaction is strengthened by the interplay between pairs of adhesion molecules.

The cognitive signal induces the expression of CD40L on T cells.CD40L ligates its receptor expressed by APC, CD40.

Crosslinking of CD40 results in the induction and/or up-regulation of the costimulatory molecules B7-1 and B7-2. These B7 molecules interact with their receptor on T cells, CD28.

Ligation of both TCR and CD28 results in the recruitment and activation of cascades of intracellular molecules leading to the transcription of the interleukin (IL)-2 gene, and secretion of IL-2 molecules.

Activation of T cells also induces the expression of a functional IL-2R, resulting in the establishment of an autocrine loop.

The final outcome is the clonal expansion of Ag-specific T cells.

Fig. 1. Sequence of events involved in the initiation of an antigen-specific T cell-mediated productive immune response. APC = antigen-presenting cell; MHC = major histocompatibility complex.

- Cognitive signal: This signal results from the recognition by a specific T-cell receptor (TCR) of the complex formed by a molecule of the major histocompatibility complex (MHC) associated with an antigenic peptide. This molecular interaction follows after the scrutiny of the TCR repertoire by APCs, to detect the T cells whose TCR are specific for the peptide–MHC complex presented by APCs. This cognitive signal is MHC restricted and confers the Ag specificity that characterizes this T cell-mediated immunity. This cell–cell contact mediated through the MHC–peptide/TCR interaction is considerably strengthened by the interplay between pairs of adhesion molecules expressed by the APC and T cells *(4,5)*. The sensitivity of T cells to their specific Ag is remarkable, as it has been demonstrated that as few as 30–100 MHC–peptide complexes are sufficient to trigger T-cell activation *(6,7)*. Nevertheless, signaling through TCR alone is not sufficient to prime naive T cells and to induce the production of optimal levels of interleukin (IL)-2 *(8,9)*. Ag processing and presentation of peptides by both MHC class I and MHC class II molecules is discussed on p. 365.
- Costimulatory signal: T-cell costimulation is delivered by accessory molecules expressed by APCs, most importantly by the molecules of the B7 family, B7-1/CD80 and B7-2/ CD86 *(10–12)*. B7-mediated costimulation is delivered through their T-cell counter-receptor, CD28 *(13)*, and must be provided within a finite time interval after presentation of the Ag *(2)*. This signal is neither MHC restricted nor Ag specific. Delivery of costimulation by itself is not sufficient to stimulate naive T cells *(14)*. This signal complements the cognitive signal delivered through TCR and leads to the production of IL-2 and ultimately to the clonal expansion of Ag-specific T cells *(15)*. The critical role of B7 costimulation in T cell-mediated immunity is evident in that delivery of a TCR signal in the absence of appropriate costimulation can result in the induction of T-cell anergy (discussed on p. 379).

Although supported by a substantial amount of evidence and its indisputable fit to the puzzle qualities, the two-signal model constitutes an oversimplification of the sequence of events that lead to T-cell activation *(16,17)*. In addition to the intrinsic variability of the cognitive (Ag affinity, specificity, quantity) and costimulatory signals, T cells must decipher these events in the context of other environmental signals, namely the presence of other accessory membrane-bound molecules and, most importantly, soluble cytokines *(17)*. The priming of naive T cells can be seen as a complex and dynamic process in which T cells receive both triggering and modulatory signals that, if appropriate in quality, intensity, and time frame, will result in the attainment of a threshold of activation and, consequently, T-cell proliferation and functional differentiation into competent effector cells.

Induction of T Cell-Mediated Productive Immunity

Under appropriate conditions, the productive activation of naive T cells will lead to the generation of sufficient numbers of differentiated effector T cells (helper, cytotoxic, suppressor) capable of mediating an appropriate response against the initiating stimuli (Fig. 1). The engagement of naive T cells with TCR specificity for the agonist peptide–MHC complex presented by APCs will lead to productive responses only if these TCR signals can be amplified. This requirement most probably derives from the restricted number of specific TCRs likely to be engaged, and from the dynamics of the TCR engagement and internalization *(6,18)*. Therefore, the amplification of the cognitive signal, which can be mediated by costimulatory molecules, plays a critical role in the profile and magnitude of the T-cell response. Consequently, it is not surprising that for optimal T-cell activation, both the cognitive and the costimulatory signals must be delivered by the same cell *(19,20)*. This stringency is of enormous biological relevance, as it prevents accidental costimulation by bystander cells that could induce undesirable effects, such as an autoimmune response.

Among the different accessory molecules reported to be capable of mediating T-cell costimulation, the B7-1/CD80 and B7-2/CD86 molecules seem to play the major role in the activation of naive T cells *(21,22)*. These two molecules deliver their signals through CD28, a glycoprotein expressed by 95% of CD4+ T cells and about 50% of CD8+ T cells *(23)*. Crosslinking of CD28 after TCR engagement results in dramatic changes in T cells that ultimately lead to *IL-2* gene transcription *(24,25)* (Fig. 1). Moreover, binding of CD28 by its cognate ligands results in the delivery of a survival signal that cannot be replaced by an increased TCR signal *(26)*. The molecular events initiated by the ligation of TCR and the costimulatory counterreceptors include the recruitment and activation of nonreceptor protein tyrosine kinases (such as lck, fyn, and ZAP-70), the phosphorylation of adaptor proteins (such as Grb2, Shc, Lnk, SLP-76, Cbl, and Crk), the influx of calcium, and the recruitment of different effector signaling pathways (such as calcium-dependent kinases and phosphatases, and serine/threonine kinases). These complex cascades of intracellular signals result in the mobilization of DNA-binding proteins that translocate to the nucleus and initiate gene transcription, such as the *IL-2* gene. More precise information on the signaling pathways involved in Ag-mediated T-cell activation can be obtained in several excellent reviews *(27–32)*.

A second counterreceptor for B7-1 and B7-2 is the CD28-related glycoprotein CTLA-4 (CD152) *(33,34)*. CTLA-4 is also a member of the immunoglobulin (Ig) gene superfamily and is expressed on primed but not naive T cells *(35)*. Its binding results in the delivery of a negative signal that inhibits T-cell responses in the presence of appropriate TCR engagement *(36,37)*. Ligation of CTLA-4 inhibits T-cell proliferation and functional differentiation, and blocks IL-2 production *(38)*. It has recently been shown that CTLA-4 associates with the TCRζ chain and inhibits its tyrosine phosphory-lation *(39)*, thereby inhibiting the signaling pathways induced by the T-cell activation at a membrane-proximal, upstream level. The capacity of CTLA-4 to compete for B7-1 and B7-2 binding and to inhibit the activation of naive T cells has broad implications for the negative regulation of T-cell function and T-cell tolerance *(39–42)* and may be an important tool for the development of novel therapies in transplantation and cancer (discussed later).

Another important player in the activation of naive T cells is the interaction between CD40 and its ligand, CD40L (CD154). CD40L plays a critical role by inducing and/or upregulating the expression of costimulatory molecules on APCs, which can then costimulate T cells more efficiently (Fig. 1). In fact, it has been demonstrated that CD40L binding by CD40 results in the priming and amplification of Ag-specific CD4+ T cells *(43,45)*, and in the activation of professional APCs such as dendritic cells (DCs), B cells, and macrophages *(46–48)*. CD40L, a member of the tumor necrosis family (TNF) family, is rapidly induced after TCR ligation (and activation of the TCR–CD3 complex) *(49)*. It has been suggested that the induction of CD40L on T cells is also mediated by the signal delivered to CD28 by B7-2 *(50)*, which is constitutively expressed at low levels by professional APCs. It has been also suggested that the CD40 pathway can as well directly costimulate T cells *(51)*. Therefore, the precise place of the CD40–

CD40L interaction in the hierarchy of stimuli required for T-cell activation is still unclear (Fig. 1).

Another major pathway involved in the activation of naive T cells is the ICAM-1:LFA-1 (CD54:CD11a-CD18) interaction. In addition to strengthening the TCR-MHC ligation by their adhesive properties, ICAM-1 binding to LFA-1 can costimulate T-cell proliferation *(52,53)*. Moreover, blockade of the ICAM-1:LFA-1 interplay results in a significant reduction of T-cell proliferation and IL-2 production *(54)*. Also, other studies suggest an important distinction between the B7 family members and ICAM-1. Although both can act as costimulators, ICAM-1 does not induce significant accumulation of IL-2 and does not seem to be capable of preventing the induction of anergy *(53,55)*.

Other molecules may also have an important impact on the induction of T cell-mediated immunity. The LFA-3:CD2 (CD58:CD2) pair represents the major adhesion interaction for resting T cells *(56)* and it has been suggested that it acts as a costimulator of naive T cells, although some controversy on whether it can induce significant T-cell proliferation and IL-2 production persists *(56,57)*. Additional molecules reported as capable costimulators of T cells include the CD70:CD27, 4-1BBL:4-1BB (CDw137), and OX40L:OX40 (CD134) pairs *(58–61)*, and the HSA, SLAM-1, and CD43 molecules *(62–64)*. It should be emphasized that soluble molecules, such as cytokines, can also regulate T-cell activation and modulate the outcome of the TCR engagement by delivering costimulatory signals and thereby preventing T-cell unresponsiveness (as is the case with IL-2) *(65)*; inhibiting T-cell reactivity (as with transforming growth factor [TGF]-β) *(66,67)*; or deviating the T-cell response to specific effector profiles (such as the induction of particular cytokine secretion patterns) *(17)*.

It is noteworthy to mention that the requirements for the activation of primed T cells are less restrictive than those for naive T cells. Memory Ag-specific and effector T cells do not require the costimulatory signal for further activation by APCs *(68,69)*. These differences have important physiologic relevance, as they allow the recognition of target cells expressing the correct agonist peptide–MHC complex even if these cells are not capable of providing costimulatory signals, and thereby allow the T cells to accomplish their effector function.

As the efficient activation of naive T cells requires the amplification of the TCR signal *(70)*, an important challenge exists in the elucidation of the mechanisms involved in the initiation of the signals leading to sustained T-cell activation. It is largely unknown whether the amplification of TCR signal occurs at a membrane-proximal level as the result of the mobilization and engagement of sufficient signaling receptors or if it occurs as a more downstream event resulting from the integration and magnification of distinct signals transduced to the cell nucleus. Studies analyzing the three-dimensional organization at the contact interface during Ag-specific T cell:APC interactions *(71–74)* shed some light on the molecular nature of these phenomena. These studies have clearly shown that the activation of T cells by APCs induces the formation of segregated clusters of receptors and intracellular proteins, such as TCR CD3 complexes, LFA-1, talin, PKCθ, Lck, and Fyn *(72)*. The formation of these supramolecular activation clusters (SMACs) is a specific and regulated process initiated by the ligation of the TCR specific to the peptide agonist *(72)*, and seems to be dependent on the presence of accessory events, as receptor engagement by itself is not sufficient to form SMACs

(72). The peptide-engaged TCR–CD3 clusters and the LFA-1 clusters were found to be organized into spatially segregated domains *(72)*. Also, it has been shown that the accumulation of pairs of both peptide–MHC:TCR and accessory molecules at the APC:T-cell contact sites can efficiently amplify weak TCR signals *(75)*. This accumulation is mediated by the movement of cytoskeleton molecules toward the APC:T-cell contact interface, which leads to an increased concentration of molecules, such as the receptor pair ICAM-1:LFA-1 *(74)*. Very importantly, this movement is modulated by B7:CD28 and ICAM-1:LFA-1 costimulatory interactions, suggesting that the amplification of the TCR signal mediated by these accessory molecules may result from the increased density (and engagement) of receptor/costimulatory molecules at the cell–cell interface *(74)*. Nevertheless, Viola and collaborators have recently demonstrated that the T cell costimulation provided by CD28 crosslinking does not result from the engagement of higher numbers of TCR but rather from an increased stability of the phosphorylation of several substrates and the recruitment and clustering of kinase-rich raft microdomains at the site of TCR engagement *(73)*. It can be expected that, in the near future, additional studies will shed more light on the precise structural and organizational mechanisms involved in the interactions of the MHC/peptide complexes with their cognate TCR.

Induction of Antigen-Specific T-Cell Anergy

An alternative functional outcome of an effective MHC–peptide recognition by T cells is the induction of a state of Ag-specific T-cell anergy (called T-cell tolerance in vivo). As predicted by the two-signal model, the occupancy of TCR by the MHC–peptide complex in the absence of appropriate costimulation would induce a state of T-cell unresponsiveness (Fig. 2). This state is characterized by the inability of Ag-specific T cells to respond and proliferate when restimulated with their primary cognitive stimuli, even if the stimulator APC delivers an appropriate costimulatory signal *(53,76)*.

Increasing evidence demonstrates the critical role of the molecules of the B7 family, B7-1 and B7-2, in preventing the induction of T-cell anergy (Fig. 2). In fact, multiple in vitro and in vivo studies have shown that the absence or functional blockade of B7-mediated costimulation prevents the production of IL-2 and results in Ag-specific T-cell unresponsiveness *(77–82)*. Most importantly, once T cells become anergic, this state of unresponsiveness cannot be reversed by signals delivered by the B7:CD28 pathway *(21,81)*. Moreover, Ag-specific T-cell anergy can be attained by the blockade of the B7:CD28 pathway through CTLA4-Ig, a soluble fusion protein formed by CTLA-4 and the heavy chain of human IgG1 that stably binds to both B7-1 and B7-2 *(21,83)*. Finally, and possibly in accordance with its critical role in mediating the expression of the B7 molecules, the blockade of the CD40L–CD40 interaction also results in the induction of T-cell anergy *(84,85)*.

Confirming the complexity of naive T-cell activation and supporting the influence of other environmental signals on the outcome of the TCR triggering, it has been shown that signaling through the IL-2R γ chain, common to the receptor complexes for IL-2, IL-4, IL-7, IL-9, and IL-15, prevents the induction of Ag-specific T-cell anergy *(65)*.

Although resulting in the functional inactivation of the T cells, induction of Ag-specific anergy is not a static process but rather involves a sequence of active signaling events. Induction of T-cell anergy results in a defective transcription of the *IL-2* gene

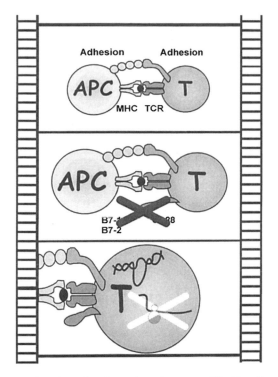

Recognition of the peptide-MHC complex by a suitable TCR. This interaction constitutes the cognitive signal, which is MHC-restricted and confers antigen (Ag)-specificity.

This interaction is strengthened by the interplay between pairs of adhesion molecules.

In the absence of B7-1 and B7-2 expression by APCs, the required costimulatory signal is not delivered to the T cells.

Absence of B7-costimulation is accompanied by defective transcription of the interleukin (IL)-2 gene, and results in the induction of T-cell anergy.

Fig. 2. Induction of antigen-specific T cell unresponsiveness (anergy in vitro; tolerance in vivo). APC = antigen-presenting cell; MHC = major histocompatibility complex.

(86,87) because of the impaired activation of critical signaling molecules such as lck, ZAP-70, and p21^{Ras} *(88,89)*. In contrast, induction of anergy is associated with activation of the Ras inhibitor Rap1, which explains the deficient production of IL-2 *(88)*. Moreover, the observed arrest of anergic cells in G_1 was recently demonstrated to be the result of a significant increase of the cyclin-dependent kinase inhibitor (CKI) p27^{kip1} *(90)*, whose down-regulation was shown to be required for entry of cells into the S-phase, and which requires Ras activity.

Another explanation for the induction of T-cell unresponsiveness was proposed in the strength-of-signal hypothesis, in which it is postulated that the presence of high levels of costimulation through CD28 coupled with TCR engagement may down-regulate the immune response *(27,80)*. This down-regulation would occur by clonal exhaustion of hyperactivated T cells or by the induction of an anergic status *(91)*.

Antigen Presentation and Antigen-Presenting Cells

The generation of T cell-mediated immunity is dependent on the recognition by specific T cells of immunogenic determinants presented by APCs. This epitope presentation takes place in the form of peptides derived from Ags that are continuously processed by the cellular catabolic machinery and further displayed by MHC molecules. MHC class I and class II molecules are proteins specialized in the capture, trafficking, and display of peptides derived from the degradation of both endogenous and exogenous molecules, thereby providing an updated representation of the molecular composition of both the intracellular and the extracellular milieu. The ontogenic evolution of the MHC proteins resulted in the development of two major processing and presenting pathways: MHC class I molecules that primarily present Ags localized in the cytosol, and MHC class II molecules that primarily present Ags localized in the endosome compartment (92) (Fig. 3).

The presentation of antigenic peptides involves the formation of hydrogen bonds between anchor residues of the MHC molecules and backbone, or terminal, residues of the associated peptide, or, alternatively, bonds between MHC polymorphic residues and specific side chains of the peptide (93–95). Multiple interactions between the peptide and the MHC-binding groove allow for a more stable and prolonged capture and presentation of the associated peptide (96). Most MHC molecules require association with two or three anchor residues for optimal peptide binding.

T lymphocytes, which exhibit a wide range of TCR rearrangements, continuously survey and sample the broad range of peptides displayed by the MHC molecules. The presentation of peptides of the same linear sequence in an equivalent conformation will likely ensure an optimal interaction with their complementary receptors on the T cells and, consequently, maximal activation and mobilization of specific T lymphocytes (97). Peptides presented by MHC class I molecules are recognized by $CD8^+$ T cells, while those displayed by MHC II are recognized by $CD4^+$ T cells. Table 1 summarizes the general characteristics of the MHC class I and MHC class II pathways.

The MHC Class I Antigen-Presentation Pathway

MHC class I proteins are formed by dimerization through noncovalent bonds of a transmembrane polymorphic heavy chain, encoded by one of the MHC I genes, and a non-MHC-encoded soluble protein, the β_2-microglobulin (β_2m). MHC I molecules primarily present peptides derived from intracellular Ags, as demonstrated by the fact that cytoplasmic and nuclear proteins are the main source of the peptides eluted from the MHC I molecules (98). These peptides result mostly from the degradation of cytosolic Ags by multicatalytic complexes, the proteasomes (99,100). Proteasomes are large protein assemblies formed by both catalytic molecules and accessory molecules that modulate their enzymatic activity (101). Translocation of the peptides suitable for binding to the MHC I into the endoplasmic reticulum (ER) lumen is mediated by the heterodimeric molecule TAP (transporter-associated with Ag processing), a member of the family of ATP-binding cassette (ABC) transporter proteins (102,103). TAP can be considered as a molecular ruler for the length of MHC I binding (97), and it has been shown that peptides with optimum length for MHC I binding are transported more efficiently. It must be emphasized that the nature of the molecular interactions of the peptides with the MHC I-binding groove restricts the peptides suitable for display by MHC I to those with 8–10 amino acids that exhibit binding residues (Table 1).

MHC class I proteins are synthesized in the ER and the formation of MHC I heterodimers displaying antigenic peptides is dependent on sequential, transient, protein–protein interactions (Fig. 3). This sequence involves:

- Interaction of newly produced, misfolded, class I heavy chains with calnexin, an ER transmembrane protein that functions as a chaperone and inhibits the traffic of peptide-free MHC molecules (104)

MHC class I

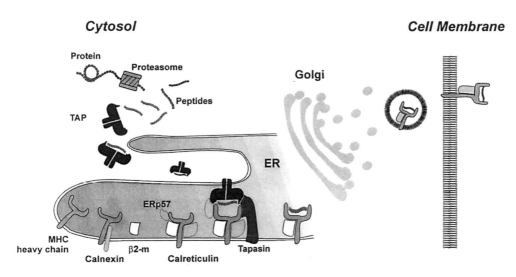

MHC class II

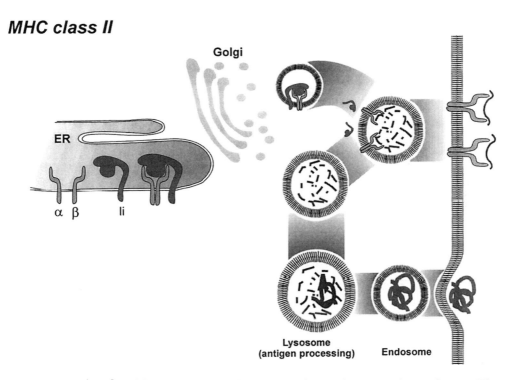

Fig. 3. MHC class I and MHC class II antigen processing and presentation pathways. The general characteristics of these pathways are summarized in Table 1.

Table 1
Structural and Functional Characteristics of MHC Class I and Class II Antigen-Processing and -Presentation Pathways

	MHC Class I	MHC Class II
Composition	45-kDa heavy chain subunit + 12-kDa β_2m	33-kDa α-subunit + 29-kDa β-subunit
Expression	Virtually all nucleated cells; higher expression on cells of the hematopoietic system	Dendritic cells, B cells, monocytes, activated T cells, some endothelium. Inducible in different cells (e.g., interferon)
Target cells	CD8+ T cells	CD4+ T cells
Peptide origin	Endogenous proteins; exogenous proteins capable of traversing membranes; proteins entering as fusion events	Exogenous molecules
Peptide binding region	Two antiparallel α-helices overlaying a platform of antiparallel β-strands	Similar to MHC I.
Antigen uptake	Largely unknown; micropinocytosis; occasional rupture of phagosomes	Receptor-mediated endocytosis, phagocytosis, macropinocytosis
Processing	Cytosol; by proteasomes	Primarily in endosomal/lysosomal system
Factors affecting antigen processing	Modulators of enzymatic activity of proteosomes (pH, temperature, interactions with other molecules); sequence of substrates (presence of particular residues)	Protease content, pH, reducing potential, Ii, interactions with MHC molecules or other molecules, polypeptide trimming by removtion of flanking residue
MHC-peptide binding	MHC : Residues at extremities of binding groove Peptide : Free N- and C-terminal residues	MHC : Main chain residues of binding site; open extremities Peptide : Backbone residues
Peptide length	8–10 residues	Variable; on average, 14–18 residues; as long as 28 residues

- Association of the thiol oxidoreductase Erp75 with the MHC heavy chain–calnexin complex *(105,106)*
- Formation of the heavy chain–β_2m dimer that is accompanied by the dissociation of calnexin, which is replaced by another ER transmembrane chaperone, the calreticulin *(107)*
- Association of the complex heavy chain–β_2m–calreticulin with the peptide-loaded transporter molecule TAP, which is mediated by the transmembrane glycoprotein tapasin *(107– 109)*
- Dissociation of peptide-loaded MHC I dimers from the chaperone molecules
- Traffic of properly folded, stable, peptide-loaded MHC I molecules to the Golgi compartment, and finally to the cell membrane through constitutive secretory vesicles (Fig. 3).

The temporal retention in the ER of MHC class I molecules is critical for the optimization of peptide binding and has been portrayed as the quality-control step in the assembly of mature MHC class I–peptide complexes *(110)*. The absence of peptide binding to the MHC heavy chain–β_2m complex results in the proteasome-mediated degradation of this heterodimer.

Some professional APCs, such as DCs and macrophages, can present Ags captured by phagocytosis or macropinocytosis through the MHC I presentation pathway *(111– 114)*. In vivo generation of cytotoxic T lymphocytes (CTLs) by soluble or particulate Ags has been documented *(115,116)*. The presentation of exogenous peptides by MHC I molecules may result in more diversified CD8$^+$ T-cell responses, as it is improbable that the phagosomal processing would reproducibly generate the same profile of T-cell epitopes generated by the proteosome/TAP system. Therefore, it is conceivable that a broader range of Ags (such as tumor Ags) can be displayed by MHC I molecules *(117)*.

The MHC Class II Antigen-Presentation Pathway

MHC class II proteins are formed by the dimerization of two transmembrane glycoproteins, the α chain and the β chain, which are synthesized and assembled as $\alpha\beta$ dimers in the ER (Fig. 3). The heterodimers then bind to the chaperone invariant chain (Ii), which is a non-MHC-encoded glycoprotein (118). This interaction leads to the formation of multimeric complexes, usually the nonameric ($\alpha\beta$-Ii)$_3$ *(119)*. Ii plays a central role in the MHC II pathway, as it facilitates the dimerization of the MHC II α and β chains and, more importantly, it occupies by its CLIP region (class II-associated invariant chain peptide), the MHC peptide-binding groove *(120)*. This occupancy of the binding groove impairs the capacity of MHC II complexes to bind peptides in the ER, thereby ensuring that the MHC II molecules do not form persistent, unproductive interactions *(121)*. Moreover, by preventing the possible binding of free peptides that are ligands for MHC I molecules, it preserves the functional separation between the two MHC pathways *(97)*. The $\alpha\beta$–Ii complex then translocates to the endosomal compartment, where the Ii is removed and the peptide binding occurs *(122)*. The release from the MHC II peptide groove of the remaining Ii CLIP region or low-affinity peptides is mediated by the MHC-linked protein HLA-DM, which facilitates the capture of high-affinity peptides *(123)*. Stable ligation of peptide to the binding groove results in a conformational change in the MHC II molecule, which increases its stability. The proteolytic degradation of Ags and the maturation of MHC II molecules in the same or in communicating compartments facilitates the assembly of mature, stable, MHC II–peptide complexes. These peptide-loaded MHC II molecules then traffic to the cell surface where they have the opportunity to be scrutinized by and interact with T cells (Fig. 3).

The peptides displayed by MHC II molecules are primarily derived from the degradation of extracellular Ags captured by phagocytosis, endocytosis, or macropinocytosis *(117,124)*. These peptides are generated in an endosomal, acidic compartment containing internalized Ag, proteases, and exocytic class II molecules *(118)*. Peptides are then loaded onto MHC II αβ dimers that enter this compartment (Fig. 3). As discussed earlier, the MHC II molecules are released from their association with their chaperone Ii before peptide binding. As MHC II molecules bind residues from the backbone of the antigenic peptide (Table 1) and their binding groove has an open design, peptides that associate with MHC II molecules can extend beyond the dimension of the binding region, allowing for the interaction with segments of intact proteins *(125)*. In contrast to the strict length-restrictive binding to MHC I molecules *(96)*, the MHC II-binding site permits the display of longer peptides *(126,127)*, which can extend by both their N- and C-terminus beyond the boundaries of the binding groove.

Professional Antigen-Presenting Cells

Professional APCs are cells specialized for the capture and degradation of Ags and for the assembly and presentation of peptides in the context of MHC molecules. These MHC molcules scrutinize the T-cell repertoire to ensure that appropriate T cell-mediated immune responses are triggered. APCs express both MHC class I and MHC class II molecules and possess the necessary machinery to efficiently display peptides derived from both endogenous and exogenous Ags. They also express molecules that serve as receptors for Ag uptake. In addition, these cells express, or can be stimulated to express, molecules required for optimal activation of naive T cells, such as costimulatory and adhesion molecules. The classical professional APCs, which fit the above description, are DCs, B cells, and macrophages.

Of these cells, DCs play the major role in the initiation, potentiation, and maturation of immune responses (reviewed in refs. *128–131*). DCs are strategically located in the organism to screen and capture Ags and, when necessary, to stimulate relevant Ag-specific cells present in T cell-dependent areas of the lymphoid tissues. The functions of DCs include transport of captured Ags to areas where reactive lymphoid cells are located, initiation of immune responses by activating both T and B cells (naive and memory), and amplification of T-cell responses. DCs also play a major role in the induction of T-cell anergy for peripheral Ags *(132–134)*. In this sense, DCs can be seen as the choreographer of an exquisite and complex, yet perfectly executed, ballet.

A critical characteristic of the DCs is that they differentiate from an immature stage, in which they are highly efficient at uptaking Ags but poorly efficient at stimulating T-cell reactivity, to a mature stage, in which are they are very potent stimulators of T-cell activation but very poor capturers of Ags. Another important property of DCs is their potency, that is, the capacity of a small number of DCs to interact with and stimulate a significant number of T cells *(135)*.

The increasing body of knowledge of the biological and molecular properties of DCs makes them prime candidates in the quest for effective T cell-mediated antitumor-specific immunotherapeutic strategies. The differentiation stage-dependent properties of DCs can be used to develop strategies for immune intervention in cancer, namely for the development of vaccination strategies (tumor cell-based and/or peptide-based). Tumor Ags can be pulsed into immature DCs, which can then be transformed into potent APCs by the induction of their maturation and activation. Therefore, the manipulation of the DC compartment, by modulating its expansion, differentiation, maturation, and stimulation, has potential impact in tumor immunity.

Other cell lineages classically defined as professional APCs are B cells and macrophages. It has been suggested that both macrophages and B cells fail to stimulate naive T cells *(130)*, so their role as initiators of T cell-mediated immunity has been questioned. In the particular case of mature B cells, some controversy arose on whether B cells could initiate responses from naive T cells or only stimulate previously primed, memory T cells *(136)*. Several properties distinguish DCs and B cells in their APC potential, including expression of different molecules and mechanisms involved in Ag uptake; expression of higher levels of MHC molecules by DCs (particularly MHC II); the significantly more potent induction of T-cell activation by DCs; and the production of higher levels of IL-12, an important cytokine in defining the differentiation (and cytokine-producing profile) of effector T cells *(128,137)*. Whether mature B cells can be used in the design of effective vaccination strategies remains to be determined.

Induction of Antitumor Immunity as Cancer Therapy

Increasing evidence shows that genetic abnormalities believed to be strictly associated with cancers can be detected in disease-free individuals, at a frequency markedly higher than the incidence of the respective malignancies in the general population *(138–141)*. These findings suggest that the presence of "tumor cells" can occur in healthy individuals without necessarily serving as predictors of the development of a full-blown cancer. It is conceivable that the establishment of cancer as a complex and ordered entity will require that the tumor cells acquire a selective advantage in their microenvironment. This likely involves a continuous process of dynamic reciprocity and positive cooperation in which tumor cells modulate their microenvironment (by producing factors that modify the composition of the stroma and the extracellular matrix [ECM]), which in turn influences the tumor cells (by the provision of survival signals, for example).

Although it is unclear whether one of the purposes of the immune system is to act as a sentinel against tumors *(142)*, it can be hypothesized that an important step for the development of a malignancy is the escape, by passive or active means, of tumor cells from surveillance by the immune system. Supporting this hypothesis is the fact that some tumors, such as Epstein–Barr-associated B-cell lymphomas, emerge more frequently in immunosuppressed patients *(143,144)*. Even if this antitumor immune surveillance does not exist for all the different malignancies (an argument based on the evidence that only a restricted type of tumors arise in immunosuppressed patients *[143]*), the mobilization of the immune system can still recognize and react against cancer, provided that tumor cells can be seen by the immune system as danger or non-self.

The conceptual framework for the development of antitumor immunotherapy is based on the assumption that tumor Ags exist; T cells with TCR specificities for the tumor Ags exist in the tumor host; tumor Ags can be efficiently presented to tumor-specific T cells; conditions that inhibit or thwart the induction of antitumor immunity can be overcome or reversed; and effective Ag-specific immune responses can be generated against tumors.

Tumor Antigens

Since the recognition of defined antigenic determinants is the central event of T cell-mediated immunity, it is evident that the development of antitumor-specific immunotherapeutic strategies is impossible without the existence of tumor Ags. The quest to solve the simple question of whether tumor Ags exist has occupied immunologists for many years and has endured waves of enthusiasm and skepticism. The initial suggestion that tumor Ags exist arose from studies showing protection against rechallenge by the parental tumor in mice whose primary carcinogen-induced tumor had been previously excised or irradiated *(145–150)*. Because this antitumor immunity was not observed in naive mice, the existence of tumor Ags (induced by the carcinogenic events) was thereby proved. The enthusiasm caused by these studies was severely hampered by the suggestion that spontaneous tumors formed in the same animal strains failed to induce an immune response, suggesting that tumor Ags did not exist in spontaneous tumors *(142,151)*. The significance of these negative results derives from the fact that spontaneous tumors represent a more accurate counterpart of human cancers, so the rationality and usefulness of an antitumor immunotherapy was questioned *(152)*.

Thierry Boon and colleagues made essential contributions to this search and have ignited new interest in tumor immunity. First, they elegantly demonstrated that tumor Ags exist in spontaneous nonimmunogenic tumors *(153,154)*. This crucial evidence was revealed by the observation that immunogenic tumor variants (tum⁻ clones) derived from mutagenesis were not only rejected by the syngeneic hosts but, most importantly, were capable of inducing protective immunity against the parental nonimmunogenic tumor cells. These findings clearly demonstrated that these spontaneous tumors possess antigenic determinants that can be recognized by the immune system. Their second major contribution was the identification, through a genetic screen, of the genes that encode for Ags specifically recognized by tumor-specific cytotoxic T cells from patients with melanoma *(155–158)*. The importance of this work derives from the demonstration that the antigenic determinants displayed by MHC molecules and recognized by antitumor-specific T cells could be identified and genetically characterized.

Different methodologies have been used to identify and characterize tumor Ags (reviewed in refs. *159–161*). Table 2 represents a list, albeit not exhaustive, of molecules identified as tumor Ags, that is, molecules from which peptides being displayed by MHC molecules and targeted by antitumor T-cell responses were identified. An important conclusion from these observations is that most of the tumor Ags identified are derived from self proteins, with nonaltered amino-acid sequences (germline encoded). Most of the Ags involved in antitumor immunity are therefore tumor-associated Ags rather than tumor-specific Ags. These tumor Ags can be divided into four categories:

- Differentiation antigens: Ags that are expressed during the normal differentiation of the tissues, such as MART-1, tyrosinase, gp100, gp75, and others. This antitumor immunity is in fact an autoimmune response, with the potential risk of damaging normal tissues that express these Ags.
- Abnormally expressed antigens or foreign antigens: Ags that are not generally expressed by the tissue in which the tumor develops, but rather by other tissues; or Ags normally expressed by the tissue but under a different form or cellular/tissular distribution; or molecules that are encoded by foreign genomes. These Ags can be ectopically expressed molecules such as the MAGE and GAGE family members, BAGE, and p15; Ags expressed

Table 2
Tumor Antigens Associated with Human Cancers (Some Examples)

Antigen	Tumor
HER–2/neu	Breast cancer
Melan-A/Mart–1	Melanoma
HOM-MEL–40	Melanoma
MAGE–1	Melanoma, gastric carcinomas, ovarian cancer (cystadenocarcinomas)
MAGE–2	Melanoma, gastric carcinomas
MAGE–3	Melanoma, gastric carcinomas
BAGE	Melanoma
GAGE–1, GAGE–2	Melanoma
Tyrosinase	Melanoma
gp100	Melanoma
MC1R	Melanoma
TRP–2	Melanoma
gp75	Melanoma
NA17A	Melanoma
Mutated β-catenin	Melanoma
COTA	Colon carcinoma
L3P40–50	Lung adenocarcinoma (cell line)
MUC–1	Adenocarcinomas (breast, pancreas, ovarian, stomach?)
PMA	Prostate carcinomas
CAG–3	Breast and melanoma
NY-ESO–1	Esophageal cancer
OFA-I	EBV-associated malignancies; EBV-transformed cells
OFA-I–2	Melanoma, glioma, neuroblastoma
BCR-ABL	Chronic myelogenous leukemia
TEL-AML1	Acute lymphoblastic leukemia
EBNA 3A, 3B, and 3C	Epstein-Barr virus-associated malignancies
HPV-E6, HPV-E7	Human papillomavirus-associated epithelial tumors

in abnormal cellular locations or in an unusual form, such as MUC-1; or viral Ags such as EBNA-3A, -3B, and -3C, HPV-E6, and HPV-E7.

- Overexpressed antigens: Ags that are expressed at lower levels by the normal tissues but become overexpressed after their malignant transformation. These Ags include oncogenes and tumor suppressor genes such as *Her-2/neu, p53,* and *p21*[Ras].

- Unique, tumor-specific antigens: These unique Ags result from mutations of normal genes (such as p53, CDK4, and β-catenin), chromosomal translocations leading to the formation of novel fusion proteins (such as p210[bcr/abl], TEL-AML1, PML/RARα), or idiotypic Ags derived from the tumor-specific rearrangement of the immunoglobulin genes.

Algorithms have been developed that predict, for any given protein, the sequences that will most likely bind to particular MHC class I and class II molecules *(162–164)*. An example of such tool can be found online at the Web site: *http://www-bimas.dcrt.nih.gov/molbio/hla_bind/index.html.* An alternative to analyzing all possible peptides derived from a large protein, which would be very expensive and time consuming, these algorithms permit the selection of a smaller number of potential optimal determinants, which can then be screened for epitope identification *(161)*. Although they constitute powerful and helpful tools, it must be mentioned that the results of these tests are predictions, and that immunogenic peptides recognized by antitumor-specific tumor-infiltrating lymphocytes (TILs) have been shown to score poorly in these algorithms.

The identification of the exact antigenic sequences that can be recognized by the antitumor-specific T cells, coupled with the demonstration that both intact proteins and peptides can be captured by APCs and presented by MHC molecules to Ag-specific T cells *(165)*, provides an important incentive for the development of antitumor immuno-therapeutic strategies. Since some professional APCs can present exogenous Ags through the MHC I presentation pathway, an attractive approach is to deliver fragments of molecules or synthesized immunogenic peptides to APCs (Fig. 4). The presentation of these exogenous epitope determinants by MHC I molecules may then induce the generation and expansion of cytotoxic $CD8^+$ T cells (CTLs) capable of lysing the specific tumor cells. Again, these strategies may allow for the generation of more diversified $CD8^+$ T-cell responses against tumors.

A large body of evidence supports the conclusion that most, and possibly all, tumors express tumor-associated Ags. Nevertheless, in spite of the successes obtained inducing antitumor-specific responses in a variety of human malignancies, particularly in in vitro studies and animal models, the antigenic peptides initiating such responses are largely unknown.

Presentation of Tumor Antigen and Strategies to Improve Immunogenicity

The inability of tumor cells to efficiently induce antitumor immunity is partially due to their inability to properly present tumor Ags to the relevant T cells. Increasing knowledge of the requirements for optimal Ag presentation and induction of productive T cell-mediated immune responses have provided critical information in the analysis of the causes associated with the poor APC capability of tumor cells. It has been demonstrated that in both human and animals, in vivo and in vitro, tumor cells are generally inefficient or ineffective Ag-presenting cells (reviewed in refs. *166,167*). Moreover, several other defects have been identified. Among the possible explanations for this failure in generating immune reactivity are:

- The tumor is not visible to the immune system. Tumor cells are seen as self and several tumor-associated Ags already identified are differentiation Ags normally expressed by the tissues. In addition, interaction of the tumor cells with their microenvironment (such as stromal elements) can render them invisible.
- Defective expression and/or presentation of MHC–peptide complexes by tumor cells, that is, inadequate cognitive signal. The down-regulation on tumor cells of MHC molecules or molecules required for the assembly of functional MHC–peptide complexes has been described *(168–173)*. Moreover, conditions may exist that hamper the capture and process-ing of tumor Ags by professional APCs.
- Inability of tumor cells to provide adequate costimulation for T cells. Most tumors lack costimulatory molecules or express them at insufficient levels *(166,168,169,174)*. This can also result in functional inactivation of T cells, with the induction of T-cell anergy to tumor Ags *(174,175)* (discussed on p. 379).

Cytosol   **Cell Membrane**

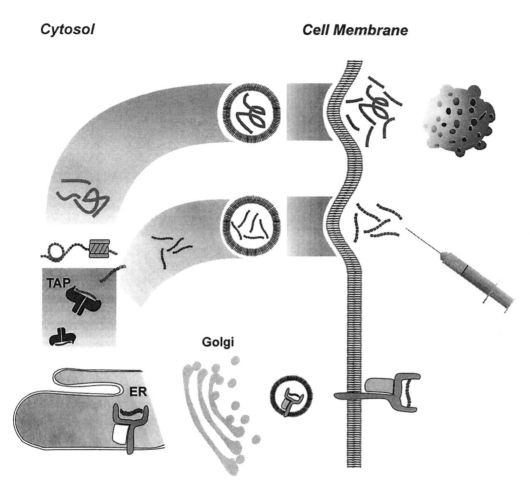

Fig. 4. Presentation of both endogenous and exogenous antigens (Ags) by the MHC class I pathways. Ags released from tumor cell death are captured, degraded, and translocated by TAP to the endoplasmic reticulum (ER), where suitable peptides are bound to MHC-I molecules. Alternatively, synthetic peptides pulsed to the APC enter the endocytic pathway and are displayed by MHC I molecules.

- Insufficient provision of T-cell help due to lack of activation of T$_{helper}$ cells or necessary accessory cells *(176)*. Alternatively, incapacity of antitumor-specific T cells to migrate and home to sites where competent tumor-presenting APCs are present, or even the incapacity of these T cells to properly respond to the antigenic stimuli (e.g., to loss of expression of signaling molecules such as TCRζ) *(177,178)*.
- Production by the tumor cells, or the tumor microenvironment, of molecules that inhibit the induction of productive immunity or that deviate the profile of this response *(67,179)*. Cytokines produced by tumor cells can also affect Ag presentation *(180)*
- Lack of accessibility of immunocompetent cells to the tumor sites, as is the case with tumors that develop at sites of immune privilege, or the creation of a state of immune privilege at the tumor site. This can be due to either a lack of professional APCs in the tumor site or local inhibitory conditions (such as the production of potent inhibitors or active T-cell apoptosis induced by tumors) *(181,182)*.

- Lack of representation on the tumor host's T-cell repertoire of lymphocytes with TCR specificities for the tumor-associated peptide Ags. Although lacking positive demonstration, this hypothesis cannot at present be excluded.

Several strategies aimed toward repairing the lack of immunogenicity of tumor cells have been designed and developed. These approaches target either the tumor cells (e.g., by attempting to improve their direct APC potential), accessory cells (e.g., by stimulating inflammation and/or professional APCs), or attempt to overcome an inhibitory microenvironment. Among the different strategies used, the most relevant include:

- Modification of tumor cells by transfection of genes encoding for MHC molecules or costimulatory molecules. The goal is to provide tumor cells with a stable expression of surface molecules required for adequate APC function and optimal stimulation of relevant T cells. This includes the transfection of MHC molecules, B7-1, B7-2, ICAM-1, etc. *(183–185).*
- Transduction of tumor cells with genes encoding soluble molecules that stimulate an antitumor response (induction and/or potentiation). This strategy allows for the local delivery, at a more relevant concentration, of cytokines that can modulate local immunologic responses to the tumor (paracrine mechanism) *(166,186–188).* These approaches include the transfection of: molecules that either directly stimulate T cells and bypass T-cell help (such as IL-2), drive the differentiation of activated T cells (such as IL-4, IL-10, or IL-12), or modulate T-cell effector function (such as TNF); molecules that can stimulate the host's professional APCs and therefore stimulate antitumor T-cell responses by an indirect mechanism (as with granulocyte-macrophage colony-stimulating factor [GM-CSF]); molecules that can directly modulate the APC's function of tumor cells by, for example, up-regulating the expression of MHC molecules (as with interferon [IFN]-γ); molecules that generate potent local inflammatory reactions with massive infiltrations of mediators of inflammation such as eosinophils and macrophages (as with GM-CSF, TNF, or IL-3).
- Modification of tumor cells by the delivery of physiologic signals that result in the induction and/or up-regulation of molecules required for the initiation of productive immunity. One such example is the conversion of APC-incompetent lymphoid leukemia cells to efficient APC by crosslinking CD40 using either a soluble form or a membrane-bound form of their natural ligand, CD40L *(20,174).*
- Delivery of antigenic tumor peptides or larger fragments of tumor Ags to professional APCs. This allows for the generation of larger numbers of competent APCs, manipulation of these cells for maximal capture of the antigenic determinants of interest, and activation of APCs for optimal expression of the molecules (adhesion, MHC, costimulation) required for effective activation of the relevant antitumor T cells *(189–191).* Among the advantages of using exogenous Ags is that, depending on the conditions of capture and processing, they can be presented by both the MHC class I and MHC II pathways, which is ideal for generating both helper (by CD4$^+$ T cells) and cytotoxic (primarily by CD8$^+$ T cells) activities.

T Cell-Mediation of Tumor-Specific Immunity

Because the ultimate goal of antitumor immunotherapy is the elimination of the tumor cells, most of the strategies that have been developed aim at the induction of Ag-specific CTL responses mediated by CD8$^+$ T cells, the classic Ag-specific cytotoxic lymphocytes. A significant part of the strategies previously described aim at the direct activation, differentiation, and expansion of cytotoxic tumor-specific CD8$^+$ T cells. In this sense, several strategies have been devised to fix potential defects, such as the transfection of tumor cells with costimulatory molecules to allow for the direct activation of CD8$^+$ T cells by the MHC I-expressing tumor cell, and/or transduction of tumor cells with cytokines such as IL-2, to circumvent the need for accessory cells such as T_{helper} cells. Nevertheless, it must be emphasized that a significant number of studies have demonstrated that the induction of optimal immunity against tumors requires the involvement of both CD4$^+$ and CD8$^+$ T cells *(192–195)*.

An important observation from multiple studies using different strategies is that the direct presentation of tumor Ag to the T cells, such as by tumor cells transduced with cell-surface stimulatory molecules (MHC, costimulatory molecules), generally results in the induction of responses mediated by CD4$^+$ T cells (Fig. 5A) rather than by CD8$^+$ T cells *(196,197)*. Modified tumor cells turn into competent APCs, thereby becoming efficient stimulators of CD4$^+$ T cells. Interestingly, increasing evidence shows that stimulation of tumor-specific CD8$^+$ T cells is, in most cases, mediated by the indirect presentation of soluble tumor Ag by professional APCs (Fig. 5B) *(198–200)*. This phenomenon, known as cross-priming, was originally described by Bevan *(201)* and is dependent on professional APCs, which must capture tumor Ags originated from dead tumor cells and then present them to T cells exhibiting TCR specificity for these Ags. This observation is of particular importance as it is possible only because endogenous Ags can also be efficiently presented through the MHC I pathway (Fig. 4). Importantly, CD4$^+$ T cells can also be activated through cross-priming. These findings have profound implications for the design of vaccination strategies aimed at the induction of tumor immunity. In fact, if cross-priming is the main pathway for the induction of CD8$^+$ CTLs, it may be of greater importance to optimize the MHC I presentation of tumor Ags by professional APCs rather to attempt modification of the tumor cells themselves. The intricacies and possible explanations for these somehow surprising findings are elegantly discussed in a review by Armstrong and colleagues *(196)*.

Another strategy used for the mobilization of antitumor T cell-mediated immunity is the redirection of the lytic activity of polyclonally activated CTLs to tumor cells. This strategy, termed T-cell retargeting, was initially developed by using antibodies (Abs) that bind simultaneously to the TCR–CD3 complex on T cells and a surface protein from tumor cells *(202–204)*. Although independent from the presence of tumor Ags (which may constitute an advantage), a serious limitation of this technique is the obvious lack of Ag specificity *(205)*.

Because the development of antitumor immunotherapy is dependent on the existence and amplification of tumor-reactive T cells, it will be of utmost utility to be able to accurately detect and enumerate tumor-specific T cells, particularly CTLs. The standard methodology consisted of the enumeration of effector T cells using limiting-dilution cytolytic assays *(206)*. However, these assays have significant limitations and it is becoming well recognized that they grossly underestimate the actual number of Ag-specific CTLs *(207–209)*. Accounting for this lack of accuracy is the fact that these techniques are indirect and require the in vitro stimulation of CTLs before the assay. Alternative methodologies have been developed and improved to quantify Ag-specific T cells more accurately. One such methodology is based on the detection of cytokines (such as IFN-γ) induced by the stimulation of tumor-specific T cells by their cognate Ag using an enzyme-linked immunospot (ELISPOT) assay *(210,211)*. This technique can be used for the identification, at the single-cell level, of CTLs reactive to either tumor cells or cells pulsed with peptides derived from tumor-associated Ags. Another approach consists of the the detection, by flow cytometry, of T cells that express the TCR

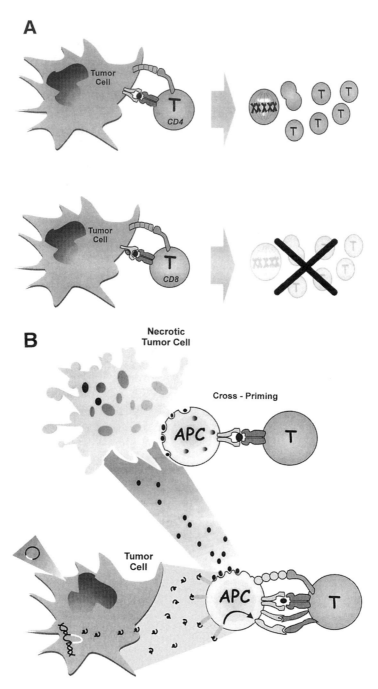

Fig. 5. (A) Direct presentation of tumor antigen (Ag) to the T cells, such as by tumor cells transduced with cell-surface stimulatory molecules (MHC, costimulatory molecules). **(B)** Indirect presentation of tumor Ag to T cells. This phenomenon, cross-priming, is dependent on professional APCs, which must capture tumor Ags originated from dead tumor cells and then present them to the relevant T cells. APC = antigen-presenting cell

specific for soluble multimerized peptide–MHC complexes, also known as tetramers *(212,213)*. Although the use of the tetramer technology is limited to the detection of T cells whose TCR recognize a known peptide bound to a particular MHC I molecule, it has important advantages. Its high sensitivity allows for the purification of these cells by cell sorting, thereby enabling the manipulation of these peptide-specific T cells. Both the ELISPOT and the tetramer technologies allow for the identification and enumeration of more Ag-specific T cells. Their use should contribute to the understanding of the mechanisms and kinetics of antitumor T cell-mediated immune responses, which may provide much needed endpoints for the design and interpretation of experimental clinical protocols.

Reversing T-Cell Tolerance

A potentially important mechanism used by tumors to escape from the immune system is the establishment of T-cell tolerance to tumor Ags *(214)*. This is an attractive hypothesis because most tumor-associated Ags are self-Ags and because several tumors develop progressively over considerable time, exposing these Ags to the immune system. This state of tolerance can result from either the clonal deletion of T cells with TCR-recognizing self-molecules presented in the thymus during T-cell development (central tolerance) or by the induction of T-cell unresponsiveness to peripheral Ags (such as extrathymic, differentiation Ags). As discussed earlier, the requirements for the initiation of a T cell-mediated immune response are very demanding, making it very unlikely that peripheral self-Ags will be targeted by the immune system *(215,216)*. Several in vivo studies in animal models have shown that different mechanisms may be involved in the protection of peripheral self-Ags from immune attack, including induction of T-cell anergy, immunological ignorance, clonal elimination, and/or immune deviation *(217–220)*. The involvement of T-cell tolerance as a mechanism conferring immune protection to the tumor, thereby providing the tumor with a selective advantage, has been demonstrated by several different studies and reviewed by different authors *(174,175,221–223)*.

Understanding the mechanisms involved in the induction and maintenance of T-cell anergy/tolerance to tumor Ags is critical for the development of reliable strategies to reverse this state of T-cell inactivation *(27,184,216,224)*. Taking this into account, different studies have shown that prolonged exposure to IL-2 may reverse T-cell anergy and drive the T cells to become responsive to the initial Ag stimuli *(80,225)*. Also, the removal of T cells from contact with tumor cells results in the reexpression of TCRζ, a result that can also be obtained by incubation with IL-2 *(21)*. Moreover, manipulation of the inhibitory signal delivered by CTLA-4, one of the counterreceptors of the B7 family molecules, may be a useful tool for reversing tolerance, as it has been demonstrated that CTLA-4 also plays an important role in the induction of T-cell anergy *(226,227)*. These findings suggest that manipulation of the B7-1/B7-2:CD28/CTLA-4 pathway has a great potential for therapeutic intervention.

Another possible mechanism is the induction by tumor cells of drastic changes in the profile of cytokines produced by T cells, such as IFN-γ, in cells that were tolerized *(175)*. Intervention at this level can also effectively reverse T-cell anergy. Finally, another mechanism that can be explored comes from the knowledge that T-cell tolerance can be broken by infectious agents *(228)*. Recombinant strategies, such as those using recombinant viruses and plasmid DNA-encoding tumor-associated Ags, are being developed to explore this mechanism for the induction of effective tumor immunity *(229,230)*.

A major concern of the strategies aiming at reversing T-cell tolerance/anergy is the potential risk of creating T-cell autoreactivity against normal tissues, which can lead to aggressive autoimmune responses. These concerns are of tremendous significance as nonspecific events, such as intercurrent infections and situations involving allogeneic contacts (transfusion, transplant, etc.), have the potential to create conditions leading to reversal of tolerance.

Clinical Strategies for Antitumor Immunotherapy

The extensive amount of information amassed over the last two decades in a variety of areas contributed to the creation of renewed and intense interest in the hypothesis of using the properties of the immune system to fight human cancer. Major advances have been achieved in, among others, the understanding of the mechanisms of Ag processing and presentation, the identification and characterization of tumor Ags, the definition of the requirements for optimal induction and amplification of T cell-mediated immune responses, and the comprehension of the development and biology of professional APCs. This progress, coupled with the development of more refined and efficient technologies for the processing and manipulation of cells, proteins, and genetic material, naturally led to the design of novel strategies for immune intervention in the treatment of human cancer. The clinical translation of the body of evidence generated in the laboratory is well represented in the variety of clinical trials already in progress. More information concerning these trials can be obtained from Web sites such as: *http://cancernet.nci.nih.gov* (National Cancer Institute, Bethesda, MD, USA). Additional information can be found in several reviews and recent manuscripts *(172,187,231–235)*.

The many therapeutic protocols developed in an autologous context, that is, using the patient's own immune system to react against his/her tumor cells, can be simplistically divided into two major strategies of intervention: the ex vivo manipulation of tumor cells to improve their immunogenicity followed by their infusion to the patient as a tumor vaccine (Fig. 6A); and 2) the ex vivo priming and/or amplification of antitumor-specific effector cells which then can be adoptively transferred to the patient (Fig. 6B).

Tumor-Cell Vaccination

Tumor-cell vaccination consist of the use of tumor cells (generally modified) as cell vaccines aimed at the initiation and mobilization of the immune system, driving a response ultimately leading to the elimination of the tumor cells. Patients' tissues are collected and tumor cells are separated using standard methodologies. Tumor cells are then cultured under optimal conditions and modified to express or produce the molecule(s) capable of inducing or enhancing immune responses. Strategies for this modification include the transduction, using recombinant viral vectors or DNA plasmids, of genes encoding for surface molecules required for optimal T-cell activation (e.g., MHC, adhesion, and costimulatory molecules); soluble molecules regulating immunity (e.g., IL-2, IL-4, IL-7, GM-CSF); tumor-associated Ags (e.g., Her-2/neu). Alternatively, tumor cells can be modified by delivering physiologic signals to them, such as by crosslinking membrane molecules naturally expressed by the tumor cells, which should

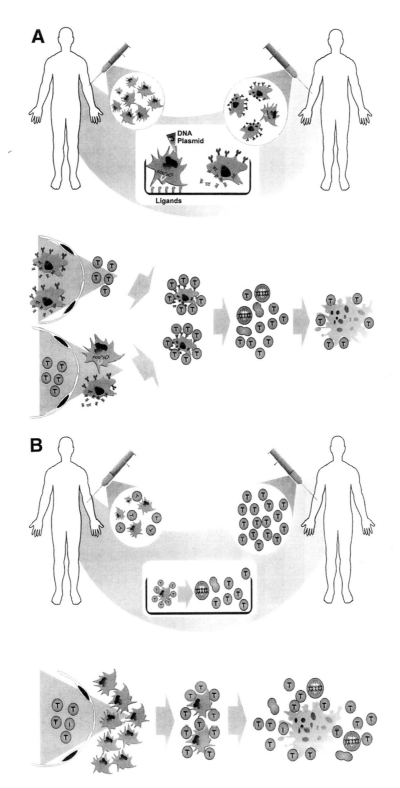

Fig. 6. Major strategies for immune intervention on human cancer: **(A)** Tumor cell vaccination. **(B)** Adoptive transfer of ex vivo primed and/or amplified antitumor specific T cells. See text for full explanation of process.

lead to the activation of these tumor cells. After this ex vivo transformation, the tumor cells are infused into the patient (Fig. 6A, *upper part*). Ideally, the tumor cells/vaccine will circulate, migrate through the endothelium, home to the sites where antitumor-reactive T cells may be present, and initiate an immune response, which, ultimately, will mediate the elimination of tumor cells (Fig. 6A, *lower part*). Concomitantly, the tumor cells may express, or be transformed to express, molecules capable of attracting T cells to the sites where the tumor vaccine will home (Fig. 6A, *lower part*). Moreover, this tumor cell lysis should result in the release of tumor Ags which can be captured and processed by local professional APCs, and presented to specific T cells, thereby amplifying the antitumor immune response. This sequence of events will hopefully lead to the activation of both $CD4^+$ and $CD8^+$ T cells, which have been suggested to be necessary components for the generation of efficient tumor immunity *(194,236)*.

Antitumor T-Cell Adoptive Transfer

In the adoptive T-cell therapy, T cells reactive against the tumor are expanded ex vivo and infused into the patient. Patients' specimens containing tumor cells and T cells are collected and cocultured ex vivo. T cells may have originated either from tumor sites (TILs) or from the peripheral blood. Tumor cells and T cells are then cultured under optimal conditions for priming and/or expansion of T cells, and cycles of restimulation with tumor cells are performed. The T cells growing in this ex vivo system are then infused to the patient (Fig. 6B, *upper part*). Ideally, after circulation and migration through endothelium, the T cells will home to the tumor site where they will recognize and lyse the tumor cells (Fig. 6B, *lower part*). As discussed earlier, this destruction of tumor cells could drive an amplification of the immune response.

The clinical use of combinatory strategies using both adoptive transfer of antitumor T cells and vaccination with modified tumors, which ideally will amplify, in vivo, the reaction mediated by the transferred T cells, can easily be devised.

Future Directions

The emergence of tumor immunology as a major area of inquiry in the quest for successful therapies for human cancer has led to the multiplication of efforts to design therapeutic strategies using the properties and potential of the immune system to fight cancer. The enormous vitality of this enterprise is well evidenced by the amplification of intellectual and financial efforts and the variety of approaches being studied and developed. The clinical translation of a substantial part of these strategies is already in progress or under protocol design. Therefore, it is reasonable to anticipate that the upcoming years should provide important, perhaps definitive, answers concerning the role of tumor immunity as anticancer therapy. These clinical studies will determine whether tumor immunotherapy will became a routine modality in the management of cancer patients and whether it will contribute to the ultimate goal of eliminating tumor cells or, at least, confining residual tumor cells to a stage of long-term, disease-free latency. The trials will also determine whether immunotherapy will allow for the reduction of the intensity of conventional therapies and consequently decrease the severity of the toxicities frequently associated with them, thereby improving the thera-peutic indices. Furthermore, lessons will be drawn from these clinical trials on how modern clinical oncology should be practiced, namely in the areas of cancer prevention, patient care, and health care costs.

Acknowledgments

I am indebted to Dr. Lee M. Nadler for his continuous support and encouragement. I thank Drs. Vassiliki Boussiotis, Paolo Ghia, and Kostas Kosmatopoulos for their critical reading of the manuscript. I also thank Pedro M. Alves for the graphics.

References

1. Bretscher P, Cohn M. A theory of self-nonself discrimination. *Science.* 1970; 169:1042–9.
2. Schwartz RH. A cell culture model for T lymphocyte clonal anergy. *Science.* 1990; 248:1349–56.
3. Schwartz RH. Costimulation of T lymphocytes: the role of CD28, CTLA-4, and B7/BB1 in interleukin-2 production and immunotherapy. *Cell.* 1992; 71:1065–8.
4. Boniface JJ, Davis MM. T-cell recognition of antigen. A process controlled by transient intermolecular interactions. *Ann NY Acad Sci.* 1995; 766:62–9.
5. Dubey C, Croft M. Accessory molecule regulation of naive CD4 T cell activation. *Immunol Res.* 1996; 15:114–25.
6. Demotz S, Grey HM, Sette A. The minimal number of class II MHC–antigen complexes needed for T cell activation. *Science.* 1990; 249:1028–30.
7. Harding CV, Unanue ER. Quantitation of antigen-presenting cell MHC class II/peptide complexes necessary for T-cell stimulation. *Nature.* 1990; 346:574–6.
8. Mueller DL, Jenkins MK, Schwartz RH. Clonal expansion versus functional clonal inactivation: a costimulatory signalling pathway determines the outcome of T cell antigen receptor occupancy. *Annu Rev Immunol.* 1989; 7:445–80.
9. Schwartz RH, Mueller DL, Jenkins MK, Quill H. T-cell clonal anergy. *Cold Spring Harb Symp Quant Biol.* 1989; 54:605–10.
10. Freeman GJ, Freedman AS, Segil JM, Lee G, Whitman JF, Nadler LM. B7, a new member of the Ig superfamily with unique expression on activated and neoplastic B cells. *J Immunol.* 1989; 143:2714–22.
11. Freeman GJ, Gribben JG, Boussiotis VA, et al. Cloning of B7-2: a CTLA-4 counter-receptor that costimulates human T cell proliferation. *Science.* 1993; 262:909–11.
12. Azuma M, Ito D, Yagita H, et al. B70 antigen is a second ligand for CTLA-4 and CD28. *Nature.* 1993; 366:76–9.
13. Linsley PS, Brady W, Grosmaire L, Aruffo A, Damle NK, Ledbetter JA. Binding of the B cell activation antigen B7 to CD28 costimulates T cell proliferation and interleukin 2 mRNA accumulation. *J Exp Med.* 1991; 173:721–30.
14. June CH, Ledbetter JA, Gillespie MM, Lindsten T, Thompson CB. T-cell proliferation involving the CD28 pathway is associated with cyclosporine resistant *interleukin 2* gene expression. *Mol Cell Biol.* 1987; 7:4472–81.
15. Gimmi CD, Freeman GJ, Gribben JG, et al. B-cell surface antigen B7 provides a costimulatory signal that induces T cells to proliferate and secrete interleukin 2. *Proc Natl Acad Sci USA.* 1991; 88:6575–9.
16. Janeway CA, Jr., Bottomly K. Signals and signs for lymphocyte responses. *Cell.* 1994; 76:275–85.
17. Paul WE, Seder RA. Lymphocyte responses and cytokines. *Cell.* 1994; 76:241–51.
18. Valitutti S, Muller S, Cella M, Padovan E, Lanzavecchia A. Serial triggering of many T-cell receptors by a few peptide-MHC complexes. *Nature.* 1995; 375:148–51.

19. Liu Y, Janeway CA, Jr. Cells that present both specific ligand and costimulatory activity are the most efficient inducers of clonal expansion of normal CD4 T cells. *Proc Natl Acad Sci USA*. 1992; 89:3845–9.

20. Cardoso AA, Seamon MJ, Afonso HM, et al. Ex-vivo generation of anti-pre-B leukemia specific autologous cytolytic T cells. *Blood*. 1997; 90:549–61.

21. Boussiotis VA, Freeman GJ, Gribben JG, Nadler LM. The role of B7-1/B7-2:CD28/CLTA-4 pathways in the prevention of anergy, induction of productive immunity and down-regulation of the immune response. *Immunol Rev*. 1996; 153:5–26.

22. Turka LA, Ledbetter JA, Lee K, June CH, Thompson CB. CD28 is an inducible T cell surface antigen that transduces a proliferative signal in $CD3^+$ mature thymocytes. *J Immunol*. 1990; 144:1646–53.

23. Chambers CA, Allison JP. Co-stimulation in T cell responses. *Curr Opin Immunol*. 1997; 9:396–404.

24. Lindstein T, June CH, Ledbetter JA, Stella G, Thompson CB. Regulation of lymphokine messenger RNA stability by a surface-mediated T cell activation pathway. *Science*. 1989; 244:339–43.

25. Thompson CB, Lindsten T, Ledbetter JA, et al. CD28 activation pathway regulates the production of multiple T-cell-derived lymphokines/cytokines. *Proc Natl Acad Sci USA*. 1989; 86:1333–7.

26. Sperling AI, Bluestone JA. The complexities of T-cell co-stimulation: CD28 and beyond. *Immunol Rev*. 1996; 153:155–82.

27. Boussiotis VA, Freeman GJ, Gribben JG, Nadler LM. The critical role of CD28 signaling in the prevention of human T-cell anergy. *Res Immunol*. 1995; 146:140–9.

28. Lai JH, Horvath G, Li Y, Tan TH. Mechanisms of enhanced nuclear translocation of the transcription factors c-Rel and NF-κ B by CD28 costimulation in human T lymphocytes. *Ann NY Acad Sci*. 1995; 766:220–3.

29. Rudd CE. Upstream-downstream: CD28 cosignaling pathways and T cell function. *Immunity*. 1996; 4:527–34.

30. Cantrell D. T cell antigen receptor signal transduction pathways. *Annu Rev Immunol*. 1996; 14:259–74.

31. Alberola-Ila J, Takaki S, Kerner JD, Perlmutter RM. Differential signaling by lymphocyte antigen receptors. *Annu Rev Immunol*. 1997; 15:125–54.

32. Berridge MJ. Lymphocyte activation in health and disease. *Crit Rev Immunol*. 1997; 17:155–78.

33. Brunet JF, Denizot F, Luciani MF, et al. A new member of the immunoglobulin superfamily-CTLA-4. *Nature*. 1987; 328:267–70.

34. Linsley PS, Brady W, Urnes M, Grosmaire LS, Damle NK, Ledbetter JA. CTLA-4 is a second receptor for the B cell activation antigen B7. *J Exp Med*. 1991; 174:561–9.

35. Linsley PS, Wallace PM, Johnson J, et al. Immunosuppression in vivo by a soluble form of the CTLA-4 T cell activation molecule. *Science*. 1992; 257:792–5.

36. Walunas TL, Lenschow DJ, Bakker CY, et al. CTLA-4 can function as a negative regulator of T cell activation. *Immunity*. 1994; 1:405–13.

37. Karandikar NJ, Vanderlugt CL, Walunas TL, Miller SD, Bluestone JA. CTLA-4: a negative regulator of autoimmune disease. *J Exp Med*. 1996; 184:783–8.

38. Bluestone JA. Is CTLA-4 a master switch for peripheral T cell tolerance? *J Immunol*. 1997; 158:1989–93.

39. Lee KM, Chuang E, Griffin M, et al. Molecular basis of T cell inactivation by CTLA-4. *Science*. 1998; 282:2263–6.

40. Mandelbrot DA, McAdam AJ, Sharpe AH. B7-1 or B7-2 is required to produce the

lymphoproliferative phenotype in mice lacking cytotoxic T lymphocyte-associated antigen 4 (CTLA-4). *J Exp Med.* 1999; 189:435–40.

41. Tivol EA, Boyd SD, McKeon S, et al. CTLA4Iγ prevents lymphoproliferation and fatal multiorgan tissue destruction in CTLA-4-deficient mice. *J Immunol.* 1997; 158: 5091–4.

42. Walunas TL, Bluestone JA. CTLA-4 regulates tolerance induction and T cell differentiation in vivo. *J Immunol.* 1998; 160:3855–60.

43. Grewal IS, Xu J, Flavell RA. Impairment of antigen-specific T-cell priming in mice lacking CD40 ligand. *Nature.* 1995; 378:617–20.

44. Grewal IS, Foellmer HG, Grewal KD, et al. Requirement for CD40 ligand in costimulation induction, T cell activation, and experimental allergic encephalomyelitis. *Science.* 1996; 273:1864–7.

45. Yang Y, Wilson JM. CD40 ligand-dependent T cell activation: requirement of B7-CD28 signaling through CD40. *Science.* 1996; 273:1862–4

46. Caux C, Massacrier C, Vanbervliet B, et al. Activation of human dendritic cells through CD40 cross-linking. *J Exp Med.* 1994; 180:1263–72.

47. Wu Y, Xu J, Shinde S, et al. Rapid induction of a novel costimulatory activity on B cells by CD40 ligand. *Curr Biol.* 1995; 5:1303–11.

48. Stout RD, Suttles J, Xu J, Grewal IS, Flavell RA. Impaired T cell-mediated macrophage activation in CD40 ligand-deficient mice. *J Immunol.* 1996; 156:8–11.

49. Armitage RJ, Fanslow WC, Strockbine L, et al. Molecular and biological characterization of a murine ligand for CD40. *Nature.* 1992; 357:80–2.

50. Van Gool SW, Vandenberghe P, de Boer M, Ceuppens JL. CD80, CD86 and CD40 provide accessory signals in a multiple-step T-cell activation model. *Immunol Rev.* 1996; 153:47–83.

51. Larsen CP, Pearson TC. The CD40 pathway in allograft rejection, acceptance, and tolerance. *Curr Opin Immunol.* 1997; 9:641–7.

52. Springer TA. Adhesion receptors of the immune system. *Nature.* 1990; 346:425–34.

53. Boussiotis V, Freeman GJ, Gray G, Gribben JG, Nadler LM. B7 but not intercellular adhesion molecule-1 costimulation prevents the induction of alloantigen-specific tolerance. *J Exp Med.* 1993; 178:1753–63.

54. de Fougerolles AR, Qin X, Springer TA. Characterization of the function of intercellular adhesion molecule (ICAM)-3 and comparison with ICAM-1 and ICAM-2 in immune responses. *J Exp Med.* 1994; 179:619–29.

55. Zuckerman LA, Pullen L, Miller J. Functional consequences of costimulation by ICAM-1 on *IL-2* gene expression and T cell activation. *J Immunol.* 1998; 160:3259–68.

56. Wingren AG, Parra E, Varga M, et al. T cell activation pathways: B7, LFA-3, and ICAM-1 shape unique T cell profiles. *Crit Rev Immunol.* 1995; 15:235–53.

57. Deckert M, Kubar J, Bernard A. CD58 and CD59 molecules exhibit potentializing effects in T cell adhesion and activation. *J Immunol.* 1992; 148:672–7.

58. Godfrey WR, Fagnoni FF, Harara MA, Buck D, Engleman EG. Identification of a human OX-40 ligand, a costimulator of CD4+ T cells with homology to tumor necrosis factor. *J Exp Med.* 1994; 180:757–62.

59. Hintzen RQ, Lens SM, Lammers K, Kuiper H, Beckmann MP, van Lier RA. Engagement of CD27 with its ligand CD70 provides a second signal for T cell activation. *J Immunol.* 1995; 154:2612–23.

60. Hurtado JC, Kim SH, Pollok KE, Lee ZH, Kwon BS. Potential role of 4–1BB in T cell activation. Comparison with the costimulatory molecule CD28. *J Immunol.* 1995; 155:3360–7.

61. Vinay DS, Kwon BS. Role of 4-1BB in immune responses. *Semin Immunol.* 1998; 10:481–9.

62. Liu Y, Jones B, Aruffo A, Sullivan KM, Linsley PS, Janeway CA Jr. Heat-stable antigen is a costimulatory molecule for CD4 T cell growth. *J Exp Med.* 1992; 175:437–45.

63. Cocks BG, Chang CC, Carballido JM, Yssel H, de Vries JE, Aversa G. A novel receptor involved in T-cell activation. *Nature.* 1995; 376:260–3.

64. Park JK, Rosenstein YJ, Remold-O'Donnell E, Bierer BE, Rosen FS, Burakoff SJ. Enhancement of T-cell activation by the CD43 molecule whose expression is defective in Wiskott-Aldrich syndrome. *Nature.* 1991; 350:706–9

65. Boussiotis VA, Barber DL, Nakarai T, et al. Prevention of T cell anergy by signaling through the γc chain of the IL-2 receptor. *Science.* 1994; 266:1039–42.

66. Ahuja SS, Paliogianni F, Yamada H, Balow JE, Boumpas DT. Effect of transforming growth factor-β on early and late activation events in human T cells. *J Immunol.* 1993; 150:3109–18.

67. Letterio JJ, Roberts AB. Regulation of immune responses by TGF-β. *Annu Rev Immunol.* 1998; 16:137–61.

68. Croft M. Activation of naive, memory and effector T cells. *Curr Opin Immunol.* 1994; 6:431–7.

69. Croft M, Bradley LM, Swain SL. Naive versus memory CD4 T cell response to antigen. Memory cells are less dependent on accessory cell costimulation and can respond to many antigen-presenting cell types including resting B cells. *J Immunol.* 1994; 152:2675–85.

70. Iezzi G, Karjalainen K, Lanzavecchia A. The duration of antigenic stimulation determines the fate of naive and effector T cells. *Immunity.* 1998; 8:89–95.

71. Monks CR, Kupfer H, Tamir I, Barlow A, Kupfer A. Selective modulation of protein kinase C-θ during T-cell activation. *Nature.* 1997; 385:83–6.

72. Monks CR, Freiberg BA, Kupfer H, Sciaky N, Kupfer A. Three-dimensional segregation of supramolecular activation clusters in T cells. *Nature.* 1998; 395:82–6.

73. Viola A, Schroeder S, Sakakibara Y, Lanzavecchia A. T lymphocyte costimulation mediated by reorganization of membrane microdomains. *Science.* 1999; 283:680–2.

74. Wulfing C, Davis MM. A receptor/cytoskeletal movement triggered by costimulation during T cell activation. *Science.* 1998; 282:2266–9.

75. Wulfing C, Sjaastad MD, Davis MM. Visualizing the dynamics of T cell activation: intracellular adhesion molecule 1 migrates rapidly to the T cell/B cell interface and acts to sustain calcium levels. *Proc Natl Acad Sci USA.* 1998; 95:6302–7.

76. Jenkins MK, Ashwell JD, Schwartz RH. Allogeneic non-T spleen cells restore the responsiveness of normal T cell clones stimulated with antigen and chemically modified antigen-presenting cells. *J Immunol.* 1988; 140:3324–30.

77. Lenschow DJ, Zeng Y, Thistlethwaite JR, et al. Long-term survival of xenogeneic pancreatic islet grafts induced by CTLA4Iγ. *Science.* 1992; 257:789–92.

78. Lin H, Bolling SF, Linsley PS, et al. Long-term acceptance of major histocompatibility complex mismatched cardiac allografts induced by CTLA4Iγ plus donor-specific transfusion. *J Exp Med.* 1993; 178:1801–6.

79. Gimmi CD, Freeman GJ, Gribben JG, Gray G, Nadler LM. Human T-cell clonal anergy is induced by antigen presentation in the absence of B7 costimulation. *Proc Natl Acad Sci USA.* 1993; 90:6586–90.

80. Boussiotis V, Freeman GJ, Griffin JD, Gray G, Gribben JG, Nadler LM. CD2 is involved in maintenance and reversal of human alloantigen specific clonal anergy. *J Exp Med.* 1994; 180:1665–73.

81. Guerder S, Meyerhoff J, Flavell R. The role of the T cell costimulator B7-1 in autoimmunity

and the induction and maintenance of tolerance to peripheral antigen. *Immunity.* 1994; 1:155–66.

82. Harlan DM, Hengartner H, Huang ML, et al. Mice expressing both B7-1 and viral glycoprotein on pancreatic β cells along with glycoprotein-specific transgenic T cells develop diabetes due to a breakdown of T-lymphocyte unresponsiveness. *Proc Natl Acad Sci USA.* 1994; 91:3137–41.

83. Tan P, Anasetti C, Hansen JA, et al. Induction of alloantigen-specific hyporesponsiveness in human T lymphocytes by blocking interaction of CD28 with its natural ligand B7/B1. *J Exp Med.* 1993; 177:165–73.

84. Hollander GA, Castigli E, Kulbacki R. Induction of alloantigen-specific tolerance by B cells from CD40-deficient mice. *Proc Natl Acad Sci USA.* 1996; 93:4994–8.

85. Blazar BR, Taylor PA, Panoskaltsis-Mortari A, et al. Blockade of CD40 ligand-CD40 interaction impairs CD4$^+$ T cell-mediated alloreactivity by inhibiting mature donor T cell expansion and function after bone marrow transplantation. *J Immunol.* 1997; 158:29–39.

86. Mondino A, Whaley CD, DeSilva DR, Li W, Jenkins MK, Mueller DL. Defective transcription of the *IL-2* gene is associated with impaired expression of c-Fos, FosB, and JunB in anergic T helper 1 cells. *J Immunol.* 1996; 157:2048–57.

87. Sundstedt A, Dohlsten M. In vivo anergized CD4$^+$ T cells have defective expression and function of the activating protein-1 transcription factor. *J Immunol.* 1998; 161:5930–6.

88. Boussiotis VA, Freeman GJ, Berezovskaya A, Barber DL, Nadler LM. Maintenance of human T cell anergy: blocking of *IL-2* gene transcription by activated Rap1. *Science.* 1997; 278:124–8.

89. Schwartz RH. T cell clonal anergy. *Curr Opin Immunol.* 1997; 9:351–7.

90. Boussiotis VA, Berezovskaya A, Appleman LJ, Freeman GJ, Nadler LM. Increased expression of p27^{Kip1} cyclin-dependent kinase inhibitor is responsible for G$_1$ arrest in alloantigen-specific helper T cell clonal anergy. *Blood.* 1998; 92:700a (abstract 2880).

91. Lenschow DJ, Walunas TL, Bluestone JA. CD28/B7 system of T cell costimulation. *Annu Rev Immunol.* 1996; 14:233–58.

92. Germain RN. The ins and outs of antigen processing and presentation. *Nature.* 1986; 322:687–9.

93. Madden DR, Gorga JC, Strominger JL, Wiley DC. The three-dimensional structure of HLA-B27 at 2.1 A resolution suggests a general mechanism for tight peptide binding to MHC. *Cell.* 1992; 70:1035–48.

94. Matsumura M, Fremont DH, Peterson PA, Wilson IA. Emerging principles for the recognition of peptide antigens by MHC class I molecules. *Science.* 1992; 257:927–34.

95. Brown JH, Jardetzky TS, Gorga JC, et al. Three-dimensional structure of the human class II histocompatibility antigen HLA-DR1. *Nature.* 1993; 364:33–9.

96. Falk K, Rotzschke O, Stevanovic S, Jung G, Rammensee HG. Allele-specific motifs revealed by sequencing of self-peptides eluted from MHC molecules. *Nature.* 1991; 351:290 6.

97. Germain RN. MHC-dependent antigen processing and peptide presentation: providing ligands for T lymphocyte activation. *Cell.* 1994; 76:287–99.

98. Hunt DF, Henderson RA, Shabanowitz J, et al. Characterization of peptides bound to the class I MHC molecule HLA-A2.1 by mass spectrometry. *Science.* 1992; 255:1261–3.

99. Goldberg AL, Rock KL. Proteolysis, proteasomes and antigen presentation. *Nature.* 1992; 357:375–9.

100. Rock KL, Gramm C, Rothstein L, et al. Inhibitors of the proteasome block the degradation of most cell proteins and the generation of peptides presented on MHC class I molecules. *Cell.* 1994; 78:761–71.

101. Driscoll J, Brown MG, Finley D, Monaco JJ. MHC-linked LMP gene products specifically alter peptidase activities of the proteasome. *Nature.* 1993; 365:262–4.
102. Neefjes JJ, Momburg F, Hammerling GJ. Selective and ATP-dependent translocation of peptides by the MHC-encoded transporter. *Science.* 1993; 261:769–71.
103. Shepherd JC, Schumacher TN, Ashton-Rickardt PG, et al. TAP1-dependent peptide translocation in vitro is ATP dependent and peptide. *Cell.* 1993; 74:577–84.
104. Degen E, Cohen-Doyle MF, Williams DB. Efficient dissociation of the p88 chaperone from major histocompatibility complex class I molecules requires both β 2-microglobulin and peptide. *J Exp Med.* 1992; 175:1653–61.
105. Hughes EA, Cresswell P. The thiol oxidoreductase ERp75 is a component of the MHC class I peptide-loading complex. *Curr Biol.* 1998; 8:709–12.
106. Lindquist JA, Jensen ON, Mann M, Hammerling GJ. ER-60, a chaperone with thiol-dependent reductase activity involved in MHC class I assembly. *EMBO J.* 1998; 17:2186–95.
107. Pamer E, Cresswell P. Mechanisms of MHC class I—restricted antigen processing. *Annu Rev Immunol.* 1998; 16:323–58
108. Lehner PJ, Surman MJ, Cresswell P. Soluble tapasin restores MHC class I expression and function in the tapasin-negative cell line .220. *Immunity.* 1998; 8:221–31.
109. Sadasivan B, Lehner PJ, Ortmann B, Spies T, Cresswell P. Roles for calreticulin and a novel glycoprotein, tapasin, in the interaction of MHC class I molecules with TAP. *Immunity.* 1996; 5:103–14.
110. Lewis JW, Elliott T. Evidence for successive peptide binding and quality control stages during MHC class I assembly. *Curr Biol.* 1998; 8:717–20.
111. Kovacsovics-Bankowski M, Clark K, Benacerraf B, Rock KL. Efficient major histocompatibility complex class I presentation of exogenous antigen upon phagocytosis by macrophages. *Proc Natl Acad Sci USA.* 1993; 90:4942–6.
112. Kovacsovics-Bankowski M, Rock KL. A phagosome-to-cytosol pathway for exogenous antigens presented on MHC class I molecules. *Science.* 1995; 267:243–6.
113. Norbury CC, Chambers BJ, Prescott AR, Ljunggren HG, Watts C. Constitutive macropinocytosis allows TAP-dependent major histocompatibility complex class I presentation of exogenous soluble antigen by bone marrow-derived dendritic cells. *Eur J Immunol.* 1997; 27:280–8.
114. Rock KL, Gamble S, Rothstein L. Presentation of exogenous antigen with class I major histocompatibility complex molecules. *Science.* 1990; 249:918–21.
115. Harding CV, Song R. Phagocytic processing of exogenous particulate antigens by macrophages for presentation by class I MHC molecules. *J Immunol.* 1994; 153:4925–33.
116. Staerz UD, Karasuyama H, Garner AM. Cytotoxic T lymphocytes against a soluble protein. *Nature.* 1987; 329:449–51.
117. Watts C. Capture and processing of exogenous antigens for presentation on MHC molecules. *Annu Rev Immunol.* 1997; 15:821–50.
118. Cresswell P, Avva RR, Davis JE, Lamb CA, Riberdy JM, Roche PA. Intracellular transport and peptide binding properties of HLA class II glycoproteins. *Semin Immunol.* 1990; 2:273–80.
119. Roche PA, Marks MS, Cresswell P. Formation of a nine-subunit complex by HLA class II glycoproteins and the invariant chain. *Nature.* 1991; 354:392–4.
120. Sanderson F, Kleijmeer MJ, Kelly A, et al. Accumulation of HLA-DM, a regulator of antigen presentation, in MHC class II compartments. *Science.* 1994; 266:1566–9.
121. Roche PA, Cresswell P. Invariant chain association with HLA-DR molecules inhibits immunogenic peptide binding. *Nature.* 1990; 345:615–8.

122. Germain RN, Rinker AG Jr. Peptide binding inhibits protein aggregation of invariant-chain free class II dimers and promotes surface expression of occupied molecules. *Nature.* 1993; 363:725–8.

123. Sherman MA, Weber DA, Jensen PE. DM enhances peptide binding to class II MHC by release of invariant chain-derived peptide. *Immunity.* 1995; 3:197–205.

124. Lanzavecchia A. Mechanisms of antigen uptake for presentation. *Curr Opin Immunol.* 1996; 8:348–54.

125. Sette A, Adorini L, Colon SM, Buus S, Grey HM. Capacity of intact proteins to bind to MHC class II molecules. *J Immunol.* 1989; 143:1265–7.

126. Hunt DF, Michel H, Dickinson TA, et al. Peptides presented to the immune system by the murine class II major histocompatibility complex molecule I-Ad. *Science.* 1992; 256:1817–20.

127. Rudensky A, Preston-Hurlburt P, Hong SC, Barlow A, Janeway CA Jr. Sequence analysis of peptides bound to MHC class II molecules. *Nature.* 1991; 353:622–7.

128. Banchereau J, Steinman RM. Dendritic cells and the control of immunity. *Nature.* 1998; 392:245–52.

129. Marland G, Bakker AB, Adema GJ, Figdor CG. Dendritic cells in immune response induction. *Stem Cells.* 1996; 14:501–7.

130. Steinman RM. The dendritic cell system and its role in immunogenicity. *Annu Rev Immunol.* 1991; 9:271–96.

131. Steinman RM, Pack M, Inaba K. Dendritic cells in the T-cell areas of lymphoid organs. *Immunol Rev.* 1997; 156:25–37.

132. Finkelman FD, Lees A, Birnbaum R, Gause WC, Morris SC. Dendritic cells can present antigen in vivo in a tolerogenic or immunogenic fashion. *J Immunol.* 1996; 157:1406–14.

133. Inaba M, Inaba K, Hosono M, et al. Distinct mechanisms of neonatal tolerance induced by dendritic cells and thymic B cells. *J Exp Med.* 1991; 173:549–59.

134. Matzinger P, Guerder S. Does T-cell tolerance require a dedicated antigen-presenting cell? *Nature.* 1989; 338:74–6.

135. Caux C, Liu YJ, Banchereau J. Recent advances in the study of dendritic cells and follicular dendritic cells. *Immunol Today.* 1995; 16:2–4.

136. Mamula MJ, Janeway CA Jr. Do B cells drive the diversification of immune responses? *Immunol Today.* 1993; 14:151–2.

137. Metlay JP, Pure E, Steinman RM. Control of the immune response at the level of antigen-presenting cells: a comparison of the function of dendritic cells and B lymphocytes. *Adv Immunol.* 1989; 47:45–116.

138. Bose S, Deininger M, Gora-Tybor J, Goldman JM, Melo JV. The presence of typical and atypical BCR-ABL fusion genes in leukocytes of normal individuals: biologic significance and implications for the assessment of minimal residual disease. *Blood.* 1998; 92:3362–7.

139. Limpens J, Stad R, Vos C, et al. Lymphoma-associated translocation t(14;18) in blood B cells of normal individuals. *Blood.* 1995; 85:2528–36.

140. Liu Y, Hernandez AM, Shibata D, Cortopassi GA. BCL2 translocation frequency rises with age in humans. *Proc Natl Acad Sci USA.* 1994; 91:8910–4.

141. Uckun FM, Herman-Hatten K, Crotty ML, et al. Clinical significance of MLL-AF4 fusion transcript expression in the absence of a cytogenetically detectable t(4;11)(q21;q23) chromosomal translocation. *Blood.* 1998; 92:810–21.

142. Fuchs EJ, Matzinger P. Is cancer dangerous to the immune system? *Semin Immunol.* 1996; 8:271–80.

143. Ioachim HL. The opportunistic tumors of immune deficiency. *Adv Cancer Res.* 1990; 54:301–17.

144. Rickinson AB, Moss DJ. Human cytotoxic T lymphocyte responses to Epstein-Barr virus infection. *Annu Rev Immunol.* 1997; 15:405–31.

145. Foley EJ. Attempts to induce immunity against mammary adenocarcinoma in inbred mice. *Cancer Res.* 1993; 313:578–80.

146. Gross L. Intradermal immunization of C3H mice against a sarcoma that originated in an animal of the same line. *Cancer Res.* 1943; 3:326–33.

147. Klein G, Sjögren H, Klein E, Hellstrom KE. Demonstration of resistance against methylcholanthrene-induced sarcomas in the primary autochthonous host. *Cancer Res.* 1960; 20:1561–72.

148. Kripke ML, Fisher MS. Immunologic parameters of ultraviolet carcinogenesis. *J Natl Cancer Inst.* 1976; 57:211–5.

149. Prehn RT, Main JM. Immunity to methylcholanthrene-induced sarcomas. *J Natl Cancer Inst.* 1957; 18:769–78.

150. Sjögren HO, Hellstrom I, Klein G. Resistance of polyoma virus-immunized mice to transplantation of established polyoma tumors. *Exp Cell Res.* 1961; 23:204–8.

151. Hewitt HB, Blake ER, Walder AS. A critique of the evidence for active host defence against cancer, based on personal studies of 27 murine tumours of spontaneous origin. *Br J Cancer.* 1976; 33:241–59.

152. Scott OC. Tumor transplantation and tumor immunity: a personal view. *Cancer Res.* 1991; 51:757–63.

153. Boon T, Van Pel A. Teratocarcinoma cell variants rejected by syngeneic mice: protection of mice immunized with these variants against other variants and against the original malignant cell line. *Proc Natl Acad Sci USA.* 1978; 75:1519–23.

154. Van Pel A, Vessiere F, Boon T. Protection against two spontaneous mouse leukemias conferred by immunogenic variants obtained by mutagenesis. *J Exp Med.* 1983; 157:1992–2001.

155. Brichard V, Van Pel A, Wolfel T, et al. The tyrosinase gene codes for an antigen recognized by autologous cytolytic T lymphocytes on HLA-A2 melanoma. *J Exp Med.* 1993; 178:489–95.

156. Traversari C, van der Bruggen P, Luescher IF, et al. A nonapeptide encoded by human gene MAGE-1 is recognized on HLA-A1 by cytolytic T lymphocytes directed against tumor antigen MZ2-E. *J Exp Med.* 1992; 176:1453–7.

157. Traversari C, van der Bruggen P, Van den Eynde B, et al. Transfection and expression of a gene coding for a human melanoma antigen recognized by autologous cytolytic T lymphocytes. *Immunogenetics.* 1992; 35:145–52.

158. van der Bruggen P, Traversari C, Chomez P, et al. A gene encoding an antigen recognized by cytolytic T lymphocytes on a human melanoma. *Science.* 1991; 254:1643–7.

159. Boon T. Toward a genetic analysis of tumor rejection antigens. *Adv Cancer Res.* 1992; 58:177–210.

160. Boon T, Cerottini JC, Van den Eynde B, van der Bruggen P, Van Pel A. Tumor antigens recognized by T lymphocytes. *Annu Rev Immunol.* 1994; 12:337–65.

161. Engelhard VH. Structure of peptides associated with class I and class II MHC molecules. *Annu Rev Immunol.* 1994; 12:181–207.

162. Rothbard JB, Taylor WR. A sequence pattern common to T cell epitopes. *EMBO J.* 1988; 7:93–100.

163. Rotzschke O, Falk K, Stevanovic S, Jung G, Walden P, Rammensee HG. Exact prediction of a natural T cell epitope. *Eur J Immunol.* 1991; 21:2891–4.

164. Parker KC, Bednarek MA, Coligan JE. Scheme for ranking potential HLA-A2 binding peptides based on independent binding of individual peptide side-chains. *J Immunol.* 1994; 152:163–75.

165. Townsend AR, Gotch FM, Davey J. Cytotoxic T cells recognize fragments of the influenza nucleoprotein. *Cell*. 1985; 42:457–67.

166. Dranoff G, Mulligan RC. Gene transfer as cancer therapy. *Adv Immunol*. 1995; 58:417–53.

167. Pardoll DM. Cancer vaccines. *Nat Med*. 1998; 4:525–31.

168. Ostrand-Rosenberg S. Tumor immunotherapy: the tumor cell as antigen-presenting cell. *Curr Opin Immunol*. 1994; 6:722–7.

169. Schultze JS, Cardoso AA, Freeman GJ, et al. Follicular lymphomas can be induced to present alloantigen efficiently: a conceptual model to improve their tumor immunogenicity. *Proc Natl Acad Sci USA*. 1995; 92:8200–4.

170. Bosshart H, Jarrett RF. Deficient major histocompatibility complex class II antigen presentation in a subset of Hodgkin's disease tumor cells. *Blood*. 1998; 92:2252–9.

171. Dohert, PC, Knowles BB, Wettstein PJ. Immunological surveillance of tumors in the context of major histocompatibility complex restriction of T cell function. *Adv Cancer Res*. 1984; 42:1–65.

172. Ellem KA, O'Rourke MG, Johnson GR, et al. A case report: immune responses and clinical course of the first human use of granulocyte/macrophage-colony-stimulating-factor-transduced autologous melanoma cells for immunotherapy. *Cancer Immunol Immunother*. 1997; 44:10–20.

173. Seliger B, Maeurer MJ, Ferrone S. TAP off–tumors on. *Immunol Today*. 1997; 18:292–9.

174. Cardoso AA, Schultze JL, Boussiotis VA, et al. Pre-B acute lymphoblastic leukemia cells may induce T-cell anergy to alloantigen. *Blood*. 1996; 88:41–8.

175. Staveley-O'Carroll K, Sotomayor E, Montgomery J, et al. Induction of antigen-specific T cell anergy: an early event in the course of tumor progression. *Proc Natl Acad Sci USA*. 1998; 95:1178–83.

176. Kern JA, Reed JC, Daniele RP, Nowell PC. The role of the accessory cell in mitogen-stimulated human T cell gene expression. *J Immunol*. 1986; 137:764–9.

177. Correa MR, Ochoa AC, Ghosh P, Mizoguchi H, Harvey L, Longo DL. Sequential development of structural and functional alterations in T cells from tumor-bearing mice. *J Immunol*. 1997; 158:5292–6.

178. Zea AH, Curti BD, Longo DL, et al. Alterations in T cell receptor and signal transduction molecules in melanoma patients. *Clin Cancer Res*. 1995; 1:1327–35.

179. Cardoso AA, Seamon M, Afonso HM, et al. Pre-B ALL cells produce functional TGF-β that inhibits both early hematopoiesis and T cell activation thereby facilitating leukemia cell growth. *Blood*. 1996; 88:666a (abstract 2652).

180. Petersson M, Charo J, Salazar-Onfray F, et al. Constitutive IL-10 production accounts for the high NK sensitivity, low MHC class I expression, and poor transporter associated with antigen processing (TAP)-1/2 function in the prototype NK target YAC-1. *J Immunol*. 1998; 161:2099–105.

181. Hahne M, Rimoldi D, Schroter M, et al. Melanoma cell expression of Fas(Apo-1/CD95) ligand: implications for tumor immune escape. *Science*. 1996; 274:1363–6.

182. Streilein JW. Unraveling immune privilege. *Science*. 1995; 270:1158–9.

183. Baskar S. Gene-modified tumor cells as cellular vaccine. *Cancer Immunopl Immunother*. 1996; 43:165–73.

184. Guinan EC, Gribbon JG, Boussiotis VA, Freeman GJ, Nadler LM. Pivotal role of the B7:CD28 pathway in transplantation tolerance and tumor immunity. *Blood*. 1994; 84:3261–82.

185. Tuting T, Storkus WJ, Lotze MT. Gene-based strategies for the immunotherapy of cancer. *J Mol Med*. 1997; 75:478–91.

186. Dranoff G, Jaffee E, Lazenby A, et al. Vaccination with irradiated tumor cells engineered

to secrete murine granulocyte-macrophage colony-stimulating factor stimulates potent, specific, and long-lasting anti-tumor immunity. *Proc Natl Acad Sci USA.* 1993; 90:3539–43.

187. Dranoff G. Cancer gene therapy: connecting basic research with clinical inquiry. *J Clin Oncol.* 1998; 16:2548–56.

188. Pardoll DM. Paracrine cytokine adjuvants in cancer immunotherapy. *Annu Rev Immunol.* 1995; 13:399–415.

189. Alijagic S, Moller P, Artuc M, Jurgovsky K, Czarnetzki BM, Schadendorf D. Dendritic cells generated from peripheral blood transfected with human tyrosinase induce specific T cell activation. *Eur J Immunol.* 1995; 25:3100–7.

190. Lee RS, Tartour E, van der Bruggen P, et al. Major histocompatibility complex class I presentation of exogenous soluble tumor antigen fused to the B-fragment of Shiga toxin. *Eur J Immunol.* 1998; 28:2726–37.

191. Zajac P, Schutz A, Oertli D, et al. Enhanced generation of cytotoxic T lymphocytes using recombinant vaccinia virus expressing human tumor-associated antigens and B7 costimulatory molecules. *Cancer Res.* 1998; 58:4567–71.

192. Baskar S, Ostrand-Rosenberg S, Nabavi N, Nadler LM, Freeman GJ, Glimcher L. Constitutive expression of B7 restores immunogenicity of tumor cells expressing truncated forms of major histocompatibility complex class II molecules. *Proc Natl Acad Sci USA.* 1993; 90:5687–90.

193. Greenberg PD, Kern DE, Cheever MA. Therapy of disseminated murine leukemia with cyclophosphamide and immune Lyt-1+,2-T cells. Tumor eradication does not require participation of cytotoxic T cells. *J Exp Med.* 1985; 161:1122–34.

194. Hung K, Hayashi R, Lafond-Walker A, Lowenstein C, Pardoll D, Levitsky H. The central role of CD4+ T cells in the antitumor immune response. *J Exp Med.* 1998; 188:2357–68.

195. Ostrand-Rosenberg S, Roby CA, Clements VK. Abrogation of tumorigenicity by MHC class II antigen expression requires the cytoplasmic domain of the class II molecule. *J Immunol.* 1991; 147:2419–22.

196. Armstrong TD, Pulaski BA, Ostrand-Rosenberg S. Tumor antigen presentation: changing the rules. *Cancer Immunol Immunother.* 1998; 46:70–4.

197. Armstrong TD, Clements VK, Ostrand-Rosenberg S. MHC class II-transfected tumor cells directly present antigen to tumor-specific CD4+ T lymphocytes. *J Immunol.* 1998; 160:661–6.

198. Cayeux S, Richter G, Noffz G, Dorken B, Blankenstein T. Influence of gene-modified (IL-7, IL-4, and B7) tumor cell vaccines on tumor antigen presentation. *J Immunol.* 1997; 158:2834–41.

199. Huang AYC, Golumbek P, Ahmadzadeh M, Jaffee E, Pardoll D, Levitsky H. Role of bone marrow-derived cells in presenting MHC class I-restricted tumor antigens. *Science.* 1994; 264:961–5.

200. Pulaski BA, Yeh KY, Shastri N, et al. Interleukin 3 enhances cytotoxic T lymphocyte development and class I major histocompatibility complex "re-presentation" of exogenous antigen by tumor-infiltrating antigen-presenting cells. *Proc Natl Acad Sci USA.* 1996; 93:3669–74.

201. Bevan MJ. Cross-priming for a secondary cytotoxic response to minor H antigens with H-2 congenic cells which do not cross-react in the cytotoxic assay. *J Exp Med.* 1976; 143:1283–8.

202. Brissinck J, Demanet C, Moser M, Leo O, Thielemans K. Treatment of mice bearing BCL1 lymphoma with bispecific antibodies. *J Immunol.* 1991; 147:4019–26.

203. Demanet C, Brissinck J, Van Mechelen M, Leo O, Thielemans K. Treatment of murine

B cell lymphoma with bispecific monoclonal antibodies (anti-idiotype × anti-CD3). *J Immunol*. 1991; 147:1091–7.

204. Staerz UD, Kanagawa, Bevan MJ. Hybrid antibodies can target sites for attack by T cells. *Nature*. 1985; 314:628–31.

205. Beun GD, van de Velde CJ, Fleuren GJ. T-cell based cancer immunotherapy: direct or redirected tumor-cell recognition? *Immunol Today*. 1994; 1:11–5.

206. Doherty PC, Topham DJ, Tripp RA. Establishment and persistence of virus-specific CD4[+] and CD8[+] T cell memory. *Immunol Rev*. 1996; 150:23–44.

207. Carmichael A, Jin X, Sissons P, Borysiewicz L. Quantitative analysis of the human immunodeficiency virus type 1 (HIV-1)-specific cytotoxic T lymphocyte (CTL) response at different stages of HIV-1 infection: differential CTL responses to HIV-1 and Epstein–Barr virus in late disease. *J Exp Med*. 1993; 177:249–56.

208. Gotch FM, Nixon DF, Alp N, McMichael AJ, Borysiewicz LK. High frequency of memory and effector gag specific cytotoxic T lymphocytes in HIV seropositive individuals. *Int Immunol*. 1990; 2:707–12.

209. Moss PA, Rowland-Jones SL, Frodsham PM, et al. Persistent high frequency of human immunodeficiency virus-specific cytotoxic T cells in peripheral blood of infected donors. *Proc Natl Acad Sci USA*. 1995; 92:57773–7.

210. Czerkinsky C, Andersson G, Ekre HP, et al. Reverse ELISPOT assay for clonal analysis of cytokine production. I. Enumeration of γ-interferon-secreting cells. *J Immunol Methods*. 1988; 110:29–36.

211. Lalvani A, Brookes R, Hambleton S, Britton WJ, Hill AV, McMichael AJ. Rapid effector function in CD8[+] memory T cells. *J Exp Med*. 1997; 186:859–65.

212. Altman JD, Moss PA, Goiulder PJ, et al. Phenotypic analysis of antigen-specific T lymphocytes. *Science*. 1996; 274:94–6.

213. Romero P, Dunbar PR, Valmori D, et al. Ex vivo staining of metastatic lymph nodes by class I major histocompatibility complex tetramers reveals high numbers of antigen-experienced tumor-specific cytolytic T lymphocytes. *J Exp Med*. 1998; 188:1641–50.

214. Antonia SJ, Extermann M, Flavell RA. Immunologic nonresponsiveness to tumors. *Crit Rev Oncogen*. 1998; 9:35–41.

215. van Parijs L, Ibraghimov A, Abbas AK. The roles of costimulation and fas in T cell apoptosis and peripheral tolerance. *Immunity*. 1996; 4:321–8.

216. van Parijs L, Abbas AK. Homeostasis and self-tolerance in the immune system: turning lymphocytes off. *Science*. 1998; 280:243–8.

217. Lo D, Burkly LC, Widera G, et al. Diabetes and tolerance in transgenic mice expressing class II MHC molecules in pancreatic beta cells. *Cell*. 1988; 53:159–68.

218. Morahan G, Allison J, Miller JF. Tolerance of class I histocompatibility antigens expressed extrathymically. *Nature*. 1989; 339:622–4.

219. Ohashi PS, Oehen S, Buerki K, et al. Ablation of "tolerance" and induction of diabetes by virus infection in viral antigen transgenic mice. *Cell*. 1991; 65:305–17.

220. Webb S, Morris C, Sprent J. Extrathymic tolerance of mature T cells: clonal elimination as a consequence of immunity. *Cell*. 1990; 63:1249–56.

221. Golumbek P, Levitsky H, Jaffee L, Pardoll DM. The antitumor immune response as a problem of self-nonself discrimination: implications for immunotherapy. *Immunol Res*. 1993; 12:183–92.

222. Levitsky HI. Tumors derived from antigen presenting cells. *Semin Immunol*. 1996; 8:281–7.

223. Liblau RS, Tisch R, Shokat K, et al. Intravenous injection of soluble antigen induces thymic and peripheral T-cells apoptosis. *Proc Natl Acad Sci USA*. 1996; 93:3031–6.

224. Robey E, Urbain J. Tolerance and immune regulation. *Immunol Today.* 1991; 12:175–7.

225. Beverly B, Kang SM, Lenardo MJ, Schwartz RH. Reversal of in vitro T cell clonal anergy by IL-2 stimulation. *Int Immunol.* 1992; 4:661–71.

226. Leach DR, Krummel MF, Allison JP. Enhancement of antitumor immunity by CTLA–4 blockade. *Science.* 1996; 271:1734–6.

227. Perez VL, Van Parijs L, Biuckians A, Zheng XX, Strom TB, Abbas AK. Induction of peripheral T cell tolerance in vivo requires CTLA-4 engagement. *Immunity.* 1997; 6:411–7.

228. Rocken M, Urban JF, Shevach EM. Infection breaks T-cell tolerance. *Nature.* 1992; 359:79–82.

229. Paterson Y, Ikonomidis G. Recombinant *Listeria monocytogenes* cancer vaccines. *Curr Opin Immunol.* 1996; 8:664–9.

230. Restifo NP. The new vaccines: building viruses that elicit antitumor immunity. *Curr Opin Immunol.* 1996; 8:658–63.

231. Abdel-Wahab Z, Weltz C, Hester D, et al. A phase I clinical trial of immunotherapy with interferon-γ gene-modified autologous melanoma cells: monitoring the humoral immune response. *Cancer.* 1997; 80:401–12.

232. Belli F, Arienti F, Sule-Suso J, et al. Active immunization of metastatic melanoma patients with interleukin-2- transduced allogeneic melanoma cells: evaluation of efficacy and tolerability. *Cancer Immunol Immunother.* 1997; 44:197–203.

233. Dranoff G, Soiffer R, Lynch T, et al. A phase I study of vaccination with autologous, irradiated melanoma cells engineered to secrete human granulocyte-macrophage colony stimulating factor. *Hum Gene Ther.* 1997; 8:111–23.

234. Nabel GJ, Gordon D, Bishop DK, et al. Immune response in human melanoma after transfer of an allogeneic class I major histocompatibility complex gene with DNA–liposome complexes. *Proc Natl Acad Sci USA.* 1996; 93:15388–93.

235. Soiffer R, Lynch T, Mihm M, et al. Vaccination with irradiated autologous melanoma cells engineered to secrete human granulocyte-macrophage colony-stimulating factor generates potent antitumor immunity in patients with metastatic melanoma. *Proc Natl Acad Sci USA.* 1998; 95:13141–6.

236. Baskar S, Glimcher L, Nabavi N, Jones RT, Ostrand-Rosenberg S. Major histocompatibility complex class II+ B7-1+ tumor cells are potent vaccines for stimulating tumor rejection in tumor-bearing mice. *J Exp Med.* 1995; 181:619–629.

15

Emerging Technologies

Molecular Targets and the Drug Discovery Process

Matthew Moyle and Michael Palazzolo

Introduction

The current paradigm of small-molecule drug discovery is based on the identification of a biological target that plays a key role in a given pathophysiological process. Large collections of small molecules are screened against a target in a search for tight-binding ligands that affect function of the target in a specific manner. Small-molecule leads, identified in this fashion, are then optimized iteratively whereby chemical variations are tested using measurements of binding, specificity, inhibitory or potentiating activity, toxicology, pharmacokinetic distribution, and clinical efficacy as the major metrics.

The emergence of genomics promises to dramatically accelerate this paradigm. Many researchers expect that high-throughput gene discovery technologies will lead to a more detailed and comprehensive molecular understanding of most diseases. The disease-associated molecules, identified using these emerging technologies, will provide a substantial increase in the number of potential targets and corresponding opportunities to develop novel small-molecule pharmaceuticals.

The earliest phases of genome analysis have resulted in physical maps, genetic maps, and large volumes of DNA sequence. In model organisms (yeast, bacteria, *Caenorhabditis elegans*, and *Drosophila*) this sequence has largely been genomic, representing partial or complete regions of individual chromosomes. In mammalian systems, the bulk of the sequencing effort has been focused on generating partial DNA-sequence information from randomly selected cDNA. An individual partial cDNA sequence is known as an EST (expressed sequence tag). The data from these partial sequences are then clustered using assembly algorithms. It has been estimated that approx 40,000 unique human genes can be associated with this fragmentary sequence data that are publicly available. The identification of larger numbers of genes have been claimed by those analyzing proprietary databases. Efforts aimed toward complete genomic sequencing of the human genome are accelerating but, to date, have finished only a small fraction (about 3%) of the entire target. The sequence data (both EST and genomic) are analyzed computationally in attempts to assign putative biochemical functions with the otherwise uncharacterized novel genes.

From: *Principles of Molecular Oncology*
Edited by: M. H. Bronchud, M. A. Foote, W. P. Peters, and M. O. Robinson © Humana Press Inc., Totowa, NJ

While sequence data are necessary components used to analyze the nature of a given gene and its product, the potential utility of a gene product as a therapeutic target increases dramatically if a given gene can be implicated in a specific pathophysiological process. Thus, the next great challenge in genomics is the need to develop and implement approaches to associate this enormous set of novel genes with specific functions. From the point of view of therapeutics development, it is extremely useful to be able to identify all (or almost all) of the molecular perturbations that underlie a given pathophysiological state and at the same time begin to determine the manner in which these molecules interact and are regulated. Owing to the large numbers of genes that reside in mammalian genomes, it is critical that these emerging technologies be conducive to implementation on high-throughput platforms.

A variety of technologies are now starting to emerge that promise to allow a detailed exploration of the molecular pathways of different pathological conditions in a high-throughput fashion. The most prominent of the new approaches can be broadly categorized into three groups. The first class are those procedures that attempt to scan the genome to characterize fluctuations, both physiological and pathophysiological, in gene expression. The second group are based on molecular pathway building protocols that use noncovalent dihybrid bi- and trimolecular protein interactions in yeast that can activate selectable pathways. The third category of pathway identification technologies are based on systems genetic approaches in model organisms including yeast, *C. elegans*, and *Drosophila*.

The different experimental approaches to large-scale gene expression analysis and pathway building are outlined in this chapter. The strengths and weaknesses of the different approaches are briefly described. Finally, the potential impact on the drug discovery paradigm will be discussed.

Genome-Wide Gene Expression Analysis

Gene expression studies (also known as transcript imaging) are being used in the study of different disease states for at least two reasons. First, it is thought that in many diseases gene expression will be significantly altered either as a proximate (complete or partial) cause of the disease or as a downstream response to a different primary initiating event. Second, many investigators suspect that transcript imaging will also be used to identify interacting molecules. This line of reasoning is based on the notion that molecules that interact are likely to be coordinately regulated at the transcriptional level. At least four different types of transcript-imaging procedures are being implemented. Each is described briefly below.

Electronic Northerns

In this method, whereby cDNA libraries are generated from two different tissues (or the same tissue in two different states), templates are randomly selected and partial cDNA sequences (or ESTs) are generated, and the frequency of appearance of each individual EST is counted and compared between the two sources.

SAGE

The serial analysis of gene expression (SAGE) technique bears a functional similarity to large-scale sequencing followed by computational comparisons. However, it is significantly different in that it is based on sequencing short gene tags (on the order of 10–13 basepairs [bps]) that are generated from each cDNA. These gene tags are arrayed tandemly within a cloning vector. The 10- to 13-bp tag is sufficient for identity because it is selected, by the cloning strategy, from a representative precise site in the cDNA molecule (i.e., the 10–13 bps immediately adjacent to a specific 4-hitter restriction site closest to the poly(A)$^+$ tail) *(1)*. The efficiency is derived from the fact that, on average, 30 tags are placed into each clone, which can then be analyzed on a single sequencing lane. Thus, the approach is approx 30-fold more efficient than large-scale sequencing. After the sequencing phase is completed, the number of each type of tag is counted and compared with the frequency of appearance of the same tag in other tissue types (similar to the electronic Northern approach).

Differential Display

Differential display strategies are all based on the notion that polyacrylamide gel electrophoresis (PAGE) can be used to identify and quantitate the expression level of every mRNA in a population if such molecules can be divided into 100–200 subgroups of 50–100 molecules each *(2,3)*. The need to subdivide the expressed sequences is based on the fact that it is likely that there are 10,000–15,000 unique mRNA species in a given cell or tissue at any given time. The large number of different molecules means that an individual molecule cannot be independently resolved by PAGE if one attempts to simultaneously analyze the entire population of molecules in a single lane on a gel. Furthermore, only 1% of the molecules are differentially transcribed and many of these are expressed at low levels. Thus, many of the differentially expressed genes would likely be obscured by the large number of unregulated genes in a given population.

There are a variety of different differential display technologies; however, they are all based on polymerase chain reaction (PCR) strategies that subdivide complex cDNA populations into unique sets of nonoverlapping fragments. These sets can be called bins. Bins that contain between 50 and 100 molecules can be analyzed by PAGE so that almost every molecule in a bin can be identified as unique as long as only one bin is run in each lane of the polyacrylamide gel *(4–8)*.

Differential display technologies commonly begin with the synthesis of cDNA wing mRNA harvested from cells or tissue as template. The cDNA is then digested with a restriction enzyme, and linkers are covalently ligated to the sticky end overhangs. Next, ligation-mediated PCR reactions are performed so that only a subset of individual molecules are amplified in a given reaction. The key reagent in the binning procedures are the PCR primers. As described previously, most approaches attempt to generate between 100 and 200 bins with a different and unique set of cDNA molecules amplified in each bin. Thus, there need to be 100–200 different PCR primer pairs. The primer pairs have three sequence components. The first part matches the linker, the second part matches the sequence of the restriction enzyme recognition site, and the third part is variable. It is this variable region that provides the sequence-dependent amplification that results in the subdivision of the cDNA population. Only those cDNA molecules that contain a sequence match for the variable region are amplified in a given PCR reaction. Each bin is then displayed in a separate lane of a polyacrylamide (sequencing) gel. The bin (lane) designation and the mobility (related to the size of the fragment) give the corresponding DNA fragment an identity. The intensity of the fragment (radioactivity or fluorescence) provides a measure of the corresponding message's prevalence. The amplifications are competitive within a given bin so that, while linear, they can be performed under conditions in which molecules present at low concentrations can still provide strong signals.

To measure differences in gene expression between samples, the cDNA molecules from the different samples are divided into bins using identical PCR strategies and analyzed on different polyacrylamide gels using identical separation parameters. Individual lanes are then compared between the different samples. As the levels of expression of most genes do not change, the invariant genes can be used as both alignment aids and quantitative controls. All lanes need to be examined to assess gene expression changes in a comprehensive fashion.

Most of the developers of this technology type believe that the results are near quantitative. Specifically, the fluorescent intensity is based not strictly only on the initial concentration of the corresponding mRNA, but also on the ability of the fragment to amplify. However, the variability introduced by the "amplifiability" of the fragment is thought to be slight as long as the PCR primers used in the amplifications are carefully characterized. Furthermore, comparisons between individual gene products in different conditions (e.g., disease states) are quantitative as long as the same binning techniques are used to examine the different mRNA preparations. Significantly, the other molecules in the bin will serve as controls to provide a baseline against which changes in gene expression can be measured for the small fraction of molecules that are differentially expressed.

Microarray

Microarray technology is based on positioning DNA fragments in compact arrays on glass slides as targets for hybridization experiments. There are two major categories of microarrays. The first includes technologies in which oligonucleotides are positioned on the glass slides. The second class is based on procedures in which cDNA (usually PCR products) are placed on the glass supports. There are a variety of applications for microarrays, including sequencing by hybridization, mutational analysis, physical mapping, and genetic mapping. However, a major use of array technology that has emerged in the past few years is transcript imaging.

A number of groups are working on oligonucleotide-based microarray technology, but the clear leader in the field is Affymetrix (South San Francisco, CA). This company has developed a photolithographic combinatorial chemical synthesis tie approach to generate oligonucleotides *in situ,* rather than synthesize the oligonucleotides off-line and array them by subsequent spotting *(9).* Each expressed sequence is represented on the chip by a series of oligonucleotides (10–20 mers) designed to hybridize to the gene based on its DNA sequence (Figure 1).

A group at Affymetrix has published a *tour de force* study of the expression of all 6200 yeast genes by hybridizing fluorescent probes derived from mRNA prepared from yeast grown under different nutrient conditions to four arrays containing a total of 260,000 different oligonucleotides *(10).* The results suggest that the technique is sensitive enough to detect messages expressed at <0.1 copies per cell, with the dynamic range to also assess quantitatively the prevalence of messages present at hundreds of copies per cell. Quantitative estimates were derived for all yeast genes under both conditions. In rich medium, for example: 13% were undetected, 6% were rare at <0.1 copies per cell, 50% were between 0.1 and 1 copy per cell, 26% were between 1 and 10 copies per cell, and 5% were at >10 copies per cell. Ninety-two genes were differentially expressed between the two growth conditions, and the range of increased expression was 4- to 70-fold.

The study was filled with a generous number of controls facilitated by the fact that the chips were reusable. For example, the chips were tested with probe generated from genomic DNA. As all genes in the genomic probe should be present in a normalized fashion, this experiment provided an assessment of the success of the synthesis, and also resulted in a correction factor with which comparative expression between genes as well as an absolute measure of gene expression under each condition. A second control was the adjacent synthesis of closely related mismatch probes that made it possible to account and adjust for some level of cross-hybridization.

The availability of the complete, interpreted sequence of yeast allowed a comprehensive approach to the problem. In addition, the approach based on design of specific oligonucleotides allowed the generation of hybridization targets that were completely gene specific allowing accurate monitoring of closely related genes. Furthermore, sequences with repeats or DNA structures that yielded anomalous hybridization results were also eliminated from consideration.

The second major class of microarrays is based on placing PCR products derived from cDNA in an ordered fashion on glass slides *(11,12)*. The techniques are essentially second-generation dot-blot hybridizations. However, it is critical to realize that essential improvements in sensitivity, signal to noise, throughput, and facility of comparative hybridization are derived from the microarray procedures. As the hybridizations are done in a relatively small area (about 1 cm^2) and on a nonporous support (compared with dot blots), the kinetics of hybridization allow sufficient hybridization of probes that represent genes expressed at extremely low levels, leading to the increases in sensitivity. Signal-to-noise ratio is improved because the glass has a lower inherent fluorescence than nylon or nitrocellulose. Throughput improvements are derived from the fact that the technology can be automated: 10,000 genes can be examined on a single slide that can be prepared in minutes to hours. Some investigators suggest that the entire complement of human genes will soon be able to be positioned on a single 1-cm^2 glass support. Finally, because probes of two different fluorescent colors can be hybridized simultaneously, direct comparative hybridization can be performed. There are many artifacts that can be generated if differential expression experiments are done in a nonsimultaneous fashion (including different amounts of target placed on the slide, support defects, dust). Simultaneous assay allows a direct comparison as long as the probes are appropriately balanced.

Evaluation of the Different Transcript-Imaging Approaches

The key metrics that can be used to contrast and compare the different transcript-imaging technologies include comprehensiveness, sensitivity, and throughput (summarized in Table 1). Comprehensiveness, in this case, refers to the fraction of the expressed sequences in a given tissue that are actually being quantitatively measured and compared. Fully comprehensive assays are those that are able to assess the concentration of every

Table 1
Metrical Comparison of Gene Expression Technologies

	Comprehensiveness	Sensitivity	Throughput
Electronic Northerns	4	3	4
SAGE	3	2	3
Differential display	1	1	2
Microarray	2	1	1

Numerical rankings are relative, with 1 being best and 4 being worst.

gene in the target tissue and compare its level of prevalence in as many situations that are relevant. Sensitivity is a measure of the limit at which genes that are expressed at extremely low levels can be detected quantitatively above background. Sensitivity includes two factors: the ability to measure the expression of rare messages as well as resolve slight changes in expression levels in different conditions. Throughput is a measure of the rapidity at which large numbers of genes can be simultaneously analyzed. High-throughput molecular genetic assays require automation. In evaluating a technique, it is important to determine how automatable that approach is. The automation does not need to cover all aspects of the process, but does need to cover those that are most labor-intensive, error-prone, or costly. An additional important consideration is the effort that is required to characterize a gene once evidence has been produced to suggest that it is differentially regulated, specifically, how much additional effort is required to obtain enough DNA sequence to make a meaningful similarity search from sequence databases.

Comparisons of Comprehensiveness

At the present time, the differential-display technologies provide the most thorough approach to a comprehensive analysis for most applications. All clones that have the appropriate restriction fragments can be amplified and analyzed. Because the amplifications are performed on cDNA populations, there is no need to construct, array, normalize, or sequence large numbers of cDNA clones. Furthermore, there is no *a priori* selection of clones based on computational assessments and subjective levels of interest. The only clones that will not be identified are those that lack appropriate restriction sites and those whose expression is obscured by clones with higher levels of expression that are localized in the same bin and have the same approximate mobility on polyacrylamide gels. It is important to note that differential-display technologies can be applied in tissues and organisms that have not been extensively characterized in a genomic sense.

Microarray is limited by the number of genes that have been uniquely identified. Current cost and throughput considerations mean that, in general, only those genes that have been characterized can be spotted onto the arrays. The Affymetrix work in yeast, however, is a good example of how microarray can become completely comprehensive if the target genome has been completely sequenced. It is reasonable to think that less than half of the human genes may be present in the public databases. Furthermore, microarray experiments make sense only in the context of those tissues that have had extensive EST-style characterization and analysis or for organisms that have been completely sequenced.

SAGE and large-scale cDNA sequence analysis are limited by the number of clones that are sequenced and the number of libraries that need to be prepared to select cDNA clones to sequence. Sequencing is still an expensive operation and comparative sequencing analysis (electronic Northerns) typically is developed largely as a byproduct of developing a large EST set. Most SAGE experiments are conducted so that 50,000–150,000 sequence tags are generated in a given comparison *(13,14)*.

Comparisons of Sensitivity of the Different Transcript-Imaging Technologies

The microarray and transcript imaging technologies all appear to be quite sensitive. The Affymetrix microarray technology is thought to be capable of measuring mRNA expression levels of molecules that are present at a level of 0.1 copies per cell *(10)*. It is important to note that these assays were performed in yeast cells that certainly have a lower message complexity than mammalian cells. Greater than 90% of all predicted yeast transcripts were detected by looking at transcription under only two different growth conditions. Microarray systems based on contact spotting of PCR is thought to be capable of detecting messages present 1 part in 100,000. Similar levels of sensitivity are claimed by those using differential display technologies.

Throughput Comparisons

The microarray approaches are probably capable of the highest throughput. Many of the aspects of microarray have been automated. Robotic systems for contact spotting of PCR products have been developed, and the photolithographic system of Affymetrix is geared toward high-throughput oligonucleotide synthesis. Thousands to tens of thousands of DNA targets can be positioned on substrates no larger than a square centimeter. Comparative hybridizations can be performed *en masse* against all the targets placed on a single chip. Similarly fluorescent scanner/detectors are capable of extracting digital data in a fashion that does not require human intervention once the slides have been loaded. Perhaps the most time-consuming aspect of microarray is the procurement and rearraying of the clones that one wishes to put on a chip. Of course, this effort is required only for the type of microarray that is based on the contact spotting of PCR products.

The initial phase of a differential display project requires a cDNA synthesis reaction, 200 individual PCR reactions, and the loading and analysis of 200 acrylamide gel lanes. The PCR reactions can be set up and performed in a completely automated environment. The loading and analysis of the acrylamide slab gels is likely to be the most costly and time-consuming step.

SAGE and electronic Northern approaches are still dependent on performing and analyzing large numbers of DNA-sequencing reactions. These procedures are still costly and labor intensive. The emergence of practical capillary electrophoresis instruments may eventually make these strategies more competitive with respect to throughput.

Additional Work

Once differential expression has been demonstrated, the immediate next set of questions focus on the nature of the gene product. From this point of view, microarray,

SAGE, and electronic Northerns have a distinct advantage in that they are based (either directly or indirectly) on DNA-sequence data. In contrast, the data set after differential display consists of bands on a gel. The fragments that correspond to the band still must be cloned, sequenced, and analyzed so that the appropriate biochemical classification can be established. In some instances, groups are trying to develop databases based on EST data in which attempts are made to correlate predicted fragment size with fragments in each bin classification. However, a large fraction of genes do not fit into predicted patterns and it is not yet clear what the error rate would be in this type of analysis. Finally, it is important to keep in mind that all EST sequences do not lead to a biochemical classification. In many cases, full-length clones must be isolated and sequenced no matter which transcript imaging technology is used, and still, in many cases, no similarities can be discerned even with full-length sequence data.

Pathway Building Based on Yeast Two-Hybrid Analysis

Classical Yeast Two-Hybrid Screens

Yeast two-hybrid assays are genetic screens that allow the identification of protein–protein interactions. The technique is based on the ability of a pair of hybrid proteins through their interaction to bring together a DNA-binding domain and a transcriptional activation domain so that a variety of reporter genes (at least one of which is selective) are activated *(15,16)*. The most common variation of the procedure uses the yeast GAL4 transcription system. A "bait" protein is expressed as a hybrid protein with the GAL4 DNA-binding domain. A cDNA library is constructed such that a large number of hybrid "prey" proteins are expressed in which protein fragments coded by the cDNA library are fused to the GAL4 transcriptional activation domain. Coexpression in the same cell of a pair of bait and prey proteins that can interact allow the cointeraction of the two GAL4 domains which, in turn, activates expression of selectable reporter genes downstream of GAL that have been placed upstream activating sequences (UAS). The transcriptional readouts are used to identify interacting bait and prey hybrids.

Significant improvements in signal-to-noise ratio have been generated by developing yeast strains with combinatorial and distinct transcriptional readouts *(17)*. For example, one yeast strain contains three reporter genes: *HIS3, ADE2,* and *lacZ.* Each gene has been placed downstream of a different promoter (GAL1, GAL2, and GAL7, respectively). All respond to the same GAL4 transcriptional activator. In these strains, the interacting hybrid has to activate all three genes to be considered "positive." The *HIS3* gene can also be used as a selective marker. The use of selection means that the system can be used in a high-throughput fashion so that millions of constructs can be selected and only surviving colonies need to be scored.

Additional improvements have come through the careful construction of prey libraries. Libraries are now typically generated so that many breakpoints in the gene are generated during library construction so that each gene product is essentially represented as a deletion series. Thus the prey is offered in many different potential contexts to the bait molecule.

Membrane-Bound Yeast Two-Hybrid Screen

A variant two-hybrid system has recently been developed called the recruitment of Sos assay (ROS) *(18)*. This yeast-based interactive screen is useful in those situations that are difficult to study in the yeast nucleus, for example, when the prey hybrid contains sequences that prevent nuclear localization. In this system, the bait is attached to a gene known as *Sos* (son of sevenless). When this gene product is attracted to the plasma membrane, the cell survives by activating a Ras-based signal transduction pathway *(19)*. The prey library is generated in a vector that generates prey hybrid fusions in which the prey open-reading frames are fused to a molecule that is localized to the membrane. Thus, if the *Sos* molecule can be recruited by the hybrid interaction to the membrane, the cell survives.

Yeast Three-Hybrid Screens

Three-hybrid screens are used in those situations in which two molecules are known to interact, but the interaction cannot be reconstituted with the two molecules alone. One hypothesis is that the interaction requires a third component. The screen is performed to find the third, stabilizing or facilitating, member of the interaction. There are at least four classes of three-hybrid screens in yeast.

In the protein three-hybrid screen *(20)*, the two known molecules are attached to one of either the DNA-binding domain or the transcription activating domain. The prey library is cloned into an expression vector (in this context the prey does not have to be covalently associated with another protein). In positive screens, the third component will combine with the two hybrids and activate the corresponding selectable markers.

Kinase three-hybrid screens are performed in those instances where a posttranslational phosphorylation event is required to allow the hybrid interaction *(21,22)*. This system has been used to identify kinase substrates in which an identified protein kinase is coexpressed. It seems reasonable to speculate that additional systems will emerge based on other types of posttranslational modifications.

Peptide ligand three-hybrid systems have been used to find peptide ligands of transmembrane receptors whose binding domains are extracellular. In these experiments, the receptor-binding domain is inserted into both halves of the hybridization scheme. Intracellular expression of the native ligand leads to dimerization and transcriptional readout.

RNA three-hybrid systems are used to identify components of protein–RNA complexes *(23)*. The RNA-binding protein is used as bait, the RNA is coexpressed, and the prey library can then be screened for hybrid interaction.

Counterselection and Reverse Two-Hybrid Systems

Classical yeast two-hybrid systems select for positive interactions. However, in many experimental situations it may be desirable to screen for a molecule that can interrupt the interaction of two proteins or peptide domains. This can be accomplished using screens in which the transcriptional readout of the two-hybrid system is associated with one or several of the yeast markers in which yeast colonies can be identified by counterselection *(24–26)*. The gene *URA3* is one example. Its expression makes the yeast sensitive to 5-fluoroorotic acid. Once established, a two-hybrid system expressing this reporter can be used, in the appropriate counterselective medium, to screen for either small molecules or mutations that disrupt the interaction of the two-hybrid proteins.

Yeast Systems in Target-Based High-Throughout Screening

At least three different types of approaches have been tested to use yeast-based systems to screen for small molecule drug candidates. In the first class, reverse two-hybrid strategies have been established. In these experiments, the screen attempts to find antagonists of protein–protein interactions (*see above*) *(27)*. Small molecules that interrupt the protein–protein interaction might qualify as lead molecules. The second category of screens involves yeast strains into which mammalian receptors have been introduced and connected to yeast signal-transduction systems whose readout is selection *(28)*. The small molecules that are successful interrupt the agonist–receptor interaction which, in turn, interrupts the signal-transduction cascade with the positive readout allowing yeast cell survival. The third category of yeast screen is one in which the molecules are endogenous yeast proteins homologous to human proteins *(29)*. It is hoped that drugs that interact directly with yeast proteins will also interact with the homologues and can be optimized in a mammalian context.

Strengths and Weaknesses of Yeast Interactive Screens

Over the past decade, yeast two-hybrid screens have become a standard tool for studying protein–protein interactions and pathway definition. A major advantage is that the screens are system independent. They can be used to study interactions between proteins from any organism. Furthermore, the selective nature of transcriptional readout makes it possible to sort through large libraries of potential interacting molecules.

The disadvantages are things that the system misses and the high number of false-positives *(30)*. The system is thought to be hard to apply to many interactions that require posttranslational modification or for interactions that occur in membranes or extracellularly *(31)*.

The high number of false-positives in the yeast screens for interactive proteins means that the positive candidates have to be subsequently followed up with verification experiments. Most common approaches are based on coimmunoprecipitation experiments in which an antibody (Ab) to the bait protein is a key reagent. If multiple proteins are pulled down, they are examined by sodium dodecyl sulfate-polyacrylamide gel electrophoresis (SDS-PAGE). In such experiments, it is likely that the development of Abs will be a rate-limiting part of the process. A second, higher throughput class of verification experiments attempt to insert epitope tags into the bait molecules, and these recombinant molecules are expressed in cultured mammalian cells. Immunocytochemical localizations and immunoprecipitations using the Abs to the epitopes confirm interaction of two proteins that was initially revealed with two-hybrid experiments *(32)*.

Pathway Building Based on Systems Genetics

Bacterial and phage geneticists established the paradigm of using classic genetic approaches to untangle complicated molecular pathways. These approaches were based on the fact that suppression of a mutant phenotype by a mutation at a second genomic site was possible because the molecules encoded by the two genes in question were interacting within the cell and the two mutations could compensate for each other *(33)*.

An example of this approach includes unraveling the molecular processes underlying phage assembly. As attention has shifted in recent years to the biological events in more complicated organisms, geneticists using yeast, *C. elegans*, and *Drosophila* have adopted this approach and added some additional tools. The techniques fall largely into four categories of genetic screening: gene knockouts, enhancer/suppressor genetics, overexpression phenotypes, and synthetic lethals. An background overview of each type of technique is described in the following section. In addition, the facility with which the techniques can be performed in each of the three model organisms is discussed.

Gene Knockouts

Gene knockout experiments aim to disrupt a single gene and generate a null allele for a selected gene of interest. Organisms homozygous for the gene can be analyzed for phenotypes in which the organism is presumably wild-type except for the single missing gene. This technique was first demonstrated in yeast using homologous recombination *(34)*. The yeast success was matched shortly thereafter in mice *(35)*. It has not yet been translated to either *Drosophila* or *C. elegans*. This is at least partly due to the fact that large numbers of mouse embryonic stem (ES) cells can be screened for the recombination event. Selected ES cell clones are then used to make fully functional organisms. There is no ES cell equivalent in either *Drosophila* and *C. elegans*.

Fly and worm geneticists have resorted to using a random knockout approach together with the development of molecular screens to identify genes that are likely to be inactivated *(36,37)*. In these experiments, mutations are generated in the target organisms (either deletions or transposition insertion) and either PCR-based or Southern blot screens are used to detect genetic regions in the selected genes. Worms have the advantage in the fact that the organism can be stored frozen, then thawed, and be fully viable. This, in turn, means that maintaining large collections of frozen stocks is relatively trivial. Thus, it is less labor intensive to use reverse-genetic gene-knockout approaches in worms compared with flies, because all of the labor can go into screens instead of stock maintenance and because the experiments can be set aside for extended periods and reactivated with little effort. Furthermore, it raises the possibility of aggressively attempting to knock out every gene in *C. elegans*. The mutations, once uncovered, can be conveniently stored as frozen stocks. It seems likely that such a comprehensive task will be undertaken by the *C. elegans* research community. In contrast, such a task will likely not happen in *Drosophila* in the foreseeable future.

Enhancer/Suppressor Genetics

As mentioned in a previous section, the ability to revert an initial mutation by a second mutation in another gene has long been an essential genetic approach to identifying protein–protein interactions. Enhancer/suppressor experiments are conducted in an organism that already bears a mutation that confers an identifiable phenotype. Genetic screens are then conducted to examine the effects of new mutations when placed in the background of the first mutation. Enhancer mutations make the phenotype more severe. Suppressor mutations minimize the severity or eliminate the phenotype. Frequently, mutations of this class display a dominant phenotype in the context of enhancing or suppressing the phenotype under observation, but will be recessive in a wild-type background (in which the first gene is wild-type). This is critically important if the second site mutation is lethal—as it is still recoverable in the context of the original mutation.

Enhancer/suppressor screens have been extended to genetic analysis in all three of the organisms under consideration in this discussion. The *Drosophila* system has two advantages. First, transgenic systems can be set up so that the screens are now being done in dosage-dependent genetic systems which makes the screens extremely sensitive. Second, the screens can be established in surface tissues such as the eye that are easy to score in large numbers. On the other hand, screens in *C. elegans* have the advantage that the organism is a hermaphrodite and both dominant and recessive modifiers can be easily recovered.

It seems likely that the slow step in the process will be cloning the corresponding mutations. This should be dramatically simplified once the genome of the organism is completely sequenced. This should happen soon for *C. elegans* but is still 3–4 yr away for *Drosophila*.

Experiments in academic laboratories using these approaches have revealed a surprising cross-species conservation of pathways *(38,39)*. In other words, it is not just molecules that are conserved but also the underlying interactions that make complicated processes possible. Screens for suppressors of individual mutations have the potential to uncover numerous different interacting molecules *(40)*. In many cases, these molecules can be used to identify corresponding elements of interacting mammalian proteins.

Overexpression and Misexpression

It is becoming clear that traditional loss of function genetic analysis (knockout mutations are the directed form of this type of analysis) frequently fails to demonstrate an easily identifiable phenotype, making functionality of the corresponding gene product difficult to decipher. It has been suggested that as many as two-thirds of the genes in worms and flies, and possibly a greater fraction in mice, fall into this category. In other words, disabling mutations in most genes are silent under laboratory conditions.

One approach being applied to systematically remedy this situation is to perform screens for genes that are conditionally overexpressed or misexpressed *(41)*. The strategy is built on the discovery of important phenotypes, that were otherwise unobserved, by natural mutations that cause overexpression or misexpression (including the homeotic genes of *Drosophila* and tumor-causing oncogenes in mammalian systems). These approaches have been used in yeast for a number of years and are now emerging in *Drosophila*. They are particularly powerful in *Drosophila* as they can be generated by moving well-characterized and regulatable gene-expression cassettes through the genome by P-element-mediated transposition. These overexpression screens can be used as a mutagenic scheme, instead of chemical mutagenesis, in situations where the readout for phenotypic analysis is the enhancement or suppression of dosage-dependent phenotypes as described previously.

Synthetic Lethals

This synthetic lethal screen has recently been developed to characterize genes for which a null alleles is silent *(30)*. A possible cause of "silence of the phenotypes" might be that many pathways are functionally redundant. DNA proofreading and repair offer a good example. There are two proofreading mechanisms involved in DNA synthesis and null mutations in either gene are nonlethal. Null mutations in both genes, simultaneously, in the same individual are lethal. Presumably the mutation rate becomes too high only in the context of the double mutant.

Synthetic lethal screens have been most extensively applied in yeast. The goal of the synthetic lethal screen is to find a situation in which the nonessential gene of interest is made essential. The manner in which it is made essential is to generate a loss of function allele in its redundant pathway. In the context of a disabled alternate pathway, the original pathway becomes essential.

Synthetic lethal screens are performed based on the notion that a situation can be generated by mutagenesis in which maintenance of the original "silent" gene is critical for yeast cell survival. Maintenance of the "silent" gene is scored by linking it to a gene that confers a phenotype, such as colony color. For example colonies will be red if they are in a genetic background in which the original silent gene is maintained, and they will be white in conditions under which the gene is lost.

The screen is performed in the following fashion. The chromosomal copy of the gene of interest is knocked out, and two plasmids are then generated. Both plasmids are unstable and easily lost unless under some type of selective pressure. Selective pressure is applied so that one of the plasmids must be maintained but not both. One plasmid carries a copy of the wild-type gene as well as a marker gene that, when present, turns the yeast cell red (under appropriate conditions). The second plasmid carries a disabled copy of the gene of interest. The yeast strain is then mutagenized. In those cells in which a mutation has knocked out the corresponding redundant pathway, the "silent" gene becomes essential, thus maintaining the plasmid with the wild-type gene linked to the chromogenic gene, and the colonies take on a red color. On the other hand, in cases where a redundant pathway is still intact (the mutation strikes elsewhere in the genome), either plasmid can be lost and they are lost in a random fashion that leads to a sectored colony that is a mixture of red and white clones.

Synthetic lethal screens are likely to emerge in experiments based on *C. elegans* and *Drosophila*. However, it is likely that *C. elegans* will prove to be the better model system for this approach because it offers an easier way to uncover recessive mutations with the use of hermaphrodites.

Summary

In the past, a major rate-limiting step in the drug discovery process has been the ability to identify molecular targets that are involved with distinct pathophysiological processes. With the development of high-throughput genomics, it is inevitable that there will be a long list of candidate targets *(42)*. It is likely two significant challenges will emerge with the application of these new critical technologies.

First, it will be important to frame the experimental questions precisely enough so that the most effective targets can be found. For example, genome-wide transcript imaging is already being used to study transcriptional differences in cancer cells compared with normal cells. Hundreds of differentially expressed genes are being discovered *(14,43)*. The critical distinction to make is that in the sea of potential targets, it is essential to seek the most optimal one. In selecting the best likely target, the biochemical nature of the protein is important because some proteins provide more facile targets for the synthesis and screening of small molecule inhibitors.

The second important criterion has to do with validation. Will inhibition of that protein provide a therapeutic effect? High-throughput approaches for validation will need to be developed to keep up with the new ability to generate hundreds or thousands of target candidates.

References

1. Velculescu V, Zhang L, Vogelstein B, Kinzler KW. Serial analysis of gene expression. *Science.* 1995; 270:484–7.
2. Liang P, Bauer D, Averboukh L, et al. Analysis of altered gene expession by differential display. *Methods Enzymol.* 1995; 254:304–21.
3. Liang P, Pardee AB. Differential display of eukaryotic messenger RNA by means of the polymerase chain reaction. *Science.* 1992; 257:967–71.
4. Bachem CW, van der Hoeven RS, de Bruijn SM, Vreugdenhil D, Zabeau M, Visser RG. Visualization of differential gene expression using a novel method of RNA fingerprinting based on AFLP: analysis of gene expression during potato tuber development. *Plant J.* 1996; 9:745–53.
5. Habu Y, Fukada-Tanaka S, Hisatomi Y, Iida S. Amplified restriction fragment length polymorphism-based mRNA fingerprinting using a single restriction enzyme that recognizes a 4-bp sequence. *Biochem Biophys Res Commun.* 1997; 234:516–21.
6. Money T, Reader S, Qu LJ, Dunford RP, Moore G. AFLP-based mRNA fingerprinting. *Nucleic Acids Res.* 1996; 24:2616–7.
7. Prashar Y, Weissman SM. Analysis of differential gene expression by display of 3′ end of restriction fragments of cDNAs. *Proc Natl Acad Sci USA.* 1996; 93:659–63.
8. Vos P, Hogers R, Bleeker M, et al. AFLP: a new technique for DNA fingerprinting. *Nucleic Acids Res.* 1995; 23:4407–14.
9. Pease AC, Solas D, Sullivan EJ, Cronin MT, Holmes CP, Fodor SP. Light-generated oligonucleotide arrays for rapid DNA sequence analysis. *Proc Natl Acad Sci USA.* 1994; 91:5022–6.
10. Wodicka L, Dong H, Mittmann M, Ho MH, Lockhart DJ. Genome-wide expression monitoring in *Saccharomyces cerevisiae. Nat Biotechnol.* 1997; 15:1359–67.
11. Schena M, Shalon D, Davis RW, Brown PO. Quantitative monitoring of gene expression patterns with a complementary DNA microarray. *Science.* 1995; 270:467–70.
12. Shalon D, Smith SJ, Brown PO. A DNA microarray system for analyzing complex DNA samples using two-color fluorescent probe hybridization. *Genome Res.* 1996; 6:639 45.
13. Velculescu V, Zhang L, Zhou W, et al. Characteristics of the yeast transcriptome. *Cell.* 1997; 88:243–51.
14. Zhang L, Zhou W, Velculescu VE, et al. Gene expression profiles in normal and cancer cells. *Science.* 1997; 276:1268–72.
15. Bai C, Elledge SJ. Gene identification using the yeast two-hybrid system. *Methods Enzymol.* 1997; 283:141–56.
16. Chien CT, Bartel PL, Sternglanz R, Fields S. The two-hybrid system: a method to identify and clone genes for proteins that interact with a protein of interest. *Proc Natl Acad Sci USA.* 1991; 88:9578–82.
17. James P, Halladay J, Craig EA. Genomic libraries and a host strain designed for highly efficient two-hybrid selection in yeast. *Genetics.* 1996; 144:1425–36.

18. Aronheim A, Zandi E, Hennemann H, Elledge SJ, Karin M. Isolation of an AP–1 repressor by a novel method for detecting protein–protein interactions. *Mol Cell Biol.* 1997; 17:3094–3102.

19. Simon MA, Bowtell DD, Dodson GS, Laverty TR, Rubin GM. Ras1 and a putative guanine nucleotide exchange factor perform crucial steps in signaling by the sevenless protein tyrosine kinase. *Cell.* 1991; 67:701–16.

20. Zhang J, Lautar S. A yeast three-hybrid method to clone ternary protein complex components. *Anal Biochem.* 1996; 242:68–72.

21. Osborne MA, Dalton S, Kochan JP. The yeast tribrid system—genetic detection of trans-phosphorylated ITAM– SH2-interactions. *Bio/Technology.* 1995; 13:1474–8.

22. Tirode F, Malaguti C, Romero F, Attar R, Camonis J, Egly JM. A conditionally expressed third partner stabilizes or prevents the formation of a transcriptional activator in a three-hybrid system. *J Biol Chem.* 1997; 272:22995–9.

23. Sen Gupta DJ, Zhang B, Kraemer B, Pochart P, Fields S, Wickens M. A three-hybrid system to detect RNA-protein interactions in vivo. *Proc Natl Acad Sci USA.* 1996; 93:8496–8501.

24. Leanna CA, Hannink M. The reverse two-hybrid system: a genetic scheme for selection against specific protein/protein interactions. *Nucleic Acids Res.* 1996; 24:3341–7.

25. Vidal M, Braun P, Chen E, Boeke JD, Harlow E. Genetic characterization of a mammalian protein–protein interaction domain by using a yeast reverse two-hybrid system. *Proc Natl Acad Sci USA.* 1996; 93:10321–6.

26. Vidal M, Brachmann RK, Fattaey A, Harlow E, Boeke JD. Reverse two-hybrid and one-hybrid systems to detect dissociation of protein-protein and DNA-protein interactions. *Proc Natl Acad Sci USA.* 1996; 93:10315–20.

27. Jansen G, Hazendonk E, Thijssen KL, Plasterk RH. Reverse genetics by chemical mutagenesis in *Caenorhabditis elegans.* *Nat Genet.* 1997; 17:119–121.

28. Huang J, Schreiber SL. A yeast system for selecting small molecule inhibitors of protein-protein interactions in nanodroplets. *Proc Natl Acad Sci USA.* 1997; 94:13396–401.

29. Superti-Furga G, Jonsson K, Courtneidge SA. A functional screen in yeast for regulators and antagonizers of heterologous protein tyrosine kinases. *Nat Biotechnol.* 1996; 14:600–5.

30. Hartwell LH, Szankasi P, Roberts CJ, Murray AW, Friend SH. Integrating genetic approaches into the discovery of anticancer drugs. *Science.* 1997; 278:1064–8.

31. Bender A, Pringle JR. Use of a screen for synthetic lethal and multicopy suppresser mutants to identify two new genes involved in morphogenesis in *Saccharomyces cerevisiae.* *Mol Cell Biol.* 1991; 11:1295–1305.

32. Luban J, Goff SP. The yeast two-hybrid system for studying protein–protein interactions. *Curr Opin Biotechnol.* 1995; 6:59–64.

33. Wong C, Naumovski L. Method to screen for relevant yeast two-hybrid-derived clones by coimmunoprecipitation and colocalization of epitope-tagged fragments—application to Bcl-xL. *Anal Biochem.* 1997; 252:33–39.

34. Jarvik J, Bolstein D. Conditional lethal mutations that suppress genetic defects in morphogenesis by altering structural proteins. *Proc Natl Acad Sci USA.* 1975; 72:2738–42.

35. Scherar S, Dawis RW. Replacement of chromosome segments with altered DNA sequences constructed in vitro. *Proc Natl Acad Sci USA.* 1979; 76:4951–5.

36. Zimmer A, Gruss P. Production of chimaeric mice containing embryonic stem (ES) cells carrying a homeobox *Hox1.1* allele mutated by homologous recombination. *Nature.* 1989; 339:150–3.

37. Plasterk RH. Reverse genetics of *Caenorhabditis elegans.* *Bioessays.* 1992; 14:629–33.

38. Jarriault S, Brou C, Logeat F, Schroeter EH, Kapan R, Isreal A. Signalling down stream of activated mammalian notch. *Nature.* 1995; 377:355–8.

39. Karim FD, Chang HC, Therrien M, Wassarman DA, Laverty T, Rubin GM. A screen for genes that function downstream of Ras1 during *Drosophila* eye development. *Genetics.* 1996; 143:315–29.

40. Verheyen EM, Purcell KJ, Fortini ME, Artavanis-Tsakonas S. Analysis of dominant enhancers and suppressors of activated Notch in *Drosophila. Genetics.* 1996; 144:1127–41.

41. Rorth P. A modular misexpression screen in *Drosophila* detecting tissue-specific phenotypes. *Proc Natl Acad Sci USA.* 1996; 93:12418–22.

42. Broach JR, Thorner J. High-throughput screening for drug discovery. *Nature.* 1996; 384:14–16.

43. DeRisi J, Penland L, Brown PO, et al. Use of a cDNA microarray to analyse gene expression patterns in human cancer. *Nat Genet.* 1996; 14:457–60.

16

Emerging Molecular Therapies for Cancer

Karol Sikora

Overview

Over the next 25 yr there will be major changes in the patterns of cancer incidence as the age distribution shifts in the population. Early detection and the ability to tailor treatments to the genetic characteristics of the tumor can be expected to improve cure rates. New diagnostic techniques involving molecular genetics will almost certainly allow the identification of high-risk groups for intensive screening and the application of preventive interventions. Early diagnosis will be enhanced by new imaging technology, based on computerized three-dimensional reconstruction together with novel tumor markers.

The main modalities of treatment will improve. Surgery will involve increasing organ preservation relying on minimally invasive techniques, computer-assisted virtual reality systems, and robots. Eventually conventional surgery, with its associated tissue destruction, will be replaced entirely with this approach. Radiotherapy will develop through multimedia imaging of tumor and normal tissues using computer optimization to obtain the best physical and biological therapeutic ratio. Designer fractionation based on individually predicted differential sensitivity to radiation will be possible through a greater understanding of the genes involved in DNA repair.

Novel systemic therapies are likely to have the greatest impact on cancer mortality. A new golden age of drug discovery is likely with the logical design of small molecules interfering with specific targets such as signal transduction, transcription control, mitosis, and apoptosis. One of the greatest challenges will be caring for people with cancer using the new technology in the face of declining organized religion and cohesive family structures. An increasing number of patients will neither die from their cancer nor be cured of it, but will have to learn to live with their disease, often being given complex therapies to control it for many years. The incidence of cancer will decrease drastically worldwide within the next 50 yr as a direct result of the application of individualized risk-reduction strategies together with genetic correction of high-risk groups. This will concentrate treatment resources for those under 70 yr who develop the disease.

From: *Principles of Molecular Oncology*
Edited by: M. H. Bronchud, M. A. Foote, W. P. Peters, and M. O. Robinson © Humana Press Inc., Totowa, NJ

**Table 1
Rare Clinical Syndromes Associated
with Increased Specific Cancer Risk**

Syndrome	Tumors
Ataxia–telangiectasia	Lymphoma, leukemia
MEN 1	Parathyroid, pancreas, pituitary
MEN 2A	Thyroid, pheochromocytoma
Familial polyposis coli	Colorectal
Von Hippel–Lindau	Renal cell, angiomas
Neurofibromatosis type 1	Neurofibroma, glioma

MEN = multiple endocrine neoplasia

Introduction

Most people who develop cancer are over 60 yr old. The biggest global demographic change predicted for the next 25 yr is a dramatic shift in the number of people over this age. Inevitably this will lead to an increase in cancer incidence. The UK Government Actuary's Department predicts that the number of people over 65 yr of age will have increased from 9.4 million in 1992 to 11.8 million in 2020 *(1)*. The World Health Organization (WHO) estimates that over the next 25 yr there will be >100% increase in the number of people older than 60 yr in 31 countries. Although health education, screening, and possibly new prevention strategies could reduce the risks of lung, skin, and oropharyngeal neoplasms, the age shift is likely to dwarf all other factors affecting cancer incidence. Cancer is thus becoming a major health problem all over the world. This year more than 10 million people will develop the disease. Half will live in countries that between them have <5% of the world's cancer treatment resources. By the year 2020 the number of new patients each year will be a frightening 20 million. Developing and implementing a strategy to reduce the untold suffering this will cause is a daunting but urgent challenge. The exciting advances in our understanding of the molecular biology of cancer are poised to transform the whole discipline of oncology.

Genetic Predisposition and Cancer

Evidence that genetic background can increase the risk of developing cancer comes from three sources. First, the risk of cancer is greater among family members of patients with cancer. This is currently the most difficult observation to examine mechanistically as the number of genes involved and their functional abnormalities are diverse. Second, there are specific families with a very high incidence of particular forms of tumors. Such cancer families may contain mutated specific genes which increase cancer risk through various mechanisms. Some of the genes have been identified such as *TP53* in the Li–Fraumeni syndrome. Finally there are specific recognizable inherited clinical syndromes associated with rare cancer types such as multiple endocrine neoplasia (MEN) 1 with its high incidence of parathyroid, endocrine pancreatic, and anterior pituitary tumors (Table 1). A common feature in all types of familial cancer is its tendency to occur at an earlier age, to be multiple, and to occur bilaterally when paired organs exist *(2)*.

Table 2
Genes in Which Mutations May Carry
an Increased Risk of Breast Cancer

BRCA1	*TP53*
BRCA2	Androgen receptor
ATM	

Until now genetic risk assessment for cancer has been confined to the relatively rare inherited syndromes. This is likely to change dramatically over the next few years *(3)*. Gene hunting has already uncovered sets of genes that if mutated may result in increased cancer risk. Table 2 lists examples of such genes for breast cancer.

The Human Genome Project continues to provide detailed sequencing data *(4)*. It is estimated that the whole genome will be completed by 2005. Novel assays for DNA mutations that can be rapidly applied to tiny samples of human tissue are being developed. Finally, advances in information technology will lead to more powerful computer storage and retrieval of sequence-based information *(5)*.

There is considerable public concern about genetic-risk assessment. The use of genetic information for life insurance, health insurance, and job selection are areas of profound ethical debate. Furthermore, preimplantation diagnosis for known inherited cancer predisposing genes is already possible *(6)*. As knowledge of the human genome increases exponentially over the next decade it is likely that selection of low cancer incidence embryos will be feasible. Genetic information will be useful in identifying individually tailored screening programs leading to specific life-style advice, and if necessary, preventive interventions for individuals. Such interventions may include gene therapy in a prophylactic setting as well as ablative surgery and chemoprevention.

As well as determining the risk of developing cancer, similar technology will be used to assess prognosis and the choice of therapy. The pathway a tumor will evolve is determined by the somatic genetic changes that led to the malignant cell in the first place. "Molecular stamp collecting" and long-term computer analysis will almost certainly revolutionize clinical decision-making, especially with regard to choosing how aggressive to be to prevent recurrence.

Chemotherapy

The major current problem in cancer treatment is undetected metastatic disease at the time of primary therapy. For many of the common tumors our systemic treatments are inadequate and there have been essentially few advances over the last 50 yr (Table 3). Table 4 examines the current status of chemotherapy in patients with a variety of metastatic tumors.

The key problem in the effective treatment of patients with solid tumors is the similarity between tumor and normal cells. Local therapies such as surgery and radiotherapy can succeed, but only if the malignant cells are confined to the area treated. This is so in approximately one-third of cancer patients. For most, some form of systemic selective therapy is required. Although many cytotoxic drugs are available, only a small proportion of patients are actually cured by their use. The success stories associated

Table 3
Advances in Chemotherapy Over the Last 25 yr

Successful cure of some rare tumors
Adjuvant chemotherapy for certain patients with breast cancer, colon cancer, sarcomas, and
  childhood tumors
Adjuvant hormone therapy for breast cancer
Hormonal treatment for prostate cancer
High-dose chemotherapy for lymphomas and leukemias
Effective supportive care during chemotherapy administration
Better organization of chemotherapy delivery

Table 4
**Effectiveness of Chemotherapy in Patients
with Metastatic Cancer**

High CR–high cure	High CR–low cure	Low CR–low cure
Acute leukemia	Ovary	Pancreas
Hodgkin's disease	Breast	Colon
Choriocarcinoma	SCLC	NSCLC
Testicular	NHL	Glioma
Burkitt's lymphoma	Sarcomas	Prostate
Childhood	Head and neck	Stomach

CR, complete response; NHL, non-Hodgkin's lymphoma; SCLC, small-cell lung
cancer; NSCLC, non-small-cell lung cancer.

with Hodgkin's disease (HD), non-Hodgkin's lymphoma (NHL), childhood leukemia,
choriocarcinoma, and germ-cell tumors have just not materialized for the common
cancers such as those of the lung, breast, or colon *(7)*. Despite enormous efforts in
new drug development, clinical trials of novel drug combinations, the addition of
cytokines, high-dose regimens, and even bone marrow rescue procedures, the gains in
survival have been marginal. Against this disappointing clinical backdrop, information
on the molecular biology of cancer has had explosive growth. Although our knowledge
of growth control is still rudimentary, we have at last had the first glimpse of its
complexity. This has brought a new vision with which to develop novel selective
mechanisms to destroy tumors *(8)*.

The next decade should see a new golden age of drug discovery. This will not be
based on empirical screening programs as in the past, but on logical drug design using
molecular graphics to produce novel structures that will interfere with specific biological
processes vital for growth. These will include blocking and stimulating therapies for
signal-transduction pathways, inactivators of oncogene products, the use of high
throughput screens to discover small molecules to mimic TSGs, transcription control
inhibitors for specific genes, selective activators of apoptosis, cell-cycle inhibitors, and
effective antimetastatic drugs *(9)* (all these topics have been discussed in detail in other
chapters of this book). These processes have evolved to use very similar pathways in

a wide range of organisms. Thus studying the molecular genetics of a specific functional process in yeast or the worm often will shed light on the human equivalent. The construction of knockout or transgenic animals, in which a specific genetic change is artificially created, allows the exploration of that gene's precise function. It is also likely that model systems will be developed to explore the use of direct genetic intervention for the treatment and perhaps even prevention of cancer before clinical trials.

Gene Therapy

Gene therapy involves the use of specific genetic sequences to treat a disease. The main problem facing the gene therapist in dealing with cancer is how to get new genes into every tumor cell. If this cannot be achieved, then any malignant cells that remain unaffected will emerge as a resistant clone. Presently no ideal vectors exist. Despite this drawback, there are already more than 300 protocols accepted for clinical trials in more than 2000 cancer patients worldwide, most in the U.S. The ethical issues are fairly straightforward, with oncology providing some of the highest possible benefit–risk ratios. Several strategies are currently under investigation.

Genetic Tagging

The use of a genetic marker to tag tumor cells may help in making decisions on the optimal treatment for an individual patient. The insertion of a foreign marker gene into cells from a tumor biopsy and replacing the marked cells into the patient before treatment can provide a sensitive new indicator of minimal residual disease after chemotherapy *(10)*. The commonest marker is the gene for neomycin phosphotransfer-ase—the *neo R* gene, an enzyme that metabolizes the aminoglycoside antibiotic G418. This gene, when inserted into an appropriate retroviral vector, can be stably incorporated into the host cell's genome. Originally detected by antibiotic resistance, it can now be picked up more sensitively by means of the polymerase chain reaction (PCR). In this way as few as one tumor cell among one million normal cells can be identified. This procedure has helped in the design of aggressive chemotherapy protocols in leukemia and neuroblastoma *(10)*. It has also proven valuable in elucidating the reasons for relapse after autologous bone marrow or stem cell transplantation where recurrent tumor samples can be examined for tagged genes inserted into donor infusions.

Enhancing Tumor Immunogenicity

The presence of an immune response to cancer has been recognized for many years. The problem is that human tumors seem to be predominantly weakly immunogenic. If ways could be found to elicit a more powerful immune stimulus, then effective immunotherapy could become a reality. Several observations from murine tumors indicate that one reason for weak immunogenicity of certain tumors is the failure to elicit a T-helper cell response. This in turn releases the necessary cytokines to stimulate the production of cytolytic T cells that can destroy tumors. The expression of cytokine genes such as interleukin-2 *(IL-2)*, tumor necrosis factor *(TNF)*, and interferon *(IFN)* in tumor cells has been shown to bypass the need for T-helper cells in mice. Similar clinical experiments are now in progress. Melanoma cells have been prepared from biopsies and infected with retrovirus containing the *IL-2* gene. These cells are being used as a vaccine to elicit a more powerful immune response *(11)*.

Table 5
Cloned Genes and Their Promoters May Be
Isolated and Coupled to Drug-Activating Genes for
Selective Expression in Either Tumors or Nonessential Tissues

Selective gene	Tumor
Carcinoembryonic antigen	Colorectal cancer, other epithelial tumors
α-Fetoprotein	Hepatoma, germ cell tumors
Neuron-specific enolase	Small-cell lung cancer
Prostate-specific antigen	Prostate cancer
Thyroglobulin	Thyroid carcinoma
Tyrosinase	Melanoma
Polymorphic epithelial mucin	Breast cancer
c-*erbB2*	Breast and gastrointestinal cancer
c-*erbB3*	Breast cancer
c-*erbB4*	Breast and gastric cancer
Tissue factor	Pancreatic
DD-PCR identified	Many types

DD-PCR, death domain polymerase chain reaction.

Vectoring Cytokines to Tumors

Cytokines such as the IFNs and ILs have been actively explored for their tumoricidal properties. Although there is evidence of cytotoxicity, their side effects are profound, which limits the dose that can safely be administered. It is possible to insert cytokine genes into cells that can potentially home in on tumors and so release a high concentration of their protein product locally. *TNF* genes have been inserted into tumor-infiltrating lymphocytes (TILs) from patients with melanoma and given systemically. These experiments are controversial for two reasons. First, it appears from in vitro studies that the amount of *TNF* expressed from such cells was unlikely to be sufficient to cause a significant cytotoxic effect, and second, the insertion of a foreign gene limits the ability of the lymphocyte to target into tumor masses *(12)*. More than 20 patients have so far been treated at the U.S. National Cancer Institute (NCI) and formal publication of the results are still awaited.

Inserting Drug-activating Genes

The main problem with existing chemotherapy is its lack of selectivity. If drug-activating genes could be inserted that would be expressed only in cancer cells then the administration of an appropriate prodrug could be highly selective. There are now many examples of genes preferentially expressed in tumors. In some cases, their promoters have been isolated and coupled to drug-activating enzymes. Examples include α-fetoprotein (AFP) in hepatoma, prostate-specific antigen (PSA) in prostate cancer, and c-*erbB2* in breast cancer *(13)* (Table 5).

These promoters can be coupled to enzymes such as cytosine deaminase or thymidine kinase, thereby producing unique retroviral vectors that are able to infect all cells but can be expressed only in tumor cells. These suicide (or Trojan horse) vectors may not have absolute tumor specificity but this may not be essential—it may be possible to

Table 6
Cancer Gene Therapy, October 1998

	US–CD	Europe
Gene marking	54	19
Immunomodulation	62	27
DNA vaccine	28	14
Drug resistance	24	19
Drug activation	29	25
Anti-oncogene	19	9
Gene replacement	29	23
Total 371	235	136

CD = Canada.

perform a genetic prostatectomy or breast ductectomy—so effectively destroying all tumor cells as well as certain normal tissue.

Suppressing Oncogene Expression

The down-regulation of abnormal oncogene expression has been shown to revert the malignant phenotype in a variety of in vitro tumor lines. It is possible to develop in vivo systems such as the insertion of genes encoding for complementary (antisense) mRNA to that produced by the oncogene. Such antigenes specifically switch off the production of the abnormal protein product. Mutant forms of the c-*ras* oncogene are an obvious target for this approach. Up to 75% of human pancreatic cancers contain a mutation in the amino acid 12 of this protein, and reversal of this change in cell lines leads to the restoration of normal growth control. Clearly the major problem is to ensure that every single tumor cell gets infected. Any cell that escapes will have a survival advantage and produce a clone of resistant tumor cells. For this reason it may be that future treatment schedules will require the repetitive administration of vectors in a similar way to fractionated radiotherapy or chemotherapy.

Replacing Defective Tumor Suppressor Genes

In cell culture, malignant properties can often be reversed by the insertion of normal TSGs such as *RB-1, TP53,* and *DCC (14)*. Although TSGs were often identified in rare tumor types, abnormalities in their expression and function are abundant in common human cancers. As with antigene therapy, the difficulty in this approach lies in the delivery of actively expressed vectors to every single tumor cell in vivo. Nevertheless clinical experiments are in progress in lung cancer in which retroviruses that encode *TP53* genes are being administered bronchoscopically. Tumor regressions have been reported *(15)*.

Gene Therapy and Cancer

More than 300 gene therapy protocols for cancer are now active (Table 6). Most of the studies are being carried out in the U.S., but many other countries are increasing their efforts in this area. Table 7 shows the geographical distribution of current protocols and Table 8 examines the tumor types being studied. The emphasis on melanoma is

Table 7
Patients in Gene Therapy Trials, October 1998

USA	3134	Egypt	21
UK	207	Poland	20
Netherlands	134	Spain	19
Germany	136	Austria	18
Italy	124	Norway	15
France	96	Sweden	9
Canada	91	China	9
Switzerland	25	Finland	7

Table 8
Cancer Gene Therapy—Tumor-Specific Protocols, October 1998

Melanoma	73	Prostate	17
Glioma	49	Colon	16
Ovary	39	Head and neck	14
Breast	31	Mesothelial	9
Renal	29	Bladder	7
Lung	23	Pancreas	6
Neuroblast	16	Cervix	4

simply a reflection of its immunogenicity and the plethora of immunogene approaches being attempted. As the field matures, it is likely that protocols will reflect the pattern of cancer incidence and therefore be developed for the three commonest cancers: lung, breast, and colon. Figure 1 shows the dominance of cancer as a target disease for global gene therapy efforts.

Immunological Approaches

The last 10 yr have seen dramatic advances in our understanding of how human T lymphocytes recognize and in some situations destroy cancer cells. Major efforts are

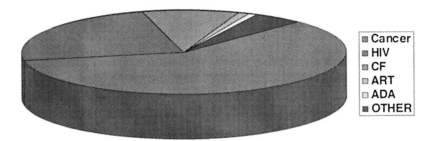

Fig. 1. Gene therapy October 1998, 4425 patients worldwide. HIV = human immunodeficiency virus; CF = cystic fibrosis; ART = arthritis; ADA = adenosine deaminase deficiency.

Table 9
Current Cancer Vaccines

Autologous cell lines	Stripped glycoproteins
Allogeneic cell lines	Peptides
Genetically modified tumor cells	Antitumor antibody idiotypes
Glycoproteins	Polynucleotides encoding tumor antigens

going into the development of various types of cancer vaccine using peptide, glycoprotein, antitumor antibody (Ab) idiotype antigens (Ags) as well as autologous or allogeneic tumor cell lines *(16)*. Polynucleotides encoding for various tumor-specific peptides have been claimed to raise a powerful immune response under certain situations.

Recently the successful cloning of cytolytic T cells (CTLs) has led to the identification of a series of antigenic peptides degraded from intracellular proteins and ending up in the clefts of major histocompatibility complex (MHC) molecules on the external surface of the cell. Three approaches have been used in their identification. Target cells transfected with cDNA libraries have been used to analyze specificity of CTL clones. This *genetic* approach was used to identify the MAGE series of melanoma Ags as well as MART, tyrosinase, and Melan-A. A *biochemical* strategy has been the separation and characterization of peptides from purified MHC molecules. A third approach has been the construction and analysis of the response to *synthetic peptides* that bind to MHC class I determinants *(17)*.

Phase 1 clinical trials are now in progress using several vaccine strategies (Table 9). Most involve direct peptide injection with immunological adjuvant but enhanced responses may be obtained by using autologous dendritic cells (DCs) pulsed with peptide Ags. Assays are available to measure immunological effectiveness of such vaccines so that optimization can be achieved before moving to larger scale phase 2 trials aimed at determining efficacy.

Conclusion

It is clear that there is tremendous potential for some very exciting advances in the prevention, diagnosis, and treatment of cancer over the next few years. Never before has so much information been available about the disease at a basic level. Looking 50 yr ahead is difficult. By then the Human Genome Project will be completed with rapid DNA sequence comparisons routinely possible by general practitioners using arrays of gene chips in their offices. Patients will seize control of their health both for prevention and treatment. The global burden of cancer will start decreasing by the year 2015, although the number of new patients will be increasing through the effects of aging. In the second half of the next century, cancer will be a relatively rare illness in the developed world although, sadly, it will continue to increase in poorer countries. The emerging molecular therapies offer considerable hope for the future not just for cancer patients but in all branches of medicine.

References

1. Our Vision for Cancer. Imperial Cancer Research Fund, London, 1995.

2. Ponder BA. Genetics of malignant disease. *Br Med Bull.* 1994; 50:517–752.

3. Markham AF, Coletta PL, Robinson PA, Clissold P, Taylor GR, Carr IM, Meredith DM. Screening for cancer predisposition. *Eur J Cancer.* 1994; 30:2015–29.

4. Strachan T. *The Human Genome.* Bios Scientific, Oxford, 1994.

5. Farzaneh F, Cooper DN. *Functional Analysis of the Human Genome.* Bios Scientific, Oxford, 1995.

6. Gullick W, Handyside A. Preimplantation diagnosis of inherited predisposition to cancer. *Eur J Cancer.* 1994; 30:2030–41.

7. Sikora K, Price P. *Treatment of Cancer.* Chapman and Hall, London, 1995.

8. Varmus H, Weinberg RA. *Genes and the Biology of Cancer.* Scientific American Library, New York, 1993.

9. Sporn M. The war on cancer. *Lancet.* 1996; 347:1377–81.

10. Brenner MK, Rill DR, Moen RC, et al. Gene marking to trace origin of relapse after autologous bone marrow transplantation. *Lancet* 1993; 341:85–86.

11. Fearon ER, Pardoll DM, Itaya T, et al. Interleukin 2 production by tumor cell bypasses the T helper cell function in the generation of an antitumor response. *Science* 1991; 254:713–6.

12. Rosenberg SA. Gene therapy for cancer. *JAMA* 1992; 268:2416–9.

13. Harris J, Guttierez A, Hurst H, Sikora K, Lemoine N. Gene therapy for cancer using tumour specific drug activation. *Gene Therapy* 1994; 1:170–7.

14. Baker SJ, Markowitz S, Fearon ER, Willson JK, Vogelstein B. Suppression of human colorectal carcinoma cell growth by wild type *p53*. *Science* 1990; 249:912–5.

15. Roth JA, Nguyen D, Lawrence DD, et al. Retrovirus-mediated wild-type *p53* gene transfer to tumors of patients with lung cancer. *Nat. Med.* 1996; 2:985–91.

16. James N, Sikora K. *Tumour Immunology,* 4th edit. (Lachmann P, Peters K, Walport M), Blackwell Scientific Publications, Oxford, 1993 pp. 1773–84.

17. Lewis JJ, Houghton AN. Definition of tumor antigens suitable for vaccine construction. *Semin Cancer Biol.* 1995; 6:321–7.

17

Emerging Molecular Therapies
Small-Molecule Drugs

Paul Workman

Introduction: The New Paradigm of Drug Discovery

The discovery and development of anticancer agents is undergoing revolutionary change. This change is characterized by the rapid transition from the classic cytotoxic and hormonal agents of the past toward drugs that are designed specifically to correct the precise molecular abnormalities that are responsible for the causation and progression of human tumors. Three major factors are contributing to this paradigm shift. The first is the recognition that further refinement of classic agents will not result in a step-jump in clinical utility. The second factor is our increasingly detailed understanding of the molecular pathology of cancer in terms of the genetic mutations, altered gene expression, and the resultant deregulation of cognate biochemical pathways. The third factor is the range of technologic breakthroughs used to accelerate contemporary drug discovery, particularly genomics, high-throughput screening, combinatorial chemistry, and modern structural biology.

The new paradigm of cancer drug discovery has been summarized *(1)* as: new genes → novel targets → innovative medicines.

The hypothesis to be tested is that greater efficacy and reduced side effects will result from the creation of therapies aimed at particular molecular targets that are responsible for driving the various key stages of cancer causation and malignant progression (Fig. 1): genetic instability, increased proliferation, aberrant cell-cycle control, reduced apoptosis, drug resistance, invasion, angiogenesis, and metastasis.

Throughout this book, one unifying theme has been presented: Cancer is a disease of faulty genes *(2)*. Genetic abnormalities in cancer range from point mutations, through small amplifications and deletions, to translocations and other gross chromosomal abnormalities *(3)*. Genetic instability and abnormality are the hallmarks of cancer cells, and the underlying mechanisms for this behavior are becoming increasingly clear *(3)*.

The mutations and pathologically deregulated gene expression changes lead to perturbations in signal transduction pathways responsible for malignancy. Thus, these cancer-causing gene and protein pathways provide the best opportunities for selective therapeutic intervention.

From: *Principles of Molecular Oncology*
Edited by: M. H. Bronchud, M. A. Foote, W. P. Peters, and M. O. Robinson © Humana Press Inc., Totowa, NJ

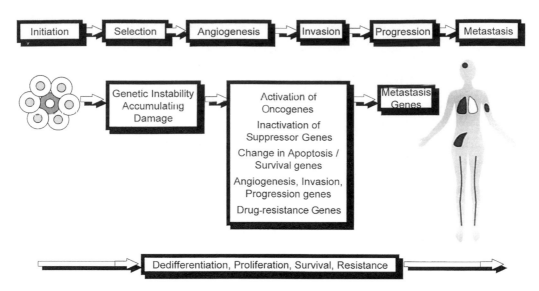

Fig. 1. Genes and potential drug targets in multistep oncogenesis.

Although this new paradigm of cancer drug discovery can also embrace antibody (Ab) targeting, gene therapy, and antisense oligonucleotide strategies, the scope of this chapter is restricted to approaches involving small molecules, commonly defined by a molecular mass cutoff of <500 kDa. Such agents hold advantages in terms of discovery, development, and pharmaceutical production *(4),* perhaps most particularly in terms of pharmacokinetics and tumor penetration *(5).* A further restriction on the scope of this chapter is the exclusive focus on proteins as molecular targets, which in turn reflects the current shift away from agents targeted at nucleic acids.

New Technologies to Overcome Bottlenecks in Small-Molecule Drug Development

There is a dual need to improve the quality of new anticancer drugs while concurrently accelerating the process of discovering and developing new drugs. Improvements in quality should result from the greater efficacy and reduced side effects expected from agents that are directed at innovative molecular targets responsible for the induction of cancer and malignant progression. Acceleration of the process of drug discovery and development will result from the extraordinary range of available new technologies.

Data for the 1990s show that it typically takes 15 yr to move the average drug (across all therapeutic areas) from initial discovery in the laboratory to marketing approval and thus to widespread patient availability *(6,7).* That average figure comprises 6.5 yr in preclinical development, 1.5 yr in phase 1 testing, 2 yr in phase 2 testing, 3.5 yr in phase 3 testing, and 1.5 yr in FDA review. The taxane antibulin agent Taxol® (paclitaxel) was discovered as a crude extract activity in 1963, but it did not obtain regulatory approval until 1992 *(8).* The aim of drug research must be to reduce discovery and development time scales to 5–7.5 yr or less, while simultaneously improving quality. In addition, the attrition rate must be reduced. Of every 5000–10,000 compounds evaluated preclinically, only 5 (0.1%) enter clinical trials, and of these, only 1 (20%)

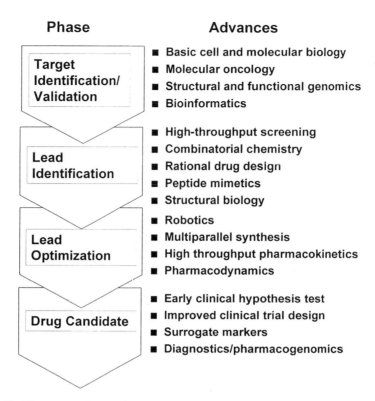

Phase

Target Identification/ Validation

Lead Identification

Lead Optimization

Drug Candidate

Advances

- Basic cell and molecular biology
- Molecular oncology
- Structural and functional genomics
- Bioinformatics

- High-throughput screening
- Combinatorial chemistry
- Rational drug design
- Peptide mimetics
- Structural biology

- Robotics
- Multiparallel synthesis
- High throughput pharmacokinetics
- Pharmacodynamics

- Early clinical hypothesis test
- Improved clinical trial design
- Surrogate markers
- Diagnostics/pharmacogenomics

- Discovery timescales will shorten
- Early bottleneck will shift from gene and target identification to assignment of function and validation
- Later bottleneck will shift from lead identification and in vitro optimization to optimization of in vivo properties
- Early clinical decision points will be key
- Pharmacogenomics will impact throughout the process

Fig. 2. Schema showing phases of small-molecule drug discovery, the technical advances impacting these phases, and the consequences arising from their implementation, particularly in terms of time scales and bottlenecks.

gains regulatory approval, at a cost of about $500 million *(6,7)*. Since development costs increase considerably during the clinical evaluation phase, an improvement in the success rate for agents entering that phase would be particularly desirable. However, advances in all stages of the drug-discovery process can contribute to enhanced overall efficiency.

Figure 2 shows the various phases of the drug discovery and development process from the identification and validation of the target, via identification and optimization of the small-molecule lead acting on that target, through to selection and development of the clinical candidate. Also shown are the technical advances that are improving the efficiency of each phase and the impact that introduction of these advances has on the bottlenecks in the system.

Table 1
Factors Affecting the Choice of Target

Frequency of pathologic deregulation (e.g., mutation or overexpression) in the disease
Linkage of target locus to disease progression (e.g., clinical outcome)
Expression and function of target locus in normal tissues
Creation of malignant phenotype by mutation or abnormal expression in a model
Reversal of malignancy by correction of the genetic abnormality
   Gene knockout/transfection
   Antisense
   Antibody
   Dominant negative
   Peptide
   Small molecules
Technical feasibility of target modulation (art of the soluble)

As a result of the activities of the Human Genome Project and the attendant improvements in high-throughput sequencing *(9)* and gene expression analysis *(10)*, all of the potential 100,000 human genes may be known by the year 2002–2005 *(11,12)*. As gene discovery gets faster and in due course genome closure is completed (i.e., all genes are identified and sequenced), the challenge and bottleneck becomes the assignment of biologic function to the cognate proteins and the validation of a proportion of these as targets for pharmacologic intervention. Validation will be aided by various improvements in genomics across all species and the use of powerful bioinformatics algorithms *(13–15)*.

In the cancer therapeutic area, molecular oncology studies are rapidly elucidating the changes in gene sequence and expression that are associated with the multistep progression of various tumors, as exemplified by colorectal cancer *(16)*. Use of gene microarrays and serial analysis of gene expression (SAGE) technologies allows the rapid elucidation of differences in gene-expression profiles in tumor vs normal cells *(10,17)* and high-throughput sequencing will enhance the rate of mutation detection *(18)*.

Of the predicted 100,000 human genes, 2000–10,000 have been projected as possibly suitable as drug targets across all major disease types *(19)*. Currently, the whole of medical treatment is based on drug action at only around 400–500 gene products. Based on an estimate of the number of key disease-related genes, say 5–10 of these for each of 100 important diseases, and multiplying this by 3–10 on the assumption that any one gene product interacts with that number of partner proteins in critical signal-transduction pathways, this predicts 3000–10,000 important drug targets, 10 times the current number of gene products. Given the number of oncogenes, tumor suppressor genes (TSGs), and the genetic-instability genes associated with cancer, it is reasonable to imagine several hundred new drug targets in oncology *(20)*.

Target validation has no absolute rules. When selecting new disease-associated genes to initiate drug-discovery projects, some simple rules of thumb can be helpful (Table 1). Those genes and pathways that are most commonly deregulated are likely to be the most fruitful *(21,22)*. An obvious example is the receptor tyrosine kinase (RTK) → Ras → Raf → MAP kinase (MAPK) pathway *(23)*. Deregulation of this pathway occurs by, for example, an overexpression of the kinase or mutation of the Kirsten *ras* (K-*ras*) gene. In fact, drugs that act on targets in this pathway already are beginning to enter the clinic. Thus RTK inhibitors and inhibitors of Ras farnesylation *(24)* are progressing through clinical trials. It should be noted that both of these are enzyme targets. Enzymes are excellent examples of pharmacologically tractable targets. The technical feasibility of finding small-molecule inhibitors of enzymes is very high because of the presence of a well-defined small molecule-binding site. By contrast, the feasibility of discovering small-molecule inhibitors of large-domain protein–protein interactions (e.g., those involving SH2 domains) is very low *(21)*. This aspect of technical feasibility should always be taken into account when selecting drug targets.

As a result of genomics and molecular oncology research, cancer targets for the development of small-molecule drugs will not be in short supply. What then are the bottlenecks downstream of target identification and validation?

As a result of remarkable improvements in combinatorial chemistry for the production of large compound libraries *(25)*, in high throughput screening *(26,27)*, and in molecular design aided by structural biology *(28)*, the discovery of leads that bind to and act on the desired target is no longer a rate-limiting step. Furthermore, optimizing small-molecule research leads to generate agents that are potent and selective and that act on the target in intact cells by the desired mechanism is in most cases no longer rate limiting. What commonly is limiting is the ability to efficiently optimize in vivo behavior in terms of pharmacokinetic and pharmacodynamic properties in the whole animal *(29)*. The current, and pragmatic, approach to overcome this serious bottleneck is to increase the throughput of pharmacokinetic and metabolic analysis (e.g., using cassette dosing of multiple compounds at low doses coupled with very sensitive high-performance liquid chromatography–mass spectrometry (HPLC–MS–MS) detection *(30)*. The accumulating database of information of quantitative structure–pharmacokinetic relationships (e.g., *31–34*) eventually should lead to the development of predictive chemoinformatics. Models giving faster in vivo readouts of pharmacodynamic activity, possibly involving reporter genes in transgenic animals, also would add value. However, the rational design of robust drug-like character is likely to remain a major roadblock for drug discovery for the next several years. The difficulties associated with working with chemically reactive leads has been emphasized *(35)* but is not sufficiently well appreciated, especially in oncology, where chemically reactive agents have found past use as DNA-damaging agents. Application of criteria, such as Lipinski's rule of five, has proved valuable in the selection of high-quality small molecular starting points for lead optimization *(36)*. Useful rules of thumb for bioavailability include molecular mass <500 kDa, number of hydrogen bond donors (OH or NH groups) ≤ 5, number of nitrogen plus oxygen atoms ≤ 10, and C log P (a measure of lipophilicity) <5. These rules can be especially useful in cases in which oral bioavailability is likely to be required, as in agents that must be given chronically as daily doses.

Although most drug-discovery groups increasingly favor the establishment of mechanism-based screens to identify small molecules that act on a chosen molecular target, the National Cancer Institute (NCI) in vitro 60 human tumor cell-line panel provides a distinct but complementary screening approach *(27,37)*. Here, a unique pattern of cellular sensitivity is sought as an indication of potential activity on a distinct cell target. Deconvolution of an unknown molecular target can be very challenging *(38,39)* but is assisted by the molecular characterization of the cell panel. Ten mechanistically interesting agents arising from the 70,000 compounds tested in the 60-cell line panel are currently being progressed through preclinical and clinical development.

After identification of a quality small-molecule lead (*see above;* also ref. *40*) and the small-molecule lead's optimization for in vivo pharmacokinetic and pharmacodynamic properties, the next important bottleneck in the drug development process (Fig. 2) is the transition from preclinical to clinical development. The selection of the optimal agent for clinical trial is not an exact science. Prediction of pharmacokinetic behavior in humans based on preclinical studies is not straightforward. Furthermore, the preclinical models for pharmacodynamics—in this case, the most commonly used are human tumor xenografts—have limited predictive value for conventional cytotoxic agents and unknown use for the new generation of molecularly targeted therapies *(41)*. Given the uncertainty surrounding the value of preclinical disease models and recognizing that new molecular targets inevitably carry high risk because of their lack of clinical precedent, the solution must be to take more agents into the clinic. This approach must be coupled concurrently with early mechanistic endpoints, so failing projects can be terminated early and resources reallocated to more promising areas.

In view of the number of targets emerging for small-molecule anticancer drugs, excellent cooperation will be needed between large pharmaceutical companies, the biotechnology industry, and academia to accelerate the discovery and development of innovative drugs. In the UK, the not-for-profit Cancer Research Campaign (CRC) has placed more than 40 new cancer drugs into phase 1 clinical trials since 1980 *(42)*, including Temodal® (temozolomide) which is now registered for the treatment of glioma *(43)*. CRC aims to progress five or more drugs annually into the clinic and move any one agent from the laboratory to the clinic in 12–18 mo. This period covers both pharmaceutical formulation and a rodent-only toxicology protocol that has proved both efficient and safe *(42)*.

Various approaches are available to improve the speed and quality of phase 1 clinical trials *(44)*, including pharmacokinetically guided dose escalation *(45,46)*, continual reassessment *(47)*, and accelerated titration designs *(48)*. Phase 1 trials of molecularly targeted therapies must involve not only the standard determination of the maximum tolerated dose, nature of the toxicity, pharmacokinetics, and possibly antitumor activity; they also must answer questions about the hypothesis being tested. In particular, is the desired pharmacodynamic effect being achieved at the target locus (e.g., kinase or farnesylation inhibition)? And is the desired biologic effect being obtained (e.g., apoptosis induction or angiogenesis inhibition)? Such assays may require biopsy followed by molecular analysis of RNA or protein. Alternatively, they may involve noninvasive methods, such as positron emission tomography (PET) or magnetic resonance imaging (MRI) *(49–52)*.

Inhibitors of Oncogenic Kinases: From Laboratory to Clinic

Kinase inhibitors are in the vanguard of agents that were developed using the new drug-discovery paradigm and that are now undergoing early clinical evaluation in humans. In many respects the development of kinase inhibitors encapsulates the generic challenges of developing small-molecule drugs against contemporary molecular targets in cancer. Because of learning points that can be picked up from the experience with

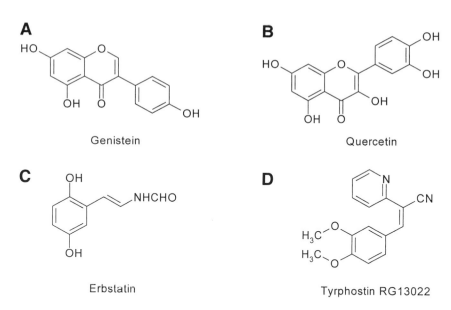

Fig. 3. Chemical structures of early tyrosine kinase inhibitors.

kinase inhibitors, their discovery and development is summarized in some detail. (For previous reviews of tyrosine kinase inhibitors, *see* refs. *53–57.)*

Why is kinase inhibition of such importance? The whole of cell biology is controlled by a series of protein–protein interactions and protein phosphorylation reactions *(58,59)*. Phosphorylation of proteins on the amino acids tyrosine, serine, threonine, and histidine changes their biologic properties. Enzymes called kinases catalyze these phosphorylation reactions. Hundreds of kinases are currently known, and an estimated 2000 (2%) of the expected 100,000 human genes may encode kinases. This number represents the largest family in the human genome. Moreover, of the 30,000 proteins expressed in the average cell, one-third will be phosphorylated. A typical kinase will phosphorylate 15 protein substrates.

Not surprisingly, evidence is accumulating that altered protein phosphorylation is involved in the pathology of many diseases, including various cancers. Many kinases function as oncogenes or are involved in the autocrine loops and signal-transduction pathways that contribute significantly to the malignant phenotype *(59)*.

Screening discovered a number of early kinase inhibitors. These inhibitors included antiproliferative natural products (e.g., erbstatin and the flavones genistein and quercetin) (Fig. 3). Such agents do inhibit protein phosphorylation in cells. On the other hand, they also exemplify the early concerns about the limitations of kinase inhibitors as potential drugs: that such agents would lack the desired potency and selectivity. Most kinase inhibitors are competitive with the ATP substrate. As a result, potency was thought to be limited by the high intracellular ATP concentration. Moreover, kinase structures were expected to be highly homologous, theoretically making it difficult to achieve a high degree of selectivity with an ATP-competitive drug. Because kinases are essential for normal cell function, lack of selectivity was seen as likely to lead to unacceptable toxicity.

The tyrphostin class of tyrosine kinase inhibitors, mainly based on the benzylidene malonitrile structure *(55)*, disproved this pessimistic prediction. For example, a high degree of selectivity could be demonstrated against the epidermal growth factor (EGF) RTK *(54)*. However, while demonstrating proof of principle for antiproliferative activity through the desired kinase inhibition mechanism in cancer cells *(60)*, tyrphostins were found deficient in drug-like properties and had many disadvantages as therapeutic agents for use in the whole animal *(54,61)*. These disadvantages *(54)* include potential for off-target effects (e.g., action on G-proteins, topoisomerases, and mitochondria); poor physiochemical properties (e.g., solubility and chemical instability); involvement of chemical reactivity (e.g., action as Michael acceptors in enzyme inhibition); potential for oxido–reduction, conjugation, and other metabolic pathways; generally poor pharma-cokinetic properties (e.g., short plasma half-life); and lack of convincing activity in vivo. The last two points are well exemplified by our studies on the relatively optimized tyrphostin RG13022 *(61)*.

A tyrphostin that shows promise is the agent AG-490 *(62)*, which exhibits selectivity toward Jak-2, a member of the Jak family of tyrosine kinases. Leukemic cells from patients acute lymphoblastic leukemia (ALL) in relapse have constitutively activated Jak-2 tyrosine kinase. AG-490 was shown to block leukemic cell growth in vitro and in vivo by induction of apoptosis, without causing adverse effects on normal hematopoiesis. Jak-Stat signaling also may be a target in certain solid tumors.

Tyrphostins led to the search for more drug-like chemical types as tyrosine kinase inhibitors. Success was achieved for combining high-throughput mechanism-based screening against chemical libraries combined with X-ray structure/modeling. A high degree of potency (nanomolar to picomolar) and selectivity (orders of magnitude) were readily achieved with a range of chemotypes, and these properties are being increasingly understood in terms of structure–activity relationships and differences in kinase three-dimensional structures *(63)*. Similarly, translating these properties on the kinase target into activity in the intact tumor cell in tissue culture proved fairly straightforward. The major hurdle was again that of antitumor activity in vivo, which required optimization of physicochemical features and pharmacokinetics. The breakthrough in whole animal properties was exemplified by the anilinoquinazoline series and related pyrimidines (discussed later).

The EGF receptor emerged as the archetypal kinase target because of its involvement in proliferative signal transduction, its participation in autocrine loops in cancer cells, its oncogenic properties in preclinical models, its overexpression (and in some cases mutation) in a range of human tumors, and the correlation of this overexpression with disease outcome (e.g., in breast, squamous cell lung, and head and neck cancers) *(61)*. These results are consistent with EGFR playing a causal role in the malignant process.

4-Anilinoquinazolines have exciting potential as inhibitors of EGF receptor and other tyrosine kinases *(54,57,64–72)*. Agents of this chemotype (e.g., those shown in Fig. 4) were identified as inhibitors of the EGF receptor tyrosine kinase by targeted screening of diverse chemical libraries. Identification was aided by three-dimensional structural searching based on a transition state model (subsequently found to be erroneous). The lead structure A was enhanced to produce compounds such as B, which is highly potent and selective for the EGF receptor kinase. Compounds of this type could be prepared in a relatively simple four-step process, and robotic multiparallel synthesis was used

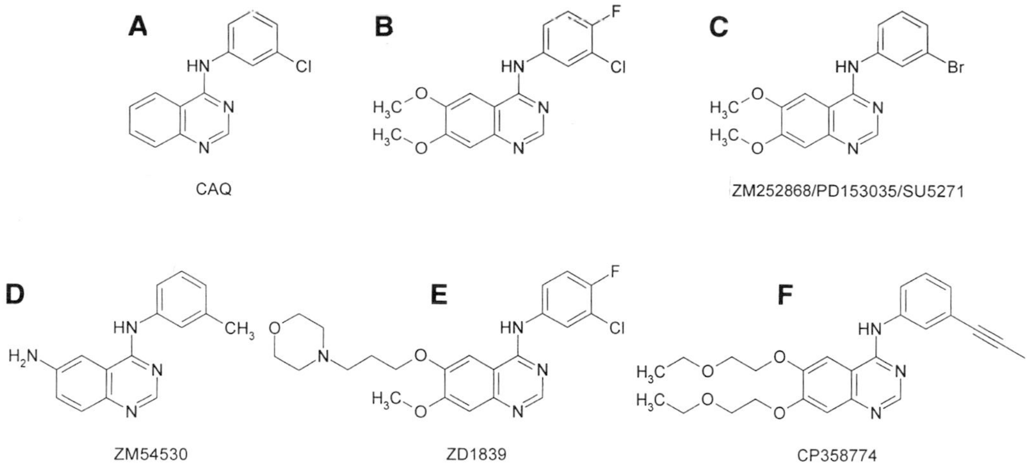

Fig. 4. Chemical structures of 4-anilinoquinazoline tyrosine kinase inhibitors.

to generate a compound library to define structure–activity relationships. The secondary amine group was essential, and substitution with electron-donating groups, such as methoxy in the 6- or 7-positions of the quinazoline ring, significantly enhanced activity. Similarly, substitution of the aniline rings with halogens in the meta position also was favorable. The combination of these, as in compound B, was supraadditive. These advantageous features also are present in ZM252868–PD153035–SU5271 (Fig. 4C). This compound was reported to have activity against xenografts in nude mice, but the physical properties of such an agent were not ideal for systemic activity in vivo. This compound, however, is being evaluated in a phase 1 trial as a topical agent for the treatment of psoriasis *(57)*.

Introduction of the 6-amino substitution gave ZM54530 (Fig. 4D). Although less potent against the kinase than several of the earlier structures, this compound had improved pharmacokinetic properties, resulting in in vivo activity in tumor models. Extensive optimization was done based on the pharmacokinetic profile. Although potency was greatest with methylamino or dimethylamino moieties in the quinazoline ring, drug absorption was preferable with the 6-aminopropoxy substitution. Excellent pharmacokinetic and antitumor properties were seen with ZD1839 (Fig. 4E), which incorporates a 7-methoxy and a solubilizing 6-morpholinylpropoxy functionality and also retains two halogens in the aniline ring. These substitutions improved physicochemical and pharmacokinetic properties, which in turn translate into impressive antitumor activity in animal models *(70)*. Studies in human volunteers showed an encouraging safety profile and oral bioavailability compatible with once-daily treatment *(71)*. This agent is now in phase 2 clinical trial. The very closely related compound CP358774 (Fig. 4F) has similar advantages and also is undergoing clinical development *(72)*.

The above-mentioned progressive improvements made in the anilinoquinazolines illustrate how limitations in potency, selectivity, and in vivo properties can be overcome. A combination of screening and modeling led to the identification of the lead series. Robotic synthesis was used to accelerate the understanding of structure–activity relationships. Achieving in vivo activity proved to be a problem, however. Improvement of

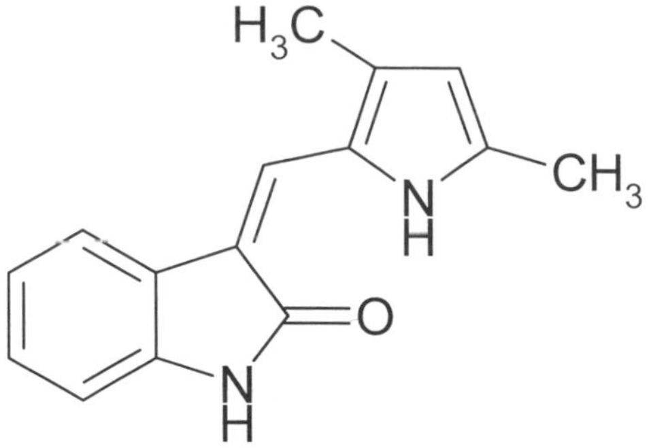

Fig. 5. Chemical structure of indolin-2-one VEGF receptor (Flk-1/KDR) tyrosine kinase SU5416.

physicochemical properties with solubilizing groups and the determination of both pharmacokinetic properties and of pharmacodynamic activity in a liver proliferation model allowed in vivo properties to be improved; xenograft tumor activity could then be achieved with sustained oral dosing. Such a regimen would be expected for an antiproliferative, cytostatic signal transduction inhibitor.

Several agents targeted to the inhibition EGFR and other tyrosine kinases are now entering phase 1 and phase 2 clinical trials *(57)*. These agents include anilinoquinazoline EGF RTK inhibitors ZD1839 and CP358,774, which have potential for activity in a wide range of tumors, including breast and non-small-cell lung cancer (NSCLC); platelet-derived growth factor (PDGF) RTK inhibitor SU101 (leflunomide) for the treatment of glioma and other cancers; substituted pyrimidine CGP57148, which inhibits the Abl and PDGF RTK and may find a place in treating leukemias as well as solid tumors; and antiangiogenic tyrosine kinase inhibitors, which have potential for broad-spectrum solid-tumor activity. This latter category includes indolinone SU5416 (Fig. 5), which blocks the Flk-1/KDR vascular endothelial growth factor (VEGF) RTK, and also a newer agent SU6668, which inhibits a wider range of kinase targets and hence has even greater potential to circumvent resistance; both agents are in phase 1 trial in the Cancer Research Campaign Centre at the Institute of Cancer Research and Royal Marsden Hospital.

Early results indicate that reasonable doses of tyrosine kinase inhibitors achieve good plasma levels without causing unacceptable toxicity. Establishment of the role of such agents in the treatment of various tumor types is ongoing. From small and unduly pessimistic beginnings, kinase inhibitor development is now a growth industry in its own right. Many pharmaceutical and biotech companies are involved in the area, including Sugen, Zeneca, Novartis, Pfizer, and Parke–Davis. Shortly, a large portfolio of inhibitors both of tyrosine kinases and of serine/threonine kinases will enter clinical trials. Interesting new kinase cancer targets include erbB2, Src, Raf, MEK, IGF1 receptor, Akt, PI3 kinase, met, JAKs, bcr-abl, and the cyclin-dependent kinases (CDKs).

Drugs that inhibit the serine/threonine CDKs are of particular interest because of their potential to restore normal cell cycle control, that has been lost through mutation or deletion of natural inhibitors (e.g., p16). Flavopiridol inhibits various CDKs and, having completed phase 1 with some evidence of activity, currently is in phase 2

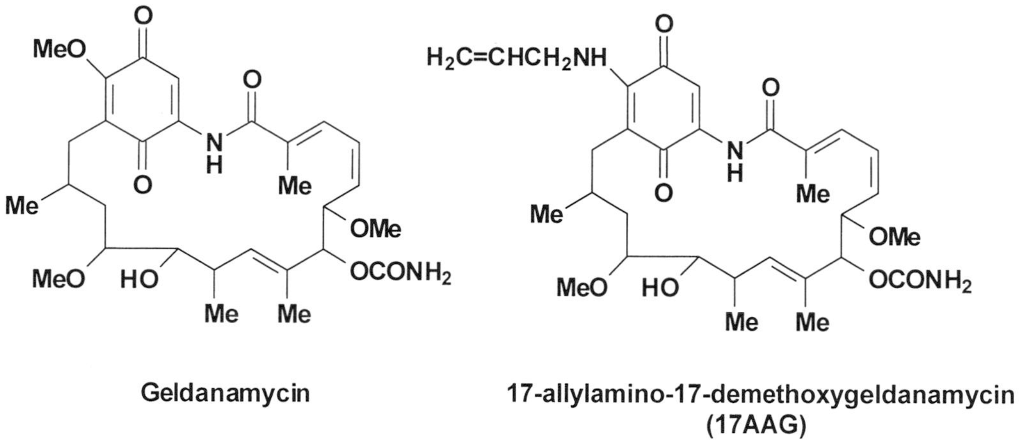

Fig. 6. Chemical structures of benzoquinone ansamycins.

clinical trial *(73)*. Aminopurine type agents related to olumoucine also are of interest because of their different spectrum of kinase selectivity *(74)*.

A recent observation has linked amplification of the chromosome region 3q26 in ovarian cancer with increased expression and activity of the pI3 kinase isotype pl10α *(75)*. This link implicates the gene as a potential oncogene in ovarian cancer and increases interest in inhibitors of the lipid kinase, which may act as inducers of apoptosis.

Geldanamycins as Depleters of Oncogenic Kinases through Hsp90 Inhibition

An interesting new approach to the blockade of kinase signaling is based on the discovery that the ansamycin benzoquinone class of agents, exemplified by the herbimycins and geldanamycins (Fig. 6), can bring about the simultaneous knockout of several important oncogenic tyrosine and serine/threonine kinases. These include Raf, erbB2, EGFR, and CDK4. This effect occurs not through inhibition of kinase catalytic activity but through degradation at the protein level by prevention of binding to the chaperone proteins Hsp90 and GRP94 *(76–78)*. Mutant p53 also is depleted. A proposed schema for the mode of action of Hsp90 inhibitors is shown in Fig. 7. A promising therapeutic ratio is seen with 17-allylamino-17-demethoxygeldanamycin (17AAG) in human tumor xenograft models. We are about to initiate a phase 1 clinical trial of the analogue 17AAG *(78)* in our center, in association with the NCI and the CRC. The phase 1 study will include molecular markers, including depletion of target oncogenic kinases and mutant p53 together with the enzymes DT-diaphorase, for which high-level expression leads to increased drug sensitivity, and the polymorphic cytochrome P450 isoform CYP3A4, which is responsible for a major metabolic route for 17AAG *(79)*.

Summary

The progressive unraveling of the mysteries of the molecular pathology of cancer is allowing an unprecedented acceleration of new therapies targeted to overcome or

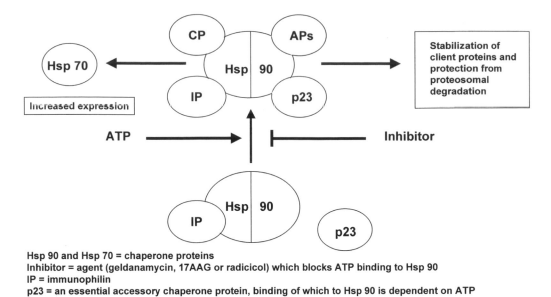

Hsp 90 and Hsp 70 = chaperone proteins
Inhibitor = agent (geldanamycin, 17AAG or radicicol) which blocks ATP binding to Hsp 90
IP = immunophilin
p23 = an essential accessory chaperone protein, binding of which to Hsp 90 is dependent on ATP
APs = other accessory proteins (eg Cdc37, Hip and Hop)
CP = client protein (eg Raf-1, erbB2, mutant p53)

Fig. 7. Proposed schema for mode of action of Hsp90 inhibitors.

exploit the precise abnormalities that are responsible for disease causation and progression. Because of their targeted mode of action, the expectation is that the successful therapies that emerge from the new paradigm of new genes → novel targets → innovative medicines will prove more effective and less toxic than traditional cancer chemotherapy.

Small-molecule drug approaches to molecular targets have many potential advantages over larger molecular-weight therapies (4). Most current medicine is based on the use of chemical agents with molecular masses <500 kDa. Small molecules are ideal for purposes such as intracellular enzyme inhibition. Higher molecular-weight agents are more likely to encounter difficulties associated with large-scale production, pharmaceutical formulation, and pharmacokinetics. Small-molecule therapeutics may have particular advantages over higher molecular-weight therapies (e.g., Abs and antisense agents) with respect to uptake into poorly vascularized regions of tumors and intracellular penetration (50). The current limiting factor in the success of gene therapy is widely recognized as delivery to the target cells. Thus small-molecule anticancer agents will continue to play an important role in new therapies directed toward novel cancer targets.

Contemporary technical breakthroughs are having a major impact on small-molecule drug development. Modern molecular biologic techniques and genomics are revolutionizing target identification and validation, although attribution of gene function probably will remain a bottleneck for some time. Robotic high-throughput screening coupled with large-compound libraries and combinatorial chemistry is revolutionizing the discovery of small-molecule leads that act on the desired target. Rational design is greatly improved by advances in modern structural biology, particularly X-ray crystallography and nuclear magnetic resonance (NMR) methods. Combinatorial chemistry together with advances in computational chemistry make the optimization of leads in terms of potency, selectivity, and drug-like properties much more efficient. Structure–activity relationships by nuclear magnetic resonance methods (SAR by NMR) have great potential. Breaking through the barrier that divides in vitro activity from activity in the intact animal remains a major rate-limiting step in drug development. Inadequate pharmacokinetics is usually the problem, and this problem is being addressed pragmatically by high-throughput cassette-dosing approaches. Eventually prediction of pharmacokinetic and in vivo behavior should be possible in a way that is not currently possible. Innovative phase 1 and 2 trial designs can accelerate safe early clinical trials. The use of both molecular and noninvasive endpoints will add value to the process and allow such clinical trials to test mechanistic hypotheses as well as fulfill the usual requirements.

Both the potential and the difficulties that are still associated with the development of small-molecule drugs are illustrated by the example of oncogenic kinase inhibitors. Agents that block the catalytic activity of kinases are leading the field of small-molecule drugs acting on novel molecular targets. Impressive anticancer activity has been demonstrated in animal models with kinase inhibitors and also with inhibitors of protein farnesylation *(24)* using sustained administration schedules. Toxicity has proved acceptable and the therapeutic margin or index is more than adequate to justify clinical studies. The well-tolerated profile of these emerging small-molecule signal-transduction inhibitors appears to have translated well into the clinical arena, suggesting that normal tissue toxicity may not be a major problem in humans.

Concluding Remarks

The era of molecularly targeted therapeutics allows us to envision a completely new approach to the treatment of cancer. We can entertain a vision of future chemotherapy in which the choice of drugs is dictated not by anatomical location and historical pragmatism but by the sequence and expression pattern of cancer-related genes and their cognate proteins in the particular patient's tumor.

Such a possibility is in fact exemplified by the recent FDA approval of a high-molecular-weight agent, namely the erbB2-targeted Ab Herceptin™ (trastuzumab) *(81)*. Approval was given for the treatment of those patients with metastatic breast cancer that have tumors overexpressing erbB2. Herceptin™ is indicated for first-line use in combination with Taxol® (paclitaxel) and as a second- or third-line single agent. This approval sets a precedent for the registration of therapeutic agents developed on the basis of gene expression abnormalities and their use in patients according to the level or nature of target expression. Whether this treatment will emerge as a general paradigm remains to be seen. It is unclear, for example, that sensitivity to small-molecule EGF RTK inhibitors is related to the level of receptor expression. At this stage it seems appropriate to collect information on target expression during early clinical studies so that any correlation can be examined. The evaluation of the genomics-based drug discovery paradigm and its subsequent application, where appropriate, will be facilitated by the development of gene microarray (e.g., chip) and proteomics technologies *(10,81)*.

Opportunities and challenges abound in the development of emerging therapies targeted to molecular abnormalities in tumor cells *(20,82)*. The opportunity is to discover a range of innovative agents that are highly effective and well tolerated. The challenge will be to develop these drugs rationally, with molecular endpoints, and to define their role in cancer and other diseases as we enter the post-genome era of molecular medicine.

Acknowledgments

This work was supported by the Cancer Research Campaign and the Institute of Cancer Research, UK. The author acknowledges the award of a Cancer Research Campaign Life Fellowship.

References

1. Workman P. Introduction: new anticancer drug design and discovery based on advances in molecular oncology. *Semin Cancer Biol.* 1992; 3:329–33.
2. Bishop JM. Molecular themes in oncogenesis. *Cell.* 1991; 64:235–48.
3. Lengauer C, Kinzler KW, Vogelstein B. Genetic instabilities in human cancers. *Nature.* 1998; 396:643–9.
4. Stevens MFG. Is there a future for the small molecule in developmental cancer therapy? In: *The Search for New Anticancer Drugs.* (Waring MJ, Ponder BAJ, eds.), Kluwer, Dordsecht, 1992, pp. 1–17.
5. Jain RK. Delivery of novel therapeutic agents in tumors: physiological barriers and strategies. *J Natl Cancer Inst.* 1989; 81:570–6.
6. PhRMA Web site. Available at: *http://www.phrma.org.* Accessed May 4, 1999.
7. Food and Drug Administration Web Site. Available at: *http://www.fda.gov/fdae/special/ne.* Accessed May 4, 1999.
8. Rowinsky EK, Donehower RC. Drug therapy: paclitaxel (Taxol®). *N Engl J Med.* 1995; 332:1004–14.
9. Lander ES. The new genomics: global views of biology. *Science.* 1996; 274:536–9.
10. *Nat* Genet. (Suppl.) 21, January 1999.
11. Collins FS, Patrinos A, Jordan E, Chakravarti A, Gesteland R, Walters L. New goals for the U.S. Human Genome Project: 1998–2003. *Science.* 1998; 282:682–9.
12. Waterston R, Sulston JE. The human genome project: reaching the finish line. *Science.* 1998; 282:53–54.
13. Anderson WF, Field C, Venter JC. Mammalian gene studies: editorial overview. *Curr Opin Biotechnol.* 1994; 5:577–8.
14. Harris TJ, Rosen CA. Editorial overview: genetics, genomics and drug discovery. *Curr Opin Biotechnol.* 1994; 5:637–8.
15. Murray-Rust P. Bioinformatics and drug discovery. *Curr Opin Biotechnol.* 1994; 5:648–53.
16. Fearon ER, Vogelstein B. A genetic model for colorectal tumorigenesis. *Cell.* 1990; 61:759–67.
17. Zhang L, Zhou W, Velculescu VE, et al. Gene expression profiles in normal and cancer cells. *Science.* 1997; 276:1268–72.
18. Hacia JG. Resequencing and mutational analysis using oligonucleotide microarrays. *Nat. Genet.* 1999; 21:42–47.
19. Drews J. Genomic sciences and the medicine of tomorrow. *Nat Biotechnol.* 1996; 14:1516–18.
20. Workman P. The potential for molecular oncology to define new drug targets. In: *New Molecular Targets for Cancer Chemotherapy* (Kerr DJ, Workman P, eds.), CRC Press, Boca Raton, FL, 1994, p. 1.
21. Gibbs JB, Oliff A. Pharmaceutical research in molecular oncology. *Cell.* 1994; 79:193–8.
22. Oliff A, Gibbs JB, McCormick F. New molecular targets for cancer therapy. *Sci Am.* 1996; September: 110–5.

23. Marshall CJ. Opportunities for pharmacological intervention in the ras pathway. *Ann Oncol.* 1995; 6(Suppl 1):S63–S67.

24. Lerner EC, Hamilton AD, Sebti SM. Inhibition of Ras prenylation: a signaling target for novel anti-cancer drug design. *Anticancer Drug Des.* 1997; 12:229–38.

25. Terrett NK, Gardner M, Gordon DW, Kobylecki RJ, Steele J. Combinatorial synthesis— the design of compound libraries and their application to drug discovery. *Tetrahedron.* 1995; 51:8135–73.

26. Bevan P, Ryder H, Shaw I. Identifying small-molecule lead compounds: the screening approach to drug discovery. *Trends in Biotechnology.* 1995; 13:115–21.

27. Workman P. Towards intelligent anticancer drug screening in the post-genome era? *Anticancer Drug Des.* 1997; 12:525–31.

28. Blundell TL. Structure-based drug design. *Nature.* 1996; 384:23–26.

29. Workman P. Pharmacokinetics and cancer: successes, failures and future prospects. *Cancer Surv.* 1993; 17:1–26.

30. Olah TV, McLoughlin DA, Gilbert JD. The simultaneous determination of mixtures of drug candidates by liquid chromatography/atmospheric pressure chemical ionization mass spectrometry as an in vivo drug screening procedure. *Rapid Commun Mass Spectrom.* 1997; 11:17–23.

31. Brown JM, Workman P. Partition coefficient as a guide to the development of radiosensitizers which are less toxic than misonidazole. *Radiat Res.* 1990; 82:171–90.

32. Workman P, Brown JM. Structure–pharmacokinetic relationships for misonidazole analogues in mice. *Cancer Chemother Pharmacol.* 1981; 6:39–49.

33. Mayer JM, van de Waterbeemd H. Development of quantitative structure–pharmacokinetic relationships. *Environ Health Perspect.* 1985; 61:295–306.

34. Rowland M. Pharmacokinetics-QSAR: definitions, concepts, and models. In *Quantitative Approaches to Drug Design* (Dearden JC, ed.), Elsevier, Amsterdam, 1983, pp. 155–61.

35. Rishton GM. Reactive compounds and in vitro false positives in HTS. *Drug Discov Today.* 1997; 2:382.

36. Current Drugs. Drug metabolism and pharmacokinetics symposium. ID *weekly highlights* Current Drugs Ltd, p. 25, September 1998.

37. Monks A, Scudiero DA, Johnson GS, Paull KD, Sausville EA. The NCI anti-cancer drug screen: a smart screen to identify effectors of novel targets. *Anticancer Drug Des.* 1997; 12:533–41.

38. Skelton LA, Ormerod MG, Titley J, Kimbell R, Brunton LA, Jackman AL. A novel class of lipophilic quinazoline-based folic acid analogues: cytotoxic agents with a folate-independent locus. *Br J Cancer.* 1999; 79:1692–701.

39. Bradshaw TD, Wrigley S, Shi DF, Schultz RJ, Paull KD, Stevens MF. 2-(4-Aminophenyl)benzothiazoles: novel agents with selective profiles of in vitro anti-tumour activity. *Br J Cancer.* 1998; 77:745–52.

40. Greengrass CW. Devising a research strategy. In: *Medicinal Chemistry: Principles and Practice* (King FD, ed.), Royal Society of Chemistry, Cambridge, 1994, pp. 179–188.

41. Gura T. Systems for identifying new drugs are often faulty. *Science.* 1997; 278:1041–2.

42. Burtles SS, Jodrell DI, Newell DR. Evaluation of "rodent only" preclinical toxicology for phase I trials of new cancer treatments—The Cancer Research Campaign (CRC) experience. *Proc Amer Assoc Cancer Res.* 1998; 39:363.

43. Newlands ES, Stevens MF, Wedge SR, Wheelhouse RT, Brock C. Temozolomide: a review of its discovery, chemical properties, pre-clinical development and clinical trials. *Cancer Treat Rev.* 1997; 23:35–61.

44. Graham MA, Kaye SB. New approaches in preclinical and clinical pharmacokinetics. *Cancer Surv.* 1993; 17:27–49.
45. Collins JM, Zaharko DS, Dedrick RL, Chabner BA. Potential roles for preclinical pharmacology in phase I clinical trials. *Cancer Treat Rep.* 1986; 70:73–80.
46. Graham MA, Workman P. The impact of pharmacokinetically guided dose escalation strategies in phase I clinical trials: clinical evaluation and recommendations for future studies. *Ann Oncol.* 1992; 3:339–347.
47. O'Quigley J, Pepe M, Fisher L. Continual reassessment method: a practical design for phase 1 clinical trials in cancer. *Biometrics.* 1990; 46:33–48.
48. Simon R, Freidlin B, Rubinstein L, Arbuck SG, Collins J, Christian MC. Accelerated titration designs for phase I clinical trials in oncology. *J Natl Cancer Inst.* 1997; 89:1138–47.
49. Maxwell RJ. New techniques in pharmacokinetic analysis of cancer drugs III: nuclear magnetic resonance. *Cancer Surv.* 1983; 17:415–423.
50. Tilsley DW, Harte RJ, Jones T, et al. New techniques in the pharmacokinetic analysis of cancer drugs. IV. Positron emission tomography. *Cancer Surv.* 1993; 17:425–42.
51. Workman P, Maxwell RJ, Griffiths JR. Non-invasive MRS in new anticancer drug development. *NMR Biomed.* 1992; 5:270–2.
52. Workman P. Bottlenecks in anticancer drug discovery and development: in vivo pharmacokinetic and pharmacodynamic issues and the potential role of PET. In: *PET for Drug Development and Evaluation* (Komar D, ed.), Kluwer, Dordrecht, 1995, p. 277.
53. Workman P, Brunton VG, Robins DJ. Tyrosine kinase inhibitors. *Semin Cancer Biol.* 1992; 3:369–81.
54. Fry DW. Protein tyrosine kinases as therapeutic targets in cancer chemotherapy and recent advances in the development of new inhibitors. *Exp Opin Invest Drugs.* 1994; 3:577–95.
55. Levitzki A, Gazit A. Tyrosine kinase inhibition: an approach to drug development. *Science.* 1995; 267:1782–8.
56. Patrick DR, Heimbrook PC. Protein kinase inhibitors for the treatment of cancer. *Drug Discov Today.* 1996; 1:325–30.
57. Strawn LM, Shawver LK. Tyrosine kinases in disease. *Exp Opin Invest Drugs.* 1998; 7:553.
58. Hunter T. A thousand and one protein kinases. *Cell.* 1987; 50:823–9.
59. Hunter T. Oncoprotein networks. *Cell.* 1997; 88:333–46.
60. Brunton VG, Carlin S, Workman P. Alterations in EGF-dependent proliferative and phosphorylation events in squamous cell carcinoma cell lines by a tyrosine kinase inhibitor. *Anticancer Drug Des.* 1994; 9:311–29.
61. McLeod HL, Brunton VG, Eckardt N, et al. In vivo pharmacology and anti-tumour evaluation of the tyrphostin tyrosine kinase inhibitor RG13022. *Br J Cancer.* 1996; 74:1714–18.
62. Meydan N, Grunberger T, Dadi H, et al. Inhibition of acute lymphoblastic leukaemia by a Jak-2 inhibitor. *Nature.* 1996; 379:645–8.
63. Mohammadi M, McMahon G, Sun L, et al. Structures of the tyrosine kinase domain of fibroblast growth factor receptor in complex with inhibitors. *Science.* 1997; 276:955–60.
64. Fry DW, Kraker AJ, McMichael A, et al. A specific inhibitor of the epidermal growth factor receptor tyrosine kinase. *Science.* 1994; 265:1093–5.
65. Ward WHJ, Cook PN, Slater AM, Davies DH, Holdgate GA, Green LR. Epidermal growth factor receptor tyrosine kinase. *Biochem Pharmacol.* 1994; 48:659–66.
66. Wakeling AE, Barker AJ, Davies DH, et al. Specific inhibition of epidermal growth factor receptor tyrosine kinase by 4-anilinoquinazolines. *Breast Cancer Res Treat.* 1996; 38:67–73.
67. Wakeling AE, Barker AJ, Davies DH, et al. New targets for therapeutic attack. *Endocrin. Rel Cancer.* 1997; 4:351–5.

68. Boyle FT, Costello GF. Cancer therapy: a move to the molecular level. *Chem Soc Rev.* 1998; 27:251–61.

69. Current Drugs. ZD-1839—an EGF receptor-tyrosine kinase inhibitor. ID *weekly highlights* Current Drugs Ltd, p. 45, April 1998.

70. Woodburn JR, Barker AJ, Gibson KH, et al. ZD 1839, an epidermal growth factor tyrosine kinase inhibitor selected for clinical development. *Proc Am Assoc Cancer Res.* 1997; 38:633 (abstr.)

71. Kelly HC, Laight A, Morris CQ, Woodburn JR, Richmond GHP. Phase I data of ZD1839— an oral epidermal growth factor receptor tyrosine kinase inhibitor. Proceedings of the 10th International NCI Symposium in New Drugs in Cancer Therapy 1998; 109.

72. Iwata K, Miller PE, Barbacci EG, Arnold L, Doty J, DiOrio CI, Pustilnik LR, Reynolds M, Thelemann A, Sloan D, Moyer JD. CP-358,774: A selective EGFR kinase inhibitor with potent antiproliferative activity against HN5 head and neck tumor cells. *Proc Am Assoc Cancer Res.* 1997; 38:633 (abstr.).

73. Senderowicz AM, Headlee D, Stinson SF, Lush RM, Kalil N, Villalba L, Hill K, Steinberg SM, Figg WD, Tompkins A, Arbuch SG, Sausville EA. Phase I trial of continuous infusion flavopiridol, a novel cyclin-dependent kinase inhibitor, in patients with refractory neoplasms. *J Clin Onc.* 1998; 16:2986–2999.

74. Gray NS, Wodicka L, Thunnissen AM, Morgan DO, Barnes G, LeClerc S, Meijer L, Kim S-H, Lockhart DJ, Schultz PG. Exploiting chemical libraries, structure and genomics in the search for kinase inhibitors. *Science.* 1998; 281:533–8.

75. Shayesteh L, Lu Y, Baldocchi R, Godfrey T, Collins C, Pinkel D, Powell B, Mills GB, Gray JW. PIK3CA is implicated as an oncogene in ovarian cancer. *Nat Genet.* 1999; 21:99–102.

76. Whitesell L, Mimnaugh EG, DeCosta B, Myers CE, Neckers LM. Inhibition of heat-shock protein HSP90-pp60v-src heteroprotein complex-formation by benzoquinone ansamycins: essential role for stress proteins in oncogenic transformation. *Proc Natl Acad Sci USA.* 1994; 91:8324–8.

77. Prodromou C, Roe SM, O'Brien R, Ladbury JE, Piper PW, Pearl LH. Identification and structural characterization of the ATP/ADP-binding site in the Hsp90 molecular chaperone. *Cell.* 1997; 90:65–75.

78. Schulte TW, Neckers LM. The benzoquinone ansamycin 17-allylamino-17-demethoxygeldanamycin binds to HSP90 and shares important biologic activities with geldanamycin. *Cancer Chemother Pharmacol.* 1998; 42:273–9.

79. Egorin MJ, Rosen DM, Wolff JH, Callery PS, Musser SM, Eiseman JL. Metabolism of 17-(allylamino)-17-demethoxygeldanamycin (NSC 330507) by murine and human hepatic preparations. *Cancer Res.* 1998; 58:2385–96.

80. Scrip No 2374 September 30th, p. 20 1998.

81. Page MJ, Amess B, Rohlff C, Stubberfield C, Parekh R. Protcomics: a major new technology for the drug discovery process. *Drug Discov Today.* 1999; 4:55–62.

82. Workman P. Cell proliferation, cell cycle and apoptosis targets for cancer drug discovery: Strategies, strengths and pitfalls. In: *Apoptosis and Cell Cycle Control. Basic Mechanisms and Implications for Treating Malignant Disease.* Bios, Oxford, 1996, p. 205.

Glossary

5-FU	5-fluorouracil
6-DMAP	6-dimethylaminopurine
Ab	antibody
ABC	ATP-binding cassette
ACTH	adrenocorticotrophic hormone
Ad	adenovirus
ADA	adenosine deaminase deficiency
AFP	α-fetoprotein
Ag	antigen
AHH	aryl hydrocarbon hydroxylase
AIDS	acquired immunodeficiency syndrome
ALCL	anaplastic large-cell lymphoma
ALL	acute lymphoblastic/lymphocytic leukemia
AML	acute myeloid/myelogenous leukemia
AP	apurinic/apyrimidic
APC	anaphase-promoting complex *or* adenomatous polyposis coli *or* antigen-presenting cell
APL	acute promyelocytic leukemia
AR	androgen receptor
Ara-C	cytosine arabinoside
ARF	alternate reading frame
ART	arthritis
ASCO	American Society of Clinical Oncology
ASO	allele-specific oligodeoxynucleotide
AST	adjuvant systemic therapy
AT	ataxia telangiectasia
ATBC	α-tocopheral, β-carotene Cancer Prevention Trial
ATF	in chapter 6
ATM	telangiectasia gene
ATRA	all *trans*-retinoic acid
ATX	autotaxin
B-CLL	B-cell chronic lymphocytic leukemia
BCPT	Breast Cancer Prevention Trial
BER	base-excision repair
BH	in chapter 9
bHLH	basic helix–loop–helix
BL	Burkitt's lymphoma
BMP	bone morphogenetic protein
BMT	bone marrow transplantation
bp	base pair
BR	benefit ratio
BRCT	breast cancer C-terminus domain
BSO	buthionine sulfoxamine
CAD	caspase-activated deoxyribonuclease
CAI	carboxyamidotriazole
CAK	CDK-activating kinase
CARET	β-Carotene and Retinol Efficacy Trial
CDGE	constant denaturant gel electrophoresis
CDK	cyclin-dependent kinase
CEA	carcinoembryonic antigen
CF	cystic fibrosis
CFTR	cystic fibrosis transmembrane receptor
CFU-GM	granulocyte-macrophage colony-forming units
CHO	Chinese hamster ovary
CIS	carcinoma *in situ*
CKI	cyclin-dependent kinase inhibitor
CLIP	class II-associated invariant chain pepetide
CLL	chronic lymphocytic leukemia
CMF	chemotherapy with cyclophosphamide, methotrexate, and fluorouracil

CML	chronic myelogenous leukemia	FSH	follicle-stimulating hormone
COX-2	cyclooxygenase-2	FUTP	5'fluorouridine triphosphate
CR	complete response	GC	gas chromatography
CRC	Cancer Research Campaign	GCF	giant cell fibroblastoma
CRS	cytoplasmic retention signal	G-CSF	granulocyte colony-stimulating factor
CS	Cockayne's syndrome		
CSF	colony-stimulating factor	GDP	guanosine diphosphate
CT	computed tomography	GEF	guanine nucleotide exchange factor
CTL	cytotoxic T lymphocyte		
D	diversity	GI	gastrointestinal
Da	daltons	GM-CSF	granulocyte-macrophage colony-stimulating factor
DAG	diacylglycerol		
DBD	DNA-binding domain	GPCR	G-protein-coupled receptor
DC	dendritic cell	GSH	glutathione
DCGE	denaturing gradient gel electrophoresis	GST	glutathione-*S*-transferase
		GTF	general transcription factor
DD	death domain	GTP	guanosine triphosphate
DES	diethylstilbestrol	GVHD	graft-vs-host disease
DHFR	dihydrofolate reductase	HAT	histone acetyltransferase
DISC	death-inducing signaling complex	Hb	hemoglobin
DLCL	diffuse large-cell lymphoma	HBD	hormone-binding domain
DP	dermafibrosarcoma protuberans	HBV	hepatitis B virus
EBV	Epstein-Barr virus	hCG	human chorionic gonadotrophin
EC	endothelial cell	HD	Hodgkin's disease
ECM	extracellular matrix	HGF	hepatocyte growth factor
EGF	epidermal growth factor	Hh	hedgehog
ELISPOT	enzyme-linked immunospot	HIV	human immunodeficiency virus
EPO	erythropoietin	HLH	helix–loop–helix
ER	estrogen receptor *or* endoplasmic reticulum	HNPCC	hereditary nonpolyposis colorectal cancer
ERAP	estrogen receptor-associated protein	HNSCC	head and neck squamous cell carcinoma
ERE	estrogen response element	HPLC-MS	high performance liquid chromatography mass spectrometry
ES	Ewing's sarcoma *or* embryonal stem		
EST	ever shorter telomeres *or* expressed sequence tag	HPRT	hypoxanthine phosphribosyl transferase
FAK	focal adhesion kinase	HPV	human papilloma virus
FAP	familial adenomatous polyposis	IBIS	International Breast Cancer Intervention Study
FdUMP	5'fluoro-2'-deoxyuridine monophosphate		
		IC_{50}	inhibitory concentration, 50%
FGF	fibroblast growth factor	ICAM	intercellular adhesion molecule
FISH	fluorescence *in situ* hybridization	ICE	interleukin-1B-converting enzyme
FITC	fluorescein isothiocynate conjugated	IFN	interferon
		Ig	immunoglobulin

IGF	insulin-like growth factor		MI	microsatellite instability
IGCCCG	International Germ Cell Cancer Collaborative Group		MIN	microsatellite instability
			MMP	matrix metalloproteinase
IHC	immunohistochemistry		MMPI	inhibitor of matrix metalloproteinase
IL	interleukin		MMR	mismatch repair
ILK	integrin-linked kinase		MOAT	multispecific organic anion transporter
IMD	intramural microvessel density			
ISEL	*in situ* end labeling		MPF	maturation-promoting factor
ITAM	immunoreceptor tyrosine-based activation motif		MRI	magnetic resonance imaging
			MRP	multidrug resistance-associated protein
IU	international unit			
IV	intravenous, intravenously		MSI	microsatellite instability
J	joining		MTC	medullary thyroid carcinoma *or* major translocation cluster
kb	kilobase			
kDa	kilodalton			
LAK	lymphokine-activated killer		MT-MMP	membrane-type metalloproteinase
LASA	lipid-associated sialic acid		MTX	methotrexate
LAT	linker for activation of T cells		NBS	Nijmegan breakage syndrome
LDH	lactate dehydrogenase		NCAM	neural cell adhesion molecule
LD-PCR	long-distance polymerase chain reaction		NCI	National Cancer Institute
			N-dMT	N-desmethyl tamoxifen
LH	leutinizing hormone		NDP	nucleoside diphosphate
LOE	level of evidence		NER	nucleotide excision repair
LOH	loss of heterozygosity		NGF	nerve growth factor
LPA	lysophosphatidic acid		NHL	non-Hodgkin's lymphoma
LPS	lipopolysaccharide		NMR	nuclear magnetic resonance
LRM	leucine-rich motif		NPC	nuclear pore complex
LRP	lung-resistance protein		NSABP	National Surgical Adjuvant Breast Project
LTC	cysteinyl leukotriene			
mAb	monoclonal antibody		NSCLC	non-small-cell lung cancer
MALT	mucosa-associated lymphoid tissue		NSE	neuron specific enolase
			ODN	oligodeoxynucleotide
MAOA	monoamine oxidase type A		PAGE	polyacrlamide gel electrophoresis
MAPK	mitogen-activated protein kinase		PAP	prostatic acid phosphatase
MBR	major breakpoint region		PBPC	peripheral blood progenitor cell
MCL	mantle-cell lymphoma			
MCR	minor cluster region		PCNA	proliferating cell nuclear antigen
MCS	myxoid chondrosarcoma		PCR	polymerase chain reaction
MDR	multidrug resistance		PDGF	platelet-derived growth factor
MEN	multiple endocrine neoplasia		PET	positron emission tomography
MGDF	megakaryocyte growth and development factor		PGK	phosphoglycerate kinase
			Pgp	permeability glycoprotein
MGMT	O^6-methylguanidine DNA methyltransferase		PH	pleckstrin homology
			Ph	Philadelphia chromosome
MHC	major histocompatibility complex		PIG	p53-induced gene

PK	protein kinase		morphism
PLAP	placental-like alkaline phosphatase	SSR	simple sequence repeat
PNET	primitive neuroectodermal tumor	SST	sequence-specific transactivation
PR	progesterone receptor	SUR	sulfonyluria receptor
PSA	prostate-specific antigen	TAP	transporter-associated with anti-
PT	permeability transition		gen processing
PTC	papillary thyroid carcinoma	TCC	transitional cell lymphoma
PTH	parathyroid hormone	TCF	ternary complex factor *or* T-cell
R	receptor		factor
RA	retinoic acid	TCR	T-cell receptor
Rb	retinoblastoma protein	TGF	transforming growth factor
RBC	red blood cell	TIL	tumor-infiltrating lymphocyte
RCC	renal cell carcinoma	TIMP	tissue inhibitor of matrix
RER	replication error repair		metalloproteinase
RFLP	restriction fragment length	TMUGS	Tumor Marker Utility Grading
	polymorphism		System
RGP	radial growth phase	TNF	tumor necrosis factor
RID	receptor-interaction domain	TNM	staging of cancer based on pri-
ROS	reactive oxygen species *or*		mary tumor, regional
	recruitment of Sos		lymph node involvement,
RTK	receptor tyrosine kinase		and distant metastases
RT-PCR	reverse transcriptase polymerase	TPO	thrombopoietin
	chain reaction	TS	thymidylate synthase
SAGE	sequential analysis of gene	TSG	tumor-suppressor gene
	expression	TSH	thyroid-stimulating hormone
SAR	structure-activity relationship	TTD	trichothiodystrophy
SCC	squamous cell carcinoma	UAS	upstream activating sequence
SCF	stem cell factor	uPA	urokinase plasminogen activator
SCID	severe combined immunodeficiency	UTR	untranslated region
SCLC	small-cell lung cancer	UV	ultraviolet
SDS-PAGE	sodium dodecyl sulfate-poly-	V	variable
	acrylamide gel electro-	VCAM	vascular cell adhesion molecule
	phoresis	VCR	variant cluster region
SERM	selective estrogen-receptor	VEGF	vascular endothelial growth
	modulator		factor
SF	scatter factor	VDAC	voltage-dependent anion channel
SMAC	supramolecular activation clusters	VGP	vertical growth phase
Sos	son of sevenless	VNR	vitronectin receptor
SRF	serum response factor	VPF	vascular permeability factor
SS	synovial sarcoma	WHO	World Health Organization
SSCP	single-strand conformation poly-	XP	xeroderma pigmentosa

Index

About the Editors

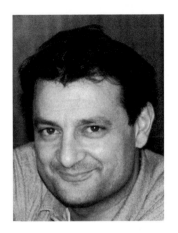

Miguel H. Bronchud graduated BM, BCh (MD) from the University of Oxford in 1983, following a BA, MA degree in Natural Sciences (Biochemistry and Molecular Biology) at the University of Cambridge, UK, in 1980. He subsequently obtained the MRCP, 1986, working at the Brompton Hospital, Guy's Hospital and Radcliffe Infirmary. His oncological training started at the Royal Marsden Hospital (1984-86), London, and continued at the Christie Hospital in Manchester (1987-89), where he conducted pioneering work on the clinical use of recombinant human growth factors, and rhG-CSF in particular. rhG-CSF (a "growth factor" or "colony-stimulating factor" that increases the production of human white blood cells) was approved by the FDA as a drug worthy of clinical use in just five years, establishing a record in pharmaceutical development. It is currently used to prevent or fight infections in cancer patients treated with chemotherapy or radiotherapy, in AIDS patients and in bone marrow transplantation. For this early work, which led to his Doctorate in Medicine (DM) from the University of Oxford in 1990 and PhD (Madrid,1991), he shared the 1988 European Society of Medical Oncology Award for Cancer Research. He was Head of Developmental Therapies at the university hospital of Sant Pau in Barcelona (1990-97), and is currently Head of Oncology at the Hospital General of Granollers (1997–) and Director of the newly founded "European Institute for Health Care S.L." in Montanyà (Barcelona). He is or has been a member of several editorial boards or panel of peer-reviewers (*European Journal of Cancer, British Journal of Cancer, The Lancet, Annals of Oncology,* and others) and is a member of several scientific societies (American Society of Clinical Oncology, American Society of Hematology, European Society of Medical Oncology, American Association for the Advancement of Science, Royal College of Physicians, European School of Oncology, European Organization for Research on Treatment of Cancer, etc). He is a member of the EORTC-Protocol Review Committee and the European School of Oncology International Advisory Committee. He has published five personal books, twenty-two co-authored books, over one hundred original articles or scientific reviews and has lectured in five continents (over 200 lectures) on cancer medicine, new drugs, history of medicine (e.g., medicine in ancient Egypt), growth factor research, gene therapy, and high-dose chemotherapy. He has been quoted over one thousand times in Scientific Search (1981–1999) and is a consultant to several biotech and pharmaceutical firms, the European Medical Evaluation Agency and Spanish health authorities; and is also involved in cultural associations (ex-president of the Catalan Jewish-Christian Society).

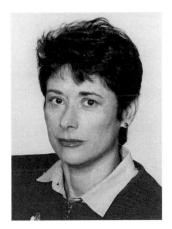

MaryAnn Foote, PhD is Department Head, Medical Writing, Amgen Inc., Thousand Oaks, California. She is the author or co-author of more than 50 journal articles and book chapters as well as a book editor. Dr. Foote is a Fellow of the American Medical Writers Association and a past president of the organization, as well as a member of the American Society of Hematology, American Society of Clinical Oncology, European Haematological Association, among others. Dr. Foote received the BS (1974) (magna cum laude) and MS (1976) degrees from Fairleigh Dickinson University, Teaneck, New Jersey, and the PhD degree (1983) from Rutgers University, New Brunswick, New Jersey.

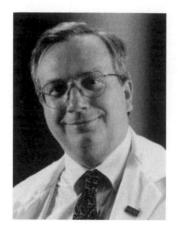

Dr. William P. Peters joined the Karmanos Cancer Institute in July 1995, as director and CEO of the Institute and Associate Dean for Cancer Programs and Professor of Medicine and Oncology at the Wayne State University School of Medicine. He is also Senior Vice President for Cancer Services at The Detroit Medical Center. Peters is widely recognized for pioneering the use of high-dose chemotherapy and autologous bone marrow transplant (ABMT) in the treatment of breast cancer, and also developing the use of transplant therapy on an outpatient basis. He established and coordinated ABMT programs at the Dana Farber Cancer Institute and the Duke University Medical Center.

Dr. Peters previously held positions at Duke University, including Professor of Medicine, Duke University Medical Center; Associate Director for Clinical Operations, Duke Comprehensive Cancer Center; Director, Bone Marrow Transplantation (BMT) Program; Director, BMT Unit; Director, BMT Support Laboratory; and Chief, Gale Gould Laboratory for Cancer Drug Pharmacology.

His faculty experience includes positions at the Harvard Medical School, Dana Farber Cancer Institute, and the Duke University Medical Center.

Dr. Peters received B.S. degrees in biochemistry and biophysics, and a B.A. in philosophy from Penn State University in 1972. He received a M.Phil. in human genetics and a PhD in human genetics/viral oncology from Columbia University in 1976, and a medical degree from the Columbia College of Physicians and Surgeons in 1978. Dr. Peters also earned an M.B.A. from the Fuqua School of Business, Duke University, in 1990.

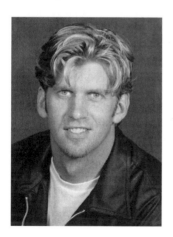

Murray Robinson, PhD is currently serving as department head for Amgen's Cancer Biology Program, Dr. Robinson has been with Amgen since 1991, where he joined after receiving his PhD from the California Institute of Technology. Amgen's cancer biology effort utilizes a systems approach to cancer, targeting properties common to cancer cells such as loss of growth control, apoptotic sensitivity, angiogenesis, and immortalization.

In addition to managing this group, Dr. Robinson maintains an active laboratory studying the biology of mammalian telomerase, having identified the first two proteins of the telomerase complex. Recently the lab published work demonstrating that telomerase inhibition can trigger a dramatic apoptotic response in human tumor cell lines.

Dr. Robinson received his bachelor's degree at UC San Diego, then moved on to graduate work at Johns Hopkins University and then to the California Institute of Technology where he received his PhD in 1991.